Recent Researches in Insulin Resistance

Recent Researches in Insulin Resistance

Edited by Frank Cohen

hayle medical

New York

Hayle Medical,
750 Third Avenue, 9th Floor,
New York, NY 10017, USA

Visit us on the World Wide Web at:
www.haylemedical.com

ISBN: 978-1-63241-602-5

Printed in China.

Cataloging-in-Publication Data

Recent researches in insulin resistance / edited by Frank Cohen.
p. cm.
Includes bibliographical references and index.
ISBN 978-1-63241-602-5
1. Insulin resistance. 2. Insulin resistance--Research. 3. Diabetes--Complications.
4. Hormone resistance. I. Cohen, Frank.

RC662.4 .R43 2019
616.399--dc23

Table of Contents

Preface

The world is advancing at a fast pace like never before. Therefore, the need is to keep up with the latest developments. This book was an idea that came to fruition when the specialists in the area realized the need to coordinate together and document essential themes in the subject. That's when I was requested to be the editor. Editing this book has been an honour as it brings together diverse authors researching on different streams of the field. The book collates essential materials contributed by veterans in the area which can be utilized by students and researchers alike.

Insulin is a hormone that is produced by the beta cells of the pancreatic islets, for the regulation of the metabolism of fats, proteins and carbohydrates. When cells fail to respond to the secretion of the hormone insulin, a pathological condition known as insulin resistance arises. In this, the body's cells are resistant to insulin and therefore unable to use it efficiently. This leads to high blood sugar. To counter that, the beta cells increase insulin production, thereby increasing the blood insulin level. These factors combine to contribute to the incidence of type 2 diabetes or latent autoimmune diabetes of adults. A high intake of carbohydrates and in particular fructose has been linked with insulin resistance. It may also develop in patients who have recently undergone bariatric or abdominal procedures. The primary treatment for this condition involves exercise and weight loss. This book is compiled in such a manner, that it will provide a clinical perspective of insulin resistance. The various advancements in the understanding of insulin resistance are glanced at and their implications as well as ramifications are looked at in detail. Students, researchers, experts and all associated with this area of research will benefit alike from this book.

Each chapter is a sole-standing publication that reflects each author´s interpretation. Thus, the book displays a multi-facetted picture of our current understanding of application, resources and aspects of the field. I would like to thank the contributors of this book and my family for their endless support.

Editor

The Association between Hematological Parameters and Insulin Resistance Is Modified by Body Mass Index – Results from the North-East Italy MoMa Population Study

Rocco Barazzoni*, Gianluca Gortan Cappellari, Annamaria Semolic, Enrico Chendi, Mario Ius, Roberta Situlin, Michela Zanetti, Pierandrea Vinci, Gianfranco Guarnieri

Internal Medicine, Department of Medical, Surgical and Health Sciences, University of Trieste, Trieste, Italy

Abstract

Objective: Increments in red blood cell count (RBC), hemoglobin (Hb) and hematocrit (Ht) levels are reportedly associated with higher insulin resistance (IR). Obesity may cause IR, but underlying factors remain incompletely defined, and interactions between obesity, hematological parameters and IR are incompletely understood. We therefore determined whether: 1) BMI and obesity per se are independently associated with higher RBC, hemoglobin and hematocrit; 2) hematological parameters independently predict insulin resistance in obese individuals.

Design and Methods: We investigated the associations between BMI, hematological parameters and insulin resistance as reflected by homeostasis model assessment (HOMA) in a general population cohort from the North-East Italy MoMa epidemiological study (M/F = 865/971, age = 49±1).

Results: In all subjects, age-, sex- and smoking-adjusted hematological parameters were positively associated with BMI in linear regression ($P<0.05$), but not after adjustment for HOMA or waist circumference (WC) and potential metabolic confounders. No associations were found between hematological parameters and BMI in lean, overweight or obese subgroups. Associations between hematological parameters and HOMA were conversely independent of BMI in all subjects and in lean and overweight subgroups ($P<0.01$), but not in obese subjects alone.

Conclusions: In a North-East Italy general population cohort, obesity per se is not independently associated with altered RBC, Hb and Ht, and the association between BMI and hematological parameters is mediated by their associations with abdominal fat and insulin resistance markers. High hematological parameters could contribute to identify insulin resistance in non-obese individual, but they do not appear to be reliable insulin resistance biomarkers in obese subjects.

Editor: Stephen L. Atkin, Weill Cornell Medical College Qatar, Qatar

Funding: This work received financial support from the European Regional Development Fund under the Regional Operational Programme of Friuli Venezia Giulia - Objective "Regional Competitiveness and Employment" 2007/2013. Friuli-Venezia Giulia Region supported biochemical analyses at Pordenone hospital. The funders had no role in study design, data collection and analysis, decision to publish, or preparation of the manuscript.

Competing Interests: The authors have declared that no competing interests exist.

* Email: barazzon@units.it

Introduction

Obesity is a major risk factor for insulin resistance [1,2], but factors linking obesity and increased insulin resistance are not completely understood [1–3]. High red blood cells and hematocrit have been hypothesized to contribute to insulin resistance through rheological alterations and impaired tissue blood flow [4,5], and red blood cell count, hematocrit and hemoglobin have been reported to be positively associated with insulin resistance [6–10]. Available studies in general population cohorts are however limited, and potential interactions between obesity, hematological parameters and insulin resistance remain undefined. In particular, evidence is lacking on the potential impact of obesity per se on hematological parameters and on potential involvement of hematological parameters in obesity-associated insulin resistance. We therefore investigated the associations between body mass index (BMI), hematological parameters and insulin resistance, calculated using the validated homeostasis model assessment (HOMA) index [11], in a cohort from the MoMa study, an epidemiological investigation aimed at assessing the prevalence of obesity in the North-East Italy Friuli-Venezia Giulia Region. In the whole cohort and in lean, overweight or obese individuals, we specifically sought to determine whether or not 1) BMI and obesity per se are independently associated with higher RBC, hemoglobin and hematocrit and 2) hematological parameters are potential independent predictors of insulin resistance in obese individuals.

Methods and Procedures

Experimental protocol and study population

The MoMa study population was recruited in the municipalities of Montereale Valcellina and Maniago, Pordenone, in the Friuli-Venezia Giulia Region in North-East Italy. The study was conducted by the University of Trieste, in collaboration with local General Practitioners and nurses in the GP outpatient clinic, in the setting of the Friuli-Venezia Giulia Region Prevention Project for Metabolic and Cardiovascular Disease. The study protocol was approved by the competent Pordenone Hospital Ethics Committee, and each subject gave written informed consent to participate before recruitment. A random sample of 2500 18–69 year-old residents in the two municipalities was invited to participate, and 1836 accepted the invitation (M/F = 865/971) and were studied between 2008–2010.

The study protocol included collection of clinical history, medical examination and blood sampling after a 10–12 hour overnight fast. Weight and height were measured and recorded to the nearest 0.1 kg and 0.5 cm, respectively. BMI was calculated as weight in kilograms divided by height in meters squared. Waist circumference was measured on bare skin during midrespiration at the natural indentation between the 10th rib and iliac crest to the nearest 0.5 cm. Blood pressure was measured on the right and left arms using a standard mercury sphygmomanometer. All variables were measured in duplicate, and the average of two measures was used for patient classification. Mean arterial pressure (MAP) was calculated as DBP + 1/3 Diff-BP, where DBP and Diff-BP are diastolic blood pressure and differential blood pressure, respectively. Collected plasma aliquots were used to measure routine biochemical profiles at the Pordenone Hospital Laboratory, and for storage at −80°C until further analyses in the Internal Medicine laboratories at the University of Trieste. For multiple regression models, definitions of metabolic alterations were based on metabolic syndrome thresholds in ATP III classification. Hypertension was therefore defined as systolic or diastolic blood pressure ≥135 and ≥85 mmHg, respectively, or use of antihypertensive medications; hypertriglyceridemia was defined as plasma triglycerides ≥150 mg/dl or use of lipid-lowering drugs; low HDL-cholesterol was defined as plasma HDL-cholesterol <50 or 40 mg/dl in female and male sex respectively; hyperglycemia was defined as plasma glucose ≥110 mg/dl or use of antidiabetic medications; high waist circumference was defined as waist circumference >88 or 102 cm in female and male sex respectively. Hypercholesterolemia was further defined as plasma total cholesterol >200 mg/dl or use of cholesterol-lowering drugs, and diabetes mellitus was diagnosed based on fasting plasma glucose higher than 126 mg/dl or antidiabetic medications.

Plasma metabolic profile and homa index

RBC count, Hb and Ht, plasma glucose, insulin, triglycerides, total and high-density lipoprotein (HDL) cholesterol were measured using standard methods. Homeostasis model assessment (HOMA) validated index of insulin resistance [11] was calculated with the following formula: HOMA = (FPG × FPI)/22.5, where FPG and FPI are fasting plasma glucose (mmol) and fasting plasma insulin (μU/ml), respectively.

Statistical analysis

Data distributions for continuous variables was assessed by Shapiro-Wilk test and appropriate transformations used for non normal data. Associations between hematological parameters and other variables were evaluated by Pearson correlation. Parameters showing univariate association ($p<0.05$) were included in stepwise multiple linear regression models in order to assess their impact in the relationship between BMI, HOMA and hematological parameters in the whole population and in BMI subgroups. Multiple linear regression analysis was validated by assessing the normality of residuals. In subgroup analysis, since neither hematological measurements nor their transformations showed normal distribution, differences were evaluated by Kruskal–Wallis tests followed by post-hoc Mann-Whitney comparisons. P values were corrected for multiple comparisons according to Benjamini and Hochberg. P values <0.05 were considered statistically significant. Analysis was performed by SPSS v.17 software (SPSS, Inc., Chicago, IL). Continuous variables are presented as mean±standard deviation.

Results

Anthropometric parameters, clinical and biochemical profile and linear regression analysis (Tables 1,2)

Anthropometric and metabolic profile, prevalence of high blood pressure and diabetes and related medications are reported in Table 1. In all subjects (n = 1836), RBC, Hb or Ht were associated with gender (r = 0.53, 0.65, 0.61; all $p<0.01$), age (r = −0.05, 0.05, 0.07; all $p<0.05$) and smoking habits (r = −0.05, 0.06, 0.09; all $p<0.05$). Sex-, age- and smoking habits-adjusted RBC, Hb and Ht were therefore used in all subsequent analyses. Sex-, age- and smoking habits-adjusted RBC, Hb and Ht were positively associated with BMI ($P<0.05$). Similar associations were observed between hematological parameters and HOMA ($P<0.001$) and WC ($P<0.01$). In addition, all hematological parameters were associated with plasma total cholesterol and blood pressure ($P<0.01$), while less strong or incomplete associations were observed with plasma glucose, triglycerides and HDL-cholesterol (Table 2).

Multiple regression analyses between BMI and hematological parameters and BMI subgroup analyses - (Figure 1, Tables 3,4)

To determine whether the associations between BMI and RBC, Hb and Ht were independent of related metabolic variables, multiple regression analyses were performed including HOMA, WC, MAP, plasma triglyceride, total and HDL-cholesterol and glucose. The associations between BMI and hematological parameters were no longer statistically significant or became substantially weaker after adjusting for HOMA (Table 3), and they were also not statistically significant after adjusting for WC or in a model including combined metabolic parameters (Table 3).

In BMI subgroup analyses, lowest RBC, Hb and Ht were observed in lean subjects ($P<0.05$), but no stepwise increments were observed from overweight to obese BMI groups (P = NS overweight vs obese, Figure 1). Similar patterns were observed for WC tertiles (P = NS Middle vs High WC, not shown). No statistically significant associations were finally observed in linear regression analysis between BMI and sex-, age- and smoking-adjusted hematological parameters in each BMI group considered separately (Table 4).

Multiple regression analyses between hematological parameters and HOMA and BMI subgroup analyses (Tables 3,5)

To determine whether the associations between hematological parameters and HOMA index were independent of BMI and waist circumference, multiple regression analyses were performed. The associations between RBC, Hb, Ht and HOMA remained

Table 1. Clinical and Biochemical profile.

Gender (M/F)	865/971
Age (years)	49±13 (18–73)
BMI (kg/m²)	26.9±5.2 (18.6–52.1)
WC (cm)	93.2±13.7 (57.0–152.0)
Prevalence (%) Metabolic Syndrome	26,7
Diabetes (Pharm. Tx)	8.8 (4.5)
Hypertension (Pharm Tx)	48.5 (24.3)
Smoking	21,4
SBP (mmHg)	135±18 (80–215)
DBP (mmHg)	81±10 (47–121)
RBC (RBC/mm³)	4.79±0.41 (3.71–7.02)
Hb (g/dl)	14.3±1.2 (9.1–18.3)
Ht (%)	42.4±3.4 (31.0–53.6)
Glucose (mmol/l)	5.55±1.33 (3.83–21.92)
Insulin (μU/ml)	10.2±7.5 (2.0–96.1)
HOMA	2.63±2.66 (0.4–63.7)
Tg (mmol/l)	1.35±0.91 (0.34–13.76)
T-Chol (mmol/l)	5.61±1.10 (2.43–10.06)
HDL-Chol (mmol/l)	1.47±0.36 (0.57–3.05)

Gender, age, body mass index (BMI), waist circumference (WC), disease (percent of pharmacological treatment. Tx) and smoking prevalence, systolic (SBP) and diastolic (DBP) blood pressure, red blood cells (RBC), hemoglobin (Hb), hematocrit (Ht), plasma glucose, insulin, homeostasis model assessment (HOMA), plasma triglycerides (Tg), total (T-Chol) and high-density-lipoprotein (HDL-Chol) cholesterol in the whole study population. Results are reported as Mean ± SD (Range).

statistically significant after adjustment for BMI or WC as well as combined metabolic variables (Table 3).

In BMI subgroup analyses, HOMA values expectedly increased from lean to overweight to obese individuals (Lean: 1.63±0.03, Overweight: 2.50±0.06, Obese: 4.57±0.22, $P<0.01$). The association between hematological parameters and HOMA remained statistically significant and independent of BMI or WC only in lean and overweight subjects ($P<0.05$) while not in the obese patient group (P = NS) (Table 5).

Multiple regression analyses between hematological parameters and blood pressure, plasma glucose, triglycerides and cholesterol (Table 6)

To further investigate the potential interactions between blood pressure, plasma glucose, plasma triglycerides, total and HDL cholesterol, as well as their potential independent association with hematological parameters, multiple regressions analyses were performed including BMI or waist circumference and HOMA. The data showed that linear association between hematological parameters and blood pressure were independent of BMI, HOMA

Table 2. Linear regression analyses.

	adj RBC	adj Ht	adj Hb
BMI	0.091***	0.046*	0.055*
WC	0.090***	0.064**	0.089***
SBP	0.061**	0.065**	0.071**
DBP	0.105***	0.105***	0.128***
MAP	0.093**	0.095**	0.111**
Glucose	0.056*	0.026	0.066**
Insulin	0.111***	0.100***	0.118***
HOMA	0.089***	0.074***	0.102***
Tg	0.042	0.053*	0.102***
T-Chol	0.071**	0.120***	0.145***
HDL-Chol	−0.082***	0.037	0.003

Linear regression analyses between age-, sex- and smoking-adjusted (adj) red blood cells (RBC), hemoglobin (Hb), hematocrit (Ht) and body mass index (BMI), waist circumference (WC), systolic (SBP), diastolic (DBP) and mean (MAP) arterial blood pressure, plasma glucose, insulin, homeostasis model assessment (HOMA), plasma triglycerides (Tg), total (T-Chol) and high-density-lipoprotein (HDL-Chol) cholesterol in the whole study population. *:$p<0.05$,**:$p<0.01$, ***:$p<0.001$.

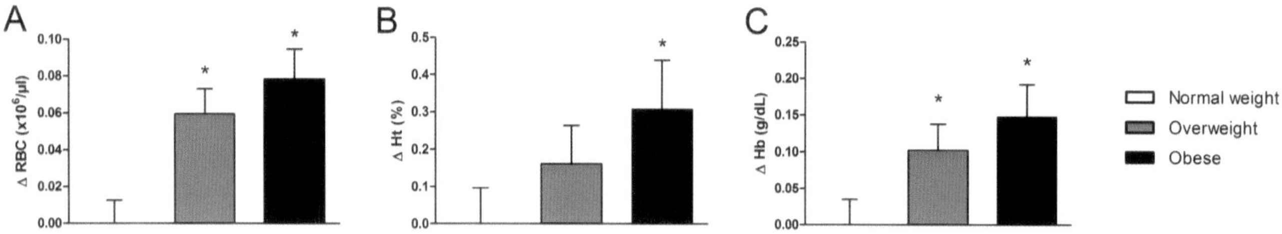

Figure 1. Changes in red blood cells (RBC) (A), hematocrit (Ht) (B) and hemoglobin (Hb) (C) in overweight (OW) and obese relative to Lean body mass index subgroups. *: $p<0.05$ vs. Lean.

or combined HOMA and BMI, and similar results were obtained when waist circumference was used instead of BMI values. Associations with plasma glucose were on the other hand not significant in any model. After adjustments, associations between hematological parameters and lipid profile were statistically significant for total cholesterol, while associations with HDL-cholesterol were only preserved for RBC, while not for Ht or Hb. No statistically significant associations were finally observed between plasma triglycerides and any hematological variable.

Discussion

The current study investigated the interactions between BMI, hematological parameters and insulin resistance. In a North-East Italy population study cohort, we demonstrated that: 1) a positive association between BMI and red blood cells, hemoglobin and hematocrit is dependent on abdominal fat distribution and insulin resistance markers, and obesity per se is not associated with altered hematological parameters; 2) hematological parameters are associated with insulin resistance independently of anthropometric variables; however, when considering separate BMI subgroups, statistically significant associations between hematological parameters and insulin resistance are observed only in lean and overweight and not in obese BMI subgroups.

The study demonstrates that BMI or obesity per se are not independently associated with higher hematological parameters. This conclusion is directly supported by lack of stepwise increments in red blood cells, hematocrit or hemoglobin in BMI subgroup analyses, and by lack of associations between hematological variables and BMI in different BMI subgroups. In the whole study cohort, red blood cells, hemoglobin and hematocrit are also not associated with BMI after adjusting for insulin resistance and abdominal fat markers, and the general association between BMI and hematological parameters appears therefore to be at least in part dependent on the higher incidence of excess abdominal fat and insulin resistance in both overweight and obese individuals.

Previous reports described positive associations between insulin resistance and red blood cells count or elevated hematocrit [6–10], but few studies investigated general population cohorts, and interactions between BMI, hematological parameters and insulin resistance had not been defined [8,9]. A direct association between insulin resistance and hematological parameters in the current general population was importantly independent of BMI and abdominal fat markers, and excess viscosity in subjects with higher red blood cells and hematocrit could indeed primarily impair insulin action through reduced blood flow in insulin target tissues [4,5]. Insulin resistance and secondary hyperinsulinemia could however also directly lead to higher red blood cells, since insulin and erythropoietin have synergistic effects in stimulating erythroid colony proliferation [12]. Based on available information, it is therefore possible that a vicious cycle mutually enhances insulin resistance and hematological parameters. The current study also investigated whether hematological parameters are associated with, and therefore represent potential markers of, insulin resistance in different BMI subgroups. BMI subgroup analyses revealed that associations between HOMA and red blood cells, hemoglobin and hematocrit remain statistically significant in lean and overweight but not in obese subjects. Since the obese individuals expectedly had markedly higher insulin resistance, it is likely that lack of associations in this group is due at least in part to a relevant negative impact on insulin action by non-hematological, obesity-associated alterations, that could include altered adipokine profiles, excess substrate availability, oxidative stress and inflammation [1–3]. The above observations have potentially relevant clinical implications since they suggest that: 1) although many important factors contribute to modulate insulin resistance, the current data suggest that, along with other parameters, higher hematological parameters may contribute to identify non-obese individuals at early stages of insulin resistance; 2) red blood cells, hemoglobin and hematocrit appear to have a less relevant metabolic impact and are unlikely to represent reliable biomarkers of insulin resistance in obese individuals.

The study provided the opportunity to directly investigate the associations between hematological parameters and obesity-associated metabolic complications. Linear associations were observed between hematological parameters and blood pressure, plasma total and HDL-cholesterol, triglycerides and glucose, with closest associations for blood pressure and lipid profile. Blood pressure remained significantly associated with hematological parameters in multiple regression models, thereby indicating that the previously reported contribution of altered rheological characteristics to enhance blood pressure [13] is at least in part independent of obesity. After adjustments, no associations were instead observed for plasma glucose, while total cholesterol retained the strongest independent association with red blood cells, hemoglobin and hematocrit among lipid variables. This pattern of associations is in general agreement with previous studies [13] and a close association between non-HDL cholesterol and hematological parameters has been recently described in a US population study [14]. The current data therefore contribute to identify an emerging cluster of cardiovascular risk factors including hematological parameters, insulin resistance, blood pressure and total cholesterol, that appears to be at least in part independent of obesity. Further studies will be needed to investigate the mechanisms underlying these relationships.

In conclusion, obesity per se is not associated with high RBC, hemoglobin and hematocrit in a North-East Italy population, and abdominal fat accumulation and insulin resistance appear to mediate a general association between BMI and hematological parameters. High RBC, hemoglobin and hematocrit could contribute to identify insulin resistance in non-obese individuals,

Table 3. Multiple regression analyses.

		RBC			Ht			Hb		
		β (95%C.I.)	F	R^2	β (95%C.I.)	F	R^2	β (95%C.I.)	F	R^2
BMI	Model 1	1.35 (0.67–2.02)***	15.3	0.01	0.08 (0–0.17)*	4.0	0.00	0.30 (0.05–0.55)*	5.7	0.00
	Model 2a	0.70 (0.11–1.28)*	306.4	0.25	0.01 (−0.05–0.09)	302.9	0.25	0.02 (−0.19–0.24)	302.9	0.25
	Model 3	0.21 (−0.14–0.56)	2582.5	0.74	−0.02 (−0.06–0.03)	2580.9	0.74	−0.11 (−0.24–0.01)	2585.7	0.74
	Model4	0.56 (−0.05–1.17)	82.0	0.21	0.03 (−0.05–0.11)	81.5	0.21	0.01 (−0.21–0.24)	81.3	0.21
	Model5	0.13 (−0.22–0.48)	762.1	0.75	−0.02 (−0.06–0.03)	762.1	0.75	0.02 (−0.2–0.25)	763.9	0.74
	Model6	0.41 (−0.11–0.93)	193.4	0.43	0.01 (−0.06–0.08)	192.9	0.43	−0.03 (−0.22–0.17)	192.8	0.43
HOMA	Model 1	0.68 (0.33–1.03)***	14.5	0.01	0.07 (0.02–0.12)**	10.2	0.01	0.28 (0.15–0.41)***	19.2	0.01
	Model 2b	0.34 (0.03–0.64)*	305.9	0.25	0.05 (0.01–0.09)*	307.2	0.25	0.21 (0.10–0.32)***	311.8	0.25
	Model 3	0.37 (0.05–0.68)*	250.7	0.22	0.05 (0.00–0.09)*	250.4	0.22	0.17 (0.06–0.29)**	252.9	0.22
	Model4	0.40 (0.10–0.70)**	124.1	0.29	0.06 (0.02–0.10)**	124.8	0.29	0.17 (0.06–0.28)**	124.7	0.29
	Model5	0.31 (0.03–0.60)*	154.3	0.37	0.05 (0.02–0.09)**	155.0	0.37	0.14 (0.04–0.25)**	154.9	0.37
	Model6	0.41 (0.09–0.72)*	69.6	0.21	0.06 (0.02–0.10)**	69.9	0.21	0.20 (0.08–0.31)**	70.4	0.21

Multiple regression analyses between red blood cells (RBC), hemoglobin (Hb), hematocrit (Ht) (independent variables) and body mass index (BMI) or homeostasis model assessment (HOMA) (dependent variables) in the whole study population (n = 1836). Similar results were observed when waist circumference (WC) was included instead of BMI (not shown). *: $p<0.05$; **: $p<0.01$; ***: $p<0.001$. P value for F test was <0.001 in all models except for Model 1 with BMI dependent variable ($P<0.05$).

Data adjustments:

Model 1: age, sex, smoking habits.

Model 2a: Model 1 + HOMA.

Model 2b: Model 1 + BMI.

Model 3: Model 1 + Waist Circumference.

Model 4: Model 1 + Triglycerides, total cholesterol, HDL cholesterol, Mean Arterial Pressure, Glucose.

Model 5: Model 4 + WC

Model 6: Model 1 + Hypertriglyceridemia, Hypercholesterolemia, Low HDL, Hypertension, Hyperglycemia, High WC.

Table 4. Multiple regression analyses.

BMI		RBC β (95%C.I.)	RBC F	RBC R^2	Ht β (95%C.I.)	Ht F	Ht R^2	Hb β (95%C.I.)	Hb F	Hb R^2
Lean	Model 1	0.29 (−0.08–0.67)	2.4	0.00	−0.02 (−0.06–0.03)	0.4	0.00	−0.02 (−0.15–0.12)	0.1	0.00
	Model 2	0.05 (−0.28–0.37)	120.1	0.25	−0.04 (−0.08–0.00)	122.3	0.25	−0.13 (−0.24–0.01)	123.0	0.25
	Model 3	0.17 (−0.20–0.54)	16.9	0.05	−0.03 (−0.08–0.02)	17.4	0.05	−0.07 (−0.21–0.06)	17.1	0.05
OW	Model 1	0.07 (−0.23–0.36)	0.2	0.00	0.00 (−0.04–0.04)	0.0	0.00	0.07 (−0.04–0.18)	1.7	0.00
	Model 2	0.09 (−0.17–0.35)	94.8	0.22	0.01 (−0.03–0.04)	94.6	0.22	0.04 (−0.06–0.14)	95.0	0.22
	Model 3	−0.01 (−0.30–0.28)	18.1	0.05	−0.01 (−0.05–0.03)	18.2	0.05	0.02 (−0.09–0.13)	18.2	0.05
Obese	Model 1	0.30 (−0.89–1.48)	0.2	0.00	0.08 (−0.07–0.23)	1.1	0.00	−0.05 (−0.48–0.38)	0.1	0.00
	Model 2	0.31 (−0.48–1.09)	273.3	0.57	−0.02 (−0.12–0.08)	272.7	0.57	−0.14 (−0.42–0.15)	273.6	0.57
	Model 3	0.07 (−1.05–1.19)	28.4	0.12	0.06 (−0.08–0.20)	28.7	0.12	−0.27 (−0.56–0.25)	28.7	0.12

Multiple regression analyses between red blood cells (RBC), hemoglobin (Hb), hematocrit (Ht) and body mass index (BMI) in normal weight (Lean, n = 725), overweight (OW, n = 688), obese (Obese, n = 423) subjects from the study population (n = 1836). P value for F test was <0.001 in all models except for Model 1.

Data adjustments:

Model 1: age, sex, smoking habits.

Model 2: Model 1 + Waist Circumference.

Model 3: Model 1 + Homeostasis Model Assessment.

Table 5. Multiple regression analyses.

		RBC			Ht			Hb		
HOMA		**β (95%C.I.)**	**F**	**R^2**	**β (95%C.I.)**	**F**	**R^2**	**β (95%C.I.)**	**F**	**R^2**
Lean	Model 1	0.31 (0.13–0.49)***	11.6	0.02	0.04 (0.02–0.06)***	10.4	0.01	0.13 (0.06–0.19)***	15.1	0.02
	Model 2	0.28 (0.11–0.46)**	21.6	0.06	0.04 (0.02–0.06)***	22.6	0.06	0.13 (0.07–0.19)***	24.9	0.07
	Model 3	0.26 (0.09–0.44)**	21.6	0.06	0.03 (0.01–0.06)**	21.6	0.06	0.11 (0.04–0.17)***	22.9	0.06
OW	Model 1	0.38 (0.03–0.73)*	4.6	0.01	0.07 (0.02–0.11)**	8.0	0.01	0.27 (0.14–0.40)***	16.0	0.02
	Model 2	0.37 (0.03–0.71)*	20.4	0.06	0.07 (0.02–0.11)**	22.5	0.06	0.25 (0.12–0.38)***	25.7	0.07
	Model 3	0.40 (0.05–0.74)*	14.0	0.04	0.07 (0.02–0.11)**	15.9	0.04	0.25 (0.13–0.38)***	19.1	0.05
Obese	Model 1	0.68 (−0.60–1.95)	1.1	0.00	0.07 (−0.09–0.23)	0.7	0.00	0.31 (−0.15–0.76)	1.7	0.00
	Model 2	0.57 (−0.63–1.77)	28.9	0.12	0.04 (−0.11–0.19)	28.5	0.12	0.33 (−0.11–0.76)	29.6	0.12
	Model 3	0.68 (−0.53–1.88)	26.6	0.11	0.02 (−0.13–0.17)	26.0	0.11	0.27 (−0.17–0.70)	26.7	0.11

Multiple regression analyses between red blood cells (RBC), hemoglobin (Hb), hematocrit (Ht) and homeostasis model assessment (HOMA) in normal weight (Lean, n = 725), overweight (OW, n = 688), obese (Obese, n = 423) subjects from the study population (n = 1836). *: $p<0.05$; **: $p<0.01$; ***: $p<0.001$. P value for F test was <0.01 in all models except for Model 1 in the Obese group.
Data adjustments:
Model 1: age, sex, smoking habits.
Model 2: Model 1 + Body Mass Index.
Model 3: Model 1 + Waist Circumference.

Table 6. Multiple regression analyses.

		RBC			Ht			Hb		
		β (95%C.I.)	F	R^2	β (95%C.I.)	F	R^2	β (95%C.I.)	F	R^2
Model 1	MAP	0.002 (0.001–0.003)**	8.8	0.02	0.016 (0.006–0.027)**	7.4	0.02	0.006 (0.002–0.009)**	11.7	0.03
	Glucose	0.000 (0.000–0.001)			0.001 (−0.005–0.006)			0.001 (0.000–0.003)		
	Tg	0.000 (0.000–0.000)			0.000 (−0.002–0.002)			0.000 (0.000–0.001)		
	T-Chol	0.001 (0.000–0.001)***			0.006 (0.003–0.010)***			0.003 (0.001–0.004)***		
	HDL-Chol	−0.003 (−0.004–0.002)***			0.002 (−0.008–0.012)			−0.001 (−0.005–0.002)		
Model 2	MAP	0.002 (0.000–0.003)*	7.9	0.03	0.015 (0.004–0.026)**	6.2	0.02	0.006 (0.002–0.009)**	9.7	0.03
	Glucose	0.000 (0.000–0.001)			0.000 (−0.005–0.006)			0.001 (0.000–0.003)		
	Tg	0.000 (0.000–0.000)			0.000 (−0.002–0.002)			0.000 (0.000–0.001)		
	T-Chol	0.001 (0.000–0.001)***			0.006 (0.003–0.010)***			0.003 (0.001–0.004)***		
	HDL-Chol	−0.003 (−0.004–0.001)***			0.003 (−0.007–0.013)			−0.001 (−0.005–0.003)		
Model 3	MAP	0.002 (0.000–0.003)*	8.4	0.03	0.015 (0.004–0.026)**	7.8	0.02	0.005 (0.001–0.009)**	11.4	0.04
	Glucose	0.000 (−0.001–0.001)			−0.003 (−0.009–0.002)			0.000 (−0.002–0.002)		
	Tg	0.000 (−0.001–0.000)			0.000 (−0.002–0.001)			0.000 (0.000–0.001)		
	T-Chol	0.001 (0.000–0.001)***			0.007 (0.003–0.010)***			0.003 (0.002–0.004)***		
	HDL-Chol	−0.003 (−0.004–0.002)***			0.004 (−0.006–0.014)			−0.001 (−0.004–0.003)		
Model 4	MAP	0.002 (0.000–0.003)*	7.3	0.03	0.014 (0.003–0.026)*	6.7	0.02	0.006 (0.002–0.01)**	10	0.04
	Glucose	0.000 (−0.001–0.001)			−0.003 (−0.009–0.002)			0.000 (−0.002–0.002)		
	Tg	0.000 (−0.001–0.000)			0.000 (−0.002–0.001)			0.000 (0.000–0.001)		
	T-Chol	0.001 (0.000–0.001)***			0.007 (0.003–0.010)***			0.003 (0.002–0.004)***		
	HDL-Chol	−0.003 (−0.004–0.001)***			0.004 (−0.006–0.014)			−0.001 (−0.005–0.003)		

Multiple regression analyses between mean arterial pressure (MAP), plasma glucose, triglycerides (Tg), total (T-Chol) or HDL-cholesterol (HDL-Chol) and red blood cells (RBC), hematocrit (Ht) and hemoglobin (Hb) in the whole study population (n = 1836). *: $p<0.05$; **: $p<0.01$; ***: $p<0.001$. P value for F test was <0.001 in all models. Similar results were observed when WC was included instead of BMI (not shown).
Data adjustments:
Model 1: age, gender, smoking habits.
Model 2: Model 1 + Body Mass Index.
Model 3: Model 1 + Homeostasis Model Assessment (HOMA).
Model 4: Model 2 + HOMA.

but they are unlikely to substantially contribute to insulin resistance and they do not appear to be reliable biomarkers of insulin resistance in obese subjects.

Acknowledgments

The authors would like to thank Ms Michela Del Mistro for skilled coordination of subject recruitment, and Drs. Paolo Comina, Fabrizio Mion, Paolo Brovedani, Michela Bruckbauer, Luigi Cerrone, Vittorio Giacomelli Battiston, Maurizio Milani for assistance in patient screening in Montereale Valcellina and Maniago. Dr. Pietro Paolo Della Putta is gratefully acknowledged for designing and creating the study database. The Azienda 6 Friuli Occidentale, Dr. Paolo Doretto and the personnel of the Clinical Pathology laboratory at Pordenone Hospital are gratefully acknowledged for their excellent work in sample collection and analyses. Dr. Manuela Boschelle, Ms Anna De Santis and Dr. Elena Franceschi, Dept of Medical, Surgical and Health Sciences, University of Trieste, are finally acknowledged for assistance in sample collection and storage.

Author Contributions

Conceived and designed the experiments: RB MI PV GG. Performed the experiments: PV RS EC AS. Analyzed the data: RB GGC MZ EC. Contributed to the writing of the manuscript: RB GGC.

References

1. Hocking S, Samocha-Bonet D, Milner KL, Greenfield JR, Chisholm DJ (2013) Adiposity and insulin resistance in humans: the role of the different tissue and cellular lipid depots. Endocr Rev 34: 463–500.
2. Lazar MA (2005) How obesity causes diabetes: not a tall tale. Science 307: 373–375.
3. Hardy OT, Czech MP, Corvera S (2012) What causes the insulin resistance underlying obesity? Curr Opin Endocrinol Diabetes Obes 19: 81–87.
4. Baron AD, Steinberg H, Brechtel G, Johnson A (1994) Skeletal muscle blood flow independently modulates insulin-mediated glucose uptake. Am J Physiol 266: E248–253.
5. Gori T (2011) Viscosity, platelet activation, and hematocrit: progress in understanding their relationship with clinical and subclinical vascular disease. Clin Hemorheol Microcirc 49: 37–42.
6. Barbieri M, Ragno E, Benvenuti E, Zito GA, Corsi A, et al. (2001) New aspects of the insulin resistance syndrome: impact on haematological parameters. Diabetologia 44: 1232–1237.
7. Catalano C, Muscelli E, Natali A, Mazzoni A, Masoni A, et al. (1997) Reciprocal association between insulin sensitivity and the haematocrit in man. Eur J Clin Invest 27: 634–637.
8. Hanley AJ, Retnakaran R, Qi Y, Gerstein HC, Perkins B, et al. (2009) Association of hematological parameters with insulin resistance and beta-cell dysfunction in nondiabetic subjects. J Clin Endocrinol Metab 94: 3824–3832.
9. Nordby G, Moan A, Kjeldsen SE, Os I (1995) Relationship between hemorheological factors and insulin sensitivity in normotensive and hypertensive premenopausal women. Am J Hypertens 8: 439–444.
10. Tamariz LJ, Young JH, Pankow JS, Yeh HC, Schmidt MI, et al. (2008) Blood viscosity and hematocrit as risk factors for type 2 diabetes mellitus: the atherosclerosis risk in communities (ARIC) study. Am J Epidemiol 168: 1153–1160.
11. Matthews DR, Hosker JP, Rudenski AS, Naylor BA, Treacher DF, et al. (1985) Homeostasis model assessment: insulin resistance and beta-cell function from fasting plasma glucose and insulin concentrations in man. Diabetologia 28: 412–419.
12. Bersch N, Groopman JE, Golde DW (1982) Natural and biosynthetic insulin stimulates the growth of human erythroid progenitors in vitro. J Clin Endocrinol Metab 55: 1209–1211.
13. Wannamethee G, Shaper AG (1994) Haematocrit: relationships with blood lipids, blood pressure and other cardiovascular risk factors. Thromb Haemost 72: 58–64.
14. Fessler MB, Rose K, Zhang Y, Jaramillo R, Zeldin DC (2013) Relationship between serum cholesterol and indices of erythrocytes and platelets in the US population. J Lipid Res 54: 3177–3188.

2

Reduced Dietary Omega-6 to Omega-3 Fatty Acid Ratio and 12/15-Lipoxygenase Deficiency Are Protective against Chronic High Fat Diet-Induced Steatohepatitis

Milos Lazic[1]❡, Maria Eugenia Inzaugarat[2]❡, Davide Povero[1], Iris C. Zhao[3], Mark Chen[4], Madlena Nalbandian[4], Yury I. Miller[4], Alejandra C. Cherñavsky[2], Ariel E. Feldstein[1], Dorothy D. Sears[4]*

1 Department of Pediatrics, University of California San Diego, La Jolla, California, United States of America, **2** Institute of Immunology, Genetics and Metabolism, CONICET-UBA, Buenos Aires, Argentina, **3** Skaggs School of Pharmacy and Pharmaceutical Sciences, University of California San Diego, La Jolla, California, United States of America, **4** Department of Medicine, University of California San Diego, La Jolla, California, United States of America

Abstract

Obesity is associated with metabolic perturbations including liver and adipose tissue inflammation, insulin resistance, and type 2 diabetes. Omega-6 fatty acids (ω6) promote and omega-3 fatty acids (ω3) reduce inflammation as they can be metabolized to pro- and anti-inflammatory eicosanoids, respectively. 12/15-lipoxygenase (12/15-LO) enzymatically produces some of these metabolites and is induced by high fat (HF) diet. We investigated the effects of altering dietary ω6/ω3 ratio and 12/15-LO deficiency on HF diet-induced tissue inflammation and insulin resistance. We examined how these conditions affect circulating concentrations of oxidized metabolites of ω6 arachidonic and linoleic acids and innate and adaptive immune system activity in the liver. For 15 weeks, wild-type (WT) mice were fed either a soybean oil-enriched HF diet with high dietary ω6/ω3 ratio (11:1, HFH), similar to Western-style diet, or a fat Kcal-matched, fish oil-enriched HF diet with a low dietary ω6/ω3 ratio of 2.7:1 (HFL). Importantly, the total saturated, monounsaturated and polyunsaturated fat content was matched in the two HF diets, which is unlike most published fish oil studies in mice. Despite modestly increased food intake, WT mice fed HFL were protected from HFH-diet induced steatohepatitis, evidenced by decreased hepatic mRNA expression of pro-inflammatory genes and genes involved in lymphocyte homing, and reduced deposition of hepatic triglyceride. Furthermore, oxidized metabolites of ω6 arachidonic acid were decreased in the plasma of WT HFL compared to WT HFH-fed mice. 12/15-LO knockout (KO) mice were also protected from HFH-induced fatty liver and elevated mRNA markers of inflammation and lymphocyte homing. 12/15-LOKO mice were protected from HFH-induced insulin resistance but reducing dietary ω6/ω3 ratio in WT mice did not ameliorate insulin resistance or adipose tissue inflammation. In conclusion, lowering dietary ω6/ω3 ratio in HF diet significantly reduces steatohepatitis.

Editor: Marcia B. Aguila, State University of Rio de Janeiro, Biomedical Center, Institute of Biology, Brazil

Funding: This work was supported by a grant from the P. Robert Majumder Charitable Foundation to DDS, NIH grants DK076852 and DK082451 to AEF, HL055798 to YIM, and CONICET PIP 051/2011 to ACC. The funders had no role in study design, data collection and analysis, decision to publish, or preparation of the manuscript.

Competing Interests: The authors have declared that no competing interests exist.

* Email: dsears@ucsd.edu

❡ These authors contributed equally to this work.

Introduction

Obesity has reached pandemic levels taking a significant toll on the health of adults and children. Obesity is associated with a range of metabolic maladies, including insulin resistance, dyslipidemia, nonalcoholic fatty liver disease (NAFLD) and hypertension, collectively grouped into the so-called metabolic syndrome [1,2,3]. Individuals with metabolic syndrome frequently exhibit pro-inflammatory metabolic profiles and have increased risk for developing type 2 diabetes and cardiovascular disease. The obesity-associated low-grade chronic inflammatory state in metabolic tissues, including adipose, liver, and muscle, contributes to insulin resistance and metabolic dysfunction that results from nutrient excess [4]. A variety of interventions to inhibit inflammatory pathways have been shown to have beneficial effects on metabolic function in rodent models of obesity and human obesity [4].

A new area of promising research in therapeutic approaches against obesity and related metabolic diseases is the use of anti-inflammatory nutrients provided through diet. The average Western-style diet is highly enriched in polyunsaturated omega-6 fatty acids (ω6) and relatively deficient in omega-3 fatty acids (ω3), reaching the estimated dietary ω6/ω3 ratio of 10–20:1 [5]. Omega-6 and ω3 fatty acids are functionally distinct and their metabolites often have the opposing physiologic functions. While diets rich in ω6 are generally pro-inflammatory and promote insulin resistance, the converse is true for ω3-enriched diets [6]. Corresponding to Western diets, standard high fat (HF) diet chows in rodent diet-induced obesity models are typically enriched for saturated fatty acids and polyunsaturated ω6 fatty acids. HF chow consumption increases tissue percentage of saturated fatty acids and polyunsaturated ω6 fatty acids, decreases tissue percentage of ω3, and directly activates pro-inflammatory toll-like receptor 4 (TLR4) signaling [7,8]. Thus, excessive amount of ω6 and a very high ω6/ω3 ratio in the diet are associated with and thought to be casual in the pathogenesis of many diseases, including cardiovascular disease, cancer and inflammatory and autoimmune diseases [5]. The reduction of ω6/ω3 ratio has also shown to be beneficial in the liver studies [9,10]. Conversely, diets enriched with ω3 have been shown to reduce hypertriglyceridemia [11], fatty liver disease [12,13], and improve renal function in type 2 diabetics [14].

Omega-6 and ω3 polyunsaturated fatty acids can be non-enzymatically oxidized and are also substrates for oxidation by lipoxygenases (LO), cyclooxygenases, and epoxygenases. In particular, 12/15-LO catalyzes the insertion of molecular oxygen into the ω6 arachidonic acid and linoleic acid; 12- and 15-hydroxy-eicosatetraenoic acids (HETE) are 12/15-LO products of arachidonic acid and 9- and 13- hydroxy-octadecadienoic acids (HODE) are 12/15-LO products of linoleic acid, all of which are pro-inflammatory. We have previously demonstrated that 12/15-LO knockout (KO) mice are protected from insulin resistance and adipose tissue inflammation induced by a short-term feeding with ω6-enriched HF diet [15].

In this study we aimed at investigating the long-term effects of altering dietary ω6/ω3 ratio in HF diet induced obesity in wild-type (WT) mice with focus on the liver and adipose tissue inflammation. We gave careful consideration on the design of the diets so that the amount of total saturated, monounsaturated and polyunsaturated fatty acids was the same in each HF diet. Moreover, the total amount of dietary fat, the ratios of ω6 to ω3, and the amount of total eicosapentaenoic acid (EPA) and docosahexaenoic acid (DHA) in our low ω6/ω3 ratio diet are more relevant to the ratios and doses used in human studies which are significantly lower in comparison to the majority of published rodent studies investigating the anti-inflammatory effects of ω3 supplementation [16,17,18,19,20]. We assessed the circulating concentration of oxidized metabolites of pro-inflammatory ω6 arachidonic and linoleic fatty acids and examined markers of both innate and adaptive immune systems in liver tissue. Lastly, we sought to delineate the effects of 12/15-LO deficiency on hepatic steatosis in the chronic ω6-enriched diet obese rodent model.

Experimental Procedures

Animal studies

All mouse procedures were performed in accordance with the *Guide for Care and Use of Laboratory Animals* of the National Institutes of Health and were approved by the University of California, San Diego, Animal Subjects Committee (protocol #S99173). All efforts were made to minimize pain and distress during animal husbandry and experimental assessments. Fourteen- to 15-week old male C57BL/6J WT mice (Jackson Laboratory, Bar Harbor, ME) were fed with normal control (NC, n = 7) rodent diet Purina 5001 (13% calories from fat; LabDiet, St. Louis, MO), high fat diet with high dietary ω6/ω3 ratio of 11:1 (HFH, n = 7; 46% calories from fat), representing typical Western diet, or high fat diet with low dietary ω6/ω3 ratio of 2.7:1 (HFL, n = 8; 46% calories from fat), Table 1. Both HF diets were custom designed and manufactured by TestDiet (PMI Nutrition International, St. Louis, MO) using their basic van Heek standard obesogenic diet 58V8. The HFH fat components were lard and soybean oil, the HFL fat components were lard, soybean oil, and Menhaden fish oil. Care was taken to ensure palatability and prevent reduced calorie intake in the HFL-fed mouse group, challenges that have been previously reported in other fish oil/ω3-enriched diet studies [19,20]. Fish oil fragrance can lead to reduced food intake, so both high fat diets were prepared with bacon flavoring and anti-oxidant t-butylhydroquinone (0.002% wt/wt) in order minimize potential odor-effects on food intake with the HFL diet. Both HFL and HFH diets were developed in pelleted form. Fifteen-week old male 12/15-LOKO mice (from our in-house colony [15] were fed with HFH diet (n = 4). Mice were housed under controlled light (12:12 light: dark) and climate conditions with unlimited access to food and water. Mouse weights and food intake were monitored daily for one week and then twice a week for the next 9 weeks on respective diets. All mice were sacrificed after 15–17 weeks into the respective diets to assess liver pathophysiology and inflammatory gene expression, plasma components, gonadal white adipose tissue (gWAT) weight and macrophage infiltration. Mouse sacrifice was performed in a matched way so that the average length of the feeding period was the same in each group. Figure 1 shows the daily intake of total ω3 FA and EPA+DHA for the mice in our study and a schematic of the study groups. For comparison with the mouse daily dose in our study, Figure 1 also shows an approximate EPA+DHA daily dose commonly prescribed to an 80 kg human.

Assessment of Insulin Resistance by HOMA-IR

Homeostatic model assessment of insulin resistance (HOMA-IR) was calculated as fasting plasma insulin (μU/mL) × fasting blood glucose (mg/dL) ÷405] [21]. Plasma insulin levels were measured using the Insulin Ultrasensitive (Mouse) EIA method (Alpco, Salem, NH). A single plasma sample with insulin level outside of the linear range of the assay was been excluded from analysis. Fasting whole blood glucose was measured using a hand-held glucometer (OneTouch Ultra2, LifeScan, Inc. Milpitas, CA).

Histology and the Assessment of Hepatic Steatosis in Mouse Livers

Livers were weighed, cut into small pieces and fixed in 10% formalin for 24 h or freshly frozen in Optimal Cutting Temperature compound (OCT). The formalin fixed tissues were embedded in paraffin and sections of 4 μm thickness were prepared. Haematoxylin and eosin stained sections were used for histopathological evaluation of hepatic injury and Oil Red O-stained frozen liver specimens was performed by the UCSD Histology Core. Samples were analyzed by light microscopy and the level of triglycerides assessed by ImageJ software (National Institutes of Health, Bethesda, MD). All photos were taken by NanoZoomer 2.0HT Slide Scanning System (Hamamatsu, Japan).

Flow cytometry

Adipose tissue stromal vascular cells (SVCs) were isolated and analyzed by FACS as previously reported [22] with minor modifications. Briefly, freshly harvested epididymal fat pads were separately rinsed and minced in DPBS +1% BSA then treated with 1 mg/mL type II collagenase (Sigma) for 25 min in a 37°C shaking water bath. Adipose tissue cell suspensions were filtered through 100 μm mesh. SVCs were separated from floating adipocytes by centrifugation, incubated in RBC lysis buffer (eBioscience) for 5 min, then re-suspended in fresh DPBS +1% BSA. SVCs were incubated with Fc Block (BD Biosciences) for 15 min and then stained for 30 min with fluorescent-conjugated antibodies against F4/80 (Ab Serotec), CD11b (BD Biosciences), and CD11c (BD Biosciences). Cells were washed two times and re-suspended in DPBS +1% BSA and propidium iodide (Sigma). Presence of the fluorescent stains in the SVCs was analyzed using a

Table 1. Composition of diets.

	HFH	HFL
Omega-6	15.9%	12.5%
LA	15.7%	12.2%
AA	0.2%	0.3%
Omega-3	1.4%	4.6%
ALA	1.4%	1.1%
EPA+DHA	0.0%	3.5%
ω6/ω3 ratio	11	2.7
SFA	40.8%	41.5%
MUFA	42.0%	41.4%
PUFA	17.3%	17.1%
Total fat	46.3%	46.3%
Protein	18.2%	18.2%
Carbohydrate	35.5%	35.5%

Fatty acid subgroup values are represented as a percent of total fat. Total fat, protein, carbohydrate values are represented as a percent of total kcal of diets. HFH, high dietary ω6/ω3 ratio; HFL, low dietary ω6/ω3 ratio; LA, linoleic acid; AA, arachidonic acid; ALA, alpha-linoleic acid; EPA, eicosapentaenoic acid; DHA, docosahexaenoic acid; SFA, saturated fatty acids; MUFA, monounsaturated fatty acids; PUFA, polyunsaturated fatty acids.

FACS Calibur flow cytometer (BD Biosciences). Control SVCs preparations, including unstained cells, PI-only stained cells, and fluorescence-minus-one (FMO) stained cells, were used to set gatings and compensation. Total macrophages were defined as F4/80$^+$CD11b$^+$ cells, while M1-type macrophages were defined as F4/80$^+$CD11b$^+$CD11c$^+$ cells.

Detection and quantification of oxidized fatty acid profile

All plasma samples for analyses contained anti-oxidant cocktail [DTPA (2 mM final) and butylated hydroxytoluene (500 μM final)]. Levels of multiple fatty acid oxidation products (free plus esterified) in plasma were quantified using liquid chromatography online electrospray ionization tandem mass spectroscopy. Preparation and analysis of plasma samples was performed as previously reported [23]. The lipid peroxidation products analyzed included structurally specific species of HETE (5-, 8-, 9-, 11-, 12-, and 15-HETE), HODE (9- and 13-HODE), oxo-octadecadienoic acids (9- and 13-oxoODE) and their precursors arachidonic acid and linoleic acid.

Gene expression

Liver tissue was preserved in RNA*later* (Invitrogen, Carlsbad, CA) and homogenized using the FastPrep 24 bead homogenization system (MP Biomedicals, Santa Ana, CA). Total RNA was isolated using RNeasy kit (Qiagen, Valencia, CA) and reverse transcribed by SuperScript III First-Strand Synthesis System RT-PCR Kit (Invitrogen) using oligodT primers according to the manufacturer instructions. The concentration and purity of RNA was assessed by NanoDrop (Thermo Scientific, Waltham, MA). The 260/280 ratio of each sample was at or slightly above 2. Additional on column DNAse digestion step was performed, and 'no template' and 'no reverse transcriptase' controls were run to ascertain purity of reagents and the lack of genomic DNA contamination, respectively. Individual samples were measured in triplicate. Data were normalized against two reference housekeeping genes: beta-2 microglobulin (B2m) and hydroxymethylbilane synthase (Hmbs) which were chosen based on stable gene expression levels, based on our pilot study. Others have also found a stable invariant expression of these genes in the livers of other high fat diet-induced obesity mouse models and hepatic cells [24,25,26]. The PCR primers used to amplify each gene are: B2m F-5′-CCCCACTGAGACTGATACATACG-3′ R-5′-CGATCCCAGTAGACGGTCTTG-3′, Ccr7 F- 5′-GTACGAGTCGGTGTGCTTCAA-3′ R-5′-GGTAGGTATCCGTCATGGTCT-3′, Ccl19 F- 5′-GTGATGGAGGGGTCAGGA-3′ R-5′-GGGATGGGACAGCCTAAACT-5′, Ccl21 F-5′-GTGATGGAGGGGGTCAGGA-3′ R-5′-GGGATGGGACAGCCTAAACT-3′, Cxcl1 (KC) F- 5′-CTGGGATTCACCTCAAGAACATC-3′ R-5′-CAGGGTCAAGGCAAGCCTC-3′, Cxcl2/3 (Mip2) F-5′-CCACCAACCACCAGGCTAC-3′ R-5′-GCTTCAGGGTCAAGGGCAAA-3′, Hmbs F-5′-TGTGGTGGCGATGCTGAAA-3′ R-5′-TTGTCTCCCGTGGACATA-3′, Ifng F-5′-ATGAACGCTACACACTGCATC-3′ R-5′-CCATCCTTTTGCCAGTTCCTC-3′, Il10 F-5′-GCTCTTACTGACTGGCATGAG-3′ R-5′-CGCAGCTCTAGGAGCATGTG-3′, Il12a F-5′-CTGTGCCTTGGTAGCATCTATG-3′ R-5′-CGCAGAGTCTCGCCATTATGAT-3′, Il12b F-5′-CTCAGAAGCTAACCATCTCCTGG-3′ R-5′-CACAGGTGAGGTTCACTGTTTC-3′, Il18 F-5′-GACTCTTGCGTCAACTTCAAGG-3′ R-5′-CAGGCTGTCTTTTGTCAACGA-3′, Srebp1 F-5′-GCAGCCACCATCTAGCCTG-3′ R-5′-CAGCAGTGAGTCTGCCTTGAT-3′, Tnfa F-5′-CCCTCACACTCAGATCATCTTCT-3′ R-5′-GCTACGACGTGGGCTACAG-3′. Quantitative Real-time PCR was performed on a CFX96 RT-PCR Detection System (BioRad, Hercules, CA, USA) by using Brilliant II SYBR Green QPCRMaster Mix (Agilent Technologies, La Jolla, CA, USA). Fold-change values were calculated using the $2^{-\Delta\Delta Ct}$ method.

Data analysis

Repeated-measures one-way ANOVA was applied to body weight with a Bonferroni post hoc test to determine significant group differences over time. Two-tailed Student's t-test was used to analyze statistical significance between groups, as indicated in the figure legends. Data are reported as mean ± standard error of the mean (SE), with significance at $P<0.05$, unless otherwise noted. GraphPad software (La Jolla, CA) was used to perform analyses and to construct graphs.

A

	ω6 : ω3 ratio	Total ω3 FA (mg/kg/day)	EPA (mg/kg/day)	DHA (mg/kg/day)	EPA+DHA (mg/kg/day)	EPA+DHA Dose for 80kg human (mg/kg/day)
HFH	11.0 : 1	240	0	0	0	0
HFL	2.7 : 1	743	203	175	378	42

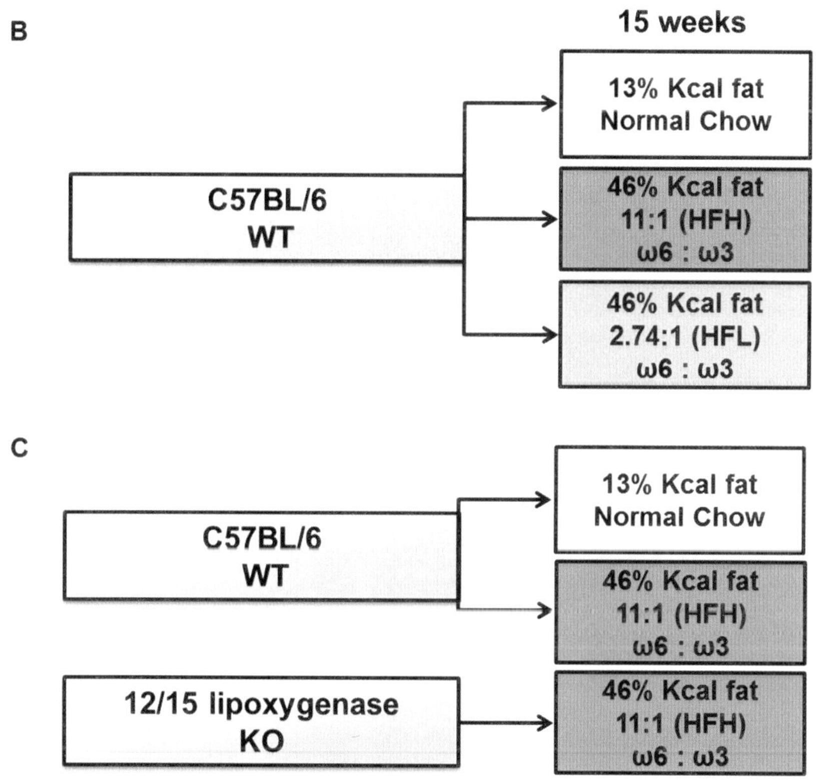

Figure 1. Schematic of diets and mouse groups. (A) Schematic illustrates the dietary ω6/ω3 fatty acid ratio, and the mg/kg/day intake of total ω3 fatty acid, EPA, DHA and EPA+DHA in the HFH and HFL diets consumed by the mice. For comparison, the approximate mg/kg/day dose of EPA+DHA for an 80 kg human taking a standard prescription of Lovaza fish oil (four 1 g capsules, containing 840 mg EPA+DHA each, per day) is shown. (B) 15-week diet regimens for WT mice: normal chow diet (13% Kcal from fat), high fat diet (46% kcal from fat) with high dietary ω6/ω3 ratio (HFH), or high fat diet (46% kcal from fat) with low dietary ω6/ω3 (HFL). (C) 15-week diet regimens for WT and 12/15-LOKO mice: high fat diet (46% kcal from fat) with high dietary ω6/ω3 ratio (HFH). FA, fatty acids; EPA, eicosapentaenoic acid; DHA, docosahexaenoic acid.

Results

Lowering dietary ω6/ω3 increases food intake, but does not significantly alter total body, liver or adipose tissue weights in high fat diet induced obesity

To assess the metabolic effects of altering dietary ω6/ω3 ratio in the context of a high fat diet, we fed WT mice isocaloric diets (46% kcal from fat) containing polyunsaturated fat contributed primarily from soybean oil (high ω6/ω3 ratio, HFH) or fish oil (low ω6/ω3 ratio, HFL), or low fat, normal chow (NC; 13% kcal from fat) (Fig. 1A and B). The high fat diets (HFH and HFL) were carefully designed to contain equivalent fat, protein and carbohydrate content as well as equivalent total saturated, monounsaturated, and polyunsaturated fatty acid content (Table 1). Both high fat diets induced significant body weight gain past week 5 as compared to NC (Fig. 2A). There was no significant difference in weight gain over the period of the first 10 weeks or in the final body weights (week 15) between WT mice fed HFH and HFL diets (Fig. 2A and Table 2). Although WT mice on HFL diet consumed significantly more calories daily, averaging over the period of the week 5 to 10 of the study ($P<0.001$) (Fig. 2B), increased food intake in the HFL group did not differentially affect liver or gonadal white adipose tissue (gWAT) weight as a percent of total body weight (Table 2). Finally, there were no differences in fasting plasma insulin and glucose levels, HOMA-IR, or proinflammatory M1-type macrophage content in gWAT between WT mice fed HFH and HFL diets (Table 2).

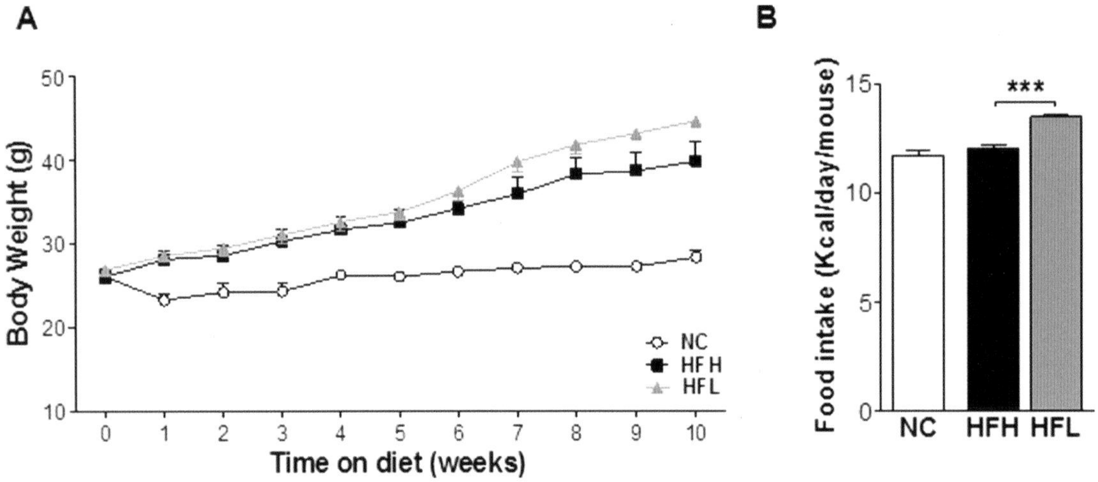

Figure 2. Body weight and food intake. The effect of varying dietary ω6/ω3 ratio in WT (NC n = 4), open circles; HFH n = 7, black squares; and HFL n = 8, gray triangles) mice on (A) body weight over fist 10 weeks of diet regimens and (B) food intake averaged over weeks 5 to 10 on the respective diets. Values are mean ±SE. ***P<0.001 HFH vs. HFL. NC, normal control (chow); HFH, high dietary ω6/ω3 ratio; HFL, low dietary ω6/ω3 ratio.

Lowering dietary ω6/ω3 reduces lymphocyte homing response in the liver and decreases hepatic inflammation and steatosis

As it was previously reported that ω3 supplemented diet reduces hepatic steatosis and inflammation [18,19], we next aimed to characterize these parameters in our animal models by measuring gene expression in liver tissue from the mouse groups. First we assessed the stimulation of Th1-mediated immune responses which generally lead to a pro-inflammatory phenotype and increased abundance of effectors IFN-γ and TNF-α. We found that HFL diet significantly reduced the mRNA levels of Il12a and b (p35 and p40 subunits) (P<0.05) and Il18 (P<0.05) as compared to HFH, thus marking attenuation of the inflammatory Th1 phenotype (Fig. 3A). Next, we assessed hepatic mRNA expression of representative pro-inflammatory (Infg and Tnfa) and anti-inflammatory pathway (Il10) genes and neutrophil chemoattractant genes, C-X-C motif ligand 1 (Cxcl1, KC) and microphage inflammatory protein 2 (Mip2; Cxcl2/3). HFL diet had a protective, anti-inflammatory effect where levels of Ifng (P<0.01) and Tnfa (P<0.001) mRNA were near to normal chow (NC) control levels, as compared to the effect of HFH diet (Fig. 3B). Levels of Il10 and Cxcl1 mRNA were both significantly lower in HFL vs. HFH diet-fed mice (P<0.05) (Fig. 3C). Next, the lymphocyte homing response was examined. When chemokine C-C motif ligands (CCL) 19 or 21 bind to lymphocyte-expressed chemokine receptor (CCR) 7, this receptor is internalized and lymphocytes stay trapped in an organ. Indeed, it has been shown that the suppression of cytokine signaling protein-1 regulates migration of $CD4^+$ T cells into peripheral tissues via changes in Ccr7 expression levels [27]. Accordingly, we observed a decrease in the expression of Ccr7 (P<0.05) and increase in the expression of Ccl19 (P<0.05) in HFH-fed animals, a phenotype that did not exist in HFL diet-fed mice, suggesting that lower dietary ω6/ω3 ratio in the context of a high fat diet protects from lymphocyte homing in the liver (Fig. 3D). Interestingly, HFL diet did not alter high fat diet-induced infiltration of M1-type inflammatory macrophages into gWAT, as determined by flow cytometry analysis (Table 2). Histological analysis of H&E and Oil Red O

Table 2. Metabolic parameters in WT mice fed NC, HFH, and HFL diets.

Parameter [unit]	NC mean±SE (n = 3–7)[a]	HFH mean±SE (n = 6–7)	HFL mean±SE (n = 7–8)	t-test[b] p-value
Final body weight (BW) [g]	29.1±0.8	41.0±2.6	45.3±0.8	0.12
Liver weight [% BW]	5.7±0.3	5.0±0.3	5.2±0.4	0.67
gWAT weight [% BW]	2.3±0.3	4.4±0.3	4.1±0.1	0.50
Fasting plasma insulin [ng/mL]	0.30±0.11	1.82±0.56	2.62±0.56	0.34
Fasting blood glucose [mg/dL]	111±8	128±20	158±12	0.21
HOMA-IR	2.0±0.8	16.0±7.4	24.0±4.1	0.33
gWAT M1-type macrophages [% total macrophages]	18.9±1.7	80.6±7.0	89.3±1.0	0.21

NC, normal chow; HFH, high dietary ω6/ω3 ratio; HFL, low dietary ω6/ω3 ratio; HOMA-IR, homeostatic model assessment of insulin resistance; gWAT, gonadal white adipose tissue.

[a]Data were not available for liver weight, fasting insulin and glucose for 4 NC mice.

[b]Student's t-test was restricted to high fat diet groups (HFH vs. HFL). NC data are shown for comparison.

stained liver specimens demonstrated significantly less hepatic steatosis in HFL as compared with HFH diet-fed mice (Fig. 3E). Correspondingly, the expression level of the sterol regulatory element-binding protein 1 gene (Srebp1) was significantly lower in HFL vs. HFH diet fed mice ($P<0.05$) (Fig. 3F).

Oxidized metabolites of arachidonic acid are significantly decreased in the plasma of HFL diet-fed mice

We have shown previously that 9- and 13-HODEs and 9- and 13-oxoODEs, products of free radical and enzymatic lipoxygenase-mediated oxidation of the ω6 linoleic acid were significantly elevated in patients with non-alcoholic steatohepatitis (NASH) [14]. Plasma concentrations of 12-, 15-, 11-, 8- and 9-HETE oxidized metabolites of the ω6 arachidonic acid were significantly lowered in HFL vs. HFH diet fed mice (all $P<0.05$) (Fig. 4A). There were no significant changes in the plasma concentrations of oxidized metabolites of linoleic acid (HODEs and oxo-ODEs) or ω6 precursor concentrations of plasma arachidonic acid or linoleic acid (Fig. 4B and C).

12/15-lipoxygenase deficiency prevents metabolic defects and liver abnormalities associated with high fat, high ω6/ω3 ratio diet

We and others have previously shown that 12/15-LOKO mice are protected from HF diet-induced insulin resistance and adipose tissue inflammation [15,28]. In this study, we were interested in additionally studying the liver phenotypes of 12/15-LOKO mice after HF feeding. 12/15-LOKO mice were subjected to HFH diet for the same duration as WT mice and compared to WT HFH mice to assess whether 12/15-lipoxygenase deficiency prevents metabolic defects associated with high fat, high ω6/ω3 ratio diet (Fig. 1C). There were no significant differences in the final total body weights or gWAT mass expressed as a percentage of total body weight among any of the groups (Fig. 5A) even though the KO mice consumed significantly less calories daily, averaged over weeks 5 to 10 of the study ($P<0.01$) (Fig. 5A). Gene expression markers of lymphocyte homing response in liver were reduced (Fig. 5B), as was expression of hepatic cytokine and chemoattractant genes (Ifng, Tnfa, Il10 and Cxcl2/3) in KO HFH as compared to WT HFH (all $P<0.05$) (Fig. 5C and D) similar to that observed in the WT HFL group (Fig. 3B and C). In addition, hepatic steatosis was also significantly less in the KO HFH as compared to WT HFH mice (Fig. 5E and F). Although plasma levels of oxidized metabolites of arachidonic acid were not individually significantly reduced in the KO mice (Fig. 5G), they were all trending lower as expected given that 12/15-lipoxygenase is an enzymatic source of 12- and 15-HETE. Levels of oxidized arachidonic acid metabolites of in the KO mice approximate those observed in the HFL-fed WT mice (Fig. 4A).

Discussion

Nonalcoholic fatty liver disease has become the most common liver disease in the United States and other developed countries. It is commonly associated with the metabolic syndrome, obesity, type 2 diabetes and dyslipidemia. With the addition of inflammation, NAFLD can progress to a more serious condition termed NASH which then can progress to cirrhosis and hepatocellular carcinoma [29]. Common causes of NAFLD, such as Western diet-induced obesity and insulin resistance, are associated with macrophage infiltration and inflammation in adipose, liver and muscle tissues of humans and rodent models where a feed-forward cycle of reciprocal adipocyte, hepatocyte, myocyte and macrophage cross-talk results in the secretion of inflammatory factors and further macrophage recruitment [4,30,31,32]. Thus, reducing this chronic inflammation may be the key to combating obesity-induced morbidities, insulin resistance and NAFLD. We aimed to identify new strategic dietary approaches for mitigating HF diet-induced inflammation and expand our knowledge of 12/15-LO activity. This study is the first to show that reducing dietary ω6/ω3 fatty acid ratio, without any other diet composition changes, is sufficient to protect WT mice from long-term HF diet-induced steatohepatitis and to reduce plasma concentration of oxidized metabolites of arachidonic acid. This reduction in dietary ω6/ω3 ratio did not protect the WT mice from HF diet-induced insulin resistance or adipose tissue inflammation. In addition, we demonstrate that 12/15-LO deficiency is sufficient to protect from ω6-enriched HF-diet induced steatohepatitis and, as we have shown previously (41), total body insulin resistance.

Published rodent studies have shown that fish oil-based, ω3-enriched HF diets do not induce insulin resistance and adipose tissue inflammation as do isocaloric ω6-enriched HF diets (same % calories from fat) [33,34,35]. Although reducing the dietary ω6/ω3 ratio in our current study prevented development of liver inflammation and steatosis, it did not prevent development of insulin resistance (HOMA-IR). The beneficial effect of ω3 fatty acid supplementation on insulin sensitivity in other rodent HF diet-induced models may have been potentiated by three factors, 1) high ratio of ω6/ω3 used in the "control" HF diets, 2) megadoses of EPA+DHA in the fish oil HF diets, and 3) reduced weight gain and food intake observed in mice consuming fish oil-containing vs. standard HF diet. The ω6/ω3 ratios of HF control diets used in several other studies are extreme, ranging from 34:1 to 86:1 [17,18]; in contrast, we used a ratio of 11:1, which is well within the estimated dietary ω6/ω3 ratio range found in the typical Western-style human diet (10-20:1) [5]. Based on our calculations using their Methods sections, other rodent studies have used extremely high EPA+DHA (long chain, anti-inflammatory ω3) doses of 1660-4370 mg/kg/day [16,36], at least 40–104X the common therapeutic dose for an 80 kg human taking a standard prescription of Lovaza fish oil (Figure 1). The EPA+DHA dose in our study was 378 mg/kg/day, approximately 9X the dose that an 80 kg human would consume taking a standard prescription of Lovaza fish oil (Figure 1). In order to minimize weight gain differences commonly attributable to reduced fish oil diet intake, we prepared both our HFH and HFL diets in pelleted form and with added bacon flavoring and anti-oxidants to mask the fragrance of the fish oil in the HFL diet. Thus, in our study, food intake and weight gain exhibited by mice in the HFL low ω6/ω3 ratio group was not reduced. In fact, HFL group mice consumed significantly more calories per day and tended to gain more weight than HFH controls. Rodents in other fish oil diet studies [17,18,19,20,37] where the fish oil-fed groups consumed less calories and had reduced body weight gain compared to controls may have experienced long-term insulin sensitizing effects that were secondary to reduced weight gain, as has been previously suggested [38]. Thus, the effects of ω3 supplementation on insulin resistance and glucose metabolism remain unclear.

Although it is known that inflammation mediated by the innate immune response plays a critical role in obesity and NAFLD, the role and importance of adaptive immune system is just beginning to be unraveled. Among adaptive cells of the immune system, T lymphocytes play a major role in the inflammatory response. Thus, we hypothesized that an unregulated function of T cells might be critical for NASH. Even though NASH is not considered a Th1-polarized disease, several studies have shown that an excessive production of Th1 proinflammatory cytokines and a deficit of anti-inflammatory cytokines are components in its

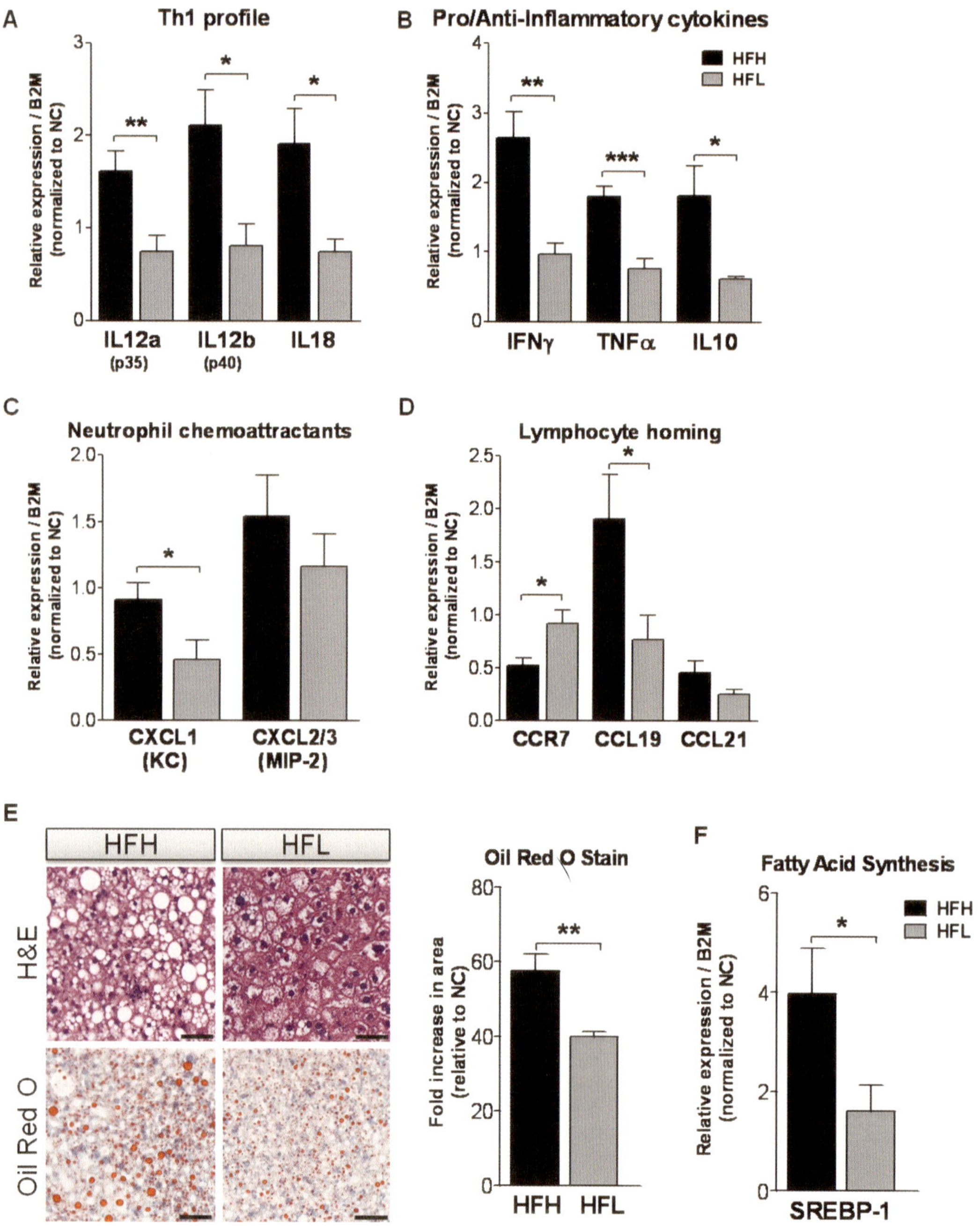

Figure 3. Assessment of hepatic inflammation and steatosis. The effect of varying dietary ω6/ω3 ratio in high fat diet-fed WT mice on the hepatic mRNA expression of (A) cytokines driving a Th1 profile, (B) pro/anti-inflammatory cytokines, (C) neutrophil chemoattractants, and (D) regulators of lymphocyte homing response, all normalized to signal in WT NC mice (n = 7). (E) Haematoxylin-eosin and Oil red O staining of paraffin-embedded liver sections. Quantitative grading scale assessing the quantity of hepatic triglycerides, normalized to signal in WT NC mice (expressed as a fold increase in stained area relative to WT NC mice). (F) The effect of varying dietary ω6/ω3 ratio in high fat diet-fed WT mice on the hepatic mRNA expression of sterol regulatory element-binding protein 1 (Srebp1) normalized to signal in WT NC mice. WT HFH: black bars; WT HFL: gray bars. Values are mean ±SE. 5-7 animals per group. *$P<0.05$, **$P<0.01$, ***$P<0.001$ HFH vs. HFL. Scale bar, 50 μm. WT NC SEs for genes Il12a (p35), Il12b (p40), Il18, Ifng, Tnfa, Il10, Cxcl1 (KC), Cxcl2/3 (Mip2), Ccr7, Ccl19, Ccl21 and Srebp1 were 0.14, 0.09, 0.14, 0.08, 0.12, 0.17, 0.14, 0.13, 0.20, 0.21, 0.15, and 0.10, respectively. WT NC SE value for oil red O stain was 0.15. NC, normal control (chow); HFH, high dietary ω6/ω3 ratio; HFL, low dietary ω6/ω3 ratio.

development [39]. CCR7, the receptor for the chemokine CCL19, is expressed on naïve T-cells, central memory T cells and Treg cells among others. CCR7 regulates trafficking and homing of lymphocytes to and within secondary lymphoid organs and nonlymphoid tissues. Lack of CCR7 expression results in accumulation of conventional T cells in diverse tissues and immediate effector function. Furthermore, it has been demonstrated that IFN-γ is exclusively produced by CCR7- T cells [40]. Herein, we report that HF diet with a high dietary ω6/ω3 ratio significantly reduced the mRNA expression of Ccr7 and increased the expression of its ligand Ccl19, suggesting that T cells are attracted to the liver and once within it, the microenvironment

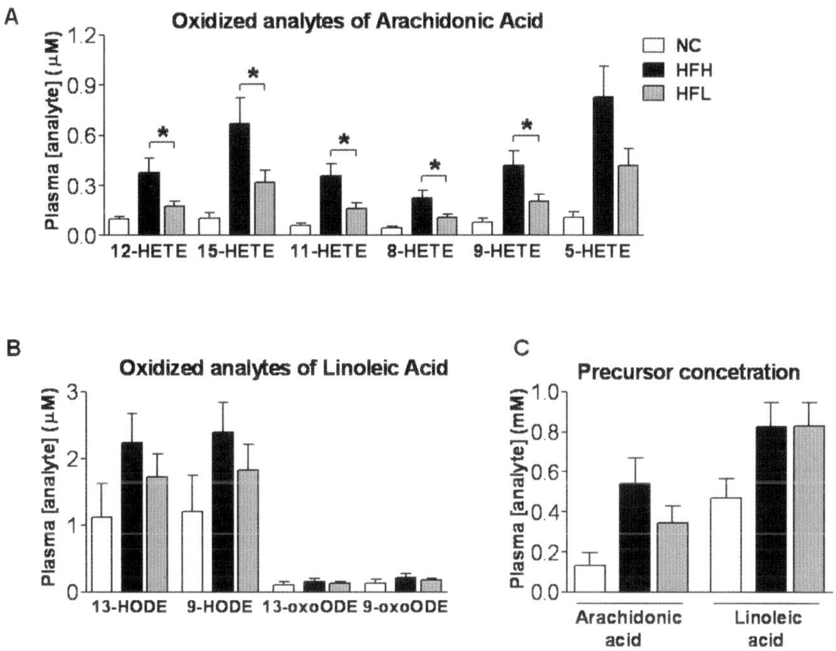

Figure 4. Plasma concentration of the major ω6 fatty acids and their corresponding pro-inflammatory metabolites. The effect of varying dietary ω6/ω3 ratio in high fat diet-fed WT mice on plasma concentrations of oxidized metabolites of (A) arachidonic acid and (B) linoleic acid. (C) Plasma concentrations of arachidonic and linoleic acids. NC n = 3 (open bars), HFH n = 7 (black bars), HFL n = 8 (gray bars). T-test analysis was restricted to HF diet animals only. Values are mean ±SE. *$P<0.05$ HFH vs. HFL. NC, normal control (chow); HFH, high dietary ω6/ω3 ratio; HFL, low dietary ω6/ω3 ratio; HETE, hydroxyeicosatetraenoic acid; HODE, hydroxyoctadecadienoic acid; oxoODE, oxooctadecadienoic acid.

triggers their differentiation into CCR7- cells and retention in the liver. Interestingly, this effect was significantly blunted in mice fed a HF diet with decreased ω6/ω3 ratio or with 12/15-LO deficiency. Lowering dietary ω6/ω3 ratio may be of clinical relevance for reducing T-lymphocyte homing to the liver.

A role for IL-18 has been postulated in the development of hepatic steatosis since both serum IL-18 concentration and hepatic Il18 mRNA expression are elevated in lipopolysaccharide-treated leptin deficient ob/ob mice and high fat diet fed-C57BL/6 mice [41]. Proinflammatory cytokines IL-18 and IL-12 are closely related and act synergistically since the administration recombinant proteins IL-12 and IL-18 concurrently induces the production of elevated levels of IFN-γ and TNF-α in mice [41]. Interestingly, exogenous administration of IL-18 with IL-12 to BALB/c mice induces fatty liver in an IFN-γ dependent manner [42], suggesting that both cytokines play an important role in the inflammatory cascade leading to NAFLD. Different experimental evidences point to an important role of IFN-γ and TNF-α in hepatic damage. The important role ascribed to IFN-γ in hepatic damage is based on its capability to prime Kupffer Cells upon the co-recruitment of monocytes and lymphocytes into the inflamed liver. Also, TNF-α contributes to insulin resistance and hepatic steatosis in diet induced obesity [43]. Accordingly, in the present study we have shown that both increased levels of Il12a, Il12b, Il18, Ifng, Tnfa, and Il10 mRNA expression seen in the liver of HFH fed mice and hepatic steatosis were reduced in HFL fed mice.

Omega-6 and ω3 polyunsaturated fatty acids are *essential* dietary components in mammals and they compete for the same enzymes for their processing, thus, the distribution of these polyunsaturated fatty acids and their metabolite products in plasma and tissue is directly influenced by dietary intake [5,6]. It has been shown that the positive effects of ω3 fatty acids are connected to modulation of eicosanoid metabolic and signaling pathways, which leads to alteration of polyunsaturated fatty acid subtypes, inflammatory responses, and direct effects on gene expression. Rodents and humans consuming diets rich in ω3 fatty acids, as a result, have reduced production of arachidonic acid and eicosanoid oxidation products of arachidonic acid including prostaglandin E_2, leukotriene B4, and HETEs [44]. Interestingly, when HETE is added to macrophages, it can cause inflammation by up-regulating proinflammatory gene expression [45]. We have previously demonstrated that 12/15-LO knockout in mice counteracts the HF diet-induced increase in proinflammatory macrophages and cytokine (IFN-γ, IL-12p40 and TNF-α) and chemokine (CXCL1) proteins in adipose tissue [15]. In this study, we demonstrate that increased mRNA expression of hepatic Ifng and Cxcl2/3 seen in HFH-fed WT mice were diminished in HFH-fed 12/15-LOKO mice. The decreased hepatic Il10 mRNA expression seen in HFL mice compared to HFH mice is not surprising. It has been demonstrated that high levels of IL-18 and IL-12 can induce IL-10 [46]. The production of IL-10 could be a mechanism for attenuating the inflammatory response mediated by IL-12. As a consequence, when IL-12 and IL-18 decreased, the attempt to reduce the proinflammatory microenvironment is no longer needed.

12/15-LO is an enzyme that catalyzes the insertion of molecular oxygen into polyunsaturated fatty acids, including the ω6 arachidonic and linoleic acids and the ω3 EPA and DHA. 12/15-LO products of ω6 substrates are involved in the signaling processes of defense response and inflammation, activating Rac, RhoA, MAP kinases, PKC, JNK and NF-κB [47,48]. We have shown that 12/15-LO oxidation products activate TLR4 in macrophages [49,50], suggesting a possible connection between 12/15-LO and TLR4 activation in the pathogenesis of insulin resistance. 12/15-LO has also been implicated with obesity.

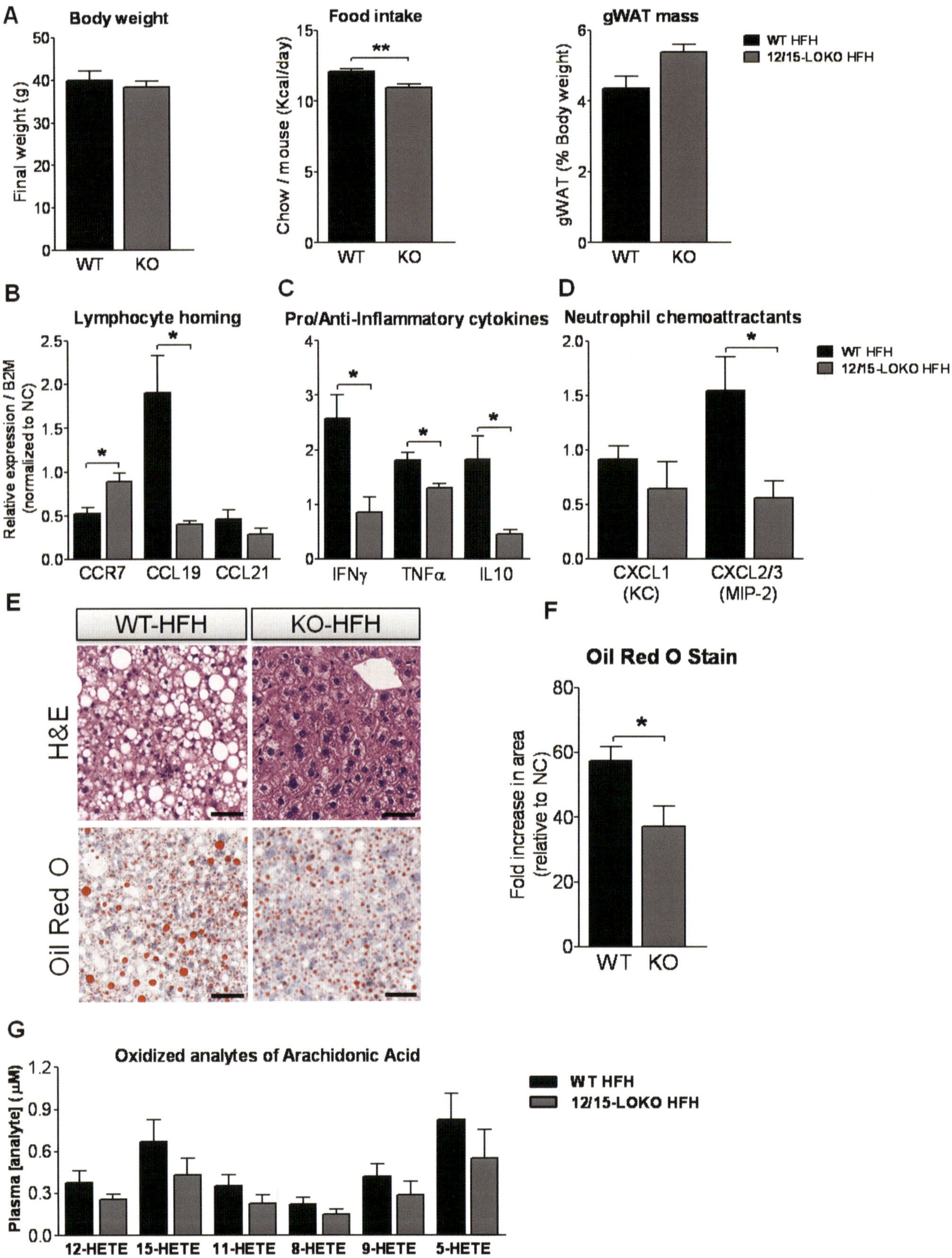

Figure 5. Assessment of hepatic inflammation and steatosis in 12/15-LOKO mice on HFH diet. The effect of 12/15-lipoxygenase deficiency on (A) terminal body weight, food intake and gonadal white adipose tissue (gWAT) weight expressed as percent total body weight, and

hepatic expression of (B) regulators of lymphocyte homing response, (C) pro/anti-inflammatory cytokines and (D) neutrophil chemoattractants. (E) Haematoxylin-eosin and Oil red O staining of paraffin-embedded liver sections to show hepatic steatosis. (F) Quantitative grading scale assessing the quantity of hepatic triglycerides, normalized to signal in WT NC (n = 7) mice (expressed as a fold increase in stained area relative to WT NC mice). (G) Plasma concentrations of oxidized metabolites of arachidonic acid in KO HFH n = 4 (dark gray bars) compared to WT HFH n = 7 (black bars) mice. Values are mean ±SE. *P<0.05, **P<0.01 WT HFH vs. 12/15-LOKO HFH. Scale bar, 50 μm. WT NC SEs for genes Ccr7, Ccl19, Ccl21, Ifng, Tnfa, Il10, Cxcl1 (KC), Cxcl2/3 (MIP-2) were 0.20, 0.21, 0.15, 0.08, 0.12, 0.17, 0.14, 0.13, respectively. WT NC SE value for oil red O stain was 0.15. KO, 12/15 lipoxygenase knockout; HFH, high dietary ω6/ω3 ratio; gWAT, gonadal white adipose tissue; HETE, hydroxyeicosatetraenoic acid.

Expression and activity of 12/15-LO is increased in liver and adipocytes after HF diet consumption in rodents [45,51]. Previously we showed that 12/15-LO deficiency protected mice from adipose tissue inflammation and, remarkably, prevented systemic insulin resistance induced after 2–4 weeks (short-term) HF diet feeding [15,28]. Longer-term (8–24 weeks) studies showed similar results and also showed that HF induces 12/15-LO activation and beta cell damage in pancreatic islets, which was prevented in 12/15-LO deficient mice [28]. In the current study, we show that 12/15-LO deficiency offers long-term (15 weeks) protection from ω6-enriched HF diet-induced fatty liver, liver inflammation and lymphocyte homing to the liver. 12- and 15-HETE are 12/15-LO oxidation products of ω6 arachidonic acid and 9- and 13-HODE are 12/15-LO products of ω6 linoleic acid, all of which are pro-inflammatory. Herein, we show that levels of oxidized metabolites of arachidonic acid in plasma were significantly reduced by lowering dietary ω6/ω3 ratio and tended to be lower with 12/15-LO deficiency. Although reducing 12/15-LO activity may seem like a potential therapeutic target for counteracting high dietary ω6/ω3 ratio, a simpler strategy would be to reduce dietary ω6/ω3 ratio which would decrease the levels of ω6-derived pro-inflammatory eicosanoids and increase the levels of ω3-derived anti-inflammatory eicosanoids produced overall by cyclooxygenases, lipoxygenases, and epoxygenases.

In this study we examined novel dietary and therapeutic approaches to reduce inflammation in obesity and metabolic syndrome-related diseases. In particular, NASH is a serious liver condition without any available treatments. These data strongly suggest that either reducing dietary ω6/ω3 ratio or inhibiting the enzymatic activity of 12/15-LO may protect against ω6-rich Western diet-induced steatohepatitis.

Acknowledgments

We thank the UCSD Neuroscience Core, especially Jennifer Santini for microscopy assistance and their grant NS047101. We thank Jachelle Ofrecio for assistance with plasma insulin assays. **GRANTS**: This work was supported by a grant from the P. Robert Majumder Charitable Foundation to DDS, NIH grants DK076852 and DK082451 to AEF, HL055798 to YIM, and CONICET PIP 051/2011 to ACC.

Author Contributions

Conceived and designed the experiments: ICZ DDS ML MEI. Performed the experiments: ML MEI DP ICZ MC MN DDS. Analyzed the data: ML MEI ICZ MC MN DDS. Contributed reagents/materials/analysis tools: MEI ACC YIM AEF DDS. Wrote the paper: ML MEI DDS.

References

1. Browning JD, Horton JD (2004) Molecular mediators of hepatic steatosis and liver injury. J Clin Invest 114: 147–152.
2. Staels B (2006) When the Clock stops ticking, metabolic syndrome explodes. Nat Med 12: 54–55; discussion 55.
3. Weiss R, Dziura J, Burgert TS, Tamborlane WV, Taksali SE, et al. (2004) Obesity and the metabolic syndrome in children and adolescents. N Engl J Med 350: 2362–2374.
4. Gregor MF, Hotamisligil GS (2011) Inflammatory mechanisms in obesity. Annual review of immunology 29: 415–445.
5. Simopoulos AP (2008) The importance of the omega-6/omega-3 fatty acid ratio in cardiovascular disease and other chronic diseases. Exp Biol Med (Maywood) 233: 674–688.
6. Schmitz G, Ecker J (2008) The opposing effects of n-3 and n-6 fatty acids. Prog Lipid Res 47: 147–155.
7. Fei H, Berliner JA, Parhami F, Drake TA (1993) Regulation of endothelial cell tissue factor expression by minimally oxidized LDL and lipopolysaccharide. 13: 1711.
8. Olefsky JM, Glass CK (2010) Macrophages, inflammation, and insulin resistance. Annu Rev Physiol 72: 219–246.
9. Valenzuela R, Espinosa A, Gonzalez-Manan D, D'Espessailles A, Fernandez V, et al. (2012) N-3 long-chain polyunsaturated fatty acid supplementation significantly reduces liver oxidative stress in high fat induced steatosis. PloS one 7: e46400.
10. Lopez-Vicario C, Gonzalez-Periz A, Rius B, Moran-Salvador E, Garcia-Alonso V, et al. (2014) Molecular interplay between Delta5/Delta6 desaturases and long-chain fatty acids in the pathogenesis of non-alcoholic steatohepatitis. Gut 63: 344–355.
11. Weitz D, Weintraub H, Fisher E, Schwartzbard AZ (2010) Fish oil for the treatment of cardiovascular disease. Cardiol Rev 18: 258–263.
12. Byrne CD (2010) Fatty liver: role of inflammation and fatty acid nutrition. Prostaglandins Leukot Essent Fatty Acids 82: 265–271.
13. Nobili V, Bedogni G, Alisi A, Pietrobattista A, Rise P, et al. (2011) Docosahexaenoic acid supplementation decreases liver fat content in children with non-alcoholic fatty liver disease: double-blind randomised controlled clinical trial. Arch Dis Child 96: 350–353.
14. Wong CY, Yiu KH, Li SW, Lee S, Tam S, et al. (2010) Fish-oil supplement has neutral effects on vascular and metabolic function but improves renal function in patients with Type 2 diabetes mellitus. Diabet Med 27: 54–60.
15. Sears DD, Miles PD, Chapman J, Ofrecio JM, Almazan F, et al. (2009) 12/15-lipoxygenase is required for the early onset of high fat diet-induced adipose tissue inflammation and insulin resistance in mice. PLoS One 4: e7250.
16. Oh DY, Talukdar S, Bae EJ, Imamura T, Morinaga H, et al. (2010) GPR120 is an omega-3 fatty acid receptor mediating potent anti-inflammatory and insulin-sensitizing effects. Cell 142: 687–698.
17. Rossmeisl M, Jilkova ZM, Kuda O, Jelenik T, Medrikova D, et al. (2012) Metabolic Effects of n-3 PUFA as Phospholipids Are Superior to Triglycerides in Mice Fed a High-Fat Diet: Possible Role of Endocannabinoids. Plos One 7.
18. Svegliati-Baroni G, Candelaresi C, Saccomanno S, Ferretti G, Bachetti T, et al. (2006) A model of insulin resistance and nonalcoholic steatohepatitis in rats: role of peroxisome proliferator-activated receptor-alpha and n-3 polyunsaturated fatty acid treatment on liver injury. The American journal of pathology 169: 846–860.
19. Buettner R, Parhofer KG, Woenckhaus M, Wrede CE, Kunz-Schughart LA, et al. (2006) Defining high-fat-diet rat models: metabolic and molecular effects of different fat types. Journal of molecular endocrinology 36: 485–501.
20. Kuda O, Jelenik T, Jilkova Z, Flachs P, Rossmeisl M, et al. (2009) n-3 fatty acids and rosiglitazone improve insulin sensitivity through additive stimulatory effects on muscle glycogen synthesis in mice fed a high-fat diet. Diabetologia 52: 941–951.
21. Matthews DR, Hosker JP, Rudenski AS, Naylor BA, Treacher DF, et al. (1985) Homeostasis model assessment: insulin resistance and beta-cell function from fasting plasma glucose and insulin concentrations in man. Diabetologia 28: 412–419.
22. Chapman J, Miles PD, Ofrecio JM, Neels JG, Yu JG, et al. (2010) Osteopontin is required for the early onset of high fat diet-induced insulin resistance in mice. PLoS One 5: e13959.
23. Feldstein AE, Lopez R, Tamimi TA, Yerian L, Chung YM, et al. (2010) Mass spectrometric profiling of oxidized lipid products in human nonalcoholic fatty liver disease and nonalcoholic steatohepatitis. Journal of lipid research 51: 3046–3054.
24. Cicinnati VR, Shen Q, Sotiropoulos GC, Radtke A, Gerken G, et al. (2008) Validation of putative reference genes for gene expression studies in human hepatocellular carcinoma using real-time quantitative RT-PCR. BMC cancer 8: 350.

25. Ding J, Loizides-Mangold U, Rando G, Zoete V, Michielin O, et al. (2013) The peroxisomal enzyme L-PBE is required to prevent the dietary toxicity of medium-chain fatty acids. Cell reports 5: 248–258.
26. Hoek-van den Hil EF, Keijer J, Bunschoten A, Vervoort JJ, Stankova B, et al. (2013) Quercetin induces hepatic lipid omega-oxidation and lowers serum lipid levels in mice. PloS one 8: e51588.
27. Yu CR, Mahdi RM, Liu X, Zhang A, Naka T, et al. (2008) SOCS1 regulates CCR7 expression and migration of CD4+ T cells into peripheral tissues. Journal of immunology 181: 1190–1198.
28. Nunemaker CS, Chen M, Pei H, Kimble SD, Keller SR, et al. (2008) 12-Lipoxygenase-knockout mice are resistant to inflammatory effects of obesity induced by Western diet. Am J Physiol Endocrinol Metab 295: E1065–1075.
29. Angulo P (2007) Obesity and nonalcoholic fatty liver disease. Nutrition reviews 65: S57–63.
30. de Luca C, Olefsky JM (2008) Inflammation and insulin resistance. Febs Letters 582: 97.
31. Matsuzawa Y (2006) The metabolic syndrome and adipocytokines. Febs Letters 580: 2917.
32. Schenk S, Saberi M, Olefsky JM (2008) Insulin sensitivity: modulation by nutrients and inflammation. J Clin Invest 118: 2992–3002.
33. Neschen S, Morino K, Rossbacher JC, Pongratz RL, Cline GW, et al. (2006) Fish oil regulates adiponectin secretion by a peroxisome proliferator-activated receptor-gamma-dependent mechanism in mice. Diabetes 55: 924–928.
34. Gonzalez-Periz A, Horrillo R, Ferre N, Gronert K, Dong B, et al. (2009) Obesity-induced insulin resistance and hepatic steatosis are alleviated by omega-3 fatty acids: a role for resolvins and protectins. Faseb J 23: 1946–1957.
35. Fedor D, Kelley DS (2009) Prevention of insulin resistance by n-3 polyunsaturated fatty acids. Curr Opin Clin Nutr Metab Care 12: 138–146.
36. Jucker BM, Cline GW, Barucci N, Shulman GI (1999) Differential effects of safflower oil versus fish oil feeding on insulin-stimulated glycogen synthesis, glycolysis, and pyruvate dehydrogenase flux in skeletal muscle: a 13C nuclear magnetic resonance study. Diabetes 48: 134–140.
37. Rossmeisl M, Jelenik T, Jilkova Z, Slamova K, Kus V, et al. (2009) Prevention and reversal of obesity and glucose intolerance in mice by DHA derivatives. Obesity (Silver Spring) 17: 1023–1031.
38. Ikemoto S, Takahashi M, Tsunoda N, Maruyama K, Itakura H, et al. (1996) High-fat diet-induced hyperglycemia and obesity in mice: differential effects of dietary oils. Metabolism: clinical and experimental 45: 1539–1546.
39. Guebre-Xabier M, Yang S, Lin HZ, Schwenk R, Krzych U, et al. (2000) Altered hepatic lymphocyte subpopulations in obesity-related murine fatty livers: potential mechanism for sensitization to liver damage. Hepatology 31: 633–640.
40. Sallusto F, Lenig D, Forster R, Lipp M, Lanzavecchia A (1999) Two subsets of memory T lymphocytes with distinct homing potentials and effector functions. Nature 401: 708–712.
41. Wang HN, Wang YR, Liu GQ, Liu Z, Wu PX, et al. (2008) Inhibition of hepatic interleukin-18 production by rosiglitazone in a rat model of nonalcoholic fatty liver disease. World journal of gastroenterology: WJG 14: 7240–7246.
42. Chikano S, Sawada K, Shimoyama T, Kashiwamura SI, Sugihara A, et al. (2000) IL-18 and IL-12 induce intestinal inflammation and fatty liver in mice in an IFN-gamma dependent manner. Gut 47: 779–786.
43. Copaci I, Micu L, Voiculescu M (2006) The role of cytokines in non-alcoholic steatohepatitis. A review. Journal of gastrointestinal and liver diseases: JGLD 15: 363–373.
44. Calder PC (2006) n-3 polyunsaturated fatty acids, inflammation, and inflammatory diseases. The American journal of clinical nutrition 83: 1505S–1519S.
45. Chakrabarti SK, Cole BK, Wen Y, Keller SR, Nadler JL (2009) 12/15-Lipoxygenase Products Induce Inflammation and Impair Insulin Signaling in 3T3-L1 Adipocytes. Obesity (Silver Spring) 17: 1657–1663.
46. O'Garra A, Vieira P (2007) T(H)1 cells control themselves by producing interleukin-10. Nature reviews Immunology 7: 425–428.
47. Bolick DT, Orr AW, Whetzel A, Srinivasan S, Hatley ME, et al. (2005) 12/15-Lipoxygenase Regulates Intercellular Adhesion Molecule-1 Expression and Monocyte Adhesion to Endothelium Through Activation of RhoA and Nuclear Factor-{kappa}B. Arteriosclerosis, Thrombosis, and Vascular Biology 25: 2301.
48. Natarajan R, Reddy MA, Malik KU, Fatima S, Khan BV (2001) Signaling mechanisms of nuclear factor-kappab-mediated activation of inflammatory genes by 13-hydroperoxyoctadecadienoic acid in cultured vascular smooth muscle cells. 21: 1408.
49. Miller YI, Viriyakosol S, Binder CJ, Feramisco JR, Kirkland TN, et al. (2003) Minimally Modified LDL Binds to CD14, Induces Macrophage Spreading via TLR4/MD-2, and Inhibits Phagocytosis of Apoptotic Cells. Journal of Biological Chemistry 278: 1561.
50. Miller YI, Viriyakosol S, Worrall DS, Boullier A, Butler S, et al. (2005) Toll-like receptor 4-dependent and -independent cytokine secretion induced by minimally oxidized low-density lipoprotein in macrophages. Arteriosclerosis, Thrombosis, and Vascular Biology 25: 1213.
51. Martinez-Clemente M, Ferre N, Titos E, Horrillo R, Gonzalez-Periz A, et al. (2010) Disruption of the 12/15-lipoxygenase gene (Alox15) protects hyperlipidemic mice from nonalcoholic fatty liver disease. Hepatology 52: 1980–1991.

3

Perinatal Exposure of Mice to the Pesticide DDT Impairs Energy Expenditure and Metabolism in Adult Female Offspring

Michele La Merrill[1,2,3]*, Emma Karey[1], Erin Moshier[2], Claudia Lindtner[3,4], Michael R. La Frano[5,6], John W. Newman[5,6,7], Christoph Buettner[3,4]

1 Department of Environmental Toxicology, University of California Davis, Davis, California, United States of America, **2** Department of Preventive Medicine, Mount Sinai School of Medicine, New York, New York, United States of America, **3** Metabolism Institute, Mount Sinai School of Medicine, New York, New York, United States of America, **4** Division of Endocrinology, Diabetes and Bone Disease, Mount Sinai School of Medicine, New York, New York, United States of America, **5** West Coast Metabolomic Center, University of California Davis, Davis, California, United States of America, **6** Department of Nutrition, University of California Davis, Davis, California, United States of America, **7** Obesity and Metabolism Research Unit, USDA-ARS-Western Human Nutrition Research Center, Davis, California, United States of America

Abstract

Dichlorodiphenyltrichloroethane (DDT) has been used extensively to control malaria, typhus, body lice and bubonic plague worldwide, until countries began restricting its use in the 1970s. Its use in malaria control continues in some countries according to recommendation by the World Health Organization. Individuals exposed to elevated levels of DDT and its metabolite dichlorodiphenyldichloroethylene (DDE) have an increased prevalence of diabetes and insulin resistance. Here we hypothesize that perinatal exposure to DDT disrupts metabolic programming leading to impaired metabolism in adult offspring. To test this, we administered DDT to C57BL/6J mice from gestational day 11.5 to postnatal day 5 and studied their metabolic phenotype at several ages up to nine months. Perinatal DDT exposure reduced core body temperature, impaired cold tolerance, decreased energy expenditure, and produced a transient early-life increase in body fat in female offspring. When challenged with a high fat diet for 12 weeks in adulthood, female offspring perinatally exposed to DDT developed glucose intolerance, hyperinsulinemia, dyslipidemia, and altered bile acid metabolism. Perinatal DDT exposure combined with high fat feeding in adulthood further impaired thermogenesis as evidenced by reductions in core temperature and in the expression of numerous RNA that promote thermogenesis and substrate utilization in the brown adipose tissue of adult female mice. These observations suggest that perinatal DDT exposure impairs thermogenesis and the metabolism of carbohydrates and lipids which may increase susceptibility to the metabolic syndrome in adult female offspring.

Editor: Barbara T. Alexander, Univ Mississippi Medical Center, United States of America

Funding: This research was supported through funding by the National Institute of Health (R00 ES019919, R03 DK082724, U24 DK092993, U24 DK097154, T32 ES007059, and P60 DK020541), the American Diabetes Association, and United States Department of Agriculture - Agricultural Research Service Intramural Project 5306-51530-019-00D. The funders had no role in study design, data collection and analysis, decision to publish, or preparation of the manuscript.

Competing Interests: The authors have declared that no competing interests exist.

* Email: mlamerrill@ucdavis.edu

Introduction

The prevalence of type 2 diabetes (T2D) is rising worldwide [1], creating a tremendous burden for health care systems in developed and developing nations. The estimated cost associated with T2D was $245 billion last year in the United States alone [2]. This rise in the incidence of T2D is largely attributed to increasing obesity rates [3]. Obesity and T2D are characterized by insulin resistance and are often associated with perturbations in energy expenditure [4,5].

Numerous epidemiological studies have suggested that exposure to persistent organic pollutants (POPs) contribute to the rising incidence of T2D [6]. For example, exposure to the organochlorine pesticide DDT has been found to be associated with increased odds of T2D [7]. Further, exposure to DDE, the primary metabolite of DDT, has also been associated with increased odds of excess body weight, insulin resistance, and dyslipidemia in people [8]. Because the World Health Organization still recommends the use of DDT for malaria control, DDT's potential contribution to the pathogenesis of T2D continues to be relevant to public health. Furthermore, obesity and T2D have increased at alarming rates in countries where DDT is still in use. For instance, the prevalence of diabetes among rural Indian adults increased 3.8 fold from 1989 to 2006 [9] and although a confluence of factors contribute to this rise, the contribution of endocrine disrupting chemicals cannot be ruled out without further study. Since epidemiological associations cannot establish causality, we tested whether exposure to DDT and DDE predisposes to T2D in mice at doses comparable to human exposures [10–13].

Both obesity and T2D are characterized by impaired energy expenditure and reduced thermogenesis, which are often the result of reduced brown adipose tissue (BAT) activity [5]. Mouse studies also suggest that impaired thermogenesis may precede insulin resistance [14]. Therefore, increasing energy expenditure by activating BAT thermogenesis may hold promise as a therapeutic strategy for managing both obesity and T2D [15–18].

Perturbations in the perinatal environment can impair metabolic programming that can consequently increase susceptibility to obesity and T2D in adulthood. A classic example of the importance of the perinatal environment on the future risk of T2D has been historically provided by the Dutch famine. Fetuses carried to term that were exposed to fetal malnutrition suffered from increased rates of the metabolic syndrome and glucose intolerance as adult offspring [19,20]. The consequences of impaired fetal development on metabolic programming can be modeled in rodents, where fetal under-nutrition results in the development of the metabolic syndrome and glucose intolerance in adult offspring [21,22]. Here we confirm the hypothesis that perinatal exposure to DDT impairs energy expenditure and metabolism leading to insulin resistance and the metabolic syndrome in adult offspring. We demonstrate for the first time that developmental exposure to DDT impairs BAT thermogenesis.

Methods

DDT exposure

To mimic the commercial formulation of DDT used as a pesticide in the US prior to its ban, 77.2% p,p′-DDT (98.5% purity neat, AccuStandard, New Haven, CT) and 22.8% o,p′-DDT (100% purity neat, AccuStandard) were dissolved at a final concentration of 0.17 g DDT mixture/L organic olive oil [23], hereafter referred to as DDT. We selected the dosing period to span liver and white- and brown- adipose tissue ontogenesis and programming [24–28]. From 11.5 days post coitus (determined by vaginal plug) to postnatal day (PND) 5, we administered 1.7 mg DDT/kg body weight (per os, n = 15 dams, 10 μL solution/g mouse), or equivalent volume of olive oil vehicle (hereafter referred to as vehicle or VEH, per os, n = 14 dams) daily to primigravid C57BL/6J mice (Jackson Laboratories, Bar Harbor, ME, Fig. S1). To determine the internal dose after transplacental and lactational transfer to pups [29], 4 additional dams were treated identically with DDT, and 24 hours after the final dose their sera was analyzed for o,p′-DDT, p,p′-DDT, and p,p′-DDE by gas chromatography using electron capture detection with detection limits of 0.36, 0.27 and 0.12 pg/μL serum respectively [30].

Study Design

We culled litters to 6 pups after the final DDT dose on PND 5, to minimize infanticide common among C57BL/6J dams while normalizing lactational transfer of DDT and maternal behavior effects (Fig. S1). We evaluated timing of puberty daily by monitoring vaginal opening (VO) and preputial separation (PPS), in all female and male mice respectively, beginning at PND 18. On PND 21 we weaned pups (1 cage/sex/litter/treatment). We assessed body composition, energy homeostasis, metabolic parameters, and glucose tolerance up to 6 months of age when we randomized mice into 2 study arms to assess: 1) energy balance or 2) the metabolic consequences of high fat feeding (Fig. S1).

For the energy balance study, 10 females from 10 litters and 8 metabolic chambers were available. Energy balance was assessed by indirect calorimetry in 1 female mouse/litter (4 mice/perinatal treatment) for 7 days after 2 days of acclimation. Cold tolerance was assessed 3 days after indirect calorimetry in 5 female mice/perinatal treatment, as described below.

For the high fat feeding study, littermates were randomized to high fat diet (HFD, 4.73 kcal/g, 20% protein, 35% carbohydrate, and 45% fat per kcal; D12451, Research Diets, New Brunswick, NJ) or a low fat diet (LFD, 3.85 kcal/g, 20% protein, 70% carbohydrate, and 10% fat per kcal; D12450B, Research Diets) feeding following their glucose tolerance test (GTT) at 6 months of age for a total of 12 weeks (n = 8 mice/sex/litter per perinatal treatment and diet combination).

All mice had access to food and water *ad libitum* (other than during stated fasting periods) in sterile ventilated cages in an American Association for the Accreditation of Laboratory Animal Care-approved facility. At the end of all the studies, mice were sacrificed by exsanguination under isoflurane anesthesia. All animal experiments were conducted under the guidelines on humane use and care of laboratory animals for biomedical research published by the US National Institutes of Health. The procedures of this study were approved by the Mount Sinai School of Medicine Institutional Animal Care and Use Committee protocol #LA11-00116.

Body composition

We measured body weight and percent fat mass by MRI (3in1-EchoMRI, Echo Medical Systems, Houston, TX) of each offspring monthly in 1–6 month old mice (n = 15 DDT- and n = 14 vehicle-exposed litters). The body mass of all mice was also measured at PND 5. During HF feeding, mice were weighed weekly and we used MRI to determine body composition at 8 months of age (n = 8 mice/sex/litter per perinatal treatment and diet combination).

Energy homeostasis

We measured food intake in mice on a monthly basis from 2–6 months (n = 15 DDT- and n = 14 vehicle- exposed litters). In 2 month old mice, each mouse/sex/litter/treatment was singly housed and food intake was assessed daily over a 5 day period. In group- housed mice aged 3–6 months, we measured food intake per cage over a 2 day period. In the HF feeding study, we measured weekly food intake of singly housed mice fed LFD or HFD. Food intake (g or kcal) was calculated as the difference in food weight divided by the number of mice that had access to it and the number of days they had access, and transformed to kcal when comparing HFD and LFD (SAS 9.2, SAS Institute, Cary, NC). We measured core temperature monthly in all mice aged 2–5 and 8 months old by inserting a thermocouple into the rectum (BAT-10, Physitemp, Clifton, NJ).

For the energy balance studies, we housed 4 females/perinatal treatment (1 mouse/litter) individually in metabolic chambers, which continuously measured oxygen consumption, carbon dioxide production, food intake, and 3 plane-locomotor activity through open-circuit, indirect calorimetry (CLAMS, Columbus Instruments, Columbus, OH). During this 9 day period, we provided mouse powdered diet (NIH 07) and water *ad libitum* while they were maintained at 21–22°C for a 12-hour light/dark cycle. The respiratory exchange ratio (RER) was calculated as the quotient of vCO_2/vO_2.

Three days after the indirect calorimetry was completed, we individually housed 5 female mice/perinatal treatment (1 mouse/litter) at 4°C with bedding enrichment. Core body temperature was measured immediately upon exposure to 4°C, and every 30 minutes thereafter until 90 minutes, when 50% of the mice reached core temperatures of <30°C after being kept for 90-minutes at 4°C. Two days later, we housed each of the 10 female mice for 1 hour at 4°C prior to sacrifice.

GTT

Glucose tolerance was assessed in 1 mouse/sex/litter/perinatal treatment aged 2, 3 and 6 months (randomized selection from n = 15 DDT- and n = 14 vehicle- exposed litters) and 1 mouse/sex/litter for each perinatal treatment and adult diet combination at eight months (randomized selection from n = 8 litters/treatment). Two-month-old mice received 2.0 mg D-glucose/g mouse body weight (i.p.), since at young age mice (as well as humans) are more glucose tolerant, and all other mice received 1.0 mg D-glucose/g mouse body weight (i.p.). For all GTT, we fasted mice for 5 hours, and collected sub-mandibular blood to determine fasting blood glucose (AlphaTrak, Abbott Laboratories, Abbott Park, IL) and fasting plasma metabolic parameters. We measured blood glucose 15, 30, 45, 60, 90, and 120 minutes after a D-glucose bolus for GTT. We determined total AUC using the trapezoidal approach (PROC SQL, SAS 9.4, SAS Institute, Cary, NC).

Metabolic parameters

Trunk blood glucose was measured in all mice culled on PND 5. Sub-mandibular blood was collected from mice fasted for 5 hours (1 mouse/sex/litter/treatment) at ages 1–6 months old (randomized selection from n = 15 DDT- and n = 14 vehicle- exposed litters) and 8 months old (randomized selection from n = 8 litters/treatment) to determine blood glucose (AlphaTrak) and plasma insulin by ELISA (Mercodia, Uppsala, Sweden). Fasting plasma triglycerides, total cholesterol, and non-esterified fatty acids (NEFA) were evaluated enzymatically (Wako Chemicals, Richmond, VA). Homeostasis model assessment- insulin resistance (HOMA-IR) was calculated as the product of fasting glucose and insulin divided by 22.5 [31].

Pathology

Livers were harvested from 1 female fed HFD per perinatal treatment group (randomized selection from n = 1 female/litter in 7 VEH and 8 DDT litters) into OCT medium, frozen 5 μM thick sections were stained with oil red O, and fields with representative staining of the sample and the least clear space (vessels, ducts, etc.) were selected. Histopathological evaluations were assessed by a veterinary pathologist who was blinded to the treatments.

Hepatic lipids

Hepatic triglycerides and cholesterol esters were measured after a modified Folch extraction (randomized selection from n = 1 female/litter in 7 VEH and 8 DDT litters fed HFD) [32]. Total cholesterol [33] and triglycerides [34] were measured enzymatically from these livers (Fisher Diagnostics, Middletown, VA).

Hepatic bile acids

A 15 mg liver sample (randomized selection from n = 1 female/litter in 7 VEH and 8 DDT litters fed HFD) was pulverized on dry ice, enriched with deuterated bile acid analogs, butylated hydroxytoluene and ethylinediaminetetraacetic acid, and extracted twice with 500 μL methanol. The combined extract was dried, reconstituted in 100 μL methanol:acetonitrile (50:50, v/v) with internal standards 1-phenyl-3-hexanoic acid urea and 1-cyclohexyl-3-dodecanoic acid urea (Sigma-Aldrich, St. Louis, MO) and filtered through 0.1 μm filters. Tissue bile acids were isolated and quantified by LC-MS/MS using modifications of a previously published method [35]. Separation of bile acids was achieved using reversed phase UPLC with a 1.7 μm, 2.1×100 mm Acquity BEH C18 column (Waters, Milford, MA) using a 16 min gradient (Solvent A = 0.1% formic acid; Solvent B = 0.1% formic acid in acetonitrile) on a Waters Acquity UPLC (Waters) and detected on an API 4000 QTrap (AB Sciex, Framingham, MA, USA) by multiple reaction monitoring (MRM) after negative mode electrospray ionization. Residues were quantified against 7 point curves of authentic standards purchased from Steraloid Inc. (Newport, RI), Sigma-Aldrich (St. Louis, MO), and Medical Isotopes, Inc. (Pelham, NH) using internal standard methodologies.

Western blot analysis

Protein expression was assessed as previously described [36]. Briefly, liver was homogenized and 10–20 μg of protein was subjected to Western blot analysis with primary antibodies against fatty acid synthase (FAS, BD Biosciences, San Jose, CA), phospho-acetyl-CoA carboxylase (ACC), ACC, phospho- adenosine triphosphate citrate lyase (ATPCL), ATPCL, adipose triglyceride lipase (ATGL), AKT Thr^{308} and Ser^{473}, AKT, phospho- glycogen synthase kinase 3 (GSK3), GSK3, phospho-ERK, and ERK (all antibodies from Cell Signaling Technology, Danvers, MA unless stated otherwise) and insulin receptor (IR) beta (Santa Cruz Biotechnology, Dallas, TX). The secondary antibody was DyLight conjugated goat anti-rabbit or anti-mouse IgG (ThermoScientific). Signal intensity of proteins of interest was divided by the intensity of the housekeeping protein HSC 70 (Santa Cruz Biotechnology) to determine fold change (Odyssey, LI-COR, Lincoln, NE). We have confirmed the specificity of ATGL in adipose tissue specific ATGL knockout vs. wild type mice, and all other antibodies have been characterized and validated in prior peer review publications [(Table S1), [37–41]].

Semi-quantitative PCR

mRNA was extracted with the RNeasy kit (Qiagen, Hilden, Germany) to synthesize cDNA using reverse transcription PCR (Applied Biosystems, Foster City, CA). Semi-quantitative PCR was performed using proprietary TaqMan primers for transcripts: peroxisome proliferative activated receptor gamma coactivator 1 alpha (*Ppargc1a*), iodothyronine type II deiodinase (*Dio2*), twist-related protein 1 (*Twist1*) and uncoupling protein 1 (*Ucp1*) in BAT using TATA box binding protein (*Tbp*) as an endogenous control; 3-hydroxy-3-methylglutaryl-Coenzyme A reductase (*Hmgcr*), low density lipoprotein receptor (*Ldlr*), and cytochrome P450 7a1 (*Cyp7a1*) in livers with glucuronidase beta (*Gusb*) as an endogenous control (Applied Biosystems). Additional semi-quantitative PCR was performed in BAT using SYBR Green with published primers: glucose transporter type 4 (*Glut4*, F: CATCCCACAAGGCACCCCTC, R: CATGCCACCCACAGAGAAGA [42]), lipoprotein lipase (*Lpl*, F:TGGAGAAGCCATCCGTGTG, R: TCATGCGAGCACTTCACCAG [42]), adipose triglyceride lipase (*Pnpla*, F: TGTTTCAGACGGAGAGAACGTC, R: TGAGAATGGGGACACTGTGATG [43]), and carnitine palmitoyltransferase 2 (*Cpt2*, F: CCAGCGGATAAACCACAACA, R: AAGCCACCGAGGCTCACTG [42]) using *Tbp* (F: GAAGCTGCGGTACAATTCCAG, R: CCCCTTGTACCCTTCACCAAT [44]) as endogenous control. Endogenous controls did not vary significantly across treatment groups. The 2^{-ddCT} method was used to approximate relative transcript fold change between treatment groups (coefficient of replicate variation <10%) [45].

Statistical analyses

Phenotypes were assessed at specific ages by modeling the fixed effect of perinatal DDT and the random effect of litter while stratifying by gender (PROC MIXED, SAS). Longitudinal analyses of body mass, fat mass, and temperature were conducted using the age-specific model as described above, with the addition of age and an age*treatment term as fixed effects, and individual mouse identifiers as random effects. To assess circadian effects during indirect calorimetry, photoperiods and a photoperiod*perinatal treatment term were included as fixed effects in the age-specific model. Body weight and fat mass were considered as potential covariates in indirect calorimetry analyses [46] but because these body composition variables were not significantly different between perinatal treatments and caused no reduction in data significance or difference in interpretation, these covariates were not included in the final indirect calorimetry models. When examining phenotypes from the HF feeding study, diet and a diet*perinatal treatment term were included as fixed effects in the age-specific and longitudinal models described above. GTTs, fasting metabolic parameters, protein expression, mRNA, lipids, and bile acids were evaluated without random effects because only one mouse per litter was included (PROC GLM, SAS). To evaluate the potential covariate behavior of hepatic bile acids and other metabolic factors which may influence or be influenced by cholesterol metabolism, imDEV v 1.4.2 [47] was employed to normalize data, transform variables to mean centers with unit variance, and conduct partial least squares discriminate analysis (PLS DA; oscores pls). The dependent variable was the perinatal treatment group while the independent variables were hepatic bile acids, *Cyp7a1* fold-change, hepatic cholesterol and triglycerides, plasma cholesterol, % body fat, and age. Measures with variable importance in projection (VIP) scores >1 were considered important discriminators of treatment [48]. Timing of puberty was evaluated using survival analysis with treatment as a fixed effect and litter as a repeated event (PROC PHREG, SAS). In all models, we used a significance threshold of $p<0.05$ for main effects and $p<0.1$ for interaction effects.

Results

Perinatal DDT exposure increases adiposity in young adults

To examine whether perinatal DDT exposure causes the metabolic syndrome in adult mouse offspring, dams were exposed to DDT from mid-gestation to PND 5. The resulting internal doses were 2.2 (±0.1) ng p,p′-DDE/mL, 51.1 (±10.2) ng p,p-DDT/mL, while o,p′-DDT was undetected [mean (± SEM)]. These exposures were sufficiently low as to have no impact on length of gestation, weight gain during gestation, or litter size (Fig. S2) and fall within the range of contemporary human exposures [10,49]. Perinatal DDT exposure decreased body weight and blood glucose in male mice (Fig. S3A–B) and decreased glucose in female mice (Fig. 1B) on PND 5. Although DDT and DDE are ligands of the estrogen and androgen receptors [50], the timing of puberty in either sex was not significantly affected by the perinatal DDT exposure (Fig. 1C, Fig S3C). Perinatal DDT exposure caused a transient increase in body weight and adiposity of young adult female mice (Fig. 2A–C) but no differences in female lean mass (Fig. 2D), or male body composition were observed (Fig. S3D–E). Further, glucose tolerance, fasting glucose, insulin, and lipid levels were not altered by perinatal DDT exposure in either sex during their first 6 months of post-weaning life (Fig. S4, Table S2). These data suggest that mice exposed to perinatal DDT manifested only subtle features of the metabolic syndrome until

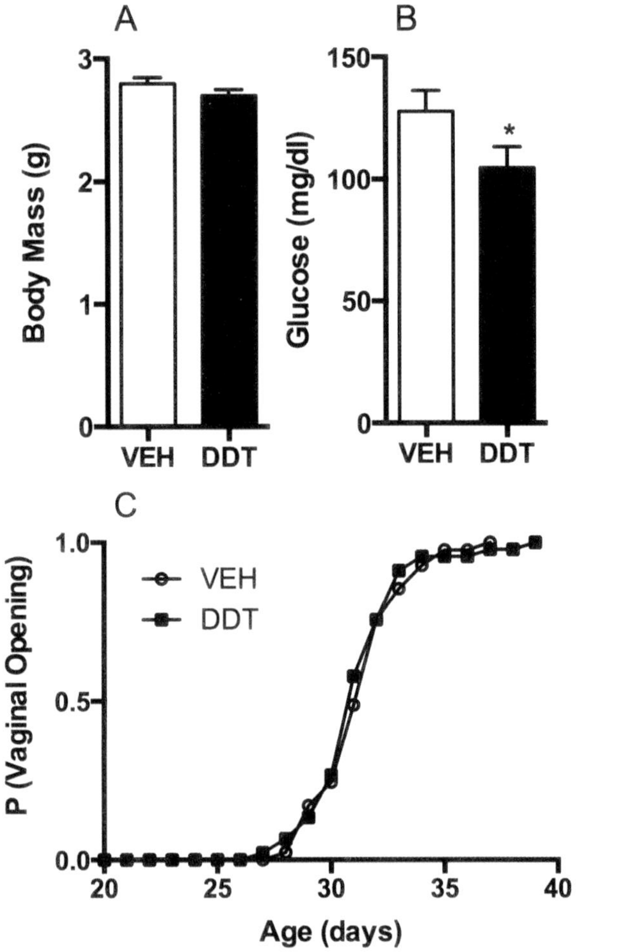

Figure 1. Effect of perinatal DDT on the development of female mice. (A) Female body mass at PND5 (n = 15 DDT- and n = 14 VEH-exposed litters). (B) Trunk blood glucose in PND5 females culled from litters >6 pups (n = 7 DDT- and n = 7 VEH- exposed litters). (C) Proportion of mice with vaginal opening as a function of age (n = 15 DDT- and n = 14 VEH- exposed litters). *$p<0.05$ DDT vs. vehicle controls. Data are represented as least squares (LS) means + SEM.

adulthood. Since perinatal DDT exposure had no effect on food intake of offspring (Fig. 2E, Fig. S3F), the increased adiposity transiently observed among young female mice exposed to DDT could have resulted from impairments in thermogenesis and energy expenditure.

Perinatal DDT exposure reduces energy expenditure

To assess thermogenesis, core body temperature was measured longitudinally. Perinatal DDT exposure did not affect the core body temperature of male mice (Fig. S3G), while it decreased the core temperature of female mice, an effect that became more pronounced with age (Fig. 2F). At 6 months, female mice perinatally exposed to DDT had decreased oxygen consumption (Fig. 3A) and a more pronounced RER reduction in the light period than in the dark period, indicative of greater fasting lipid utilization (Fig. 3B), although food intake appeared equivocal across treatment groups (Fig. 3C). Female mice perinatally exposed to DDT also had decreased energy expenditure, while physical activity was not altered (Fig. 3D–E), suggesting that decreased energy expenditure was the result of decreased

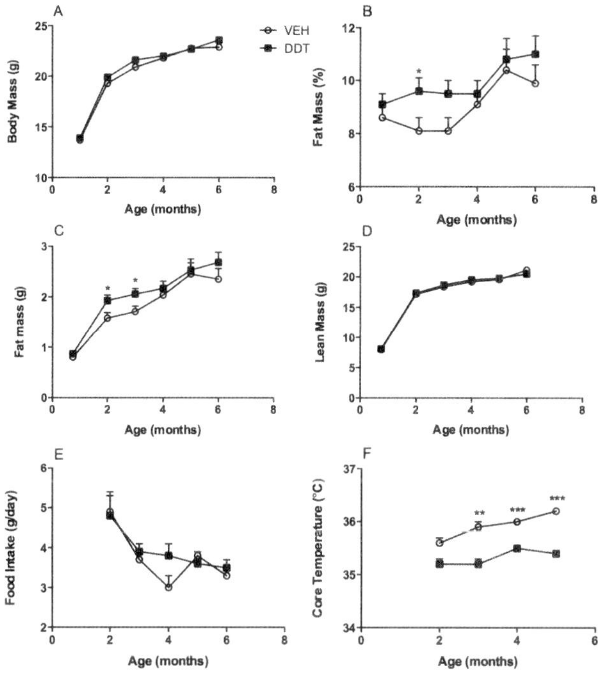

Figure 2. Effect of perinatal DDT on body composition and energy balance in female mice. Monthly (A) body mass (p = 0.05 at 2 months, p = 0.08 at 3 months), (B) percent adiposity (p = 0.05 at 3 months), (C) fat mass, (D) lean mass, and (E) food intake (A–E: n = 15 DDT- and n = 14 VEH- exposed litters). (F) Monthly core temperature (1 female/litter at 2 month time point, all females/litter thereafter, p = 0.07 at 2 months, age*DDT pi = 0.07). *p<0.05, **p<0.001, ***p<0.0001 DDT vs. vehicle controls. Data are represented as LS means + SEM.

thermogenesis. To further establish that female mice perinatally exposed to DDT had compromised thermogenesis, we evaluated cold tolerance in female mice exposed to 4°C. Female mice with perinatal DDT exposure exhibited marked cold intolerance, necessitating the termination of the cold tolerance test after 90 minutes (Fig. 3F).

To determine if high fat feeding, a commonly used metabolic stressor to model human obesity, could unveil a metabolic phenotype caused by perinatal DDT exposure, mice were fed either LFD or HFD for 12 weeks beginning at 6 months of age. HF feeding increased caloric intake, adiposity, and body mass equally in all groups (Fig. 4A–C, Fig. S5), indicating that any metabolic alterations observed in HF fed mice that were perinatally exposed to DDT occurred independently of caloric intake and/or body composition.

Perinatal DDT exposure reduced core temperature in 9 month old female mice (Fig. 4D). HFD feeding led to higher body core temperatures in non-exposed mice, however this thermogenic adaptation to HFD was absent in mice perinatally exposed to DDT (Fig. 4D). Perinatal DDT exposure paradoxically reduced body core temperature by more than 1°C in mice fed HFD ($p< 0.0001$). Thus, perinatal DDT impairs thermogenesis which is further worsened by HFD, indicating that developmental DDT exposure increases susceptibility to HFD induced- impairment in energy balance.

We next examined if perinatal DDT exposure altered molecular mechanisms controlling thermogenesis in BAT of 9 month old female mice (Fig. 5). Compared to LFD-fed control mice, adult HF feeding and perinatal DDT exposure caused a reduction in mRNA expression of *Ppargc1a* (Fig. 5A), a master regulator of thermogenesis. Indeed HFD and DDT exposures reduced the expression of *Dio2* (Fig. 5B), which encodes an enzyme that locally activates thyroid hormone by deiodinating T4 to T3 to stimulate thermogenesis in BAT. However there was no significant change in *Ucp1* RNA expression (Fig. 5C), a protein that uncouples respiration to increase thermogenesis [51,52]. Consistent with the regulatory role of PGC1A in substrate utilization [14,53–56], perinatal DDT exposure and adult HF feeding decreased the expression of glucose transporter *Glut4*, lipoprotein transporter *Lpl* (no diet effect), lipolysis rate-limiting *Pnpla*, and the fatty acid oxidation shuttle *Cpt2* (Fig. 5D–G). Because transcription of *Ppargc1a* and its downstream targets was suppressed, we investigated negative regulation of *Ppargc1a* across DDT and HFD treatments. Indeed, expression of *Twist1*, a negative regulator of *Ppargc1a* [57], was increased in BAT of 9 month old mice exposed perinatally to DDT and fed a HFD during adulthood (Fig. 5H).

Perinatal exposure to DDT increases susceptibility to HFD- induced insulin resistance

Female mice maintained on a LFD and exposed perinatally to DDT had equivocal glucose tolerance compared to vehicle treated controls (Fig. 6A). However, after HF feeding for 12 weeks, female mice exposed perinatally to DDT developed glucose intolerance and insulin resistance as evidenced by higher AUC during GTT, fasting hyperinsulinemia, and increased HOMA-IR (Fig. 6A–C). Of note, this constellation is often observed in prediabetic patients that commonly have the metabolic syndrome. Further, the expression and activation states of AKT and ERK, proteins involved in insulin signaling, were moderately decreased in female mice perinatally exposed to DDT and fed a HFD (Fig. 6D–E), although it remains unclear how much these moderate decreases in hepatic insulin signaling contribute to the observed glucose intolerance and insulin resistance. However, male mice perinatally exposed to DDT developed glucose intolerance when fed LFD, but not HFD (Fig. S8A–B). Thus, perinatal exposure to DDT increases the susceptibility to HFD- induced glucose intolerance in female but not male mice (Fig. 6, Fig. S6). The sex differences will require further studies in the future to test if this is estrogen dependent, but of note, female mice (and humans) are somewhat protected from HF feeding- induced glucose intolerance [58].

Perinatal DDT exposure and high fat feeding cause mild dyslipidemia in female mice

To evaluate whether perinatal DDT exposure impaired lipid metabolism in adult HFD fed- mice, we measured fasting triglycerides, cholesterol, and NEFAs (Fig. 7, Fig. S6). Perinatal DDT exposure significantly increased fasting cholesterol in female mice fed HFD, although it had a negligible effect on cholesterol in female mice fed LFD (Fig. 7A). A similar, but non-significant trend was observed in fasting triglycerides levels in female mice (Fig. 7B), whereas NEFAs were not altered by perinatal DDT or HFD in female mice (Fig. 7C). Thus perinatal DDT exposure combined with HFD caused mild dyslipidemia in female (Fig. 7A) but not male mice (Fig. S6E-G). We also examined whether perinatal DDT exposure altered the expression of mRNA and proteins associated with the regulation of lipid homeostasis in livers from female mice fed HFD. mRNA expression of *Ldlr*, a cholesterol transporter, was significantly decreased, whereas that of *Cyp7a1*, the rate limiting enzyme in the synthesis of bile acids from cholesterol, was significantly increased by perinatal DDT exposure (Fig. 7D). Changes in hepatic bile acid metabolism among females fed HFD were consistent with these changes in *Cyp7a1* expression

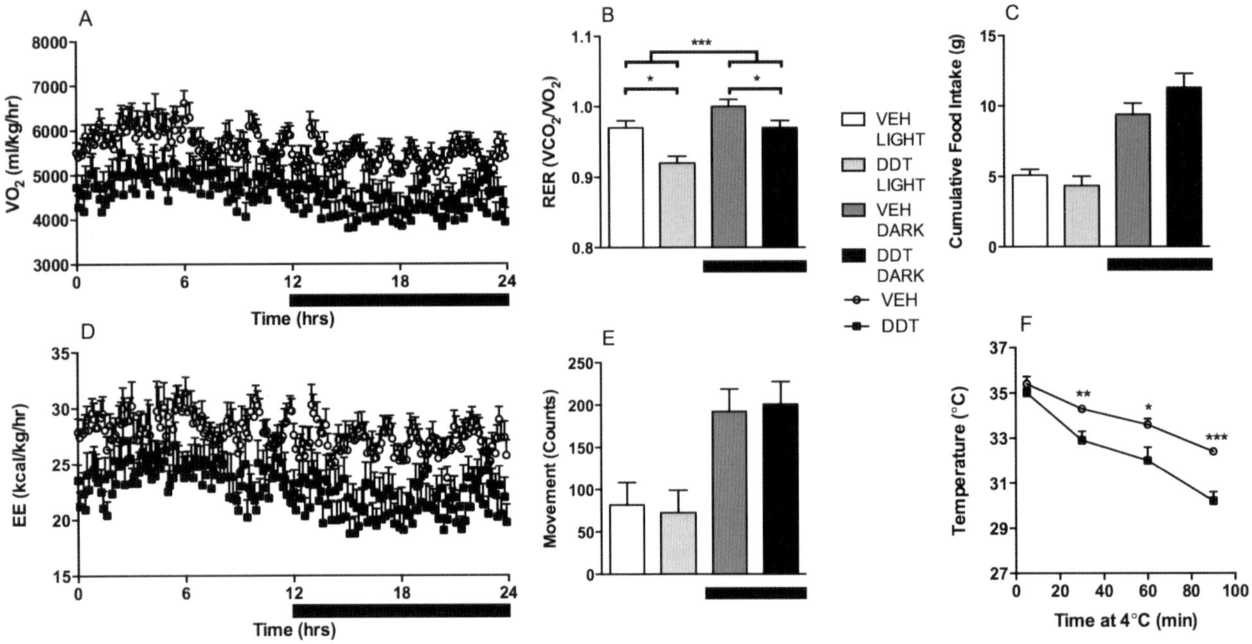

Figure 3. Effect of perinatal DDT on energy expenditure and cold tolerance in six month old female mice. (A) Oxygen consumption, (B) RER (period*DDT $p_{interaction}<0.0001$), (C) cumulative food intake, (D) energy expenditure, and (E) movement (over 5 day period and 4 female/treatment, 1 mouse/litter). (F) Core temperature (5 females/treatment, 1 female/litter). *p<0.05, **p<0.01, ***p<0.001 DDT vs. vehicle controls. Data are represented as LS means + SEM.

due to perinatal DDT exposure. Specifically, conjugated bile acids, including GLCA, TLCA, and TDCA, and the C27 precursor TriHCA, increased with DDT treatment and these conjugated bile acid changes were closely correlated with hepatic *Cyp7a1* expression and plasma cholesterol (VIP>1, Fig. 7E, Fig. S7, Table S3). Conversely, unconjugated bile acids, including HCA, HDCA, and β-MCA, were relatively lower in the DDT exposed versus control groups and were closely associated with hepatic lipids (VIP>1, Fig. 7E, Fig. S7, Table S3). Hepatic protein expression of two lipogenic enzymes ACC and ATPCL was also increased, consistent with increased hepatic lipogenesis as a consequence of perinatal DDT exposure (Fig. 7F). This did not appear to contribute to steatosis, as hepatic lipid content was not increased due to perinatal DDT exposure among female mice fed HFD (Fig. S8).

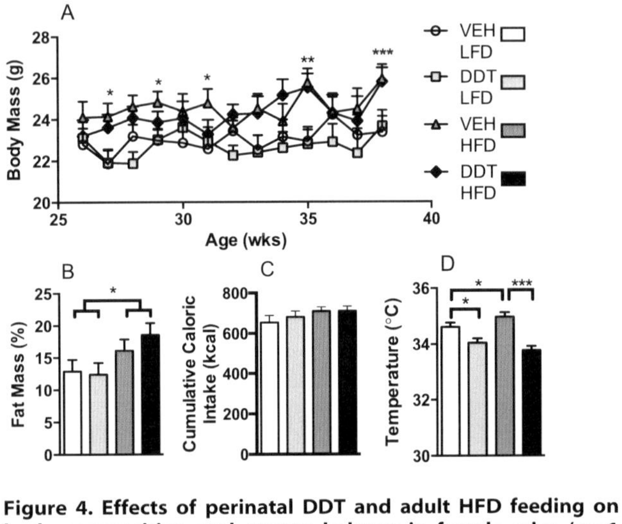

Figure 4. Effects of perinatal DDT and adult HFD feeding on body composition and energy balance in female mice (n = 1 female/litter in 7 VEH and 8 DDT litters). (A) Weekly body mass (HFD*age pi<0.0001). (B) Percent adiposity in 8 month old mice. (C) Cumulative caloric intake over 12 weeks of HFD or LFD feeding. (D) Core temperature in 8 month old mice (DDT*HFD pi = 0.01). *p<0.05, **p<0.01, ***p<0.0001 A–B) LFD vs. HFD only; D) significance between groups indicated by bars. Data are represented as LS means + SEM.

Discussion

Here we investigated the hypothesis that perinatal DDT exposure impairs energy expenditure and metabolism in adult mice. Our results suggest that perinatal DDT exposure decreases energy expenditure, and impairs the regulation of thermogenesis, glucose-, and lipid- homeostasis, which contribute to the development of insulin resistance and the metabolic syndrome in adult female mice.

Obesity and thermogenesis

Perinatal DDT exposure increased adiposity in young adult female mice. This transient increase in adiposity may have resulted from the profoundly impaired thermogenesis we observed after DDT exposure, which was greater than what was observed in UCP1 knock-out mice [59]. Impaired thermogenesis may have been a consequence of reduced energy supply and utilization in BAT as perinatal DDT exposure significantly decreased expression of lipolytic *Pnpla* and substrate transporters (*Glut4*, *Lpl*, *Cpt2*) [14,53–56]. Because food intake and physical activity were equal among groups, the reduced energy expenditure would be predicted to increase fat mass more profoundly than what we observed. Whether increased caloric content in feces accounts for this discrepancy will require further study [60].

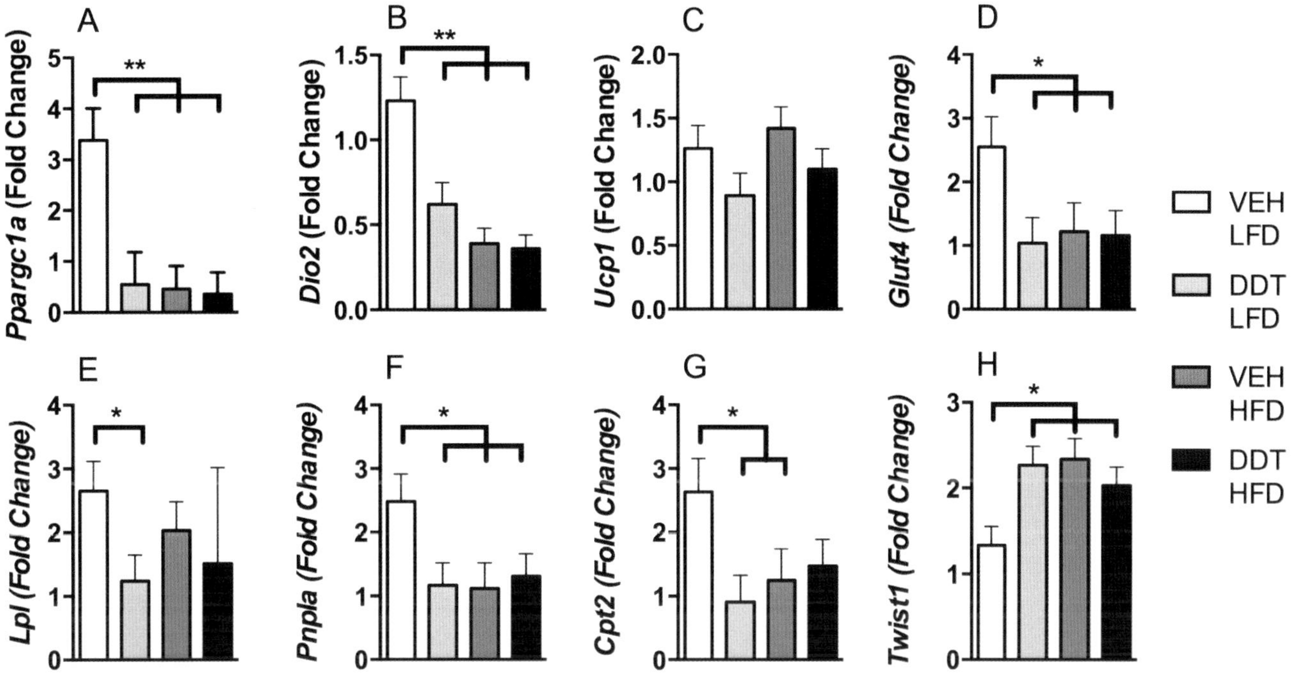

Figure 5. Effects of perinatal DDT and adult HFD feeding on RNA expression in BAT from 9 month old female mice (n = 1 female/litter in 8 VEH + LFD, 8 DDT + LFD, 7 VEH + HFD and 8 DDT + HFD litters). (A) *Ppargc1a*- (DDT*HFD pi$<$0.01), (B) *Dio2*- (DDT*HFD pi$<$0.01), (C) *Ucp1*-, (D) *Glut4*- (DDT*HFD pi$<$0.05), (E) *Lpl*- (DDT*HFD pi$<$0.05), (F) *Pnpla*- (DDT*HFD pi$<$0.05), (G) *Cpt2*- (DDT*HFD pi$<$0.05), and (H) *Twist1*- (DDT*HFD pi$<$0.1) fold change (relative to LFD + VEH and adjusted by *Tbp*). *p$<$0.05, **p$<$0.01 significance between groups indicated by bars. Data are represented as LS means + SEM.

Insulin resistance and thermogenesis

Epidemiological studies have demonstrated associations between adult DDT and DDE exposures and diabetes in humans [7,8,61,62]. Similarly, adult rodents exposed to high doses of DDT had impaired insulin secretion, glucose intolerance, and elevated gluconeogenesis [63,64]. Here we find that female mice perinatally exposed to low doses of DDT and subsequently fed a HFD in adulthood developed impaired glucose tolerance, increased fasting insulin, and HOMA-IR, indicative of insulin resistance and increased risk for T2D. We have observed that *Ppargc1a* expression in BAT of adult female offspring was reduced after perinatal DDT exposure. *Ppargc1a* plays an important role linking thermogenesis to risk of T2D as illustrated by genetic ablation studies of *Ppargc1a* in mice, after which thermogenesis was impaired and susceptibility to HFD-induced insulin resistance, but not obesity, was increased [14]. Whether the reduced *Ppargc1a* expression in BAT of DDT-exposed mice accounts for their reduced thermogenesis and insulin resistance needs further study. It is plausible that the effects of perinatal DDT on thermogenesis and insulin resistance in mice may be relevant to humans who suffered elevated DDT exposure perinatally.

Lipid homeostasis and adaptive energy metabolism

We also observed that perinatal DDT exposure caused a modest increase in circulating lipids after HFD feeding, which may in part be due to increased hepatic de novo lipogenesis as suggested by the increased protein expression of key lipogenic enzymes in the liver. Previous studies suggest that acute DDT administration increases hepatic cholesterol and triglyceride synthesis, resulting in their increased circulation in both rats and monkeys [65,66]. It is plausible that DDT and HFD exposures caused higher hepatic de novo lipogenesis, which was compensated for by increased lipid utilization, as evidenced by reduced RER, and increased hepatic bile acid conjugation, to prevent the development of hepatic steatosis in the female mice here [67,68].

Developmental origins of metabolic disruption

Several lines of evidence implicate developmental origins in DDT-induced metabolic syndrome. First, when the developmental stage of newborn mice was equivalent to that of a human fetus at term, pups exposed to DDT exhibited reduced body weights and glucose levels. This may contribute to their increased susceptibility to the metabolic syndrome since human studies have demonstrated that low birth weight and low neonatal glucose can be associated with the metabolic syndrome in adulthood [20,69,70]. Second, perinatal DDT exposure was associated with early-adult obesity in female offspring here and across generations in other rodent studies [71,72]. While sex differences are common in mouse models of metabolic disease [73], and both DDT and DDE have estrogenic and anti-androgenic properties [50] the basis for the sex differences observed in our study will have to be delineated in future studies. Further, these data corroborate a prospective study of women where higher cord blood levels of DDE were associated with significantly increased BMI of the adult daughters in a dose dependent manner [74].

Conclusions

Our study is the first to establish a link between developmental exposure to DDT and a moderately increased risk for the metabolic syndrome in adult offspring. Further, we know of no other studies implicating impaired thermogenesis in toxicant-induced insulin resistance and the metabolic syndrome. Given that circulating DDT and DDE levels in our mice fell within the range of DDT and DDE found in serum of contemporary people living

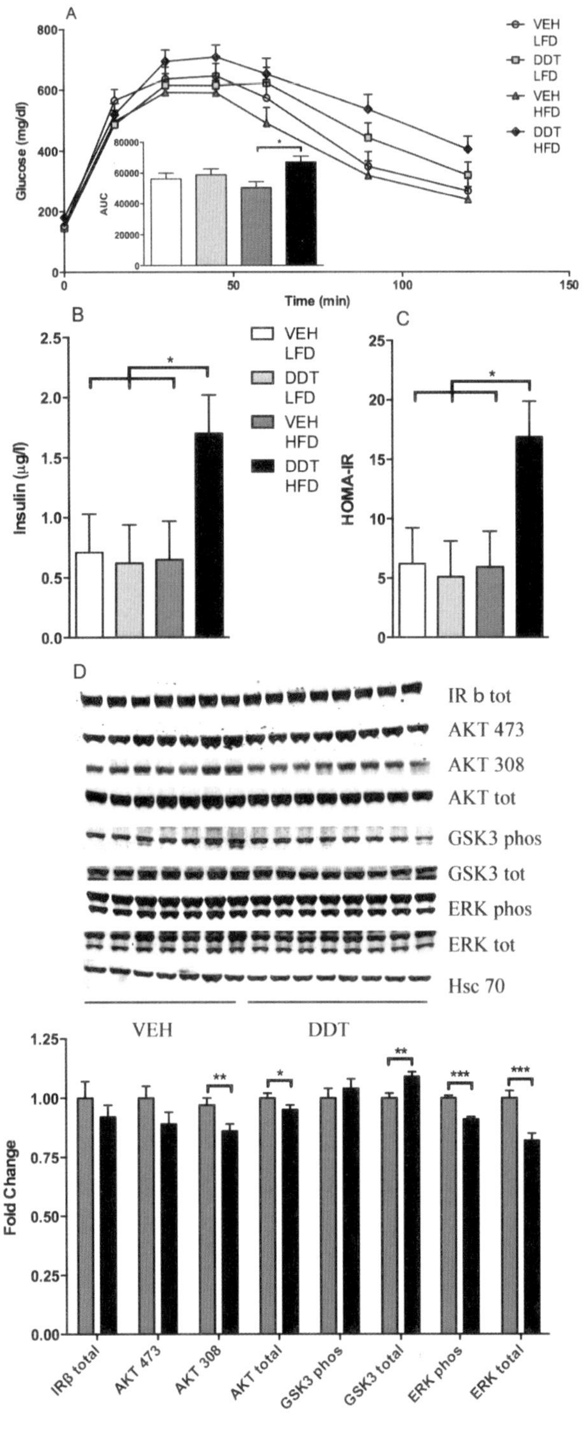

Figure 6. Effects of perinatal DDT and adult HFD feeding on glucose homeostasis in adult female mice (n = 1 female/litter in 8 VEH + LFD, 8 DDT + LFD, 7 VEH + HFD and 8 DDT + HFD litters). (A) Glucose tolerance test and resulting AUC (DDT*HFD pi = 0.08), (B) fasting insulin (DDT*HFD pi = 0.08) and (C) HOMA-IR (DDT*HFD pi = 0.07) in 8 month old mice. (D) Hepatic IRβ total, AKT 473 phosphorylation, AKT 308 phosphorylation, AKT total, GSK 3 phosphorylation, GSK 3 total, ERK phosphorylation, and ERK total fold change (relative to LFD + VEH and adjusted by HSC 70) as assessed by Western blot analysis (n = 1 female/litter in 7 VEH and 8 DDT litters) in 9 month old mice fed HFD. *p<0.05, **p<0.01, ***p<0.001 significance between groups indicated by bars. Data are represented as LS means + SEM.

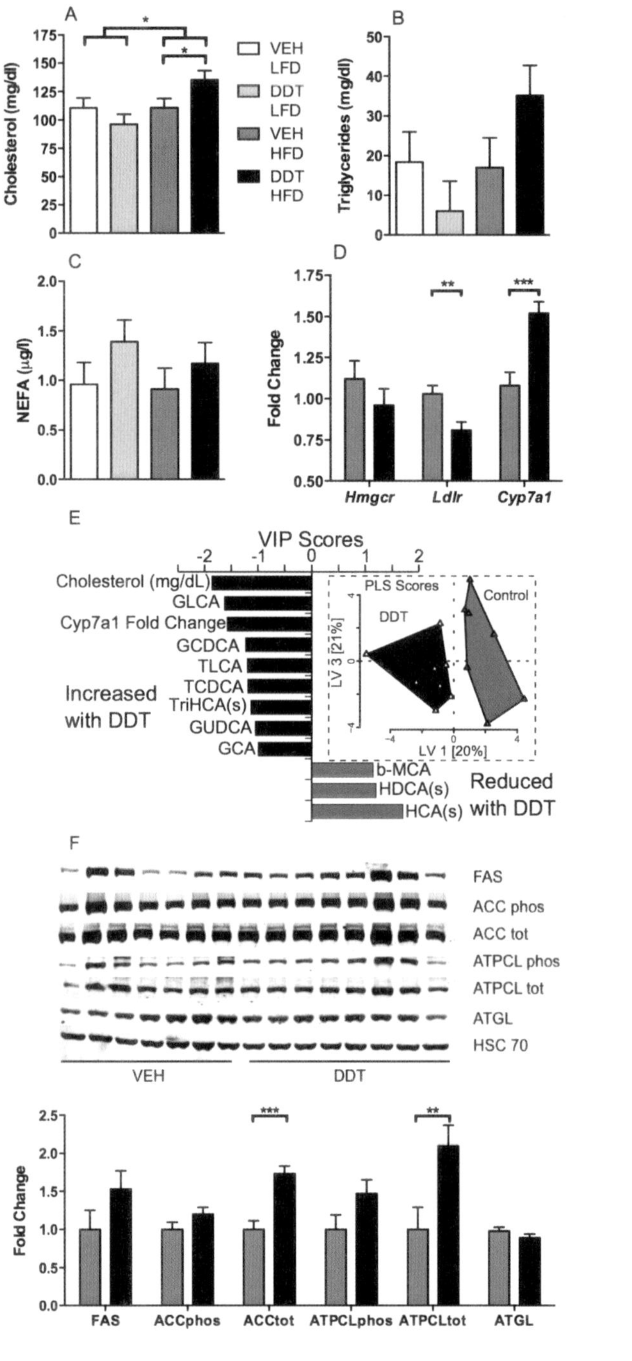

Figure 7. Effects of perinatal DDT and adult HFD feeding on lipid homeostasis in adult female mice (n = 1 female/litter in 8 VEH + LFD, 8 DDT + LFD, 7 VEH + HFD and 8 DDT + HFD litters). Fasting- (A) total cholesterol (HFD*DDT pi = 0.02), (B) triglycerides (HFD*DDT pi = 0.16), and (C) NEFA in 8 month old mice. (D) Hepatic *Hmgcr-*, *Ldlr-*, and *Cyp7a1-* fold change (relative to LFD + VEH and adjusted by *Gusb*) in 9 month old female mice fed HFD. (E) Bile acid metabolites discriminated by DDT or VEH exposure (VIP>1). Inset: The PLS-DA Scores Plot demonstrates clear discriminatory separation of mice with or without perinatal DDT exposure along latent variable 1 (LV1). Symbols represent individual animals. Metabolite abbreviations followed by "(s)" indicate "screening" data without the benefit of authentic calibration standards. F) Hepatic FAS- (p = 0.14), ACC phosphorylation - (p = 0.13), ACC total-, ATPCL phosphorylation - (p = 0.07), ATPCL total-, and ATGL- (p = 0.22) fold change (relative to LFD + VEH and adjusted by HSC 70) in 9 month old female mice fed HFD. *p<0.05, **p<0.01, ***p<0.001 significance between groups indicated by bars. Data are represented as LS means + SEM.

in northern Europe and in malaria-infested regions, and of the pregnant mothers of US adults who are currently in their mid-fifties [7,49,75,76] this is an important observation. Thus, it is likely that perinatal DDT exposure represents a risk factor for reduced energy expenditure in adult humans, even decades after DDT usage had ceased. The exact mechanism of this metabolic toxicity is unknown and how much it contributes to insulin resistance and dyslipidemia in the current obesity and diabetes epidemic will require further studies. But even small dysmetabolic effects of DDT and DDE are likely to be important from a public health perspective due to the ubiquity of these exposures among aging US and European populations as well as current populations of some developing and circumpolar countries. Given that the ban of DDT has reduced DDT exposure among the US population by about 100 fold [77], replacing DDT in malaria control should decrease DDT exposures over time and may reduce the susceptibility to the metabolic syndrome in future generations.

Supporting Information

Figure S1 Schematic of study design. 1.7 mg DDT/kg body weight was administered to dams daily on gestational day 11 through postnatal day 5 and litters were culled to 6 mice at postnatal day 6. Mice were metabolically screened from 2–6 months when they were randomized into 2 independent study arms: energy balance and HFD or LFD feeding. Indirect calorimetry and cold tolerance were assessed in 6-month-old mice. Metabolic parameters (e.g. body composition, fasting lipids, glucose, and insulin, GTT) were assessed during 12 weeks of HFD or LFD feeding until mice were sacrifice at 9 months of age.

Figure S2 Effect of prenatal DDT on gestation. (A) Gestation length, (B) gestation weight gain, and (C) litter size (n = 15 DDT litters and n = 14 VEH litters). Data are represented as LS means ± SEM.

Figure S3 Effect of perinatal DDT on body composition and energy balance in male mice. (A) Body mass at PND5 (n = 15 DDT- and n = 14 vehicle- exposed litters). (B) Trunk glucose in PND5 males culled from litters >6 pups (n = 7 DDT and n = 7 VEH litters). (C) Proportion of males with preputial separation as a function of age (n = 15 DDT and n = 14 VEH litters). Monthly (D) body mass and (E) percent adiposity, (F) food intake, and (G) rectal temperature ((n = 15 DDT and n = 14 VEH litters, 1 mouse/litter at 2 month time point, all males/litter thereafter). Data are represented as LS means ± SEM. *$p<0.05$ DDT vs. vehicle controls.

Figure S4 Effects of perinatal DDT on glucose tolerance. GTT in (A) female and (B) male 2 month old mice (2.0 mg glucose/kg body mass, 1.5 mg glucose/kg body mass, n = 15 DDT-exposed litters and n = 14 oil-exposed litters, 1 mouse/litter), in (C) female and (D) male 3 month old mice (1.0 mg glucose/kg body mass, 1.5 mg glucose/kg body mass, n = 12 litters/treatment, 1 mouse/litter), and in (E) female and (F) male 6 month old mice (1.0 mg glucose/kg body mass, n = 15 DDT-exposed litters and n = 14 oil-exposed litters, 1 mouse/litter). Data are represented as LS means ± SEM.

Figure S5 Joint effects of perinatal DDT and HFD on body composition and energy balance in male mice. (A) Weekly body mass (n = 8 litters/treatment, 1 mouse/litter, HFD*age pi<0.0001). (B) Percent adiposity in 8 month old mice (n = 8 litters/treatment, 1 mouse/litter). (C) Cumulative food intake over 12 week HFD and LFD feeding period (n = 8 litters/treatment, 1 mouse/litter). (D) Rectal temperature in 8 month old mice (n = 8 litters/treatment, 1 mouse/litter). *$p<0.05$, **$p<0.01$, ***$p<0.0001$ LFD vs. HFD. Data are represented as LS means ± SEM.

Figure S6 Joint effects of perinatal DDT and HFD on glucose and lipid homeostasis in male mice. (A) Glucose tolerance test at 1 mg glucose/kg body mass and (B) corresponding AUC, in 8 month old mice (n = 8 litters/treatment, 1 mouse/litter). (C) Insulin, (D) HOMA-IR, (E) total cholesterol, (F) triglycerides, and (G) NEFA (µg/l plasma) in 8 month old mice fasted for 5 hrs (n = 8 litters/treatment, 1 mouse/litter). LFD vs. HFD. *$p<0.05$ significance between groups indicated by bars. Data are represented as LS means ± SEM.

Figure S7 Partial Least Squares Discrimination Analysis (PLS-DA) of hepatic bile acids, triglycerides, and other metabolic factors which may influence or be influenced by cholesterol metabolism segregate treatment groups. (B) Relative weight of independent variable to this segregation are shown in the PLS Loadings Plot. Hierarchical cluster analyses were used to segregate variables and 4 unique clusters are displayed with unique colors. Variables with the variable importance in projection VIP scores >0.8 or <−0.8 are labeled, >1 or <−1 shown as triangles. (C) All LV1 VIP scores. Metabolite abbreviations followed by "(s)" indicate "screening" data relative areas generated from the expected precursor > product ion mass transition in the LC-MS/MS system, without the benefit of authentic calibration standards.

Figure S8 Lipid content of adult female mice fed HFD. (A) Oil red O stained liver from 9 month old female mice fed HFD for 12 weeks with exposure to perinatal vehicle (top) or DDT (bottom, bar = 50 microns). (B) Hepatic triglycerides and cholesterol in 9 month old female mice fed HFD. Data are represented as LS means + SEM.

Table S1 Table of Information about Western Blot Antibodies.

Table S2 Effects of perinatal DDT on metabolic parameters in mice fed regular chow. LS Means (± SEM) shown.

Table S3 Liver Bile Acid concentrations (nmol/g). Values are reported as mean ± SEM).

Acknowledgments

We wish to thank Leslie Roteta for help with parts of the animals studies and Drs. Gary Schwartz and Derek LeRoith for sharing their BAT-10 and Echo-MRI respectively; Drs. Myrto Petreas and June-Soo Park for quantitating sera DDTs; Drs. James Godbold, Philip Landrigan, and Michael Gallo for their comments. The USDA is an equal opportunity provider and employer.

Author Contributions

Conceived and designed the experiments: MLM. Performed the experiments: MLM EK CL MLF. Analyzed the data: MLM EK EM CL MLF JN. Contributed reagents/materials/analysis tools: MLM JN CB. Contributed to the writing of the manuscript: MLM EK EM CL MLF JN CB.

References

1. Shaw JE, Sicree RA, Zimmet PZ (2010) Global estimates of the prevalence of diabetes for 2010 and 2030. Diabetes Res Clin Pract 87: 4–14.
2. American Diabetes A (2013) Economic costs of diabetes in the U.S. in 2012. Diabetes Care 36: 1033–1046.
3. InterAct C, Langenberg C, Sharp SJ, Schulze MB, Rolandsson O, et al. (2012) Long-term risk of incident type 2 diabetes and measures of overall and regional obesity: the EPIC-InterAct case-cohort study. PLoS Med 9: e1001230.
4. Gallagher EJ, Leroith D, Karnieli E (2010) Insulin resistance in obesity as the underlying cause for the metabolic syndrome. Mount Sinai Journal of Medicine 77: 511–523.
5. Ouellet V, Routhier-Labadie A, Bellemare W, Lakhal-Chaieb L, Turcotte E, et al. (2011) Outdoor temperature, age, sex, body mass index, and diabetic status determine the prevalence, mass, and glucose-uptake activity of 18F-FDG-detected BAT in humans. Journal of Clinical Endocrinology and Metabolism 96: 192–199.
6. Taylor KW, Novak RF, Anderson HA, Birnbaum LS, Blystone C, et al. (2013) Evaluation of the association between persistent organic pollutants (POPs) and diabetes in epidemiological studies: a national toxicology program workshop review. Environ Health Perspect 121: 774–783.
7. Cox S, Niskar AS, Narayan KM, Marcus M (2007) Prevalence of self-reported diabetes and exposure to organochlorine pesticides among Mexican Americans: Hispanic health and nutrition examination survey, 1982–1984. Environ Health Perspect 115: 1747–1752.
8. Lee DH, Steffes MW, Sjodin A, Jones RS, Needham LL, et al. (2011) Low Dose Organochlorine Pesticides and Polychlorinated Biphenyls Predict Obesity, Dyslipidemia, and Insulin Resistance among People Free of Diabetes. PLos One 6: e15977.
9. Ramachandran A, Snehalatha C, Shetty AS, Nanditha A (2012) Trends in prevalence of diabetes in Asian countries. World J Diabetes 3: 110–117.
10. Herrera-Portugal C, Ochoa H, Franco-Sanchez G, Yanez L, Diaz-Barriga F (2005) Environmental pathways of exposure to DDT for children living in a malarious area of Chiapas, Mexico. Environmental Research 99: 158–163.
11. Bouwman H, Becker PJ, Cooppan RM, Reinecke AJ (1992) Transfer of DDT used in malaria control to infants via breast milk. Bull World Health Organ 70: 241–250.
12. Kreiss K, Zack MM, Kimbrough RD, Needham LL, Smrek AL, et al. (1981) Cross-sectional study of a community with exceptional exposure to DDT. JAMA 245: 1926–1930.
13. Farhang L, Weintraub JM, Petreas M, Eskenazi B, Bhatia R (2005) Association of DDT and DDE with birth weight and length of gestation in the Child Health and Development Studies, 1959–1967. American Journal of Epidemiology 162: 717–725.
14. Kleiner S, Mepani RJ, Laznik D, Ye L, Jurczak MJ, et al. (2012) Development of insulin resistance in mice lacking PGC-1alpha in adipose tissues. Proc Natl Acad Sci U S A 109: 9635–9640.
15. Fisher FM, Kleiner S, Douris N, Fox EC, Mepani RJ, et al. (2012) FGF21 regulates PGC-1alpha and browning of white adipose tissues in adaptive thermogenesis. Genes Dev 26: 271–281.
16. Hondares E, Gallego-Escuredo JM, Flachs P, Frontini A, Cereijo R, et al. (2013) Fibroblast growth factor-21 is expressed in neonatal and pheochromocytoma-induced adult human brown adipose tissue. Metabolism.
17. Zhao Y, Dunbar JD, Kharitonenkov A (2012) FGF21 as a therapeutic reagent. Adv Exp Med Biol 728: 214–228.
18. Hinoi E, Nakamura Y, Takada S, Fujita H, Iezaki T, et al. (2013) Growth differentiation factor-5 promotes brown adipogenesis in systemic energy expenditure. Diabetes.
19. Ravelli AC, van der Meulen JH, Michels RP, Osmond C, Barker DJ, et al. (1998) Glucose tolerance in adults after prenatal exposure to famine. Lancet 351: 173–177.
20. Hult M, Tornhammar P, Ueda P, Chima C, Bonamy AK, et al. (2010) Hypertension, diabetes and overweight: looming legacies of the Biafran famine. PLoS One 5: e13582.
21. Dahri S, Snoeck A, Reusens-Billen B, Remacle C, Hoet JJ (1991) Islet function in offspring of mothers on low-protein diet during gestation. Diabetes 40 Suppl 2: 115–120.
22. Fernandez-Twinn DS, Wayman A, Ekizoglou S, Martin MS, Hales CN, et al. (2005) Maternal protein restriction leads to hyperinsulinemia and reduced insulin-signaling protein expression in 21-mo-old female rat offspring. Am J - Physiol Regul Integr Comp Physiol 288: R368–373.
23. Ecobichon DJ, Saschenbrecker PW (1968) Pharmacodynamic study of DDT in cockerels. Canadian Journal of Physiology and Pharmacology 46: 785–794.
24. Nnodim JO, Lever JD (1985) The pre- and postnatal development and ageing of interscapular brown adipose tissue in the rat. Anat Embryol (Berl) 173: 215–223.
25. Asahina K, Tsai SY, Li P, Ishii M, Maxson RE, Jr., et al. (2009) Mesenchymal origin of hepatic stellate cells, submesothelial cells, and perivascular mesenchymal cells during mouse liver development. Hepatology 49: 998–1011.
26. Han J, Lee JE, Jin J, Lim JS, Oh N, et al. (2011) The spatiotemporal development of adipose tissue. Development 138: 5027–5037.
27. Lee JS, Ward WO, Knapp G, Ren H, Vallanat B, et al. (2012) Transcriptional ontogeny of the developing liver. BMC Genomics 13: 33.
28. Wang QA, Tao C, Gupta RK, Scherer PE (2013) Tracking adipogenesis during white adipose tissue development, expansion and regeneration. Nat Med 19: 1338–1344.
29. You L, Gazi E, Archibeque-Engle S, Casanova M, Conolly RB, et al. (1999) Transplacental and lactational transfer of p,p′-DDE in Sprague-Dawley rats. Toxicology and Applied Pharmacology 157: 134–144.
30. Sholtz RI, McLaughlin KR, Cirillo PM, Petreas M, Park JS, et al. (2011) Assaying organochlorines in archived serum for a large, long-term cohort: implications of combining assay results from multiple laboratories over time. Environ Int 37: 709–714.
31. Matthews DR, Hosker JP, Rudenski AS, Naylor BA, Treacher DF, et al. (1985) Homeostasis model assessment: insulin resistance and beta-cell function from fasting plasma glucose and insulin concentrations in man. Diabetologia 28: 412–419.
32. Folch J, Lees M, Sloane Stanley GH (1957) A simple method for the isolation and purification of total lipides from animal tissues. Journal of Biological Chemistry 226: 497–509.
33. Allain CC, Poon LS, Chan CS, Richmond W, Fu PC (1974) Enzymatic determination of total serum cholesterol. Clinical Chemistry 20: 470–475.
34. Trinder P (1969) Determination of blood glucose using an oxidase-peroxidase system with a non-carcinogenic chromogen. Journal of Clinical Pathology 22: 158–161.
35. Garcia-Canaveras JC, Donato MT, Castell JV, Lahoz A (2012) Targeted profiling of circulating and hepatic bile acids in human, mouse, and rat using a UPLC-MRM-MS-validated method. J Lipid Res 53: 2231–2241.
36. Lindtner C, Scherer T, Zielinski E, Filatova N, Fasshauer M, et al. (2013) Binge drinking induces whole-body insulin resistance by impairing hypothalamic insulin action. Sci Transl Med 5: 170ra114.
37. Hou X, Xu S, Maitland-Toolan KA, Sato K, Jiang B, et al. (2008) SIRT1 regulates hepatocyte lipid metabolism through activating AMP-activated protein kinase. J Biol Chem 283: 20015–20026.
38. Scherer T, O'Hare J, Diggs-Andrews K, Schweiger M, Cheng B, et al. (2011) Brain insulin controls adipose tissue lipolysis and lipogenesis. Cell Metab 13: 183–194.
39. Novo CL, Polese C, Matheus N, Decottignies A, Londono-Vallejo A, et al. (2013) A new role for histone deacetylase 5 in the maintenance of long telomeres. FASEB J 27: 3632–3642.
40. Green HF, Nolan YM (2012) GSK-3 mediates the release of IL-1beta, TNF-alpha and IL-10 from cortical glia. Neurochem Int 61: 666–671.
41. Zaytseva YY, Rychahou PG, Gulhati P, Elliott VA, Mustain WC, et al. (2012) Inhibition of fatty acid synthase attenuates CD44-associated signaling and reduces metastasis in colorectal cancer. Cancer Res 72: 1504–1517.
42. Yu XX, Lewin DA, Forrest W, Adams SH (2002) Cold elicits the simultaneous induction of fatty acid synthesis and beta-oxidation in murine brown adipose tissue: prediction from differential gene expression and confirmation in vivo. FASEB J 16: 155–168.
43. Qiao A, Liang J, Ke Y, Li C, Cui Y, et al. (2011) Mouse patatin-like phospholipase domain-containing 3 influences systemic lipid and glucose homeostasis. Hepatology 54: 509–521.
44. Bostrom P, Wu J, Jedrychowski MP, Korde A, Ye L, et al. (2012) A PGC1-alpha-dependent myokine that drives brown-fat-like development of white fat and thermogenesis. Nature 481: 463–468.
45. Livak KJ, Schmittgen TD (2001) Analysis of relative gene expression data using real-time quantitative PCR and the 2(-Delta Delta C(T)) Method. Methods 25: 402–408.
46. Butler AA, Kozak LP (2010) A recurring problem with the analysis of energy expenditure in genetic models expressing lean and obese phenotypes. Diabetes 59: 323–329.
47. Grapov D, Newman JW (2012) imDEV: a graphical user interface to R multivariate analysis tools in Microsoft Excel. Bioinformatics 28: 2288–2290.
48. Mevik BH, Wehrens R (2007) The pls package: Principal component and partial least squares regression in R. Journal of Statistical Software. 18: 1–23.
49. Rylander C, Sandanger TM, Brustad M (2009) Associations between marine food consumption and plasma concentrations of POPs in a Norwegian coastal population. J Environ Monit 11: 370–376.
50. Sohoni P, Sumpter JP (1998) Several environmental oestrogens are also anti-androgens. Journal of Endocrinology 158: 327–339.
51. Uldry M, Yang W, St-Pierre J, Lin J, Seale P, et al. (2006) Complementary action of the PGC-1 coactivators in mitochondrial biogenesis and brown fat differentiation. Cell Metab 3: 333–341.
52. Hall JA, Ribich S, Christoffolete MA, Simovic G, Correa-Medina M, et al. (2010) Absence of thyroid hormone activation during development underlies a permanent defect in adaptive thermogenesis. Endocrinology 151: 4573–4582.
53. CR B, JG N, J L, XX H, GP H, et al. (2007) Modest PGC-1alpha overexpression in muscle in vivo is sufficient to increase insulin sensitivity and palmitate oxidation in subsarcolemmal, not intermyofibrillar, mitochondria. J Biol Chem 283: 4228–4240. Epub 2007 Dec 4212.
54. Koves TR, Sparks LM, Kovalik JP, Mosedale M, Arumugam R, et al. (2013) PPARgamma coactivator-1alpha contributes to exercise-induced regulation of intramuscular lipid droplet programming in mice and humans. J Lipid Res 54: 522–534.

55. Bastin J, Lopes-Costa A, Djouadi F (2011) Exposure to resveratrol triggers pharmacological correction of fatty acid utilization in human fatty acid oxidation-deficient fibroblasts. Hum Mol Genet 20: 2048–2057.
56. Rohas LM, St-Pierre J, Uldry M, Jager S, Handschin C, et al. (2007) A fundamental system of cellular energy homeostasis regulated by PGC-1alpha. Proc Natl Acad Sci U S A 104: 7933–7938.
57. Jun HJ, Gettys TW, Chang JS (2012) Transcriptional Activity of PGC-1alpha and NT-PGC-1alpha Is Differentially Regulated by Twist-1 in Brown Fat Metabolism. PPAR Res 2012: 320454.
58. Clegg DJ (2012) Minireview: the year in review of estrogen regulation of metabolism. Mol Endocrinol 26: 1957–1960.
59. Stefl B, Janovska A, Hodny Z, Rossmeisl M, Horakova M, et al. (1998) Brown fat is essential for cold-induced thermogenesis but not for obesity resistance in aP2-Ucp mice. Am J Physiol 274: E527–533.
60. Kim JY, Moon KD, Seo KI, Park KW, Choi MS, et al. (2009) Supplementation of SK1 from Platycodi radix ameliorates obesity and glucose intolerance in mice fed a high-fat diet. J Med Food 12: 629–636.
61. Rylander L, Rignell-Hydbom A, Hagmar L (2005) A cross-sectional study of the association between persistent organochlorine pollutants and diabetes. Environ Health 4: 28.
62. Patel CJ, Bhattacharya J, Butte AJ (2010) An environment-wide association study (EWAS) on Type 2 Diabetes Mellitus. PLos One 5: e10746.
63. Yau DT, Mennear JH (1977) The inhibitory effect of DDT on insulin secretion in mice. Toxicology and Applied Pharmacology 39: 81–88.
64. Kacew S, Singhal RL (1974) Role of cyclic adenosine 3′:5′-monophosphate in the action of 1,1,1-trichloro-2,2-bis-(p-chlorophenyl)ethane (DDT)on hepatic and renal metabolism. Biochemical Journal 142: 145–152.
65. Nagaoka S, Masaki H, Aoyama Y, Yoshida A (1986) Effects of excess dietary tyrosine or certain xenobiotics on the cholesterogenesis in rats. Journal of Nutrition 116: 726–732.
66. Sanyal S, Agarwal N, Dudeja PK, Mahmood A, Subrahmanyam D (1982) Effect of a single oral dose of DDT on lipid metabolism in protein-calorie malnourished monkeys. Indian Journal of Biochemistry and Biophysics 19: 111–114.
67. Rolo AP, Palmeira CM, Wallace KB (2002) Interactions of combined bile acids on hepatocyte viability: cytoprotection or synergism. Toxicol Lett 126: 197–203.
68. Attili AF, Angelico M, Cantafora A, Alvaro D, Capocaccia L (1986) Bile acid-induced liver toxicity: relation to the hydrophobic-hydrophilic balance of bile acids. Med Hypotheses 19: 57–69.
69. Bazaes RA, Salazar TE, Pittaluga E, Pena V, Alegria A, et al. (2003) Glucose and lipid metabolism in small for gestational age infants at 48 hours of age. Pediatrics 111: 804–809.
70. Barker DJ, Hales CN, Fall CH, Osmond C, Phipps K, et al. (1993) Type 2 (non-insulin-dependent) diabetes mellitus, hypertension and hyperlipidaemia (syndrome X): relation to reduced fetal growth. Diabetologia 36: 62–67.
71. Tomatis L, Turusov V, Day N, Charles RT (1972) The effect of long-term exposure to DDT on CF-1 MICE. International Journal of Cancer 10: 489–506.
72. Skinner MK, Manikkam M, Tracey R, Guerrero-Bosagna C, Haque M, et al. (2013) Ancestral dichlorodiphenyltrichloroethane (DDT) exposure promotes epigenetic transgenerational inheritance of obesity. BMC Medicine 11: 228–244.
73. Guarner-Lans V, Rubio-Ruiz ME, Perez-Torres I, Banos de MacCarthy G (2011) Relation of aging and sex hormones to metabolic syndrome and cardiovascular disease. Exp Gerontol 46: 517–523.
74. Karmaus W, Osuch JR, Eneli I, Mudd LM, Zhang J, et al. (2009) Maternal levels of dichlorodiphenyl-dichloroethylene (DDE) may increase weight and body mass index in adult female offspring. Occupational and Environmental Medicine 66: 143–149.
75. Bouwman H, Cooppan RM, Becker PJ, Ngxongo S (1991) Malaria control and levels of DDT in serum of two populations in Kwazulu. Journal of Toxicology and Environmental Health 33: 141–155.
76. La Merrill M, Cirillo PM, Terry MB, Krigbaum NY, Flom JD, et al. (2013) Prenatal Exposure to the Pesticide DDT and Hypertension Diagnosed in Women before Age 50: A Longitudinal Birth Cohort Study. Environ Health Perspect 121: 594–599.
77. Eskenazi B, Chevrier J, Rosas LG, Anderson HA, Bornman MS, et al. (2009) The Pine River statement: human health consequences of DDT use. Environ Health Perspect 117: 1359–1367.

4

Partial Deletion of eNOS Gene Causes Hyperinsulinemic State, Unbalance of Cardiac Insulin Signaling Pathways and Coronary Dysfunction Independently of High Fat Diet

Cecilia Vecoli[1], Michela Novelli[2], Anna Pippa[3], Daniela Giacopelli[1], Pascale Beffy[1], Pellegrino Masiello[2], Antonio L'Abbate[1,3], Danilo Neglia[1,4]*

1 Istituto di Fisiologia Clinica-CNR, Pisa, Italy, **2** Dipartimento di Ricerca Traslazionale e delle Nuove Tecnologie in Medicina e Chirurgia, Università di Pisa, Pisa, Italy, **3** Institute of Life Sciences, Scuola Superiore Sant'Anna, Pisa, Italy, **4** Fondazione Toscana G. Monasterio-CNR, Pisa, Italy

Abstract

Abnormalities in eNOS gene, possibly interacting with high fat diet (HFD), affect peripheral vascular function and glucose metabolism. The relative role of eNOS gene, HFD and metabolic derangement on coronary function has not been fully elucidated. We test whether eNOS gene deficiency per se or in association with HFD modulates coronary function through mechanisms involving molecular pathways related to insulin signaling. Wild type (WT), eNOS$^{-/-}$ and eNOS$^{+/-}$ mice were studied. WT and eNOS$^{+/-}$ mice were fed with either standard or HF diet for 16 weeks and compared with standard diet fed eNOS$^{-/-}$. Glucose and insulin tolerance tests were performed during the last week of diet. Coronary resistance (CR) was measured at baseline and during infusions of acetylcholine (Ach) or sodium-nitroprusside (SNP) to evaluate endothelium-dependent or independent vasodilation, in the Langendorff isolated hearts. Cardiac expression of Akt and ERK genes as evaluation of two major insulin-regulated signaling pathways involved in the control of vascular tone were assessed by western blot. HFD-fed mice developed an overt diabetic state. Conversely, chow-fed genetically modified mice (in particular eNOS$^{-/-}$) showed a metabolic pattern characterized by normoglycemia and hyperinsulinemia with a limited degree of insulin resistance. CR was significantly higher in animals with eNOS gene deletions than in WT, independently of diet. Percent decrease in CR, during Ach infusion, was significantly lower in both eNOS$^{-/-}$ and eNOS$^{+/-}$ mice than in WT, independently of diet. SNP reduced CR in all groups except eNOS$^{-/-}$. The cardiac ERK1-2/Akt ratio, increased in animals with eNOS gene deletions compared with WT, independently of diet. These results suggest that the eNOS genetic deficiency, associated or not with HFD, has a relevant effect on coronary vascular function, possibly mediated by increase in blood insulin levels and unbalance in insulin-dependent signaling in coronary vessels, consistent with a shift towards a vasoconstrictive pattern.

Editor: You-Yang Zhao, University of Illinois College of Medicine, United States of America

Funding: Scuola Superiore Sant'Anna and IFC-CNR internal funding. The funders had no role in study design, data collection and analysis, decision to publish, or preparation of the manuscript.

Competing Interests: The authors have declared that no competing interests exist.

* Email: dneglia@ifc.cnr.it

Introduction

Major risk factors for coronary artery disease (CAD) include a cluster of conditions such as obesity, dyslipidemia, hypertension and insulin resistance that is also referred to as metabolic syndrome. Unbalanced, fat-rich diet, which is a recognized cause of the metabolic syndrome, has been reported to have direct effects on vascular tone mainly by interfering with activation of eNOS [1], [2]. Thus, abnormal endothelial function is a common feature of the syndrome and is usually considered to be secondary to the metabolic abnormalities.

More recently, it has been hypothesized that endothelial dysfunction may precede or even cause metabolic deregulation. Nitric oxide (NO), a major factor in the regulation of vascular function, is believed to also exert a significant role in the maintenance of glucose homeostasis, by contributing to modulation of peripheral insulin sensitivity [3], [4] and possibly insulin secretion [5], [6]. Both arterial hypertension and insulin resistance have been documented in either endothelial NO synthase (eNOS) null mice [7], [8], [9] or mice with partial deletion of the eNOS gene when challenged with a nutritional stress such as high fat diet (HFD) [10]. In the clinical setting, polymorphic variants of the eNOS gene are associated with arterial hypertension and insulin resistance in various populations [11]–[13]. In particular, in a recent paper from our group, we showed that the CC polymorphic variant of eNOS −786 T/C polymorphism was associated with a significant increase in arterial blood pressure and impairment of glucose metabolism in a population of cardiomyopathic patients [13]. These recent experimental and clinical evidences suggest that eNOS gene abnormalities, possibly interacting with HFD, may contribute to endothelial/vascular dysfunction as well as to deregulation of glucose metabolism. Whether eNOS genetic determinants and metabolic abnormalities might interact to affect coronary circulatory function has not been fully elucidated.

In the present study, we measured coronary function in $eNOS^{-/-}$ mice as well as in $eNOS^{+/-}$ partially deficient mice, with or without HFD. Specifically, baseline coronary resistance and coronary response to vasodilating stimuli were measured in isolated hearts from total or partial eNOS knockout mice fed or not with HFD for 16 weeks, after in vivo assessment of glucose tolerance and insulin sensitivity. In addition we tested whether eNOS gene deficiency directly modifies insulin-dependent cardiac molecular pathways involved in the control of coronary tone. NOS expression, insulin-dependent triggering of PI3K/Akt pathway, resulting in eNOS phosphorylation and activation, as well as stimulation of (MAPK)/ERK pathway, that leads to production of the vasoconstrictor factor endothelin (ET)-1 [14], [15], were evaluated in the cardiac tissue in the same groups.

Methods

Experiments were carried out in wild-type (WT) C57BL/6 mice and in mice with B6/129 $eNOS^{-/-}$ genotype backcrossed onto the C57BL/6 strain [8], [16]. C57-Bl/6J female wild type (WT) and male $eNOS^{-/-}$ mice were mated to generate $eNOS^{+/-}$ mice. To assess genotype, genomic DNA was extracted from mouse tail biopsies and genotyped by polymerase chain reaction (PCR) according to a protocol provided by the Jackson Laboratory [http://www.jax.org]. For this study, male mice only were included in the experimental groups (WT, $eNOS^{-/-}$ and $eNOS^{+/-}$). Starting at the age of 4 weeks, WT and $eNOS^{+/-}$ mice were fed for 16 weeks either a standard diet (chow food, containing protein 23%, fat 5%, carbohydrate approximately 60%, fiber 5% and ash 5.5%, with 10% energy deriving from fat), or a high-fat diet (HFD) containing protein 23%, fat 34%, carbohydrate approximately 30%, fiber 5% and ash 5.5%, with 60% energy deriving from fat. Both diets were purchased from Mucedola, Settimo Milanese, MI, Italy). $eNOS^{-/-}$ mice, being per se insulin resistant and hypertensive, were nursed only with standard diet. Therefore, five groups of animals were studied: 1) WT (n = 16); 2) HFD-fed WT (n = 18); 3) $eNOS^{+/-}$ (n = 15); 4) HFD-fed $eNOS^{+/-}$ (n = 16) and 5) $eNOS^{-/-}$ (n = 10).

Body weight and blood glucose levels (measured by a glucometer, Glucocard GT-1610, Menarini Diagnostic, Firenze, Italy) were measured weekly in animals left without food 4 h before testing.

Experimental protocols were approved by the Animal Care Committee of the Italian Ministry of Health and conformed to the "Guiding Principles for Research Involving Animals and Human Beings" approved by the Council of the American Physiological Society. Throughout the study period, the mice were housed under controlled 12/12 h light/dark cycle and given food and water ad libitum. To avoid oxidation and organoleptic alteration of HFD, this food was added fresh every other day.

Intraperitoneal glucose tolerance test

After 15 weeks of diet, glucose (1.5 g/kg body weight as 16.5% solution) was given intraperitoneally to 4-h-fasting conscious animals. Drops of blood taken from the tail vein before and 15, 60, 120 and 180 min after the glucose injection were immediately used for glucose determination by a glucometer. Some blood samples (at 0, 15 and 60 min) were also collected in EDTA-treated tubes and centrifuged at 4°C; plasma was stored at −20°C for subsequent insulin measurement. Insulin was determined by radioimmunoassay (RIA), according to Herbert et al. [17], using anti-insulin antibody and ^{125}I-labeled insulin obtained from Linco (Linco Research, INC. St. Charles, MO, USA).

Intraperitoneal insulin tolerance test

After 16 weeks of diet, human insulin (0.75 U/kg body weight, Humulin R, Eli Lilly, Indianapolis, IN, USA) was administered to conscious animals by intraperitoneal route. Blood glucose was measured by a glucometer in drops of blood taken from the tail vein before and 15, 30, 60 and 120 min after insulin administration.

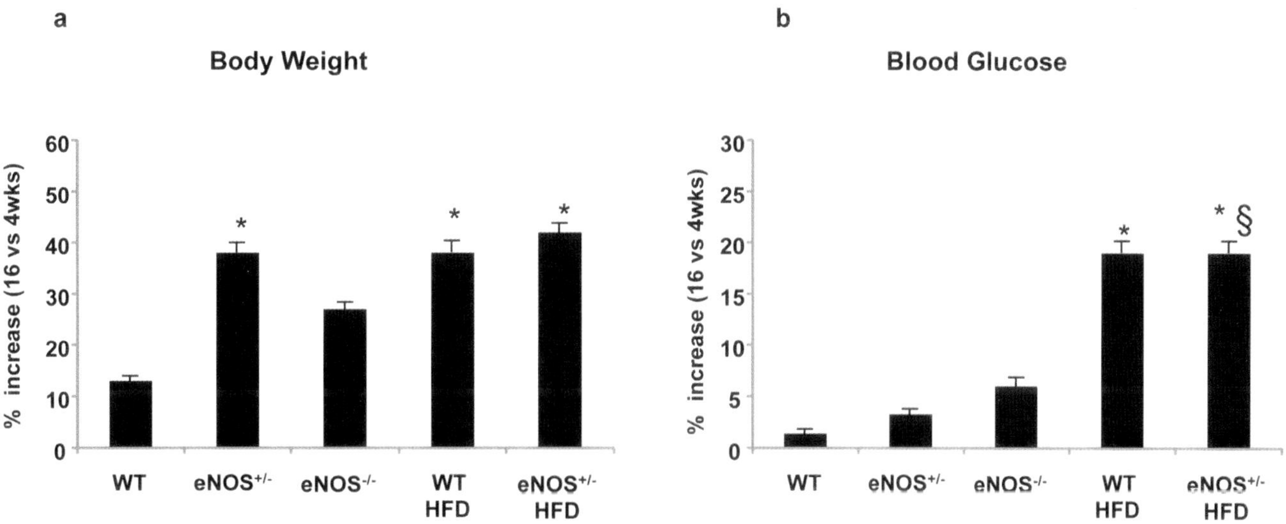

Figure 1. Percent increase (16 versus 4 weeks) of body weight (a) and blood glucose levels (b) during the 16 weeks of monitoring in all groups of animals, indicated as follows: WT, healthy controls fed with standard diet; $eNOS^{+/-}$, partial knockout eNOS mice fed with standard diet; $eNOS^{-/-}$, total knockout eNOS mice fed with standard diet; WT HFD, healthy controls fed with high-fat diet (HFD); $eNOS^{+/-}$ HFD, partial knockout eNOS mice fed with HFD. Mean ± SEM of 15–18 mice for each group, except $eNOS^{-/-}$ mice (n = 10). *$p<0.05$, at least, *vs* WT; §$p<0.05$, at least, *vs* $eNOS^{+/-}$.

Table 1. Body weight and basal blood glucose levels during the 16 weeks of controlled diet in all groups of animals.

	4 wks	8 wks	12 wks	16 wks
Body Weight (g)				
WT	25.8±1.1	27.8±1.4	28.±1.0	29.2±0.9
eNOS$^{+/-}$	23.3±0.9	26.9±1.0	30.6±1.2	32.3±0.8
eNOS$^{-/-}$	26.0±1.8	28.1±1.5	31.4±1.0	32.7±1.7
WT HFD	26.3±0.9	32.0±1.2*	35.1±1.3*	36.4±0.6*
eNOS$^{+/-}$ HFD	24.5±1.5	29.0±1.2*§	32.4±0.9*§	34.9±1.3*§
Blood Glucose (mg/dL)				
WT	144±5	148±5	147±4	146±4
eNOS$^{+/-}$	148±5	151±5	150±5*	153±4*
eNOS$^{-/-}$	145±8	152±10	148±7	154±6*
WT HFD	160±10*	168±10*	179±15*	190±9*
eNOS$^{+/-}$ HFD	160±8*§	174±9*§	185±5*§	192±8*§

WT: wild type controls HFD: high fat diet.
*$p<0.05$, at least, vs WT;
§$p<0.05$, at least, vs eNOS$^{+/-}$.
Just before starting diet regimens (at 4 weeks of age), body weights of animals' groups were: WT, 22.1±0.9 g; eNOS$^{+/-}$, 21.7±1.2 g; eNOS$^{-/-}$, 22.0±1.3 g; blood glucose levels were: WT, 142±4 mg/dL; eNOS$^{+/-}$, 138±9 mg/dL; eNOS$^{-/-}$, 140±8 mg/dL.

Isolated heart preparation

At the end of the experiment, after 16 weeks of diet, at least 6 mice of each group were anaesthetized with pentobarbital i.p. injection and heparinized via the left femoral vein (500 U i.m.). The heart was rapidly excised, weighed and placed in cold perfusion medium. The isolated hearts were immediately attached to the Langendorff apparatus and retrogradely perfused at constant pressure (at 37°C), as previously described [18]. The perfusion medium consisted of oxygenated Krebs-Henseleit buffer (NaCl 118.5; $NaHCO_3$ 25.0; KCl 4.7; $MgSO_4$ 1.2; KH_2PO_4 1.2; glucose 11.0; $CaCl_2$ 1.4 mmol/L) and gassed with 95% O_2 and 5% CO_2 (pH 7.4). Coronary flow was continuously monitored while collecting the cardiac effluent. Coronary resistance (CR) was measured as input pressure divided by coronary flow per gram of myocardial tissue (mmHg*min*g/mL).

Isolated hearts were studied according to one of two protocols: after a stabilization period (30 min, baseline), the heart was perfused either with acetylcholine (Ach, 10 µmol/L) to measure the degree of endothelium-dependent vasodilation (at least 6 mice for each group) or with nitroprusside (SNP, 10 µmol/L) to measure the degree of endothelium-independent vasodilation (at least 6 mice for each group). Ach and SNP were infused into the aortic cannula for 3 minutes at infusion rates ranging from 0.2% to 1% of coronary flow. Injection of vehicle alone did not cause changes in coronary flow. The concentrations of Ach and SNP were selected on the basis of pilot experiments aimed at assessing the concentrations giving the maximum degree of vasodilation.

Western blot analysis of cardiac tissue for Akt, pAKT, ERK1-2, pERK1-2, eNOS, peNOS

From at least four randomly chosen animals in each group, hearts were immediately frozen in liquid nitrogen and subsequently pulverized. Lysates were prepared using lysis buffer (50 mM Tris HCl pH 7.5, 150 mM NaCl, 1 mM EDTA, 1% Triton X-100, 1 mM PMSF, 2 mM Na_3VO_4, 2 mM NaF), containing Protease Inhibitor Cocktail. Protein concentration in supernatant was determined using the Bio-Rad protein assay (Bio-Rad Laboratories, Hercules, CA, USA). Equal amounts of protein (30 µg of heart tissue lysate) were submitted to 10% SDS/polyacrylamide gel electrophoresis and transferred to a nitrocellulose membrane. The membranes were blocked and then incubated overnight al 4°C with the primary antibody, followed by an appropriate secondary antibody. Secondary antibody binding was visualized using the ECL detection kit (Euroclone, Milan, Italy), according to the manufacturer's instructions. Densitometric analysis of developed blots was performed with the ImmageJ program. Protein bands were quantified and values were normalized to those of α-tubulin (Sigma, St. Louis, MO, USA). Antibodies to Akt and pAkt were purchased from Cell Signaling Technology (Beverly, MA, USA); antibodies to eNOS, peNOS, ERK1-2, and pERK1-2 were purchased from Santa Cruz Biotechnologies (Santa Cruz, CA, USA). The pERK/pAkt ratio was calculated as double ratio between phosphorylated and not phosphorylated form of ERK1-2 (pERK1-2/ERK1-2) and phosphorylated and not phosphorylated form of Akt (pAkt/Akt).

RT-PCR analysis of cardiac tissue for iNOS

The mRNA expression levels of iNOS were determined by semi-quantitative PCR method. RNA was extracted from myocardial tissue using the RNeasy Mini Kit (Qiagen, Milan, Italy). RNA was quantified by measuring absorbance at 260 nm and stored at −80°C until use. One microgram of total RNA was reversed transcribed using iScriptTM cDNA Synthesis Kit (Bio-Rad, Milan, Italy). Quantification of mRNA for these PCR products was accomplished by using GoTaqGreen Master Mix Kit (Promega, Madison, WI) with the Applied Biosystems 2720 Thermal Cycler (Life Technologies, Foser City, CA). The forward and reverse primers were purchased from QIAGEN (QuantiTect Primer Assay). The PCR products were then subjected to agarose gel electrophoresis (1%), pre-stained with GelRedTM (Biotium, Hayward, CA), and photographed. Data analysis were performed using ImmageJ program. PCR results were normalized to ribosomal gene Rn18S as housekeeping gene.

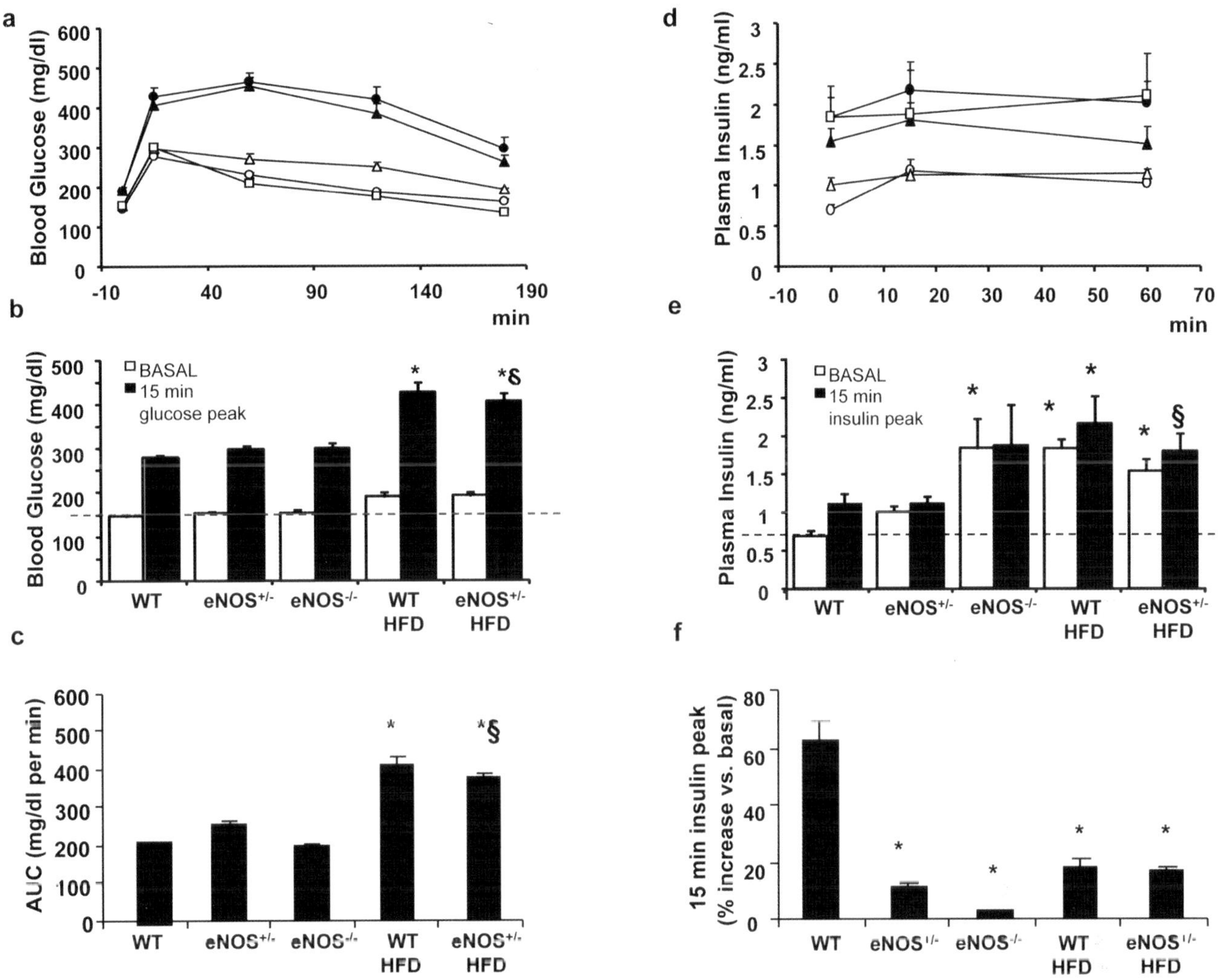

Figure 2. Blood glucose and plasma insulin levels during glucose tolerance test. Abbreviations are defined in Fig. 1. a) Blood glucose levels were determined during a glucose tolerance test (glucose 1.5 g/kg i.p.) performed after 15 weeks of HFD diet. b) values of blood glucose at baseline and 15 minutes after the glucose load. c) the area under the curve (AUC) for glycaemic values. d) Plasma insulin levels were determined during a glucose tolerance test (glucose 1.5 g/kg i.p.) performed after 15 weeks of HFD diet. e) Plasma insulin levels at baseline and 15 minutes after the glucose load (insulin peak). f) % increase of 15-min post-loading plasma insulin level with respect to the corresponding basal value. Abbreviations are as in Fig. 1. In the panels a) and d) empty circles are WT mice, empty triangles are eNOS$^{+/-}$ mice, empty squares are eNOS$^{-/-}$ mice, filled circles are WT HFD mice, and filled triangles are eNOS$^{+/-}$ HFD. Mean ± SEM of 15–18 mice for each group, except for eNOS$^{-/-}$ mice (n = 4). *p<0.05, at least, vs WT; §p<0.05, at least, vs eNOS$^{+/-}$.

Statistical analysis

Results are presented as mean ± SEM of the number (n) of replicate determinations. Statistical significance between different experimental groups was determined by using a two-way ANOVA followed by the Fisher's exact test as post-hoc test. A p<0.05 was considered significant.

Results

Body weight and basal glycemic levels

During the experimental period, body weight increased progressively in all groups of animals, with some differences in the growth rate and final weight attained at the end of the 16 weeks of diet (Table 1). As expected, HFD-fed mice gained significantly higher body weight than corresponding standard diet groups. The percent increase in body weight from 4 to 16 weeks of diet was significantly higher not only in HFD-fed mice but also in eNOS$^{+/-}$, as compared with WT group (Fig. 1a). No differences in the daily amount of food and water intake were observed (not shown). In chow-fed WT, eNOS$^{+/-}$ and eNOS$^{-/-}$ mice, basal blood glucose levels changed very little during the 16 weeks of observation, whereas in both the HFD-fed groups they were significantly higher than those of controls already after 4 weeks of diet and progressively increased thereafter (Table 1 and Fig. 1b).

Glucose tolerance and insulin sensitivity

The intraperitoneal glucose tolerance test revealed that both groups of animals fed with HFD (WT and eNOS$^{+/-}$ mice), which already had significantly higher basal glucose levels than controls, were clearly glucose intolerant (Fig. 2a). Indeed, they had the highest post-loading glucose peaks at 15 minutes (Fig. 2b) and the largest areas under the curve (Fig. 2c) as compared to the other groups. The corresponding post-loading insulin profile (Fig. 2d) showed that the HFD-fed mice, which had significantly higher

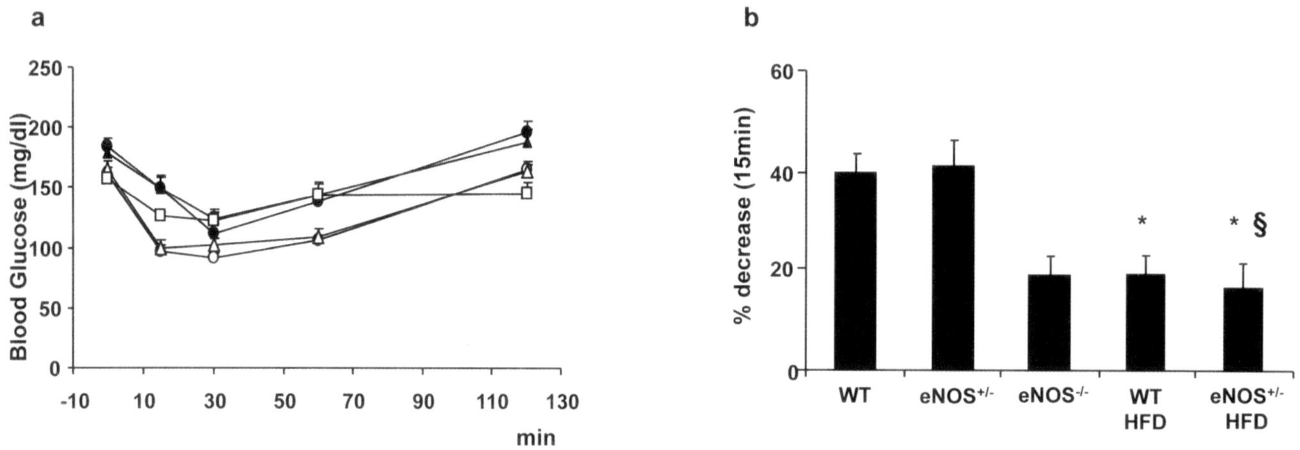

Figure 3. Blood glucose levels during insulin tolerance test. Abbreviations are as in Fig. 1. a) Blood glucose levels were determined during an insulin tolerance test (insulin 0.75 U/kg i.p.) performed after 16 weeks of diet. b) percent decrements of blood glucose values with respect to basal at 15 minutes after the insulin administration.. Abbreviations are as in Fig. 1. Empty circles are WT mice, empty triangles are eNOS$^{+/-}$ mice, empty squares are eNOS$^{-/-}$ mice, filled circles are WT HFD mice, and filled triangles are eNOS$^{+/-}$ HFD Mean ± SEM of 15–18 mice for each group, except for eNOS$^{-/-}$ mice (n = 4). *$p<0.05$, at least, *vs* WT; §$p<0.05$, at least, *vs* eNOS$^{+/-}$.

basal insulin levels than chow-fed WT, slightly augmented these levels at 15 and 60 min after the glucose load, although the percent increase over basal at the 15 min peak was limited as compared to controls (Fig. 2e). Interestingly, despite normoglycemia, eNOS$^{-/-}$ mice had increased insulin levels at baseline, that remained high after the load, without any further increase in response to glucose (Fig. 2f).

An intraperitoneal insulin tolerance test (Fig. 3) showed that the HFD-fed groups were insulin resistant, as indicated by a significantly lower glucose clearance from the bloodstream in response to administered insulin.

In chow-fed eNOS$^{+/-}$ mice the hypoglycaemic effects of exogenous insulin administration were super-imposable to those of controls, while eNOS$^{-/-}$ mice showed a different trend, as the early limited reduction of blood glucose (Fig. 3b) and the subsequent glycemic values until 60 min were closer to HFD-fed animals than to controls (Fig. 3a).

Coronary vascular resistance

Coronary vascular resistance (CR) was significantly higher in animals with eNOS gene deletions than in WT mice, independently of diet (Fig. 4a). In particular, as compared with WT, CR was increased by 21%, 20% and 14% in eNOS$^{+/-}$, eNOS$^{-/-}$ and HFD-fed eNOS$^{+/-}$, respectively. Percent decrease in CR, during endothelium-dependent vasodilating stimulus by Ach, was significantly lower in eNOS genetically modified mice than in WT, again independently of diet ($p<0.05$) (Fig. 4b). Conversely, the endothelium-independent vasodilator SNP was effective in all groups of animals except eNOS$^{-/-}$. This latter group showed negligible reduction in CR after SNP (~5% decrement), suggesting the occurrence of irreversible coronary vascular abnormalities (Fig. 4c).

NOS expression in the heart

As expected, western blot analysis documented that eNOS protein expression was reduced by approximately a half in eNOS$^{+/-}$ mice compared with WT and was absent in eNOS$^{-/-}$ (Fig. 5). HFD did not alter eNOS expression. The ratio peNOS/eNOS was affected neither by partial eNOS deletion nor by HFD. Inducible NOS isoform (iNOS) was over-expressed in all groups with respect to WT controls (Fig. 6). The up-regulation of iNOS was more evident in the eNOS genetically modified animals, but HFD per se (in WT mice) was also able to moderately increase the levels of this enzyme.

ERK and Akt signaling pathways in the heart

eNOS genetic abnormalities were associated with a moderate activation of ERK1-2 pathway (as implied by a tendency to an increased pERK/ERK1-2 ratio, that attained statistical significance in the eNOS$^{-/-}$ group), concomitantly with a small deactivation of the Akt pathway, as indicated by a slight decrease in the pAkt/Akt ratio (Fig. 7). As a result, the double ratio of pERK/pAkt showed a clear trend to increase in all eNOS-genetically modified groups as compared with WT (statistical significant in eNOS$^{-/-}$ and HFD-fed eNOS$^{+/-}$), pointing out a definite imbalance between the two molecular pathways downstream the insulin receptor. HFD did not modify the trend in eNOS$^{+/-}$ group, while moderately decreasing the pERK/pAkt ratio mainly due to a significant reduction in the pERK/ERK1-2 ratio.

Discussion

In the present experimental study, deletion of eNOS gene, either partial or total, results in a significant impairment in coronary vasodilating capability. Genetically modified mice also show a peculiar abnormality of glucose homeostasis characterized by a normoglycemic/hyperinsulinemic state with partial preservation of peripheral insulin sensitivity. In the myocardium of these animals, the molecular pathways downstream the insulin receptor are altered leading to a shift of the ERK1-2/Akt balance towards a prevalent vasoconstrictive pattern. HFD, while causing overt diabetes and marked insulin resistance, does not independently affect coronary tone and the balance of cardiac molecular pathways downstream insulin receptor. A diagrammatic representation of proposed mechanisms of interaction between eNOS deficiency, metabolic stress and insulin- dependent signaling pathways in endothelial cells is shown in Figure 8.

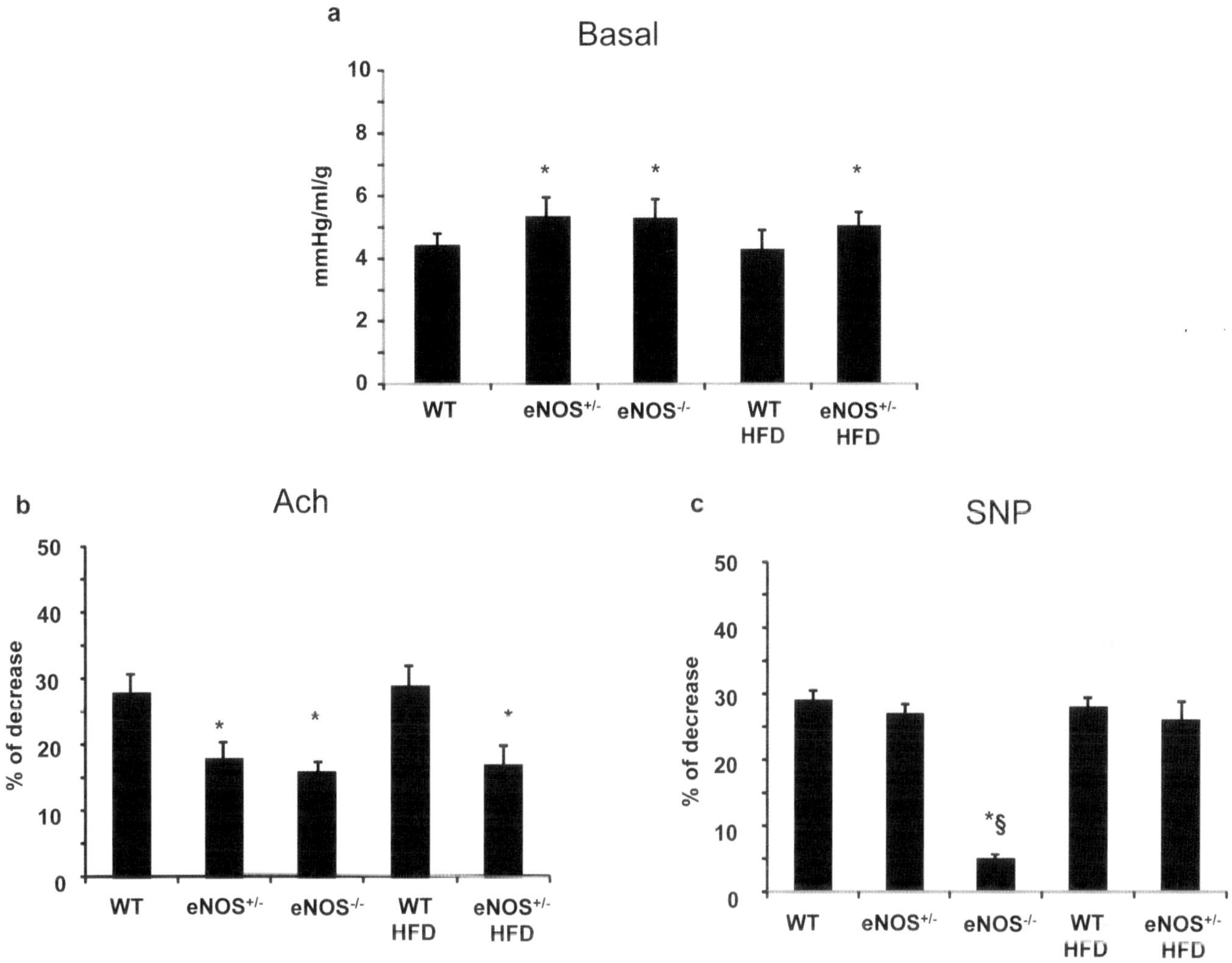

Figure 4. Coronary resistance (CR) in Langendorff configuration in basal conditions (a); b) Percent change in CR during 3 minutes of acetylcholine (Ach) infusion with respect to the corresponding basal value; c) percent change in CR during 3 minutes of sodium nitroprusside (SNP) infusion. Abbreviations are as in Fig. 1. Mean ± SEM of at least 6 mice for each group. *$p<0.05$, at least, *vs* WT; §$p<0.05$, at least *vs* eNOS$^{+/-}$.

Effects of eNOS gene deletions and HFD on coronary vascular tone

Our findings demonstrate that partial or total deletion of eNOS gene is able per se to impair coronary vascular tone. Gödecke et al [19] firstly studied coronary hemodynamics in eNOS$^{-/-}$ mice by Langendorff-perfused hearts, showing no changes in basal coronary flow. Possible differences in animal models could account for such discrepancy. Indeed, in our study, eNOS deficiency was associated with increased coronary resistance both at baseline and during Ach infusion as compared with WT and HFD-WT groups. Both eNOS$^{-/-}$ and eNOS$^{+/-}$ had the same impaired response to endothelium-dependent vasodilation, suggesting that NO bioavailability is insufficient when 50% of the enzyme is lacking. Interestingly, the endothelium independent vasodilation capability (assessed by SNP infusion) was still preserved in eNOS$^{+/-}$, whereas it was totally blunted in eNOS$^{-/-}$. It can be hypothesized that in total knockout mice, severe eNOS gene abnormalities affect coronary function with additional mechanisms besides the impaired endothelium dependent vasodilating capability. Structural alterations of the coronary arterioles are most likely involved, as observed in the systemic microvasculature of adult hypertensive eNOS$^{-/-}$mice [20], [21].

In the present study, HFD caused a somewhat expected overt diabetic state concomitantly with basal hyperinsulinemia, indicative of insufficient compensation of a quite relevant insulin resistance, but such metabolic alteration was neither associated per se with abnormal coronary vascular function nor induced synergistic changes at coronary level when used in eNOS-deficient animals. In previous studies performed in partially eNOS-deficient mice subjected to HFD, the two conditions were additive in causing an increase in systemic vascular resistance and hypertension [10]. It is conceivable that different vascular districts may have different behaviors. Moreover, while systemic resistance is measured in vivo, coronary resistance can be only measured ex-vivo, in the absence of the in vivo circulating milieu, which in turn may differently affect vascular function.

In genetic (db/db mice) or chemically-induced animal models of diabetes with marked hypoinsulinemia, we have previously shown the occurrence of increased coronary resistance ex-vivo, associated with decreased cardiac expression of eNOS [18], [22], [23]. In the same models, pharmacological treatments able to restore the

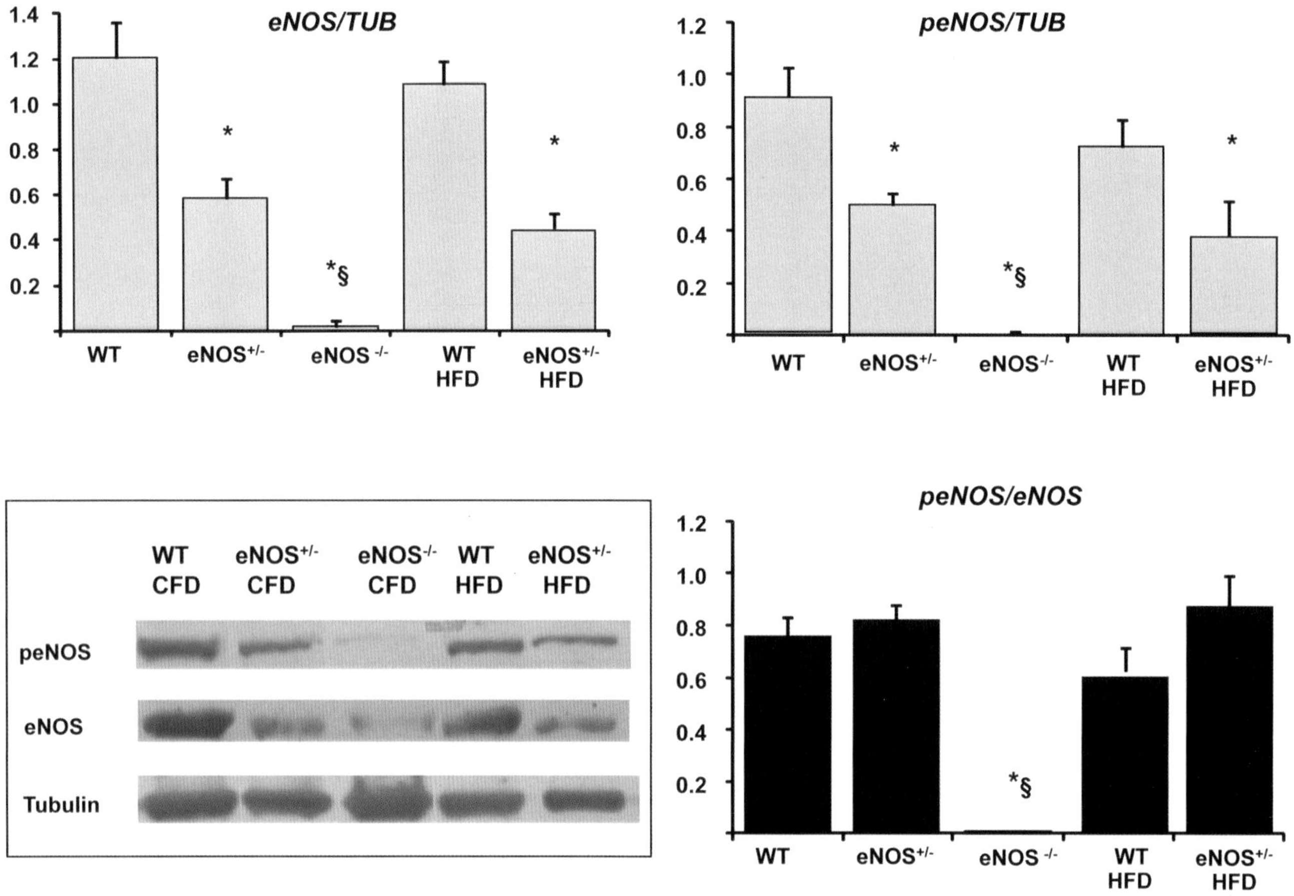

Figure 5. eNOS expression in cardiac tissue of experimental animals. Cardiac tissue homogenates were subjected to Western blotting for eNOS, peNOS and α-tubulin protein determination. Representative immunoblots (inferior left panel) are shown for all groups of mice. Abbreviations are defined in Fig. 1. Mean ± SEM of 4–6 mice for each group. *$p<0.05$, at least, *vs* WT; §$p<0.05$, at least, *vs* eNOS$^{+/-}$.

eNOS expression were also able to reduce coronary resistance, leading to improvement of cardiac function [18], [23]. Differences in the animal models employed may account for the apparent difference between previous and present results. In particular, in the genetic model of db/db mice, diabetes and obesity are the result of a deficit in the leptin receptor, while the beta-cytotoxic agent streptozotocin causes a severe hyperglycemic/hypoinsulinemic state. In the present experiments, diabetes associated with insulin resistance and partially compensatory hyperinsulinemia was induced by HFD; however, HFD per se was unable to interfere with coronary resistance.

Effects of eNOS gene deletions on insulin/glucose homeostasis

Both partial and total deletion of the eNOS gene were able to affect insulin/glucose homeostasis causing hyperinsulinemia but not the overt insulin resistant state induced by HFD. Indeed, mainly the total deletion of eNOS gene (the partial deletion had a minor effect) was associated with increased circulating insulin levels in the basal state and during the glucose tolerance test, in the absence of basal hyperglycemia or glucose intolerance. This metabolic impairment is somewhat different from the clear-cut insulin resistant state produced by HFD, as the high circulating levels of insulin in eNOS-deficient animals maintained normoglycemia in basal condition and allowed a normal glucose clearance during glucose tolerance test, despite the lack of a definite post-loading insulin peak.

A generic insulin resistant state has been already described in eNOS$^{-/-}$ [7], [24] and in eNOS$^{+/-}$ mice fed with HFD [10], [25]. The exact mechanism by which eNOS gene deficiencies lead to increased circulating insulin awaits further investigations, although several authors suggest that the increased peripheral vascular resistance and the consequent reduction of blood flow might reduce glucose uptake by skeletal muscle, thereby favouring a trend to increased blood glucose levels which on turn stimulate insulin secretion [7], [10], [24] [25]. This is also interpreted as a compensatory mechanism that in physiological/healthy conditions aids to maintain vascular homeostasis, by means of the vasodilating effects of insulin, during temporary stresses.

Whichever the mechanism involved, partially or totally eNOS-deficient mice had normal glycemia and increased circulating levels of insulin, although to a different extent. Interestingly, eNOS$^{+/-}$ mice showed an approximate 40% increase in body weight (from 4 to 16 weeks of diet) that was significantly higher than in WT and comparable to that of HFD-fed mice. It is conceivable that the presence of even a slight hyperisulinemic state early in life in these mice, not associated with a true insulin resistance, would probably induce increased weight gain. This pattern might not apply to eNOS$^{-/-}$ mice, as the total deletion of the enzyme would likely induce multiple additional effects limiting body growth.

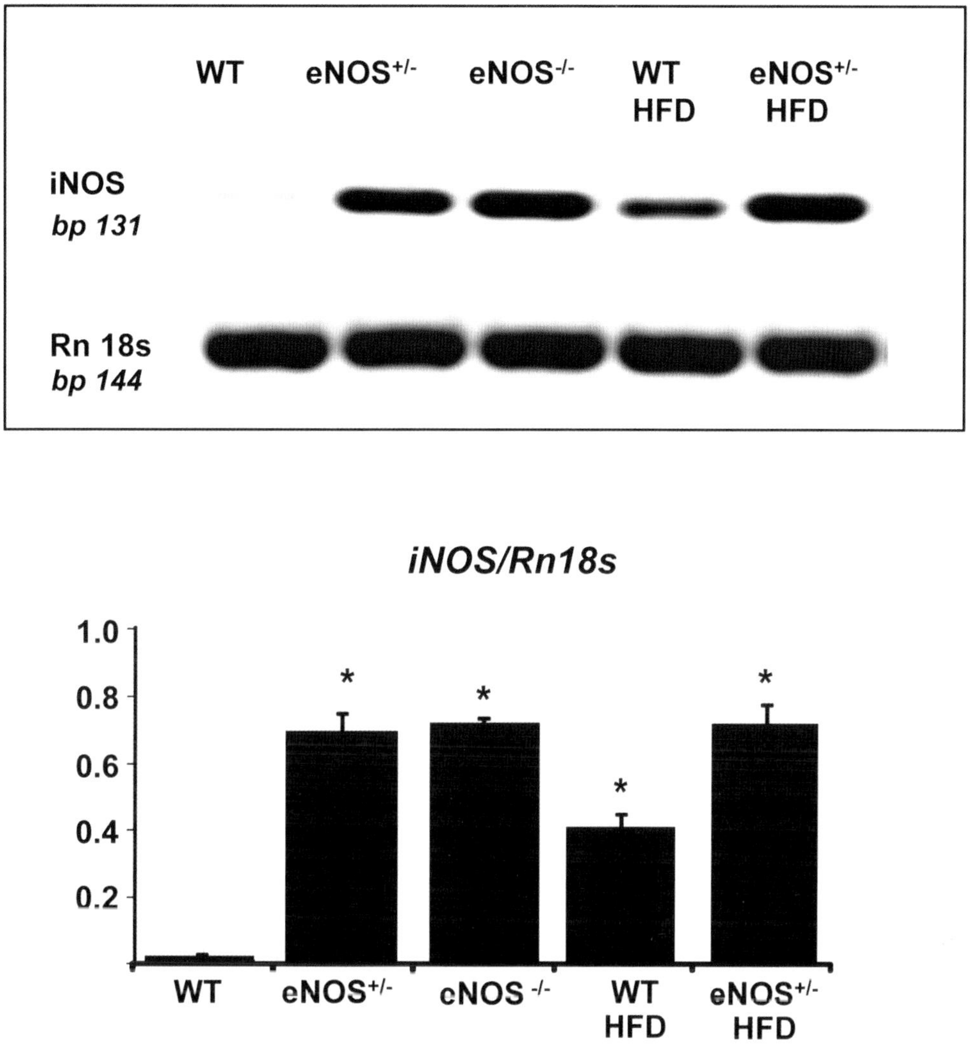

Figure 6. iNOS gene expression in cardiac tissue of experimental animals. Cardiac tissue homogenates were subjected to RT-PCR. Results were normalized to ribosomal gene Rn18S as housekeeping gene. Abbreviations are defined in Fig. 1. Mean ± SEM of 4–6 mice for each group. $^*p < 0.05$, at least, *vs* WT.

Cardiac molecular changes and pathways downstream insulin

The cardiac molecular analysis of eNOS protein showed a roughly 50% reduction of the enzyme in $eNOS^{+/-}$ mice and its absence in $eNOS^{-/-}$ animals, as expected from the experimental model used. HFD did not influence the expression of this protein or its activation, as the levels of protein and its phosphorylated forms were balanced in all groups of animals. As a consequence, the ratio between peNOS/eNOS was similar in all groups. These results suggest that the link between genetic eNOS abnormalities and increased coronary vascular tone is related to the decreased levels of eNOS protein caused by the genetic background rather than to its phosphorylation/activation.

Insulin binding to its receptor triggers a phosphorylation cascade that on the one hand activates eNOS through PI3K/Akt pathway and on the other hand activates the pro-atherogenic MAPK/ERK1-2 pathway which is associated with mitogenesis, cell growth and the production of ET-1 [26], [27]. Accordingly, insulin may have a vasodilating effect through stimulation of NO production and a vasoconstrictive effect through stimulation of synthesis and release of ET-1 [15].

In our study, there was no significant difference in Akt activation (pAkt) among the experimental groups. Since pAkt is recognized as a major protein involved in eNOS phosphorylation [28], our finding is consistent with the documented normal ratio peNOS/eNOS. Conversely, in all eNOS-genetically modified groups there was a clear trend towards activation of ERK1-2 (as documented by higher pERK/ERK1-2 ratio as compared with the WT group). As a consequence, in these animals, the ratio between ERK1-2 and Akt was unbalanced towards the vasoconstrictive pathway. Our data confirm and expand previous evidence [20], [21], [29]–[32] that a primary genetically determined eNOS deficiency directly impairs endothelial function, possibly resulting in increased coronary resistance, and decreases coronary vasodilating capability. In addition we demonstrated that this condition was associated with an increase in ERK1-2 phosphorylation. Further studies are required to elucidate the specific signaling pathways involved. It is conceivable that the association of an altered eNOS expression with the imbalance of the downstream insulin-dependent molecular signals could be further detrimental to coronary function. In fact, together with lower NO bioavailability, the altered signal transduction pathways could cause

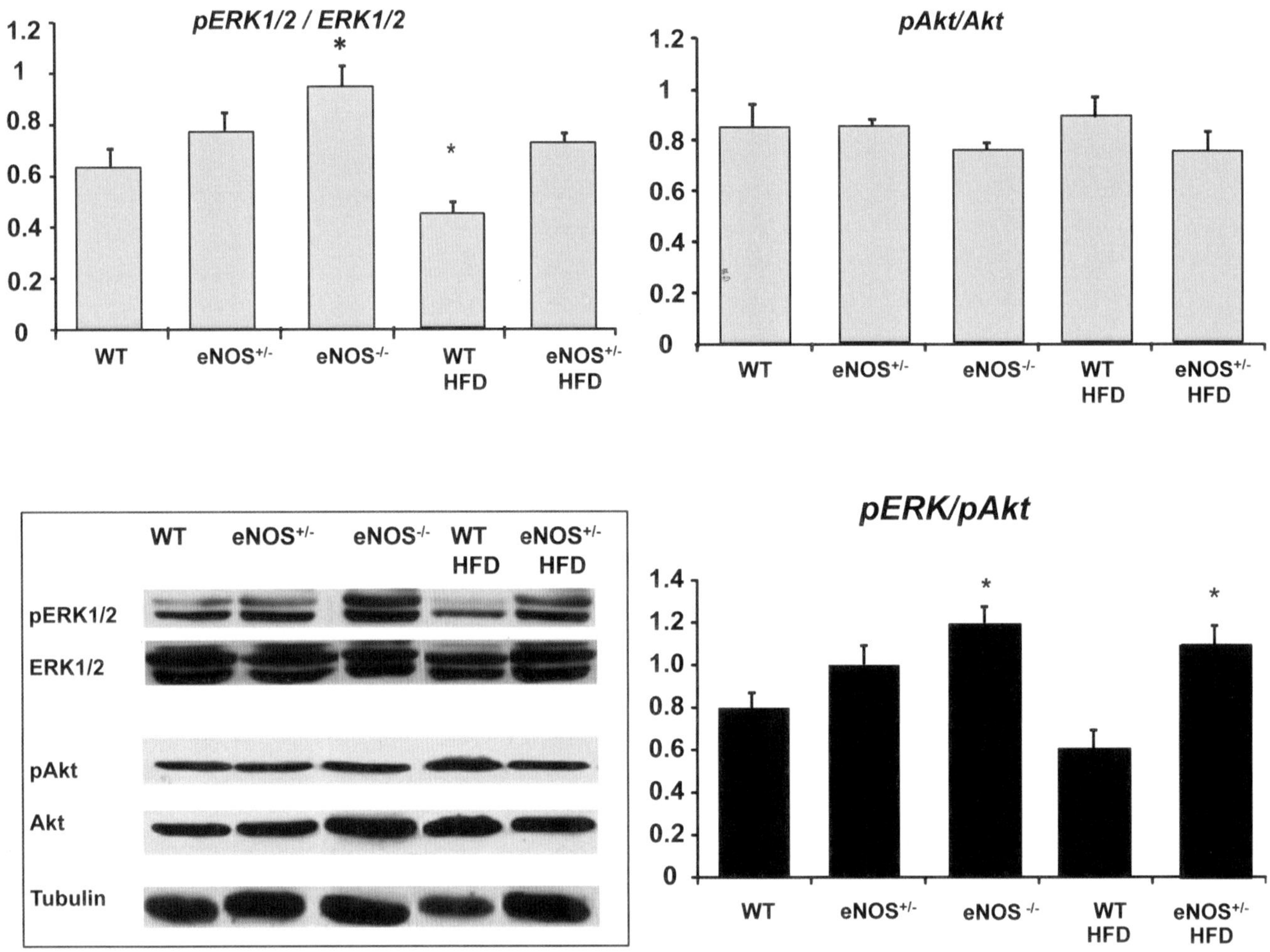

Figure 7. Expression of ERK1-2 and Akt in cardiac tissue of experimental animals. Cardiac tissue homogenates were subjected to Western blotting for Akt, pAkt, ERK1-2, and pERK1-2 protein determination. Representative immunoblots (inferior left panel) are shown for all groups of mice. Abbreviations are defined as in Fig. 1. Histograms showing the double pERK/p-Akt ratio have been reported. Mean ± SEM of 4–6 mice for each group. *$p<0.05$, at least, *vs* WT; §$p<0.05$, at least *vs* eNOS$^{+/-}$.

increased production of ET1. Moreover, since circulating insulin increases as a side effect of eNOS deficiency, its interaction with insulin receptor would further activate a pro-vasoconstrictive environment. HFD did not affect the balance of cardiac molecular pathways downstream insulin receptor, consistently with the lack of effects on coronary tone. Previous experimental studies showed that HFD may actually affect the Akt/eNOS signal in peripheral arteries. For instance, in HFD-fed mice, a FFA-mediated impairment of both basal and insulin-induced eNOS phosphorylation has been reported in peripheral vessels [1] and associated with endothelial dysfunction and hypertension. However, different results have been obtained in coronary arteries of diet-induced obese rats, as the endothelial NO vasorelaxation in response to insulin and the underlying PI3K/Akt/eNOS pathway were preserved [33] even though the pERK/ERK/ET-1 pathway seemed activated. The differential effects of HFD on insulin molecular pathways in peripheral arteries as compared with coronary vessels and cardiac tissue might explain the negligible effect of diet on coronary vascular resistance documented in the present study.

Together with eNOS, the cardiac expression of the inducible isoform of the enzyme was measured. In previous studies we have reported an increased expression of iNOS in cardiac tissue in animal models of metabolic impairment and secondary reduction of eNOS expression [18], [22], [23]. Decreased levels of eNOS and augmented expression of iNOS, together with enhanced oxidative stress, have been implicated in the pathogenesis of abnormal coronary function and potential myocardial damage [34]. The stress-induced iNOS isoform is able to produce an abnormal amount of NO, which, in an oxidative environment, reacts with superoxide, producing peroxynitrite and thus losing its vasodilating properties. Furthermore, peroxynitrite causes vasoconstriction and nitrosylation of cardiac proteins potentially resulting in functional coronary and myocardial damage. Accordingly, we have previously shown that a pharmacological treatment able to restore eNOS/iNOS ratio and counteract oxidative stress resulted in an increase of NO bioavailability associated to improvement of coronary vascular tone and myocardial function [18], [22], [23]. In the present study, iNOS expression in cardiac tissue was elevated in all eNOS deficient mice. Whether this pattern could further contribute to the abnormal coronary function and could potentially be reversed by treatment is an interesting matter of future investigation.

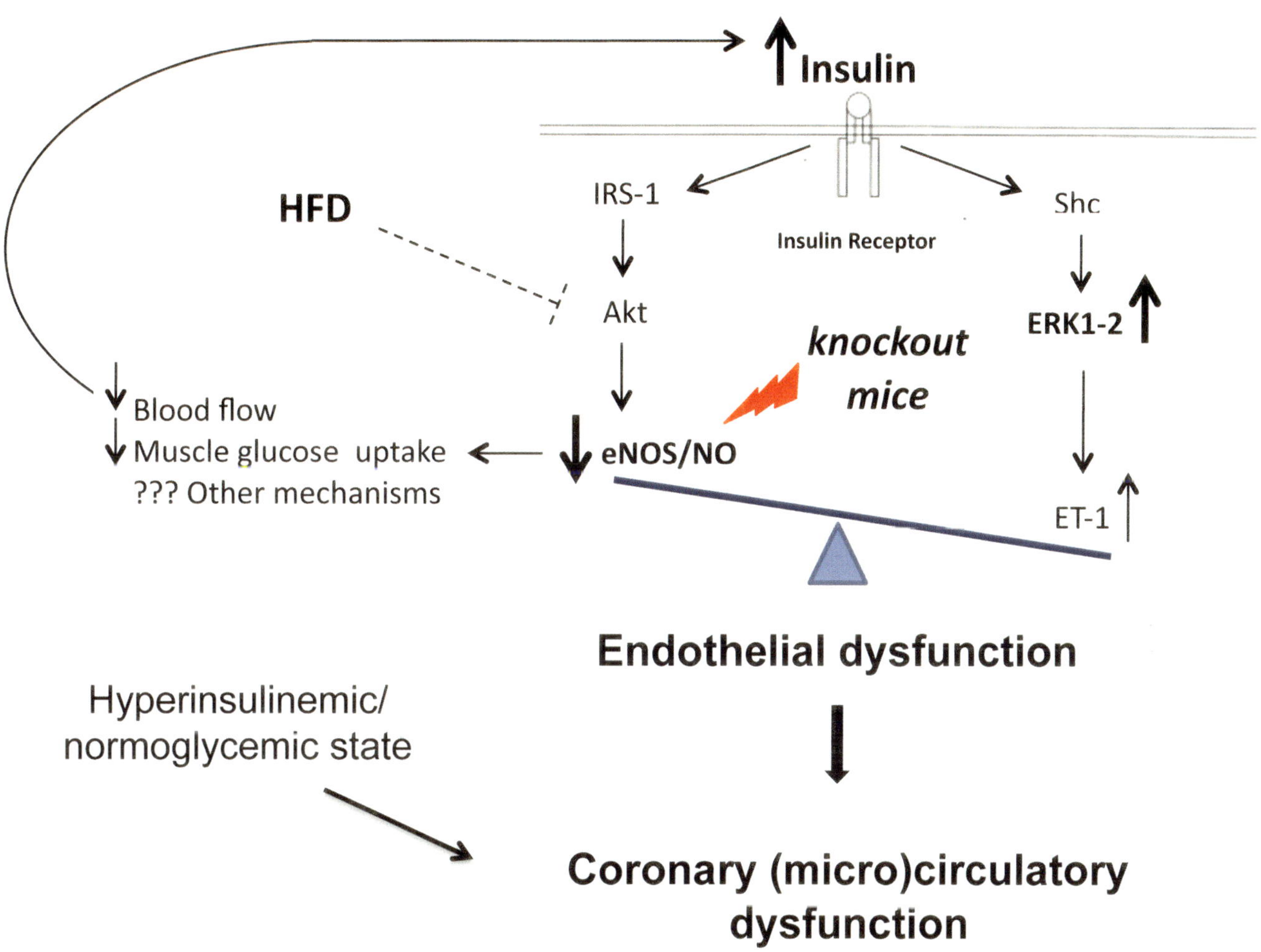

Figure 8. Diagrammatic representation of proposed mechanisms of interaction between eNOS deficiency, metabolic stress and insulin-dependent signaling pathway in coronary endothelial cells.

Clinical implications and conclusion

While there is no evidence on genetic variants leading to a total eNOS deficiency in humans, some polymorphic variants of the gene encoding eNOS, such as Glu298Asp and −786 T/C SNPs, have been shown to alter the function or the expression of the enzyme [12], [35]. These variants have been associated with coronary disease, hypertension, insulin resistance and obesity in clinical populations [11]–[13], [36]–[40]. In this study partial eNOS knockout mice have been used to mimic this clinical condition of reduced eNOS expression and to study the interaction with HFD, while eNOS total knockout mice represented a reference extreme condition (not found in the clinical setting) with more marked abnormalities in all the parameters related with eNOS complete deficiency. Altogether, the results of the present experimental study, although not immediately translatable to humans, strongly highlight a role of eNOS gene both as a key regulator of, and a link between metabolism and coronary function. These findings could be clinically relevant, taking into account that in human populations the prevalence of eNOS polymorphism ranges from 5 to 35% [41]–[46]. It is intriguing to speculate that known or still unknown genetic abnormalities of the eNOS gene can be a common substrate of major abnormalities predisposing to coronary disease.

Acknowledgments

We thank Prof. Flavio Coceani for providing the mutant mice used in this study. We thank Dr. Francesca Scebba for helping us in the initial mouse genotyping. We are grateful to Mrs. Cecilia Ciampi for her daily care of the animals.

Author Contributions

Conceived and designed the experiments: CV ALA DN. Performed the experiments: CV MN AP DG PB. Analyzed the data: CV MN PM. Contributed reagents/materials/analysis tools: PM DN. Wrote the paper: CV MN PM ALA DN.

References

1. Symons JD, McMillin SL, Riehle C, Tanner J, Palionyte M, et al. (2009) Contribution of insulin and Akt1 signaling to endothelial nitric oxide synthase in the regulation of endothelial function and blood pressure. Circ Res 104: 1085–1094.
2. Wang XL, Zhang L, Youker K, Zhang MX, Wang J, et al. (2006) Free fatty acids inhibit insulin signaling stimulated endothelial nitric oxide synthase activation through upregulating PTEN or inhibiting Akt kinase. Diabetes 55: 2301–2310.

3. Huang PL (2009) eNOS, metabolic syndrome and cardiovascular disease. Trends Endocrinol Metab 20: 295–302.
4. Wu G, Meininger CJ (2009) Nitric oxide and vascular insulin resistance. Biofactors 35: 21–27.
5. Lajoix AD, Reggio H, Chardès T, Péraldi-Roux S, Tribillac F, et al. (2001) A neuronal isoform of nitric oxide synthase expressed in pancreatic beta cells controls insulin secretion. Diabetes 50: 1311–1323.
6. Kaneko YK, Ishikawa T (2013) Dual role of nitric oxide in pancreatic beta cells. J Pharmacol Sci 123: 295–300.
7. Duplain H, Burcelin R, Sartori C, Cook S, Egli M, et al. (2001) Insulin resistance, hyperlipidemia, and hypertension in mice lacking endothelial nitric oxide synthase. Circulation 104(3): 342–345.
8. Shesely EG, Maeda N, Kim HS, Desai KM, Krege JH, et al. (1996) Elevated blood pressures in mice lacking endothelial nitric oxide synthase. Proc Natl Acad Sci U S A 93: 13176–13181.
9. Huang PL, Huang Z, Mashimo H, Bloch KD, Moskowitz MA, et al. (1995) Hypertension in mice lacking the gene for endothelial nitric oxide synthase. Nature 377: 239–242.
10. Cook S, Hugli O, Egli M, Ménard B, Thalmann S, et al. (2004) Partial gene deletion of endothelial nitric oxide synthase predisposes to exaggerated high-fat diet-induced insulin resistance and arterial hypertension. Diabetes 53(8): 2067–2072.
11. Niu W, Qi Y (2011) An updated meta-analysis of endothelial nitric oxide synthase gene: three well-characterized polymorphisms with hypertension. PLoS One 6(9): e24266.
12. Monti LD, Barlassina C, Citterio L, Galluccio E, Berzuini C, et al. (2003) Endothelial nitric oxide synthase polymorphisms are associated with type 2 diabetes and the insulin resistance syndrome. Diabetes 52(5): 1270–1275.
13. Vecoli C, Andreassi MG, Liga R, Colombo M G, Coceani M, et al. (2012) T−786→C polymorphism of the endothelial nitric oxide synthase gene is associated with insulin resistance in patients with ischemic or non-ischemic cardiomyopathy. BMC Medical Genetics 13: 92.
14. Montagnani M, Chen H, Barr VA, Quon MJ (2001) Insulin-stimulated activation of eNOS is independent of Ca2+ but requires phosphorylation by Akt at Ser(1179). J Biological Chem 276(32): 30392–30398.
15. Kim J, Montagnani M, Kon KK, Quon MJ (2006) Reciprocal relationships between insulin resistance and endothelial dysfunction. Molecular and pathophysiological mechanisms. Circulation 113: 1888–18904.
16. Leuwerke SM, Kaza AK, Tribble CG, Kron IL, Laubach VE (2002). Inhibition of compensatory lung growth in endothelial nitric oxide synthase-deficient mice. Am J Physiol 282: L1272–L1278.
17. Herbert V, Lau KS, Gottlieb CW, Bleicher SJ (1965) Coated charcoal immunoassay of insulin. J Clin Endocrinol Metab 25: 1375–1384.
18. Vecoli C, Cao J, Neglia D, Inoue K, Sodhi K, et al. (2011) Apolipoprotein A-I mimetic peptide L-4F prevents myocardial and coronary dysfunction in diabetic mice. J Cell Biochem 112(9): 2616–2626.
19. Gödecke A, Decking UK, Ding Z, Hirchenhain J, Bidmon HJ, et al. (1998) Coronary hemodynamics in endothelial NO synthase knockout mice. Circ Res 82(2): 186–194.
20. Kubis N, Richer C, Domergue V, Giudicelli JF, Lévy BI (2002) Role of microvascular rarefaction in the increased arterial pressure in mice lacking for the endothelial nitric oxide synthase gene (eNOS3pt$^{-/-}$). J Hypertens 20(8): 1581–1587.
21. Kubis N, Besnard S, Silvestre JS, Feletou M, Huang PL, et al. (2002) Decreased arteriolar density in endothelial nitric oxide synthase knockout mice is due to hypertension, not to the constitutive defect in endothelial nitric oxide synthase enzyme. J Hypertens 20(2): 273–280.
22. L'Abbate A, Neglia D, Vecoli C, Novelli M, Ottaviano V, et al. (2007) Beneficial effect of heme oxygenase-1 expression on myocardial ischemia-reperfusion involves an increase in adiponectin in mildly diabetic rats. Am J Physiol Heart Circ Physio 293(6): H3532–3541.
23. Cao J, Vecoli C, Neglia D, Tavazzi B, Lazzarino G, et al. (2012) Cobalt-Protoporphyrin Improves Heart Function by Blunting Oxidative Stress and Restoring NO Synthase Equilibrium in an Animal Model of Experimental Diabetes. Front Physiol 3: 160.
24. Shankar RR, Wu Y, Shen HQ, Zhu JS, Baron AD (2000) Mice with gene disruption of both endothelial and neuronal nitric oxide synthase exhibit insulin resistance. Diabetes 49: 684–687.
25. Cook S, Hugli O, Egli M, Vollenweider P, Burcelin R, et al. (2003) Clustering of cardiovascular risk factors mimicking the human metabolic syndrome X in eNOS null mice. Swiss Med Wkly 133: 360–363.
26. Zeng G, Nystrom FH, Ravichandran LV, Cong LN, Kirby M, et al. (2000) Roles for insulin receptor, PI3-kinase, and Akt in insulin-signaling pathways related to production of nitric oxide in human vascular endothelial cells. Circulation 101(13): 1539–1545.
27. Cardillo C, Nambi SS, Kilcoyne CM, Choucair WK, Katz A, et al. (1999) Insulin stimulates both endothelin and nitric oxide activity in the human forearm. Circulation 100: 820–825.
28. Dimmeler S, Fleming I, Fisslthaler B, Hermann C, Busse R, et al. (1999) Activation of nitric oxide synthase in endothelial cells by Akt-dependent phosphorylation. Nature 399: 601–605.
29. Nathan C, Xie Q (1994) Nitric oxide synthases: Roles, tolls, and controls. Cell 78: 915–918.
30. Radomski MW, Moncada S (1993) Regulation of vascular hemostasis by nitric oxide. Thromb Haemost 70: 36–41.
31. Mashimo H1, Goyal RK (1999) Lessons from genetically engineered animal models. IV. Nitric oxide synthase gene knockout mice. Am J Physiol. 277(4 Pt 1): G745–750.
32. Huang PL (2000) Mouse models of nitric oxide synthase deficiency. J Am Soc Nephrol. Suppl 16: S120–S123.
33. Contreras C, Sánchez A, García-Sacristán A, Martínez MC, Andriantsitohaina R, et al. (2011) Preserved insulin vasorelaxation and up-regulation of the Akt/eNOS pathway in coronary arteries from insulin resistant obese Zucker rats. Atherosclerosis 217(2): 331–339.
34. Nagareddy PR, Xia Z, McNeill JH, MacLeod KM (2005) Increased expression of iNOS is associated with endothelial dysfunction and impaired pressor responsiveness in streptozotocin-induced diabetes. Am J Physiol Heart Circ Physiol. 289(5): H2144–H2152.
35. Modan M, Halkin H, Almog S, Lusky A, Eshkol A, et al. (1985) Hyperinsulinemia: a link between hypertension, obesity, and glucose intolerance. J Clin Invest. 75: 809–817.
36. Lucas CP, Estigarribia JA, Darga LL, Reaven GM (1985) Insulin and blood pressure in obesity. Hypertension 7: 702–706.
37. Kapur S, Bédard S, Marcotte B, Côté CH, Marette A (1997) Expression of nitric oxide synthase in skeletal muscle: a novel role for nitric oxide as a modulator of insulin action. Diabetes 46: 1691–1700.
38. Sartori C, Scherrer U (1999) Insulin, nitric oxide and the sympathetic nervous system: at the crossroads of metabolic and cardiovascular regulation. J Hypertens 17: 1517–1525.
39. Scherrer U, Sartori C (2000) Defective nitric oxide synthesis: a link between metabolic insulin resistance, sympathetic overactivity and cardiovascular morbidity. Eur J Endocrinol 142: 315–323.
40. Matsa LS, Rangaraju A, Vengaldas V, Latifi M, Jahromi HM, et al. (2013) Haplotypes of NOS3 gene polymorphisms in dilated cardiomyopathy. PLoS One 29; 8(7): e70523.
41. Miyamoto Y, Saito Y, Kajiyama N, Yoshimura M, Shimasaki Y, et al. (1998) Endothelial nitric oxide synthase gene is positively associated with essential hypertension. Hypertension 32: 3–8.
42. Hingorani AD, Liang CF, Fatibene J, Lyon A, Monteith S, et al. (1999) Stephens NG, O'Shaughnessy KM, Brown MJ: A common variant of the endothelial nitric oxide synthase (Glu298–Asp) is a major risk factor for coronary artery disease in the UK. Circulation 100: 1515–1520.
43. Shimasaki Y, Yasue H, Yoshimura M, Nakayama M, Kugiyama K, et al. (1998) Association of the missense Glu298Asp variant of the endothelial nitric oxide synthase gene with myocardial infarction. J Am Coll Cardiol 31: 1506–1510.
44. Cai H, Wilcken DE, Wang XL (1999) The Glu-298 >Asp (894G–>T) mutation at exon 7 of the endothelial nitric oxide synthase gene and coronary artery disease. J Mol Med 77: 511–514.
45. Wang XL, Sim AS, Badenhop RF, McCredie RM, Wilcken DE (1996) A smoking dependent risk of coronary artery disease associated with a polymorphism of the endothelial nitric oxide synthase gene. Nat Med 2: 41–45.
46. Shoji M, Tsutaya S, Saito R, Takamatu H, Yasujima M (2000) Positive association of endothelial nitric oxide synthase gene polymorphism with hypertension in northern Japan. Life Sci 66: 2557–2562.

Mitogen-Activated Protein Kinase-Activated Protein Kinase 2 Deficiency Reduces Insulin Sensitivity in High-Fat Diet-Fed Mice

Jan Freark de Boer[1], Arne Dikkers[1], Angelika Jurdzinski[1], Johann von Felden[2], Matthias Gaestel[3], Udo Bavendiek[2], Uwe J. F. Tietge[1]*

1 Department of Pediatrics, Center for Liver, Digestive and Metabolic Diseases, University of Groningen, University Medical Center Groningen, Groningen, The Netherlands, **2** Clinic of Cardiology and Angiology, Hannover Medical School, Hannover, Germany, **3** Institute of Biochemistry, Hannover Medical School, Hannover, Germany

Abstract

Adipose tissue inflammation is considered an important contributor to insulin resistance. Mitogen-activated protein kinase-activated protein kinase 2 (MK2) is a major downstream target of p38 MAPK and enhances inflammatory processes. In line with the role of MK2 as contributor to inflammation, $MK2^{-/-}$ mice are protected against inflammation in different disease models. Therefore, MK2 is considered an attractive therapeutic target for the treatment of chronic inflammatory diseases. This study tested the impact of MK2-deficiency on high-fat diet (HFD)-induced adipose tissue inflammation and insulin resistance. After feeding $MK2^{-/-}$ and WT control mice a HFD (60% energy from fat) for 24 weeks, body weight was not different between groups. Also, liver weight and the amount of abdominal fat remained unchanged. However, in $MK2^{-/-}$ mice plasma cholesterol levels were significantly increased. Surprisingly, macrophage infiltration in adipose tissue was not altered. However, adipose tissue macrophages were more skewed to the inflammatory M1 phenotype in $MK2^{-/-}$ mice. This differerence in macrophage polarization did however not translate in significantly altered expression levels of *Mcp-1*, *Tnfα* and *Il6*. Glucose and insulin tolerance tests demonstrated that $MK2^{-/-}$ mice had a significantly reduced glucose tolerance and increased insulin resistance. Noteworthy, the expression of the insulin-responsive glucose transporter type 4 (GLUT4) in adipose tissue of $MK2^{-/-}$ mice was reduced by 55% ($p<0.05$) and 33% ($p<0.05$) on the mRNA and protein level, respectively, compared to WT mice. *In conclusion*, HFD-fed $MK2^{-/-}$ display decreased glucose tolerance and increased insulin resistance compared to WT controls. Decreased adipose tissue expression of GLUT4 might contribute to this phenotype. The data obtained in this study indicate that clinical use of MK2 inhibitors has to be evaluated with caution, taking potential metabolic adverse effects into account.

Editor: Makoto Kanzaki, Tohoku University, Japan

Funding: This study was funded by the Groningen Expert Center for Kids with Obesity (GECKO, to U.J.F.T.), by a grant from the Netherlands Organization for Scientific Research (VIDI Grant 917-56-358, to UJFT) and the Deutsche Forschungsgemeinschaft (SFB 566 B12 to M.G.). The funders had no role in study design, data collection and analysis, decision to publish, or preparation of the manuscript.

Competing Interests: The authors have declared that no competing interests exist.

* Email: u_tietge@yahoo.com

Introduction

As a result of the present obesity epidemic, prevalence of insulin resistance and type 2 diabetes mellitus is increasing rapidly in developed countries [1]. Inflammation most likely contributes to the development of insulin resistance. Altough inflammation might not impact on insulin sensitivity in the onset phase of obesity [2], inflammation within adipose tissue has been shown to have deleterious effects on systemic insulin sensitivity in models of chronic obesity [3–5]. Although many diffent types of immune cells are present in inflamed adipose tissue, macrophages are the major cell type associated with adipose tissue inflammation [4]. Interestingly, not only the amount of macrophages present in the adipose tissue increases with obesity, their phenotype also shifts. While anti-inflammatory M2 macrophages predominate in lean adipose tissue, the balance shifts towards more inflammatory M1 macrophages with increasing obesity [6]. Moreover, M1 macrophages are reported to negatively impact on insulin sensitivity compared to macrophages of the M2 phenotype [7]. Amelioration of adipose tissue inflammation might conceivably improve insulin sensitivity and thereby lead to a reduction of morbidity and mortality associated with type 2 diabetes.

A potential candidate pathway suitable for therapeutic intervention is the p38 mitogen-activated protein kinase (p38 MAPK, p38) pathway. Inhibition of p38 itself has potent anti-inflammatory effects. However, the wide range of biological effects of this signaling mediator hampers the clinical use of p38 inhibitors. Since p38 has numerous down-stream targets, inhibition of one of these targets might reduce adipose tissue inflammation without inducing substantial adverse effects. Mitogen-activated protein kinase-activated protein kinase 2 (Mapkapk2 or MK2) is a direct target of p38, enhances inflammatory processes and is essential for sustained activation of NF-κB, a central transcription factor in inflammation that has been shown to be involved in the development of insulin resistance [8,9]. Furthermore, MK2 increases the mRNA stability of key proinflammatory cytokines, including TNFα, by phosphorylating tristetraprolin (TTP) which normally binds to the 3′-UTR of certain mRNA molecules and directs their deadenylation. However, upon phosphorylation by MK2, TTP is unable to recruit the deadenylation machinery, resulting in decreased mRNA degradation [10], and is replaced in RNA binding by the mRNA-stabilizing and -translation-stimulating factor HuR [11].

MK2 deficiency has been shown to result in a potent reduction of inflammation in several disease models and, so far, no severe side effects have been reported. It has for instance been shown that $MK2^{-/-}$ mice are resistant to endotoxic shock because of reduced production of TNFα after injection of lipopolysaccharide/D-galactosamine [12]. Furthermore, it has been demonstrated that $MK2^{-/-}$ mice have a reduced susceptibility for the development of collagen-induced rheumatoid arthritis (RA) [12] and that $MK2^{-/-}$ mice on a $Ldlr^{-/-}$ background are protected against the development of atherosclerosis despite a pro-atherogenic lipoprotein profile [13]. The atheroprotective effect of MK2-deficiency observed in this study could be explained in part by a reduced expression of adhesion molecules and monocyte chemoattractant protein-1 (Mcp-1), factors that also play key roles in adipose tissue inflammation.

Therefore, the present study explored the effects of MK2-deficiency on the development of adipose tissue inflammation and insulin resistance in high-fat diet (HFD-) fed mice. In contrast to our hypothesis, no effect was observed in the amount of macrophages that had infiltrated the adipose tissue. The balance between M1 and M2 macrophages appeared, however, to be more skewed towards the M1 phenotype in $MK2^{-/-}$ mice. HFD-fed $MK2^{-/-}$ mice were more insulin resistant compared to wild-type (WT) controls. Decreased expression of the glucose transporter GLUT4 in adipose tissue might contribute to the glucose intolerant, insulin resistant, phenotype observed in HFD-fed $MK2^{-/-}$ mice.

Materials and Methods

Animals

Male $MK2^{-/-}$ mice [12] were obtained from the breeding colony of Hannover Medical School and were backcrossed to the C57BL/6J genetic background for >10 generations using mice from Charles River (Sulzfeld, Germany). For the reported experiments littermate controls were used. All mice were exposed to a 12 hour light-dark cycle, were housed under climate-controlled conditions and had free access to food and water. Mice were fed a hypercaloric high-fat diet (HFD) containing 60% (energy) fat (AB-diets, Woerden, The Netherlands) for 24 weeks. After this period, experiments were carried out as indicated below. All animal experiments were performed according to the national law on animal welfare, and experimental procedures were approved by the responsible local ethics committee of the University of Groningen (Permit Number: 5997).

Plasma lipid and lipoprotein analysis

Blood samples were obtained at the end of the study by cardiac puncture after 4 h of fasting using heparinized syringes, and were immediately placed on ice. Blood was centrifuged at 8000 rpm for 10 min at 4°C and plasma was stored at −80°C until further analysis. Plasma triglycerides, free fatty acids, glycerol, and cholesterol were determined using commercially available kits (Roche Diagnostics, Mannheim, Germany and Diagnostic Systems, Holzheim, Germany). Plasma insulin levels were measured with an ultrasensitive mouse insulin ELISA kit (Alpco, Salem, NH, USA). Pooled plasma samples were subjected to fast protein liquid chromatography (FPLC) gel filtration using a superose 6 column (GE Healthcare, Uppsala, Sweden) as described [14]. Individual fractions were assayed for cholesterol and triglyceride concentrations as detailed above.

Analysis of gene expression

Gene expression was analyzed by real-time qPCR. Briefly, RNA was extracted from tissue samples with Tri-reagent (Sigma, St. Louis, MO, USA) and quantified with a NanoDrop ND-100 UV-Vis spectrophotometer (NanoDrop Technologies, Wilmington, DE, USA). One μg of RNA was reverse transcribed using M-MLV reverse transcriptase (Sigma) according to the manufacturer's instructions. Real-time qPCR analysis was performed on a 7900 HT Fast Real-Time PCR system (Applied Biosystems, Darmstadt, Germany) using multi-exon spanning primer/probe sets synthesized by Eurogentec (Seraing, Belgium). Gene expression levels were normalized to cyclophilin and further normalized to the mean expression level of the control group. Gene expression levels of the macrophage polarization markers *Mgl-1* and *Mgl-2* were normalized to *Cd68* to correct for the amount of macrophages present in the adipose tissue.

Glucose and insulin tolerance tests

Mice were fasted for 4 hours in the morning before the start of the glucose or insulin tolerance test. For the glucose tolerance test, mice were intraperitoneally (i.p.) injected with 1.25 g/kg glucose. Blood glucose levels were assessed by tail bleeding before injection and at 15, 30, 60 and 120 minutes after injection using a Onetouch Ultra glucose meter (LifeScan Benelux, Beerse, Belgium). The procedure for the insulin tolerance test was the same as described for the glucose tolerance test except that mice were injected with 0.6 U/kg insulin (i.p.) instead of glucose and blood glucose levels were measured at 15, 30, 45, 60 and 90 minutes after injection.

Western blot

Adipose tissue samples were homogenized and sodium dodecyl sulfate (SDS) was added to a final concentration of 2%. Next, 25 μg protein of each sample was loaded onto a polyacrylamide gel for electrophoresis. Subsequently, semi-dry blotting was applied to transfer the proteins to a 0.45 μm nitrocellulose membrane (Schleicher & Schuell). Blocking of the membrane was performed overnight using 5% BSA in PBS after which the blot was incubated with an anti-GLUT4 antibody (Ab654, Abcam, Cambridge, UK) at a 1:1500 dilution in PBS supplemented with 2% BSA and 0.1% Tween-20 for 2 h. A horseradish peroxidase-conjugated secondary goat anti-rabbit antibody (DAKO, Glostrup, Denmark) was then added at a 1:2000 dilution for 45 min. Bands were visualized using chemiluminescence (GE Healthcare, Chalfont St Giles, UK). Band intensity was quantified using the freely available ImageJ software (http://rsbweb.nih.gov/ij/).

Statistics

Statistical analyses were performed using the Statistical Package for Social Sciences (SPSS, SPSS Inc., Chicago, IL). Data are presented as means ± SEM. Differences between groups were compared using the Mann-Whitney U-test. For comparison between more than two groups, significance of differences was assessed using the Kruskal-Wallis test and Conover *post-hoc* analysis. P values <0.05 were considered statistically significant.

Results

MK2-deficiency does not affect body weight, but causes dyslipidemia in HFD-fed mice

After feeding a HFD for 24 weeks, *MK2*$^{-/-}$ mice and WT controls were sacrificed and blood and tissues were collected for analysis. Body weight of the mice did not differ between the groups and also liver weight was not different (Table 1). Furthermore, there was no effect of MK2 deficiency on the abdominal fat content of the mice (Table 1). However, plasma cholesterol levels were about 25% higher in *MK2*$^{-/-}$ mice compared to WT controls (Table 1). Plasma triglyceride levels tended to be increased as well in *MK2*$^{-/-}$ mice albeit this difference did not reach statistical significance (Table 1). Plasma free fatty acid levels were slightly decreased in *MK2*$^{-/-}$ mice (Table 1), whereas plasma glycerol levels remained unchanged (0.18±0.03 vs. 0.16±0.02 mmol/l). To identify which lipoproteins were responsible for the elevation of plasma lipids, lipoprotein subclasses were fractionated using Fast Protein Liquid Chromatography (FPLC). The cholesterol profile revealed that *MK2*$^{-/-}$ mice had a somewhat higher HDL peak. Furthermore, a shoulder was observed in the profile of *MK2*$^{-/-}$ mice, likely representing LDL particles (Fig. S1A). The triglyceride profile confirmed an increased amount of LDL particles and showed an increase in VLDL in the *MK2*$^{-/-}$ mice (Fig. S1B).

Impact of MK2-deficiency on adipose tissue inflammation

Adipose tissue samples from 24 weeks HFD-fed mice were analyzed to assess the degree of inflammation. Compared to chow-fed animals, expression levels of macrophage markes (*Cd68* and *F4/80*) in adipose tissue were increased in both genotype (table S1), however there was no significant increase in the expression of macrophage markers between genotypes (Fig. 1A), indicating that the amount of adipose tissue macrophages was similar in both groups. Interestingly, the subpopulation of Cd11c-positive macrophages, which has been linked to insulin resistance, appeared to be increased in the adipose tissue of HFD-fed *MK2*$^{-/-}$ mice (Fig. 1A). Higher expression of *Cd3e* in the *MK2*$^{-/-}$ mice (Fig. 1A) suggests an increased presence of T cells in the adipose tissue of those mice. The polarization of adipose tissue macrophages appears to be altered in *MK2*$^{-/-}$ mice. HFD-feeding induced a shift in macrophage polarization towards the M1 phenotype as suggested by the decreased expression of the macrophage-specific M2-markers *Mgl-1* and *Mgl-2* (table S1). Specifically in the HFD-fed MK2$^{-/-}$ mice, the expression of those markers was decreased compared to HFD-fed WT mice, suggestive of an altered macrophages polarization state in the adipose tissue of those mice. An increased M1/M2 macrophage balance is reported to result in more inflammation and to negatively impact insulin sensitivity [7]. The apparent increase in the M1/M2 balance did however not result in significantly altered expression levels of pro- as well as anti-inflammatory cytokines (Fig. 1A and table S1). Adipose tissue histology showed identical amounts of characteristic crown-like stuctures in the adipose tissue of the respective mouse models (Fig. 1B). In addition, no major differences in size distribution of adipocytes was observed (Fig. 1C). Analysis of liver histology did not reveal any difference in the degree of steatosis (Fig. S2). In addition, hepatic gene expression analysis did not show major differences in hepatic inflammation, although the amount of T cells might be somewhat higher in MK2$^{-/-}$ mice compared to WT as indicated by the increased expression of the T cell marker *Cd3e*.

MK2 deficiency results in impaired glucose tolerance and insulin resistance

Chow-fed MK2$^{-/-}$ mice displayed a moderately decreased glucose tolerance compared to WT controls but with identical fasting glucose levels (Fig. S3A). In the HFD-fed mice, fasting blood glucose levels were higher in MK2-deficient mice compared to WT (14.0±1.0 vs. 11.5±0.4 mmol/l, $p<0.05$, Fig. 2A). *MK2*$^{-/-}$ mice and WT controls were then injected i.p. with a glucose bolus (1.25 g/kg) to assess glucose tolerance. As indicated by the higher glucose levels during the glucose tolerance test, HFD-fed *MK2*$^{-/-}$ mice have an impaired glucose tolerance compared to WT controls (Fig. 2A), with significant differences at time points 15 and 30 minutes (both $p<0.05$). The difference in glucose tolerance remained significant when corrected for baseline glucose levels (Fig. S3B). Several days later, the mice were subjected to an insulin tolerance test to explore whether the impaired glucose tolerance in *MK2*$^{-/-}$ mice could be ascribed to insulin resistance. Higher blood glucose levels during the insulin tolerance test indicated that *MK2*$^{-/-}$ mice were indeed insulin resistant (Fig. 2B). Differences reached significance at time points 15, 30, 45 and 90 minutes (all $p<0.05$) and also the area under the curve (ΔAUC) was 38% reduced ($p<0.01$, Fig. 2B insert). Increased fasting plasma insulin levels in *MK2*$^{-/-}$ mice (+55%, $p<0.05$, Fig. 2C) further indicated that those mice were more insulin resistant compared to WT controls. Taken together, these data show that HFD-fed *MK2*$^{-/-}$ mice have a glucose intolerant, insulin resistant phenotype.

Table 1. Basal characteristics of HFD-fed WT and MK2$^{-/-}$ mice.

	WT	MK2$^{-/-}$
Body weight (g)	46.1±1.2	45.4±1.0
Liver weight (g)	2.8±0.3	2.4±0.2
Abdominal fat content (g)	4.9±0.2	4.7±0.1
Total plasma cholesterol (mM)	3.65±0.20	4.52±0.18**
Plasma triglycerides (mM)	0.46±0.03	0.68±0.08
Plasma free fatty acids (mM)	0.42±0.03	0.35±0.01*

*$p<0.05$,
**$p<0.01$ vs. WT controls.
Data are presented as means ± SEM (n = 8 animals per group).

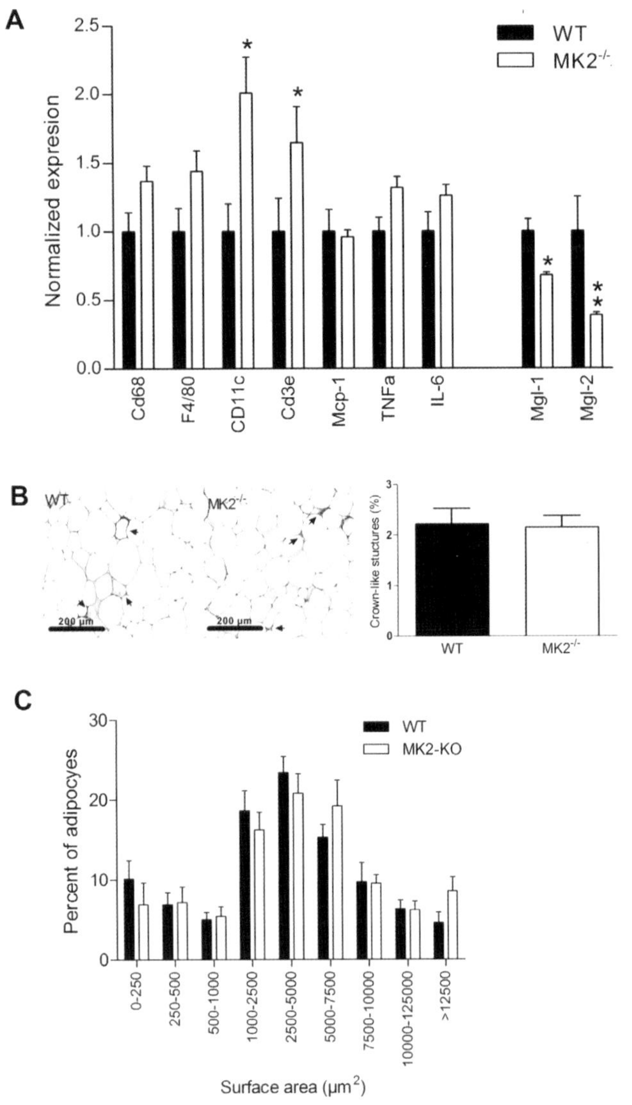

Figure 1. Impact of MK2-deficiency on adipose tissue inflammation. Abdominal fat was excised from mice that were fed a high-fat diet (HFD) for 24 weeks (n = 8 mice per group). Real-time qPCR was performed to measure mRNA expression of inflammation-related genes in adipose tissue (A). Formalin-fixed paraffin-embedded tissue sections were stained with hematoxyline and eosine to assess infiltration of immune cells in adipose tissue and sections from 5 randomly selected animals of each group were used to quantify the amount of crown-like structures. At least 300 adipocytes were counted per animal (B). Adipocyte size distribution was assessed by measuring the surface of ~100 adipocytes per animal using freely available ImageJ software (imagej.nih.gov) and sections from 5 randomly selected animals of each group were used for quantification of adipocyte size (C).

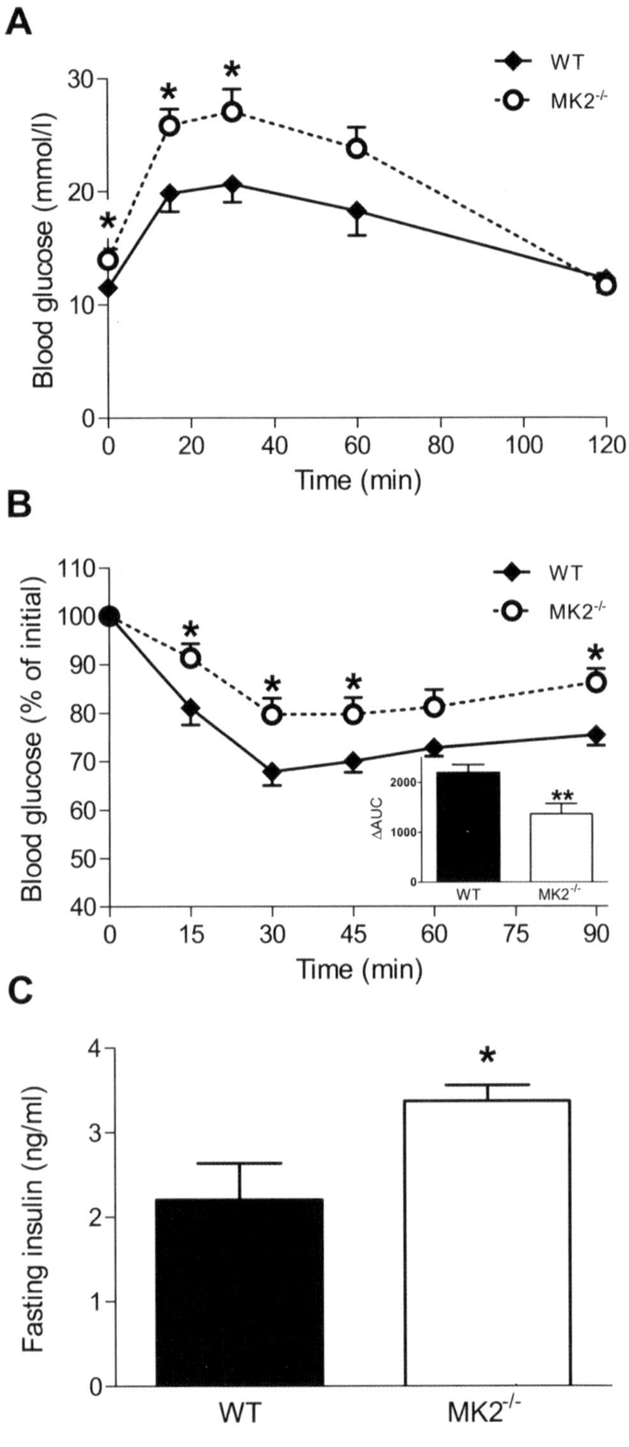

Figure 2. High-fat diet-fed *MK2*$^{-/-}$ mice are insulin resistant. High-fat diet (HFD) fed wild-type (WT) and *MK2*$^{-/-}$ mice were injected intraperitoneally (i.p.) with glucose (1.25 g/kg) and blood glucose levels were measured at the indicated time points (A). Several days later, mice were injected i.p. with insulin (0.6 U/kg) and blood glucose levels were determined at the indicated time points. Blood glucose levels during the insulin tolerance test (ITT) are depicted as percentage of initial blood glucose levels (B). ΔArea under the curve was calculated by subtracting the area under the curve of an individual mouse by the area under a hypothetical curve that remained at 100% throughout the duration of the test (B, insert). Fasting insulin levels were determined using an ultra-sensitive mouse insulin ELISA (C). *$p<0.05$, **$p<0.01$ compared to WT mice (n = 8 mice per group).

GLUT4 expression is reduced in adipose tissue of HFD-fed MK2$^{-/-}$ mice

To explore the underlying basis for the decreased glucose tolerance and increased insulin resistance in the *MK2*$^{-/-}$ mice, expression of the insulin-responsive glucose transporter GLUT4 was determined in the tissues that account for the major part of glucose disposal within the body, namely muscle and adipose tissue. Whereas no difference was found for expression of *Glut4* in muscle (data not shown), *Glut4* mRNA expression was 55% ($p< 0.05$) lower in adipose tissue of *MK2*$^{-/-}$ mice (Fig. 3A). Also,

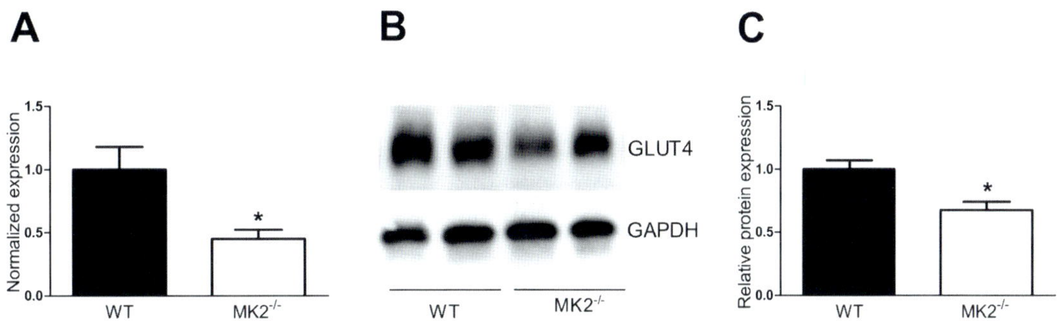

Figure 3. High-fat diet-fed *MK2*$^{-/-}$ mice have reduced adipose tissue expression of the insulin-responsive glucose transporter GLUT4. Adipose tissue *Glut4* mRNA expression (n = 8 mice per group) was measured by real-time qPCR (A). Western blot was performed (n = 5 mice per group) to determine GLUT4 protein expression in adipose tissue; GAPDH served as loading control (B); band intensities were quantified using ImageJ software and normalized to the mean intensity of the wild-type (WT) control mice (C). *p<0.05 compared to WT control mice.

GLUT4 protein expression was reduced in the adipose tissue of *MK2*$^{-/-}$ mice compared to WT controls (−33%, P<0.05, Fig. 3B and C). Decreased expression of GLUT4 in adipose tissue might therefore represent a contributing factor to the glucose intolerant, insulin resistant phenotype of HFD-fed *MK2*$^{-/-}$ mice.

Discussion

This study demonstrates that HFD-fed *MK2*$^{-/-}$ mice are more glucose intolerant and insulin resistant compared to the respective WT controls. Although these results were unexpected considering the important role of MK2 in various animal models of inflammatory disease, *MK2*$^{-/-}$ mice were found to have decreased adipose tissue expression of the insulin-responsive glucose transporter GLUT4, which might contribute to the observed glucose intolerant, insulin resistant, phenotype in these mice.

Since the observation that TNFα production is increased in adipose tissue of obese individuals [15], the contribution of adipose tissue inflammation to systemic insulin resistance gained substantial interest. Subsequently, macrophages have been identified as major effector cells of adipose tissue inflammation. Obesity is associated with an increased infiltration of macrophages into adipose tissue [4,5,16,17] and an inverse correlation between the number of macrophages present in the adipose tissue and insulin sensitivity was shown [18–20]. Intracellular signal transduction plays a decisive role in inflammatory responses and MAPKs are central in many of these signal transduction pathways. p38 belongs to the MAPK superfamily and has important functions in apoptosis as well as transcriptional regulation, but is also a key mediator of inflammatory signaling [21]. p38 can be activated by inflammatory cytokines but, interestingly, also by free fatty acids and high concentrations of glucose [22], factors that are usually elevated in patients with type 2 diabetes. As p38 has many downstream targets, its activity affects a wide range of biological processes, which is exemplified by the fact that *p38α*$^{-/-}$ mice die in utero [23]. Furthermore, hepatotoxicity has been demonstrated for many p38-inhibitors [24], hampering the clinical use of such compounds. Inhibiting more downstream mediators in the p38 signaling cascade is likely to increase the specificity of the effects and is therefore considered a more attractive therapeutic option [25]. MK2 is a direct target of p38 and is essential for sustained NF-κB activation [26]. Of note, in contrast to *p38α*$^{-/-}$ mice, *MK2*$^{-/-}$ mice are viable and do not display any obvious health problems [12]. *MK2*$^{-/-}$ mice are resistant to LPS-induced endotoxic shock [12] and studies using these mice have indicated that MK2 inhibition might be a good treatment option for a variety of chronic inflammatory diseases [13,26,27]. Using a mouse model of collagen-induced RA, it was shown that *MK2*$^{-/-}$ mice were protected against disease development [27]. In another study, we previously demonstrated that *MK2*$^{-/-}$ mice on the *Ldlr*$^{-/-}$ background were protected against atherosclerosis when fed an atherogenic diet [13]. Decreased foam cell formation but also a reduction of macrophage recruitment were identified as mechanisms accountable for the anti-atherogenic phenotype [13]. Since diet-induced obesity as well as insulin resistance coincide with chronic inflammation, and macrophage recruitment to adipose tissue is a critical step in the development of insulin resistance [28,29], we tested whether MK2-deficiency would ameliorate diet-induced adipose tissue inflammation and would thereby improve insulin sensitivity. Surprisingly, adipose tissue expression of inflammatory cytokines was not markedly different between HFD-fed *MK2*$^{-/-}$ and WT mice. Also, the amount of adipose tissue macrophages remained unchanged. However, the subpopulation of Cd11c macrophages, reported to be recruited to adipose tissue in obesity and to have deleterious effects on insulin sensitivity [30], appeared to be increased in the adipose tissue of MK2$^{-/-}$. In adition, the M1/M2 balance seems to be more skewed towards the M1 phenotype in those mice. Expression levels of the polarization markers were normalized to *Cd68* rather than cyclophilin to correct for the number of macrophages present in the adipose tissue. This is justifiable because expression of *Mgl-1* and *Mgl-2* is barely detectable in adipocytes (data not shown). The altered characteristics of adipose tissue macrophages could contribute to the glucose intolerant, insulin resistant phenotype in MK2$^{-/-}$ mice. However, the analysis of macrophage polarization was limited to mRNA expression in the current study. As bone marrow-derived MK2$^{-/-}$ macrophages did not show differences in macrophage polarization (unpublished observations), the results of this study indicate that the specific environment of adipose tissue impacts on macrophage skewing. Additional information could be obtained by studying the characteristics of macrophages isolated from adipose tissue. In addition, adipose tissue contains a wide variety of immune cells that were not quantified in this study. Detailed analysis of all immune cells present in the adipose tissue, e.g. using flow cytometry, could further increase our knowledge regarding the impact of MK2-deficiency on adipose tissue inflammation.

Interestingly, glucose tolerance tests revealed that HFD-fed *MK2*$^{-/-}$ mice had impaired glucose tolerance compared to WT controls. In addition, the response during the insulin tolerance test indicated that HFD-fed *MK2*$^{-/-}$ mice were significantly more insulin resistant. Fasting hyperglycemia and more than 50% elevated plasma fasting insulin levels further substantiated the conclusion that these mice were insulin resistant. This unexpected phenotype suggests that MK2 not only plays a role in inflammation, but also is a mediator of metabolism. We identified decreased expression of the insulin-responsive glucose transporter GLUT4 in adipose tissue as a mechanism likely contributing to the glucose intolerant, insulin resistant phenotype. With respect to human pathophysiology, GLUT4 expression was found to be decreased in adipose tissue, but importantly not in muscle, of obese individuals and in insulin resistant and type 2 diabetic patients [31,32]. In addition, the pivotal role of adipose tissue GLUT4 in maintaining insulin sensitivity is emphasized by the fact that adipose tissue-specific *Glut4*$^{-/-}$ mice develop insulin resistance [33] whereas mice overexpressing GLUT4 specifically in the adipose tissue have enhanced glucose tolerance and reduced fed insulin levels, indicative of improved insulin sensitivity [34]. Furthermore, overexpression of GLUT4 in adipose tissue of mice that lack GLUT4 expression in muscle corrected the insulin resistant phenotype in those mice [35]. Combined these studies identify adipose tissue GLUT4 expression as a central mediator of whole body glucose tolerance. Accordingly, decreased adipose tissue expression of GLUT4 in *MK2*$^{-/-}$ mice conceivably offers an explanation for the glucose intolerant, insulin resistant phenotype observed in our present study. However, as decreased expression of GLUT4 in adipose tissue likely leads to insulin resistance in other organs, insulin signaling and uptake of 2-deoxyglucose in multiple tissues, including muscle and liver, could be assessed in future studies. Furthermore, it remains to be explored how MK2-deficiency leads to decreased adipose tissue GLUT4 expression. In that respect, it is important to point out that only total body MK2-deficient mice were used in the current study. More mechanistic insights might be gained from tissue-specific knock-out mice and/or bone marrow transplantation studies.

The fact that plasma cholesterol levels were increased in *MK2*$^{-/-}$ mice further indicates that, in addition to its role in inflammation, MK2 also impacts metabolism. The more dyslipidemic phenotype observed in the HFD-fed *MK2*$^{-/-}$ mice in our study is in accordance with our previous data obtained in Western diet-fed *MK2*$^{-/-}$ *Ldlr*$^{-/-}$ mice that had increased plasma levels of apoB-containing lipoproteins [13]. The mechanistic basis underlying the decreased circulating free fatty acids in the HFD-fed *MK2*$^{-/-}$ mice remains to be elucidated. As the phenotype of adipose tissue macrophages seems to be different in MK2$^{-/-}$ mice, it is tempting to speculate that they might have an altered capacity to buffer excess circulating lipids. This property of adipose tissue macrophages was recently described [36]. Moreover, it has been demonstrated that p38, the MAPK that activates MK2, has ample effects on glucose and lipid metabolism [22,37]. Part of these effects might be mediated via MK2, however, the effects of MK2 on metabolic pathways have thus far barely been explored and warrant more detailed investigation.

In conclusion, HFD-fed *MK2*$^{-/-}$ mice have increased plasma triglyceride and cholesterol levels and display a glucose intolerant, insulin resistant phenotype. Decreased adipose tissue expression of GLUT4 and an altered macrophage polarization balance in adipose tissue might contribute to this unfavorable metabolic profile. These data indicate that the clinical use of MK2 inhibitors for the treatment of chronic inflammatory diseases has to be evaluated with caution, taking potential metabolic adverse effects into account.

Supporting Information

Figure S1 High-fat diet-fed MK2$^{-/-}$ mice have increased apoB-containing lipoproteins. Blood was collected at time of sacrifice after 4 hours of fasting and pooled plasma fractions (n = 8 mice per group) were subjected to fast protein liquid chromatography (FPLC) gel filtration using a Superose 6 column as detailed in materials and methods. Subsequently, individual fractions were assayed for cholesterol (A) and triglyceride (B) content. The black line represents the wild-type (WT) mice and the dashed line the MK2$^{-/-}$ mice.

Figure S2 Liver histology of high-fat diet-fed MK2-KO mice and controls shows no obvious difference in steatosis. Formalin-fixed paraffin-embedded sections were stained with hematoxylin and eosin and images were aquired using the Aperio scanning system. Four representative images are shown out of n = 8 mice per group.

Figure S3 Tendency towards decreased glucose tolerance in chow-fed MK2$^{-/-}$ mice. Chow-fed wild-type (WT) and MK2$^{-/-}$ mice were injected intraperitoneally (i.p.) with glucose (1.25 g/kg) and blood glucose levels were measured at the indicated time points (A). Baseline-substracted calculation of the area under the curve (AUC) of the glucose levels during the glucose tolerance test (B). *$p<0.05$ vs WT control.

Table S1 Expression of inflammation-related genes in chow- and high-fat diet-fed MK2-KO mice and controls.

Table S2 Hepatic expression of inflammation-related genes in High-fat diet-fed MK2-KO mice and controls.

Author Contributions

Conceived and designed the experiments: JFDB UJFT UB. Performed the experiments: JFDB AD AJ JVF. Analyzed the data: JFDB UJFT. Contributed reagents/materials/analysis tools: MG UB. Contributed to the writing of the manuscript: JFDB UJFT.

References

1. Centers for Disease Control and Prevention National Diabetes Surveillance System.
2. Lee YS, Li P, Huh JY, Hwang IJ, Lu M, et al. (2011) Diabetes 60: 2474–2483.
3. Bouloumie A, Curat CA, Sengenes C, Lolmede K, Miranville A, et al. (2005) Role of macrophage tissue infiltration in metabolic diseases. Curr Opin Clin Nutr Metab Care 8: 347–354.
4. Neels JG, Olefsky JM (2006) Inflamed fat: what starts the fire? J Clin Invest 116: 33–35.
5. Shoelson SE, Lee J, Goldfine AB (2006) Inflammation and insulin resistance. J Clin Invest 116: 1793–1801.
6. Lumeng CN, Bodzin JL, Saltiel AR (2007) Obesity induces a phenotypic switch in adipose tissue macrophage polarization. J.Clin.Invest 117: 175–184.
7. Kang K, Reilly SM, Karabacak V, Gangl MR, Fitzgerald K, et al (2008) Adipocyte-derived Th2 cytokines and myeloid PPARdelta regulate macrophage polarization and insulin sensitivity. Cell Metab 7: 485–495.
8. Cai D, Yuan M, Frantz DF, Melendez PA, Hansen L, et al. (2005) Local and systemic insulin resistance resulting from hepatic activation of IKK-beta and NF-kappaB. Nat Med 11: 183–190.
9. Goldfine AB, Silver R, Aldhahi W, Cai D, Tatro E, et al. (2008) Use of Salsalate to Target Inflammation in the Treatment of Insulin Resistance and Type 2 Diabetes. Clin Transl Sci 1: 36–43.
10. Clement SL, Scheckel C, Stoecklin G, Lykke-Andersen J (2011) Phosphorylation of tristetraprolin by MK2 impairs AU-rich element mRNA decay by preventing deadenylase recruitment. Mol Cell Biol 31: 256–266.

11. Tiedje C, Ronkina N, Tehrani M, Dhamija S, Laass K, et al. (2012) The p38/MK2-driven exchange between tristetraprolin and HuR regulates AU-rich element-dependent translation. PLoS Genet 8: e1002977.
12. Kotlyarov A, Neininger A, Schubert C, Eckert R, Birchmeier C, et al. (1999) MAPKAP kinase 2 is essential for LPS-induced TNF-alpha biosynthesis. Nat Cell Biol 1: 94–97.
13. Jagavelu K, Tietge UJ, Gaestel M, Drexler H, Schieffer B, et al. (2007) Systemic deficiency of the MAP kinase-activated protein kinase 2 reduces atherosclerosis in hypercholesterolemic mice. Circ Res 101: 1104–1112.
14. Nijstad N, Wiersma H, Gautier T, van der Giet M, Maugeais C, et al. (2009) Scavenger receptor BI-mediated selective uptake is required for the remodeling of high density lipoprotein by endothelial lipase. J Biol Chem 284: 6093–6100.
15. Hotamisligil GS, Arner P, Caro JF, Atkinson RL, Spiegelman BM (1995) Increased adipose tissue expression of tumor necrosis factor-alpha in human obesity and insulin resistance. J Clin Invest 95: 2409–2415.
16. Anderson EK, Gutierrez DA, Hasty AH (2010) Adipose tissue recruitment of leukocytes. Curr Opin Lipidol 21: 172–177.
17. Weisberg SP, McCann D, Desai M, Rosenbaum M, Leibel RL, et al. (2003) Obesity is associated with macrophage accumulation in adipose tissue. J Clin Invest 112: 1796–1808.
18. Apovian CM, Bigornia S, Mott M, Meyers MR, Ulloor J, et al. (2008) Adipose macrophage infiltration is associated with insulin resistance and vascular endothelial dysfunction in obese subjects. Arterioscler THromb Vasc Biol 28: 1654–1659.
19. Kloting N, Fasshauer M, Dietrich A, Kovacs P, Schon MR, et al. (2010) Insulin-sensitive obesity. Am J Physiol Endocrinol Metab 299: E506–E515.
20. Xu H, Barnes GT, Yang Q, Tan G, Yang D, et al. (2003) Chronic inflammation in fat plays a crucial role in the development of obesity-related insulin resistance. J Clin Invest 112: 1821–1830.
21. Sabio G, Davis RJ (2014) TNF and MAP kinase signalling pathways. Semin Immunol 26: 237–245.
22. Liu Z, Cao W (2009) p38 mitogen-activated protein kinase: a critical node linking insulin resistance and cardiovascular diseases in type 2 diabetes mellitus. Endocr Metab Immune Disord Drug Targets 9: 38–46.
23. Allen M, Svensson L, Roach M, Hambor J, McNeish J, et al. (2000) Deficiency of the stress kinase p38alpha results in embryonic lethality: characterization of the kinase dependence of stress responses of enzyme-deficient embryonic stem cells. J Exp Med 191: 859–870.
24. Hammaker D, Firestein GS (2010) "Go upstream, young man": lessons learned from the p38 saga. Ann Rheum Dis 69 Suppl 1: i77–i82.
25. Gaestel M, Mengel A, Bothe U, Asadullah K (2007) Protein kinases as small molecule inhibitor targets in inflammation. Curr Med Chem 14: 2214–2234.
26. Gorska MM, Liang Q, Stafford SJ, Goplen N, Dharajiya N, et al. (2007) MK2 controls the level of negative feedback in the NF-kappaB pathway and is essential for vascular permeability and airway inflammation. J Exp Med 204: 1637–1652.
27. Hegen M, Gaestel M, Nickerson-Nutter CL, Lin LL, Telliez JB (2006) MAPKAP kinase 2-deficient mice are resistant to collagen-induced arthritis. J Immunol 177: 1913–1917.
28. Kamei N, Tobe K, Suzuki R, Ohsugi M, Watanabe T, et al. (2006) Overexpression of monocyte chemoattractant protein-1 in adipose tissues causes macrophage recruitment and insulin resistance. J Biol Chem 281: 26602–26614.
29. Kanda H, Tateya S, Tamori Y, Kotani K, Hiasa K, et al. (2006) MCP-1 contributes to macrophage infiltration into adipose tissue, insulin resistance, and hepatic steatosis in obesity. J Clin Invest 116: 1494–1505.
30. Patsouris D, Li PP, Thapar D, Chapman J, Olefsky JM, et al. (2008) Ablation of CD11c-positive cells normalizes insulin sensitivity in obese insulin resistant animals. Cell Metab 8: 301–309.
31. Carvalho E, Jansson PA, Nagaev I, Wenthzel AM, Smith U (2001) Insulin resistance with low cellular IRS-1 expression is also associated with low GLUT4 expression and impaired insulin-stimulated glucose transport. FASEB J 15: 1101–1103.
32. Shepherd PR, Kahn BB (1999) Glucose transporters and insulin action–implications for insulin resistance and diabetes mellitus. N Engl J Med 341: 248–257.
33. Abel ED, Peroni O, Kim JK, Kim YB, Boss O, et al. (2001) Adipose-selective targeting of the GLUT4 gene impairs insulin action in muscle and liver. Nature 409: 729–733.
34. Shepherd PR, Gnudi L, Tozzo E, Yang H, Leach F, et al. (1993) Adipose cell hyperplasia and enhanced glucose disposal in transgenic mice overexpressing GLUT4 selectively in adipose tissue. J Biol Chem 268: 22243–22246.
35. Carvalho E, Kotani K, Peroni OD, Kahn BB (2005) Adipose-specific overexpression of GLUT4 reverses insulin resistance and diabetes in mice lacking GLUT4 selectively in muscle. Am J Physiol Endocrinol Metab 289: E551–E561.
36. Kosteli A, Sugaru E, Haemmerle G, Martin JF, Lei J, et al. (2010) Weight loss and lipolysis promote a dynamic immune response in murine adipose tissue. J Clin Invest 120: 3466–3479.
37. Gehart H, Kumpf S, Ittner A, Ricci R (2010) MAPK signalling in cellular metabolism: stress or wellness? EMBO Rep 11: 834–840.

6

Glucose Kinetics in the Collagen-Induced Arthritis Model: An All-in-One Model to Assess Both Efficacy and Metabolic Side Effects of Glucocorticoids

Erik J. M. Toonen[1*], Anke J. Laskewitz[2], Theo H. van Dijk[3], Aycha Bleeker[2], Aldo Grefhorst[4], Annelies E. Schouten[5], Ellen A. J. Bastiaanssen[5], Dov B. Ballak[1], Marije I. Koenders[6], Cindy van Doorn[5], Monique A. J. van der Vleuten[5], Marie-Jose C. van Lierop[5], Albert K. Groen[2,3], Wim H. A. Dokter[5¤]

1 Department of Internal Medicine, Radboud University Medical Centre, Nijmegen, The Netherlands, **2** Department of Pediatrics, University of Groningen, University Medical Center Groningen, Groningen, The Netherlands, **3** Department of Laboratory Medicine, University of Groningen, University Medical Center Groningen, Groningen, The Netherlands, **4** Department of Internal Medicine, Erasmus MC, University Medical Center Rotterdam, Rotterdam, The Netherlands, **5** Department of Immune Therapeutics, MSD Research Laboratories, Oss, The Netherlands, **6** Department of Experimental Rheumatology, Radboud Institute for Molecular Life Sciences (RIMLS), Radboud University Medical Centre, Nijmegen, The Netherlands

Abstract

Prednisolone and other glucocorticoids (GCs) are potent anti-inflammatory drugs, but chronic use is hampered by metabolic side effects. Therefore, there is an urgent medical need for improved GCs that are as effective as classical GCs but have a better safety profile. A well-established model to assess anti-inflammatory efficacy is the chronic collagen-induced arthritis (CIA) model in mice, a model with features resembling rheumatoid arthritis. Models to quantify undesired effects of glucocorticoids on glucose kinetics are less well-established. Recently, we have described a model to quantify basal blood glucose kinetics using stably-labeled glucose. In the present study, we have integrated this blood glucose kinetic model in the CIA model to enable quantification of both efficacy and adverse effects in one animal model. Arthritis scores were decreased after treatment with prednisolone, confirming the anti-inflammatory properties of GCs. Both inflammation and prednisolone induced insulin resistance as insulin secretion was strongly increased whereas blood glucose concentrations and hepatic glucose production were only slightly decreased. This insulin resistance did not directly resulted in hyperglycemia, indicating a highly adaptive compensatory mechanism in these mice. In conclusion, this 'all-in-one' model allows for studying effects of (novel) GC compounds on the development of arthritis and glucose kinetics in a single animal. This integrative model provides a valuable tool for investigating (drug-induced) metabolic dysregulation in an inflammatory setting.

Editor: Kang Sun, Shanghai Jiaotong University School of Medicine, China

Funding: This research is supported by Dutch Top Institute Pharma; project T1-106 (www.tipharma.nl). The authors AS, EB, CvD, MvdV and MJvL and WD were previously employed by MSD and received salary from MSD to fund part of this study. The funders had no role in study design, data collection and analysis, decision to publish, or preparation of the manuscript.

Competing Interests: The authors have declared that no competing interests exist. AS, EB, CvD, MvdV and MJvL were previously employed by MSD. WD is employed at Synthon Biopharmaceuticals B.V.

* Email: eriktoonen@hotmail.com

These authors contributed equally to this work.

¤ Current address: Synthon Biopharmaceuticals B.V., Nijmegen, The Netherlands

Introduction

Prednisolone and other glucocorticoids (GCs) are very potent immunosuppressive and anti-inflammatory compounds that are among the top 10 most prescribed drugs [1]. Exogenous GCs are used in daily clinical practice to treat (chronic) inflammatory, autoimmune and allergic disorders, to attenuate organ rejection after transplantation, to treat brain edema, shock and various blood cancers [2]. Most of the effects of GCs are mediated through binding of GCs to the glucocorticoid receptor (GR), which is found in almost all human tissues.

Although very effective in reducing inflammation, prolonged treatment at medium or high dose of GCs is hampered by a wide range of metabolic side effects such as derangements of glucose metabolism, induction of insulin-resistance, beta-cell dysfunction, hyperlipidemia, fat redistribution and central obesity that are all strongly associated with elevated risk for cardiovascular disease and type 2 Diabetes mellitus in humans [3–5]. The mechanisms of action underlying these metabolic side effects are largely unknown.

Seen this wide range of GC-induced side effects, there is a high medical need for improved anti-inflammatory drugs that are as effective as classical GCs but show less metabolic side effects. This type of experimental compounds are often referred to as selective GR modulators (SGRMs) [4]. Given the complexity of glucocorticoid actions, the use of animal models is required to investigate these mechanisms and several animal models have been applied to study the efficacy and/or

Table 1. The formulas used to calculate the concentration *vs.* time curves and the kinetic parameters in a first order absorption process in an one-compartment model.

Eq. 1	Tracer Concentration at time point t	$C_t = M_t \times [glc]_t$
Eq. 2	Single-pool first-order kinetics	$C_t = C_0^{el} e^{-k^{el} t} - C_0^{ab} e^{-k^{ab} t}$
Eq. 3	Bioavailability	$F = 1 - \left(\frac{C_0^{ab} \times k^{el}}{k^{ab} \times C_0^{el}}\right)$
Eq. 4	Area under the curve	$AUC = \frac{C_0^{el}}{k^{el}} - \frac{C_0^{ab}}{k^{ab}}$
Eq. 5	Metabolic clearance rate	$MCR = \frac{F \times D}{AUC}$
Eq. 6	Apparent volume of distribution	$V = \frac{MCR}{k^{el}}$
Eq. 7	Turnover rate	$Ra = MCR \times BG$
Eq. 8	Pool size	$A = \frac{Ra}{k^{el}}$

C_t, D-[6,6-^{2}H]-glucose concentration at time point t; M_t, fractional contribution of D-[6,6-^{2}H]-glucose at time point t; $[glc]_t$, blood glucose concentration at time point t. $C(0)^{ab}$, initial concentration of D-[6,6-^{2}H]-glucose determined by extrapolation of the absorption period; $C(0)^{el}$, initial concentration of D-[6,6-^{2}H]-glucose determined by extrapolation of the elimination period; k^{ab}, absorption rate constant; k^{el}, absorption rate constant. D, dose D-[6,6-^{2}H]-glucose administrated; BG, average blood glucose concentration during the test; Ra = EGP.

metabolic side effects of new pharmaceutical compounds *in vivo* [6,7]. Preclinical efficacy of experimental GCs is often measured in collagen-induced arthritis (CIA) mice, a chronic inflammatory model with features resembling rheumatoid arthritis (RA) [8,9]. Arthritis can be induced in susceptible strains of mice by immunization with type II collagen, the major component of articular cartilage, and has histopathologic and serological features in common with RA [10,11]. Regarding *in vivo* investigation of (compound-induced) metabolic dysregulation, such as insulin resistance, a number of methods have been developed to measure glucose and insulin kinetics, of which the hyperinsulinemic euglycemic clamp (HIEC) is considered as the 'gold standard'. With respect to mice studies, the HIEC is difficult to use for longitudinal studies, since it can only be performed once in a single animal [12]. In addition, arthritic mice in the CIA model are severely ill, with highly inflamed joints and therefore these mice can not be subjected to the invasive HIEC protocol. To overcome these drawbacks, a new method was developed in which stably-labeled glucose (D [6,6-$^2H_2$]-glucose) was used in combination with a single-pool, first order kinetic model to determine blood glucose kinetics [13]. This model is especially of interest for longitudinal studies, due to the ability of repeated measurements.

Currently, an animal model to study both efficacy and glucocorticoid-induced metabolic side effects in a chronic inflammatory setting is not available. Therefore, the aim of the present study is to develop a chronic inflammatory model which can be used to investigate both efficacy *and* metabolic safety of GCs in the same animal at the same time. To do so, we have integrated the newly developed blood glucose kinetics model into the CIA mice model.

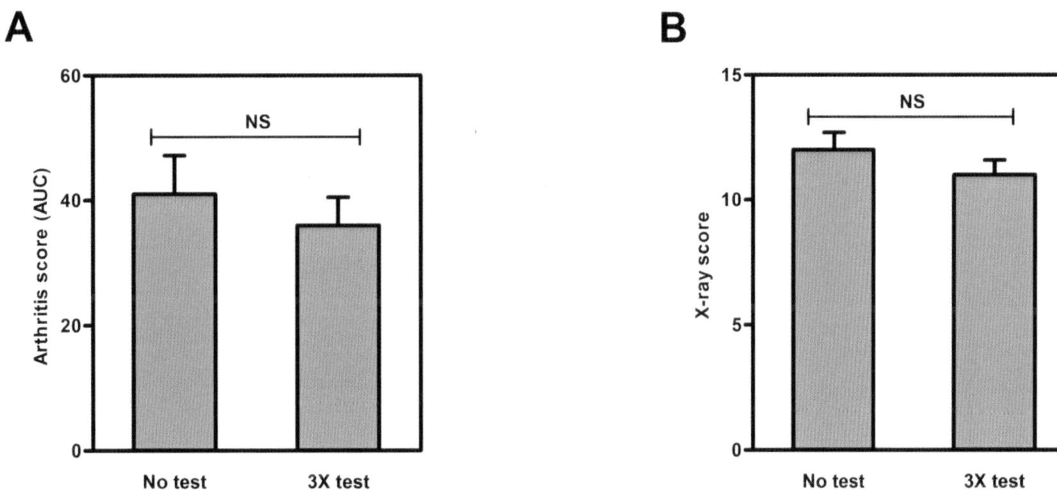

Figure 1. Arthritis development. Arthritis development in mice subjected to blood glucose kinetics three times and in mice in which no experiments were performed. (**A**) AUC of the overall arthritis score, corrected for base line, after 21 days. (**B**) X-ray analysis to assess bone destruction. Results are presented as mean ± SEM (n = 20). No significant differences between the two groups was observed. NS = not significant.

To validate this model and to investigate the mechanisms involved in GC-induced metabolic dysfunction in a chronic inflammatory setting, we performed two consecutive CIA experiments. First, we assessed the effects of several doses of prednisolone (0, 1.5, 10 and 30 mg/kg/day) on efficacy and metabolic safety after 0, 7 and 21 days of treatment. Next, in order to distinguish between direct effects of prednisolone and indirect effects on glucose kinetics resulting from its anti-inflammatory efficacy, we compared effects of prednisolone to those of ORG 37663. This compound is a steroid which has previously been described to be effective for the treatment of arthritis in CIA mice, but mediates its effect through the estrogen receptor alpha (ERα) instead of the GR (6). Comparing the results from the prednisolone-treated subgroup to the subgroup treated with the anti-inflammatory compound ORG 37663 allowed us to distinguish between direct effects of prednisolone on glucose and insulin kinetics and indirect effects induced by the anti-inflammatory properties of prednisolone.

The results from this study reveal that it was possible to measure both efficacy and metabolic side effects of prednisolone in one experimental set-up. Arthritis scores were dose-dependently decreased in arthritic mice after treatment with both prednisolone and ORG 37663. Concerning effects on glucose metabolism, there was a decrease in insulin sensitivity in both arthritic and non-arthritic control mice after treatment with prednisolone for three weeks, while ORG 37663 unexpectedly increased insulin sensitivity in both groups. These prednisolone-mediated effects on insulin sensitivity were mainly reflected by an increased insulin secretion.

Overall, the integration of these two models provides a valuable tool for studying both the efficacy *and* metabolic side-effects of experimental glucocorticoids at the same time in one model.

Methods

Animals

All experiments were approved by the Animal Welfare Committee of MSD Oss, The Netherlands. Male DBA1/J mice were obtained from Bomholtgard (Ry, Denmark). Animals were housed and maintained at 23°C with *ad libitum* access to water and food in a 12 hour-12 hour light-dark cycle (lights on 6 am-6 pm).

Therapeutic murine collagen-induced arthritis

The murine CIA model was performed as previously described [14]. In brief, DBA1/J mice were immunized at the base of the tail at the age of eight weeks with 200 µg bovine type II collagen in complete Freud's adjuvant enriched with 2 mg/ml *M. tuberculosis* (H37Ra). Three weeks after immunization the animals were boosted with an intraperitoneal injection of 200 µg collagen type II, dissolved in saline. Earlier experiments have taught us that, after immunization, mice will drop-out due to an early aggressive arthritis or fail to develop arthritis. About 60–70% of the mice develop the necessary arthritis. Therefore, the total amount of mice that are immunized and boosted for the experiment is 40% above the actual number of mice needed for the experiment. The clinical severity of arthritis (arthritis score) was graded per inflamed digit (a scale of 0 to 2 for each paw). Mice were scored on alternative days, resulting in mean scores with an overall maximum of 8 per animal. To assess the effects of treatment, the area under curve (AUC) of the mean arthritis of each animal with baseline correction (subtracting baseline AUC of arthritis score on day 0) was used. After disease onset, animals with an arthritis score ranging from 2 to 4 were divided into separate groups of 12 mice so that the mean arthritis score of all experimental groups was comparable at the start of the treatment (day 0). Mice were considered to have arthritis when significant changes in redness and/or swelling were noted in the digits or in other parts of the paws.

Treatment and experimental regimes

For the first experiment, a total of 40 arthritic animals were divided into an experimental and a control group of 20 mice each. Both groups were orally treated once a day for 21 days with placebo (0.5% gelatin and 5% mannitol in water) and arthritis development was monitored. In the experimental group (n = 20) mice were subjected to a blood glucose kinetics test three times (on day 0, 7 and 21) while mice in the control group were not subjected to the blood glucose kinetics tests.

For the second experiment, arthritic animals were treated orally once a day for 21 days with either 1.5, 10 or 30 mg/kg prednisolone in vehicle (0.5% gelatin and 5% mannitol in water) or vehicle alone as placebo. In total, 48 arthritic mice (12 per treatment group) were included. For non-arthritic control groups, mice were mock immunized with saline at the base of the tail at the age of eight weeks and three weeks later mock boosted with saline. Mice were further treated according the same experimental protocol and handled exactly the same as the mice that developed arthritis. In this study, these mice are referred to as non-arthritic control mice.

For the third experiment, arthritic mice were treated orally once a day for 21 days either with prednisolone (10 mg/kg) or ORG 37663 (12 mg/kg) in vehicle (0.5% gelatin and 5% mannitol in water) or vehicle alone as placebo. The dose of 12 mg/kg/day for ORG 37663 was selected because this dose is comparable to a dose of 10 mg/kg/day prednisolone regarding efficacy [6]. In total, 36 arthritic mice (12 per treatment group) and 36 non-arthritic control mice, like described above, were included in this consecutive experiment.

All experimental treatments were conducted in a blinded fashion. At the end of the experiment, serum samples and hind knees and paws were obtained. Hind knees and paws were evaluated using X-ray analysis to assess bone destruction [15]. X-ray photographs were examined with a Faxitron X-ray MX-20 (0.02 mm resolution) and bone destruction was scored on a scale from 0 to 5 ranging from no damage to complete destruction [16].

Blood glucose kinetics

The fasted blood glucose kinetic test was performed three times; at day 0 (before treatment, but after disease onset) and after 7 and 21 days of treatment. For each experiment, mice were fasted for 9 hours overnight (11.00 pm–8.00 am), body weights were measured and mice were injected intraperitoneally with a small volume of 2.0 mg D-[6,6-$^2H_2$]glucose in 0.20 ml by intraperitoneal injection (~450 µmol/kg BW) which did not cause changes in blood glucose and plasma insulin concentrations. Before and at 10, 20, 30, 40, 50, 60, 75 and 90 minutes after D-[6,6-$^2H_2$]-glucose administration, blood glucose concentrations were measured in a blood drop collected by tail tip bleeding using a glucocard X-meter (A. Menarini Diagnostics; Valkenswaard; The Netherlands). At the same time points, a small blood spot was taken on filter paper (FT-2-460-210297, Sartorius, Goettingen, Germany) and stored at room temperature until further analysis of D-[6,6-$^2H_2$]-glucose label distribution. After the last test (day 21) a blood sample (15 µl) was taken by tail tip bleeding for C-peptide measurements.

Table 2. Treatment parameters for both non-arthritic and arthritic mice treated with prednisolone for 21 days.

	Non-arthritic mice				Arthritic mice			
Prednisolone (mg/kg/d)	**0**	**1.5**	**10**	**30**	**0**	**1.5**	**10**	**30**
Bodyweight (g) day 0	23.0±1.9	24.3±1.9	24.3±2.0	24.8±1.7	21.0±1.5#	20.7±2.5	20.5±1.5	20.3±1.6
Bodyweight (g) day 7	22.5±1.4	23.3±2.3	22.8±2.4	23.5±1.5	20.4±2.2#	20.1±2.1	20.7±1.8	20.2±1.6
Bodyweight (g) day 21	23.1±2.6	23.2±2.4	22.7±2.7	23.0±3.1	20.8±1.5#	20.1±2.1	20.4±2.6	21.6±1.8
Glucose (mM) day 0	5.2±1.4	4.9±1.5	5.9±1.9	6.3±2.5	5.0±1.1	4.4±1.1	5.1±1.2	4.7±2.0
Glucose (mM) day 7	6.5±1.6	5.1±1.2	4.6±1.1*	4.3±1.1*	5.4±1.0	4.7±1.0	4.7±0.9	4.3±1.7
Glucose (mM) day 21	6.7±1.2	5.9±1.0	5.6±1.2	4.9±0.7*	5.5±0.9	4.6±0.7*	4.7±1.0*	5.1±0.3
MCR (ml/kg/min) day 0	14.4±3.2	15.2±2.6	13.4±3.5	11.7±2.2	19.1±3.3#	19.2±3.2	19.0±1.8	17.9±3.4
MCR (ml/kg/min) day 7	15.9±2.2	15.3±2.8	16.1±2.6	17.4±1.5	17.2±2.4	18.4±3.0	17.6±1.5	16.8±2.9
MCR (ml/kg/min) day 21	11.5±1.6	12.1±1.6	11.5±1.5	12.5±1.2	14.4±1.4#	14.1±1.2	14.3±1.1	14.0±1.3
EGP (µmol/kg/min) day 0	71.2±10.9	72.5±22.1	75.3±24.1	72.0±27.7	94.3±24.7#	82.0±12.2	95.8±19.5	90.7±7.5
EGP (µmol/kg/min) day 7	100.9±18.6	78.8±23.1	73.0±15.6*	73.1±15.2*	92.0±14.7	84.7±19.2	80.8±9.7	81.3±14.2
EGP (µmol/kg/min) day 21	76.7±13.5	66.8±10.3	61.9±7.3*	58.5±10.2*	84.1±13.9	68.0±7.5*	65.8±10.1*	71.0±7.7*

Both non-arthritic and arthritic mice are treated with prednisolone (0, 1.5, 10 and 30 mg/kg/day) for 21 days. Each experimental group consists of 12 mice; in total 48 non-arthritic and 48 arthritic mice were included. Values represent means ± SD during the blood glucose kinetics test except BW, which is represented as means ± SD before the test.

* Significant difference ($p \leq 0.05$) when compared to the placebo-treated group of that same parameter.

\# Significant difference ($p \leq 0.05$) when compared to the placebo-treated non-arthritic mice.

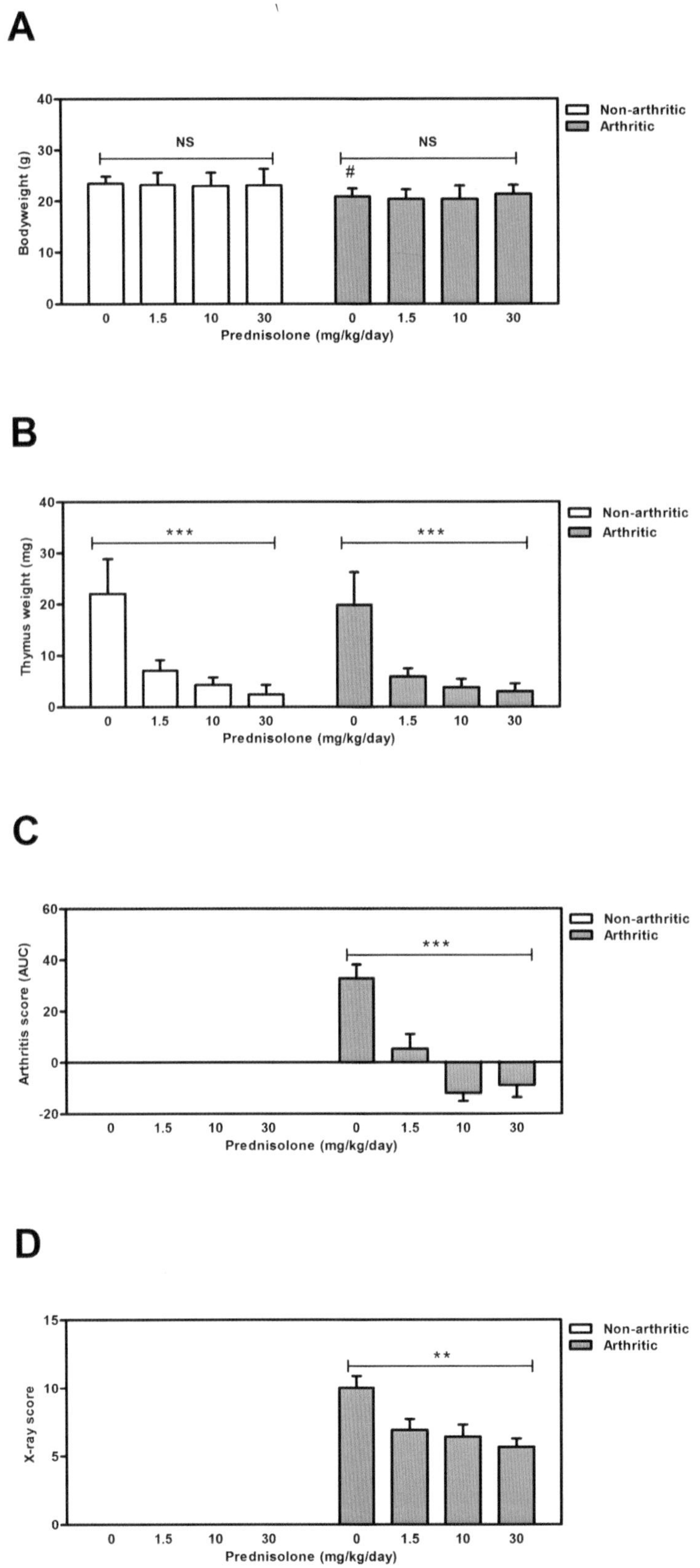

Figure 2. Effects of prednisolone on bodyweight, thymus weight and arthritis development after 21 days of treatment. (**A**) Bodyweight (**B**) thymus weight (**C**) AUC of the overall arthritis score (**D**) X-ray analysis to assess bone destruction. Results are represented as means ± SD for bodyweight and thymus weight and as mean ± SEM for AUC arthritis score and X-ray score and are outlined for each experimental group (n = 12). * Significant difference p≤0.05, ** significant difference p≤0.01, *** significant difference p≤0.001, NS = not significant.

Measurements of mass isotopomer distribution by GC-MS

Whole body glucose turnover and clearance were calculated by kinetic analysis from the wash-out of injected D-[6,6-$^{2}H_2$]-glucose from circulation for which blood spots on filter paper were taken. Extraction of glucose from filter paper, derivatization of the extracted compounds and gas chromatography-mass spectrometry (GC-MS) measurements of blood glucose was performed as previously described by Van Dijk and colleagues [17]. In short, a disk was punched out of the blood spots, glucose was extracted from the disk by incubation in ethanol/water (10:1 v/v) and glucose was derivatized to its pentaacetate-ester. Samples were analyzed by GC-MS with positive ion chemical ionization with ammonia. The fractional isotopomer distribution measured by GC-MS (m_0-m_6) was corrected for the fractional distribution due to natural abundance of ^{13}C by multiple linear regression as described by Lee *et al.* [18] to obtain the excess fractional distribution of mass isotopomers (M_0-M_6) due to dilution of infused labeled compounds.

Calculation of blood glucose kinetics

For calculating the blood glucose kinetics parameters EGP (Endogenous Glucose Production) and MCR (Metabolic Clearance Rate), a single-pool, first-order kinetic model was assumed [19–21]. The excess fractional distribution of mass isotopomers (M_2) was used to calculate the first order absorption process in an one-compartment model using SAAM-II software (version 1.2.1; SAAM Institute, University of Washington, Seattle, WA, USA) [13]. The formulas used to calculate the concentration *vs.* time curves and the kinetic parameters are outlined in Table 1.

C-peptide measurements

In this study C-peptide concentrations as a marker for insulin production, since the half life of C peptide is longer than that of insulin. Thereby, by measuring C-peptide we can focus on de novo synthesis of insulin and not just circulating insulin that might also be released/taken up by cells. Peripheral blood samples obtained after each experiment were centrifuged and the retrieved serum samples were stored at −20°C until analyzed. C-peptide concentrations were measured using a commercially available ELISA kit (mouse C-peptide ELISA; Alpco immunoassays, Salem, NH, USA).

Calculation of HOMA-IR

The Homeostasis Model Assessment for Insulin Resistance (HOMA-IR) combines fasting glucose and insulin concentrations to calculate insulin resistance [22]. Besides using insulin, it is also possible to calculate the HOMA-IR using C-peptide concentrations [23]. The HOMA-IR expresses changes in insulin sensitivity and β-cell function relative to a population in which these parameters are considered to be normal. However, although the HOMA-IR has been used for mice studies previously, it was developed based upon human values. Therefore we adjusted the HOMA-IR for mice in which the healthy mice, treated with placebo, had an insulin resistance (IR) of 1 (no insulin resistance). This group is used as the reference group. The reference value can be calculated from median blood glucose concentration (6.6 mM) during the blood glucose kinetics protocol and the mean plasma C-peptide concentration (221 pM) at the end of the test. For this study, the value was 1459. In this manuscript, the HOMA-IR was therefore calculated as:

$$\text{HOMA-IR} = \frac{[\text{Glu}]*[\text{C-peptide}]}{1459}$$

In which [Glu] is the blood glucose concentration in mM and [C-peptide] is the C-peptide plasma concentration in pM. An HOMA-IR >1 indicates induction of insulin resistance and an HOMA-IR <1 indicates improved insulin sensitivity.

Insulin tolerance test

For the insulin tolerance test, mice were fasted for 4 hours before i.p. injection with insulin (0,75 U/kg bodyweight). Blood samples were taken by tail-cut at baseline and after 15, 30, 45, 60, 90 and 120 minutes of insulin administration. Blood glucose concentration were measured with a blood glucose meter (Accu-Chek Avia; Roche Diagnostics, Almere, The Netherlands).

Statistical analysis

All data are represented as mean ± SD except for the arthritis data which, is represented as mean ± SEM. Data were analyzed using, where appropriate, the Student's t-test, ANOVA or 2-way ANOVA followed by the Tukey *post hoc* test (SPSS, Chicago, IL, USA). A p-value <0.05 was considered significant.

Results

The blood glucose kinetics test does not interfere with arthritis development

Before reliable statements could be made regarding prednisolone-induced effects on arthritis development and glucose kinetics in mice, we wanted to confirm that the blood glucose kinetics protocol itself did not influence arthritis development. Therefore, we first investigated if performing this protocol three times in arthritic mice would affect arthritis development. Figure 1 shows that a triple blood glucose kinetic test in three weeks time did not affect AUC of arthritis scores and X-ray scores in the CIA mouse model.

Assessing the effects of both arthritis development and prednisolone treatment on glucose kinetics

Blood glucose kinetics was used to assess both arthritis-induced and prednisolone-induced metabolic dysfunction and was performed three times: at day 0 (before prednisolone treatment) and after 7 and 21 days of treatment. Before treatment, bodyweights were significantly lower in arthritic mice when compared to non-arthritic mice ($p<0.0001$) (Table 2). This decrease in bodyweight is caused by the active inflammatory state of these arthritic mice as was previously reported [24]. Even though arthritic mice have lower bodyweights compared to control mice, treatment with several doses of prednisolone for 21 days did not have any effect on bodyweight in both groups compared to vehicle treated mice (Table 2 and Fig. 2A).

Prednisolone treatment induced apoptosis of thymocytes, thereby severely reducing thymus weight dose dependently [25]. No differences in thymus weight were observed between arthritic and non-arthritic mice. Treatment with 1.5, 10 or 30 mg/kg prednisolone per day significantly reduced thymus weight in a dose-dependent manner respectively with 68%, 80% and 89% ($p<0.0001$) in the non-arthritic control group and with 70%, 81% and 85% ($p<0.0001$) in the arthritic group (Fig. 2B). These reductions are indicative for sufficient prednisolone exposure in

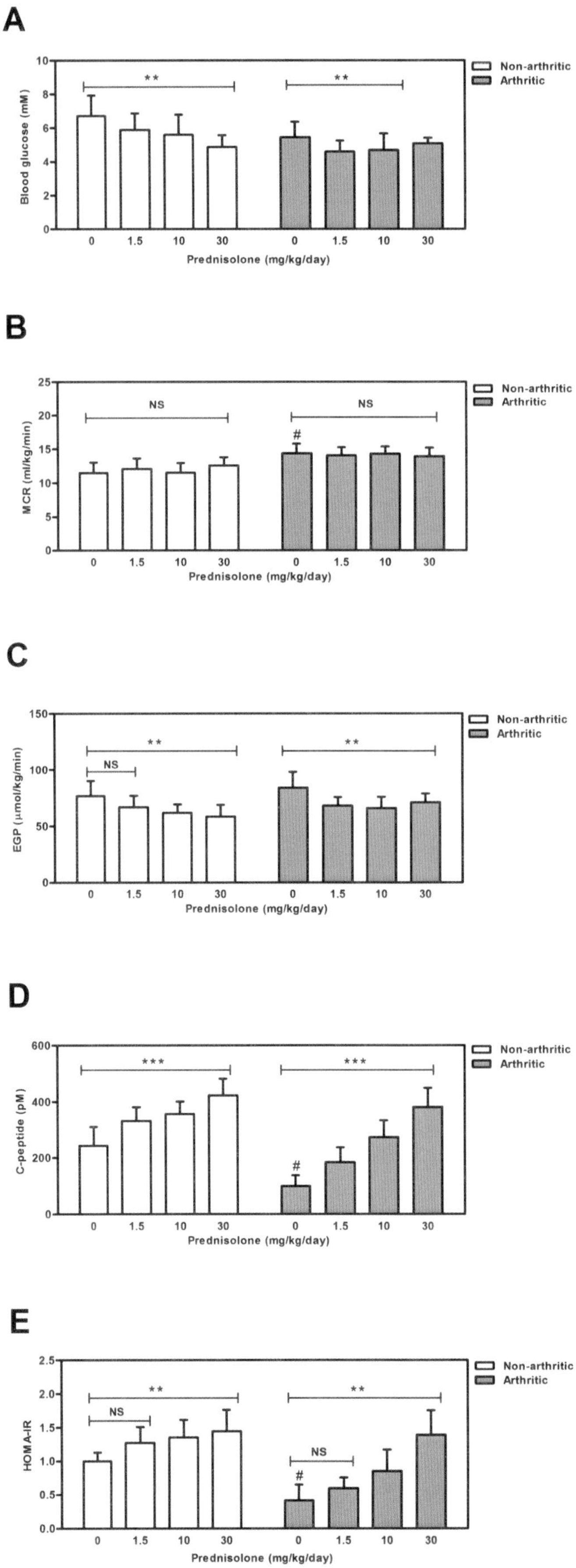
A
Blood glucose (mM)
Non-arthritic
Arthritic
**
**
0 1.5 10 30 0 1.5 10 30
Prednisolone (mg/kg/day)
B
MCR (ml/kg/min)
Non-arthritic
Arthritic
NS
NS
#
0 1.5 10 30 0 1.5 10 30
Prednisolone (mg/kg/day)
C
EGP (μmol/kg/min)
Non-arthritic
Arthritic
**
NS
**
0 1.5 10 30 0 1.5 10 30
Prednisolone (mg/kg/day)
D
C-peptide (pM)
Non-arthritic
Arthritic
***
***
#
0 1.5 10 30 0 1.5 10 30
Prednisolone (mg/kg/day)
E
HOMA-IR
Non-arthritic
Arthritic
**
NS
**
NS
#
0 1.5 10 30 0 1.5 10 30
Prednisolone (mg/kg/day)

Figure 3. Effects of prednisolone on glucose kinetics after 21 days of treatment. (**A**) Blood glucose concentrations (**B**) MCR (**C**) EGP levels MCR (**D**) C-peptide concentrations (**E**) C-peptide HOMA-IR. Results represent means ± SD and are outlined for each experimental group (n = 12). * Significant difference p≤0.05, ** significant difference p≤0.01, *** significant difference p≤0.001, #significant difference (p≤0.05) when compared to the placebo-treated non-arthritic mice, NS = not significant.

these treatment groups. No differences in thymus weight reduction between arthritic and non-arthritic mice was observed.

To confirm the anti-arthritic properties of prednisolone, arthritic mice were monitored for arthritis score and X-ray score. Prednisolone dose-dependently reduced disease severity since a significant reduction of the AUC arthritis score covering the entire treatment period was observed ($p<0.0001$) (Fig. 2C). X-ray analysis of the arthritic joints indicate severe cartilage and bone destruction in the placebo-treated arthritic animals. In line with previous results [6], prednisolone significantly reduced the rate of cartilage and bone destruction in a dose-dependent manner ($p = 0.0029$) (Fig. 2D). As expected, the non-arthritic control mice that were mock immunized with saline and three weeks later mock boosted with saline, did not develop arthritis.

No differences were observed in blood glucose concentrations between arthritic and non-arthritic mice before treatment (Table 2), and after 21 days placebo treatment ($p = 0.1$). (Fig. 3A). A minimal but significant decrease in blood glucose concentrations was observed in non-arthritic mice after treatment with several doses of prednisolone for three weeks ($p = 0.0064$) (Fig. 3A). Also a slightly but significant decrease in blood glucose concentrations was observed in arthritic mice after treatment with several doses of prednisolone ($p = 0.0012$) (Fig. 3A).

The glucose kinetics parameters MCR (Metabolic Clearance Rate) and EGP (Endogenous Glucose Production) were calculated by modeling the wash-out of injected D-[6,6-$^2H_2$]-glucose. MCR was increased in arthritic mice when compared to non-arthritic before treatment started ($p<0.0001$) (Table 2). Prednisolone did not affect MCR in both non-arthritic or arthritic mice (Fig 3B). Interestingly, even though no effects were seen upon three weeks of prednisolone treatment between the groups, MCR is lowered in the arthritic group over time. For the non-arthritic group, MCR is increased at day 7 but decreased at day 21 when compared baseline (Table 2 and Fig. 3B)

Before treatment started the EGP in arthritic mice was significantly higher than in non-arthritic mice ($p<0.0001$), but decreased after 21 days of placebo treatment (Table 2), leveling the difference between placebo-treated arthritic and placebo-treated non-arthritic mice after 21 days of treatment ($p = 0.2$) (Table 2 and Fig. 3C). Prednisolone treatment for 21 days significantly decreased EGP in both non-arthritic ($p = 0.006$) and arthritic mice ($p = 0.002$) (Fig. 3C).

Surprisingly, after three weeks of treatment, plasma C-peptide concentrations of placebo treated arthritic mice were significant lower than those of placebo-treated non-arthritic mice ($p = 0.0006$). C-peptide concentrations were strongly increased in a dose-dependent manner by prednisolone in both non-arthritic ($p<0.0001$) and arthritic mice ($p<0.0001$) implying increased insulin production (Fig. 3D).

From the fasting blood glucose and C-peptide concentrations, the HOMA-IR was calculated to evaluate insulin resistance. Remarkably, the HOMA-IR showed that placebo-treated arthritic mice are 2.4 times more insulin sensitive than placebo-treated non-arthritic animals (p-value = 0.0007) (Fig. 3E). According to the HOMA-IR data, prednisolone treatment significantly reduced insulin sensitivity in a dose-dependent manner in both non-arthritic ($p = 0.028$) and arthritic mice ($p = 0.0001$ after correction for differences in arthritis scores between the groups). After treatment with prednisolone (30 mg/kg/d) for 21 days, both groups were equally sensitive to insulin (Fig. 3E).

Validating the blood glucose kinetics results by using the insulin tolerance test.

As described above, results from the blood glucose kinetic model showed that prednisolone treatment significantly reduced insulin sensitivity in both non-arthritic and arthritic mice. To validate these results, we repeated the experiment and assessed insulin resistance by the use of a insulin tolerance test (ITT). Both non-arthritic and arthritic mice were treated either with prednisolone (30 mg/kg/day) in vehicle or with vehicle alone for 21 days. After treatment, an ITT was performed. Prednisolone reduced disease severity as shown by a significant reduction of the AUC arthritis score ($p<0.0001$) (Fig. 4A). Fasting glucoses were not significant different between groups (Fig. 4B). Results from the ITT demonstrated that non-arthritic mice treated with vehicle were more insulin sensitive than non-arthritic mice treated with prednisolone (Fig. 4C). The area under the curve showed that differences between prednisolone- and vehicle treated animals was significant ($p - 0.012$) (Fig. 4D). In arthritic animals, a clear trend is visible suggesting that vehicle-treated mice are more insulin sensitive than prednisolone-treated mice (Fig. 4E). However, the AUC shows that differences are not significant (Fig. 4F). Taken together, data from the glucose kinetics test and the ITT showed that prednisolone treatment most likely reduces insulin sensitivity in both non-arthritic and arthritic mice.

Assessing the effects of ORG 37663 treatment on glucose kinetics

To distinguish between the direct effect of prednisolone on metabolic processes versus indirect effects on metabolism via the suppressed inflammatory condition by prednisolone, we performed an experiment in which arthritic and non-arthritic mice were treated with prednisolone or ORG 37663. The latter compound is a steroid that was previously shown to have anti-inflammatory properties and effectively reduces arthritis in the CIA model. ORG 37663 mediates its effects through a mechanism that is independent of GR binding [6]. Therefore, ORG 37663 was used in a head-to-head comparison to prednisolone in one experiment to study to what extent effects of prednisolone on glucose kinetics are due to its anti-inflammatory properties or due to a direct effect through GR on metabolic pathways.

Similar to the previous experiment, bodyweights before treatment were significantly lower in arthritic mice compared to non-arthritic mice ($p = 0.0001$) (Table 3). Non-arthritic mice were found to have significant lower bodyweights after treatment with ORG 37663 but not after treatment with prednisolone (Fig. 5A).

In the non-arthritic control group, treatment with 10 mg/kg prednisolone or 12 mg/kg ORG 37663 per day reduced thymus weight respectively with 84% ($P<0.0001$) and 78% ($P<0.0001$) (Fig. 5B). In the arthritic group thymus weight was reduced with 86% ($P<0.0001$) and 76% ($P<0.0001$), again indicative for sufficient compound exposure. In arthritic mice, both arthritic score and X-ray score were significantly decreased ($P<0.0001$ and $p = 0.0279$ respectively) after treatment with either prednisolone or ORG 37663 (Fig. 5C-D).

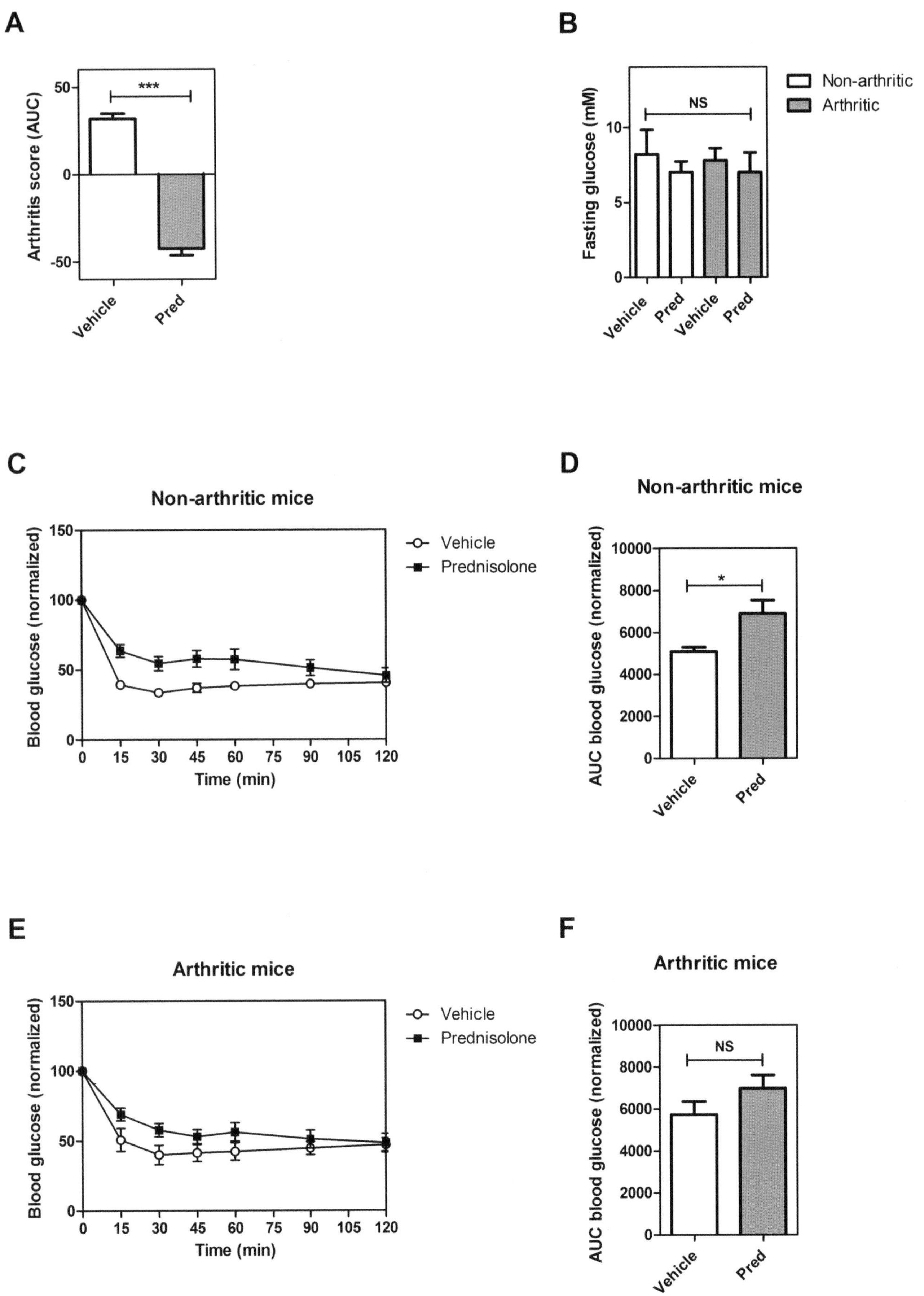
A
Arthritis score (AUC)
50
0
-50
***
Vehicle
Pred
B
Fasting glucose (mM)
10
5
0
NS
Non-arthritic
Arthritic
Vehicle
Pred
Vehicle
Pred
C
Non-arthritic mice
Blood glucose (normalized)
150
100
50
0
0 15 30 45 60 75 90 105 120
Time (min)
Vehicle
Prednisolone
D
Non-arthritic mice
AUC blood glucose (normalized)
10000
8000
6000
4000
2000
0
*
Vehicle
Pred
E
Arthritic mice
Blood glucose (normalized)
150
100
50
0
0 15 30 45 60 75 90 105 120
Time (min)
Vehicle
Prednisolone
F
Arthritic mice
AUC blood glucose (normalized)
10000
8000
6000
4000
2000
0
NS
Vehicle
Pred

Figure 4. Assessment of insulin sensitivity by the use of the insulin tolerance test (ITT). (**A**) AUC of the overall arthritis score, corrected for base line, after 21 days. (**B**) Blood glucose concentrations of non-arthritic and arthritic mice treated with prednisolone or vehicle. (**C**) Blood glucose values during the ITT of non-arthritic mice treated with prednisolone or vehicle. (**D**) ITT AUC values of non-arthritic mice treated with prednisolone or vehicle. (**E**) Blood glucose values during the ITT of arthritic mice treated with prednisolone or vehicle. (**F**) ITT AUC values of arthritic mice treated with prednisolone or vehicle.). * Significant difference $p \leq 0.05$, *** significant difference $p \leq 0.001$, NS = not significant.

Arthritic mice showed slight but significant lower blood glucose concentrations after ORG 37663 treatment in comparison to placebo treatment ($p = 0.036$). In both the non-arthritic and arthritic groups of mice, no effect of prednisolone on blood glucose concentrations was detected (Fig. 6A). Non-arthritic mice treated with prednisolone or ORG 37663 both had a significant lower MCR compared to placebo treated mice ($p < 0.0001$), while this effect was not observed in the arthritic mice after treatment (Fig. 6B). This is probably caused by the fact that MCR was already decreased in arthritic mice after 21 days of treatment with placebo compared to non-arthritic mice treated with placebo ($p < 0.0001$). The same effect was observed for EGP: in non-arthritic mice the EGP levels decreased by prednisolone ($p = 0.0006$) or ORG 37663 treatment ($p = 0.036$) (Fig.6C) and a same trend was visible in arthritic mice, but due to the fact that the placebo-treated arthritic mice already showed some neutralization of the increased EGP levels, the effects of prednisolone and ORG 37663 on EGP in these mice was less obvious (as was seen in the previous experiment).

As was observed in the prednisolone dose-response experiment, C-peptide concentrations from arthritic mice treated with placebo were significant lower compared to the non-arthritic mice treated with placebo after three weeks of treatment (p-value = 0.0047) (Fig. 6D). The ORG 37663 compound caused a decrease in C-peptide concentrations in both non-arthritic ($p < 0.0001$) and arthritic mice ($p < 0.0001$) when compared to prednisolone (Fig. 6D). As a consequence of the low C-peptide concentrations after treatment with ORG 37663, both arthritic ($p = 0.0022$) and non-arthritic mice ($p = 0.0002$) showed a tremendous increase in insulin sensitivity as calculated by the HOMA-IR (Fig. 6E). These data indicate that treatment with ORG 37663 improved insulin sensitivity in mice compared to prednisolone-treated mice.

Discussion

There is an urgent need for improved GCs that are as effective as classical GCs, but have a better safety profile. However, a chronic *in vivo* inflammatory model in which (experimental) GCs can be studied for both their effectiveness and the induction of metabolic side effects is currently unavailable. Goal of the present study was to develop such an *in vivo* inflammatory model for efficacy and metabolic adverse effects at the same time. Therefore we have integrated a single-pool, first order kinetic protocol to examine blood glucose kinetics, in the well-established collagen-induced arthritis (CIA) mice model, a chronic inflammatory model which is often used to monitor efficacy of experimental anti-inflammatory compounds. We were able to measure effects on glucose kinetics without influence on arthritis development. Importantly, this indicates that we have successfully performed blood glucose kinetics in the CIA model enabling the quantification of both efficacy and effects on glucose metabolism in a single animal.

The 'gold standard' to investigate and quantify insulin resistance is the hyperinsulinemic euglycemic clamp (HIEC) [26]. However, seen from the perspective of laboratory animal welfare, performing such clamp studies within an inflammatory mouse model such as the CIA model is impossible. Measuring glucose kinetics by

Table 3. Treatment parameters for both non-arthritic and arthritic mice treated with placebo, prednisolone (10 mg/kg) or ORG 37663 (12 mg/kg) for 21 days.

	Non-arthritic mice			Arthritic mice		
	Placebo	**Prednisolone**	**ORG 37663**	**Placebo**	**Prednisolone**	**ORG 37663**
Bodyweight (g) day 0	23.5±1.5	23.2±1.0	25.0±2.4	20.9±1.3#	21.5±2.9	20.8±1.3
Bodyweight (g) day 7	24.3±1.6	22.6±1.2	23.7±1.6	21.4±2.2#	21.4±2.7	21.7±1.9
Bodyweight (g) day 21	25.1±1.9	22.9±1.2	20.5±1.6*	21.6±1.7#	22.4±2.9	18.7±1.2*
Glucose (mM) day 0	3.5±1.1	4.6±1.7	3.6±1.8	4.8±1.0	5.0±1.1	4.5±0.9
Glucose (mM) day 7	5.3±1.9	4.4±1.2	5.2±1.4	5.7±0.7	4.6±1.0	6.0±0.8
Glucose (mM) day 21	5.2±1.4	4.9±0.9	4.6±1.5	5.9±1.3	5.2±0.8	4.7±0.7*
MCR (ml/kg/min) day 0	17.8±9.4	18.6±8.3	15.6±10.2	19.0±4.1	18.9±2.8	13.4±10
MCR (ml/kg/min) day 7	11.6±5.6	14.1±4.9	9.8±6.3	17.0±1.9#	16.7±2.6	8.8±6.9*
MCR (ml/kg/min) day 21	16.5±1.8	12.0±1.1*	13.2±1.9*	12.3±1.4#	12.9±1.8	13.6±2.4
EGP (μmol/kg/min) day 0	71.1±13.3	84.6±16.1	68.5±19.5	92.3±25.5#	95.1±21.5	89.9±15.9
EGP (μmol/kg/min) day 7	72.7±25.6	65.5±13.2	65.9±9.8	94.1±14.3#	74.0±7.7*	70.7±12.2*
EGP (μmol/kg/min) day 21	84.4±19.4	58.4±8.3*	58.6±12.9*	73.7±19.4	66.0±10.8	63.6±16.4

Both non-arthritic and arthritic mice are treated with placebo, prednisolone (10 mg/kg/day) or ORG 37663 (12 mg/kg/day) for 21 days. Each experimental group consists of 12 mice; in total 36 non-arthritic and 36 arthritic mice were included. Values represent means ± SD during the blood glucose kinetics test except BW, which is represented as means ± SD before the test.
* Significant difference ($p \leq 0.05$) when compared to the placebo-treated group of that same parameter.
#Significant difference ($p \leq 0.05$) when compared to the placebo-treated non-arthritic mice.

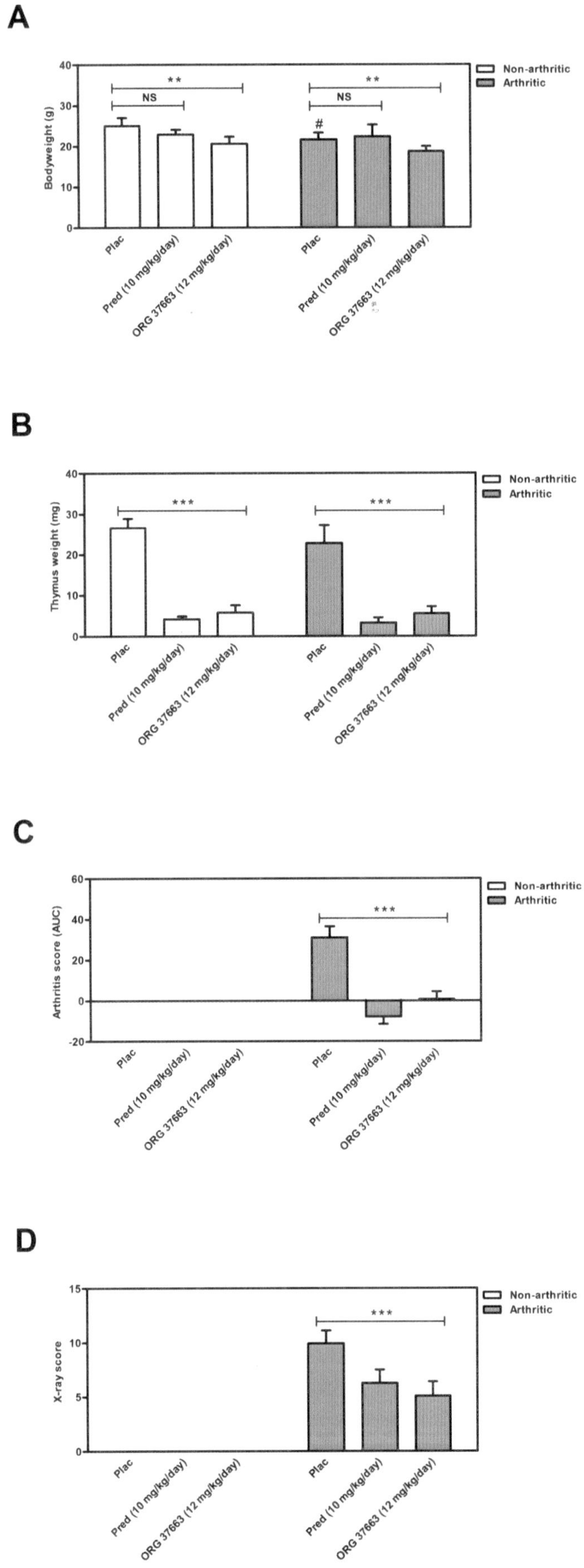
A
Bodyweight (g)
Non-arthritic
Arthritic
**
NS
#
Plac
Pred (10 mg/kg/day)
ORG 37663 (12 mg/kg/day)
B
Thymus weight (mg)
***
C
Arthritis score (AUC)
D
X-ray score

Figure 5. Effects of ORG 37663 and prednisolone on bodyweight, thymus weight and arthritis development after 21 days of treatment. (**A**) Bodyweight (**B**) thymus weight (**C**) AUC of the overall arthritis score (**D**) X-ray analysis to assess bone destruction. Results are represented as means ± SD for bodyweight and thymus weight and as mean ±SEM for AUC arthritis score and X-ray score and are outlined for each experimental group (n = 12). * Significant difference p≤0.05, ** significant difference p≤0.01, *** significant difference p≤0.001, #significant difference (p≤0.05) when compared to the placebo-treated non-arthritic mice, NS = not significant.

modeling the wash-out of *ip* injected D-[6,6-$^2H_2$]-glucose is performed under fasted conditions whereas the HIEC utilizes steady-state insulin concentrations that are supraphysiological [13,27,28]. Thus, the wash-out of ip-injected glucose presumably reflects a more physiological relevant situation. In addition, unlike the HIEC the blood glucose kinetics test can be applied repeatedly and is therefore applicable in longitudinal studies, such as the CIA model described here.

This study showed that prednisolone decreased disease severity and joint destruction in arthritic mice, thereby confirming the anti-inflammatory properties of this compound. Regarding the induction of metabolic effects, prednisolone slightly decreased fasted glucose concentrations and EGP, but strongly increased insulin production (as measured by the increase in C-peptide concentrations) at the same time in both non-arthritic and arthritic mice. This resulted in an increased HOMA-IR after prednisolone treatment, indicating the induction of insulin resistance. To validate these results, we repeated the experiment and measured insulin sensitivity by the use of an ITT. Results from the ITT showed that prednisolone induced insulin resistance in both non-arthritic and arthritic mice, thereby confirming our previous results obtained by the blood glucose kinetic model. Although the ITT is a more classical model to assess insulin resistance, it is only capable of measuring glucose metabolism in peripheral tissues. The additive value of the applied blood glucose kinetic model, *i.e.*, the injection of D [6,6 $^2H_2$]-glucose, is that this allowed for discrimination of the changes in glucose metabolism in peripheral tissues and the liver since the MCR reflects peripheral glucose metabolism and EGP reflects hepatic glucose production in fasted conditions. To our knowledge, no animal model was previously described which enables quantification of both anti-arthritic efficacy and longitudinal tissue-specific metabolic adverse effects in one animal in one chronic treatment protocol. In the field of GCs and the search for compounds with improved efficacy/safety profiles (SGRMs), such a model is of great value since it closely mimics the clinical RA practice. Interestingly, our results show that the overall effects of prednisolone on glucose kinetics were similar in both arthritic and non-arthritic animals indicating that the disease state in this model did not influence regulation of glucose homeostasis.

One reason to include both non-arthritic and arthritic mice in this study was to be able to distinguish between inflammation-induced and GC-induced metabolic dysfunction. Our results showed that arthritic mice produce less insulin than non-arthritic mice after treatment with placebo. It is known that arthritic mice have elevated circulating levels of the pro-inflammatory cytokines TNFα and IL-1β [14]. Proinflammatory cytokines have been shown to induce beta cell dysfunction [29]. In addition, chronic inflammation may reduce beta cell mass by stimulating apoptosis of beta cells [30]. Also factors related to the disease status may play a role in the difference in C-peptide production between arthritic and non-arthritic mice. For example, mice suffering from arthritis eat less and have to be more efficient with energy which might affect glucose metabolism. Nonetheless, based upon the fact that glucose concentrations did not change, the untreated arthritic mice in our study were still able to compensate for the inflammation-induced reduction of insulin secretion. Both severely arthritic mice and mice treated with a high dose of prednisolone are able to compensate for reduced insulin secretion and reduced insulin sensitivity respectively by keeping the MCR steady and even reduce EGP, which indicates a highly adaptive compensatory mechanism in both groups of mice.

Regarding GC-induced insulin resistance in mice, many conflicting results have been reported [27,31–38]. Also the results described in this paper show discrepancies in results when compared to previously reported studies. For instance, we report a minimal decrease in glucose levels after treatment with prednisolone whereas other studies reported an increase of glucose levels after treatment with glucocorticoids [27,31–34]. One reason explaining (at least partly) these differences in results is that different strains of mice were used. We used DBA1/J mice since this strain showed to be highly susceptible for inducing collagen-induced arthritis [39]. However, most studies use C57BL/6 mice to investigate GC-induced insulin resistance [27,36–38,40] and DBA1/J mice are hardly ever used in diabetic or metabolic model systems. Other reasons for differences in results between studies might be explained by differences in study design (e.g. fasting conditions), administered dose, treatment duration and/or route of administration.

In humans, GCs are well known to negatively affect glucose metabolism. Short-term clinical trials in healthy individuals have shown that GCs reduce hepatic and peripheral insulin sensitivity [5] and impair beta cell function [41]. Population-based studies showed that GC use was associated, in a cumulative dose-dependent manner, with the incidence of diabetes [42]. However, studies investigating the metabolic effects of GCs in RA patients yielded conflicting results. On the one hand, in cross-sectional studies in RA patients showed that GC exposure was related to impaired fasting insulin sensitivity [43] and tended to predict development of type 2 diabetes [44,45]. On the other hand, the use of GCs by patients with chronic inflammatory conditions may improve glucose tolerance via anti-inflammatory effects, as has been demonstrated in a number of studies [46,47]. Our results regarding glucose and C-peptide levels are in line with the results reported by den Uyl and co-workers. These authors investigated the dose-related effects of short-term GC treatment on glucose tolerance, beta cell function and insulin sensitivity in patients with early active RA. They showed that fasting C-peptide levels increased significantly after treatment with prednisolone while fasting glucose levels did not change [48]. These results regarding C-peptide and glucose levels are also observed in our experiments, indicating reduced insulin sensitivity. However, both the non-arthritic and arthritic mice were, after 21 days of prednisolone treatment, still able to compensate for their prednisolone-induced reduction in insulin sensitivity, resulting ultimately in no change in blood glucose concentrations. Most likely, the treatment period (3 weeks) in this combined model is too short to study a next stage in the development of diabetes, *i.e.*, hyperglycemia and beta-cell dysfunction. These results, together with the results reported by den Uyl and coworkers point to a delicate balance between the anti-inflammatory and diabetogenic effects in which dose and duration of GC treatment are crucial. Further studies will be needed to challenge this.

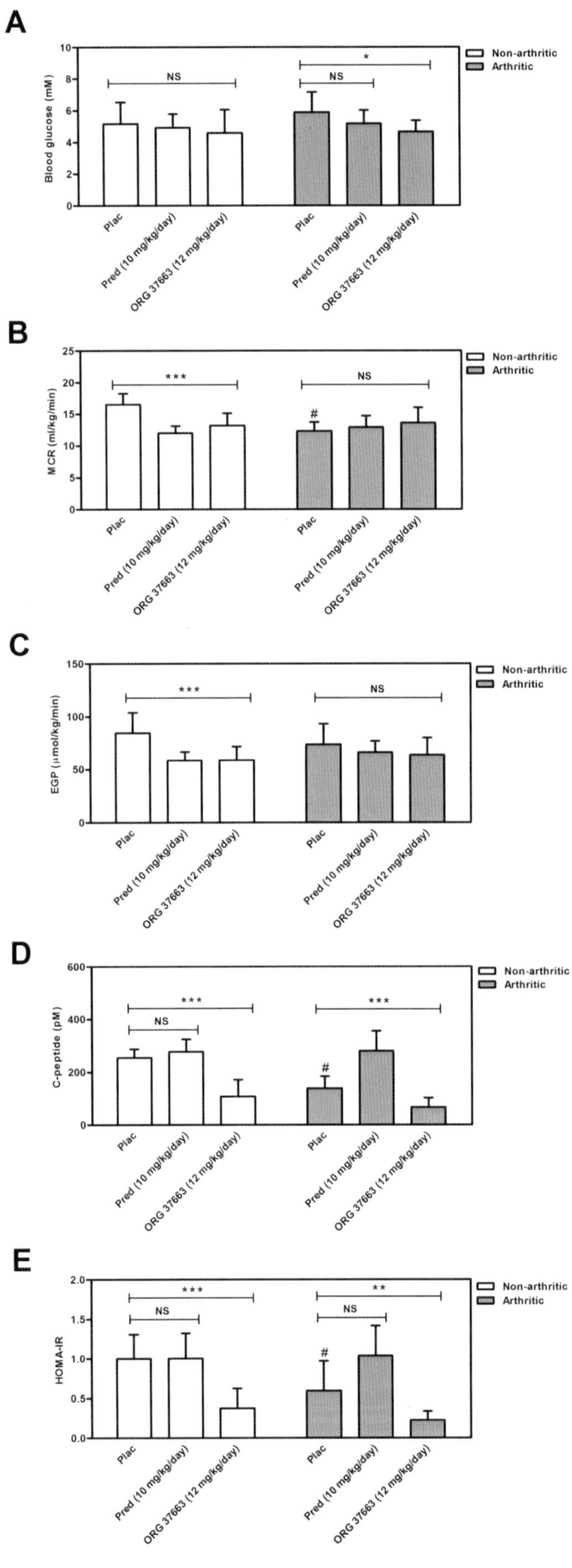
A
Blood glucose (mM)
Non-arthritic
Arthritic
NS
*
NS
Plac
Pred (10 mg/kg/day)
ORG 37663 (12 mg/kg/day)
B
MCR (ml/kg/min)
***
NS
#
C
EGP (μmol/kg/min)
***
NS
D
C-peptide (pM)
***
NS
***
#
E
HOMA-IR
***
NS
**
NS
#

Figure 6. Effects of ORG 37663 and prednisolone on glucose kinetics after 21 days of treatment. (**A**) Blood glucose concentrations (**B**) MCR (**C**) EGP levels (**D**) C-peptide concentrations (**E**) C-peptide HOMA-IR. Results represent means ± SD and are outlined for each experimental group (n = 12). * Significant difference p≤0.05, ** significant difference p≤0.01, *** significant difference p≤0.001, #significant difference (p≤0.05) when compared to the placebo-treated non-arthritic mice, NS = not significant.

To be able to study to what extent the effects of prednisolone on glucose kinetics are due to its anti-inflammatory properties or due to a direct effect on glucose kinetics, mice were also treated with ORG 37663, a non-GC anti-inflammatory compound, and directly compared to prednisolone. This compound was chosen because of its strong anti-inflammatory effects that are not mediated through the GR. Although it is reported that this compound lacks anti-rheumatic activity in humans [49], Dulos and co-workers showed that treatment with ORG 37663 suppressed clinical arthritis score, reduced inflammatory infiltrates and decreased pro-inflammatory cytokines in collagen-induced arthritis mice [6]. Also our own data showed that the clinical arthritis score was strongly decreased after treatment with this compound. Therefore, we believe that this compound is suitable to compare GR- and non-GR-mediated effects in this in-vivo model. Treatment with ORG 37663 resulted in lower C-peptide concentrations when compared to prednisolone treatment in both non-arthritic and arthritic mice. This indicates that prednisolone mediates its effects on insulin production directly and not via indirect anti-inflammatory effects. However, the effects on glucose kinetics (MCR) and metabolism (EGP) seem to be due to the anti-inflammatory activity of prednisolone as treatment with another (non-GR agonistic) anti-inflammaroy drug (ORG 37663) showed the same effects. However, ORG 37663 also influenced glucose kinetics in non-arthritic mice, decreasing C-peptide levels. This indicate that the observed effects of ORG 37663 are not only mediated indirectly by suppressing inflammation but might also by directly influencing glucose kinetic pathways.

To conclude, we successfully integrated the whole body glucose test in the CIA mice model, which enabled us to measure both efficacy and metabolic (adverse) effects of (experimental) GCs in a chronic *in vivo* inflammatory setting. Thereby, it may prove a useful translational model for compound-induced metabolic derangements in patients suffering from RA or other (auto)immune diseases. This study showed that both inflammation and glucocorticoids affect insulin secretion and sensitivity but this did not lead immediately to the development of hyperglycemia and type 2 Diabetes Mellitus. Data from this study emphasizes the highly adaptive character of these mice and the complex network of several integrated mechanisms underlying the development of GC-induced and/or inflammation-induced metabolic dysfunction.

Acknowledgments

We would like to thank Monique Helsen and Birgitte Walgreen of the department of Experimental Rheumatology of the Radboudumc for their help during the CIA experiments in Nijmegen. This research was performed within the framework of project T1-106 of the Dutch Top Institute Pharma.

Author Contributions

Conceived and designed the experiments: ET AL AG MVDV MJVL AKG WD. Performed the experiments: ET AL AG AB AS EB CVD MVDV DB. Analyzed the data: ET AL TVD AG MJVL AKG WD. Contributed reagents/materials/analysis tools: MK. Wrote the paper: ET AL AKG WD.

References

1. Hillier SG (2007) Diamonds are forever: the cortisone legacy. JEndocrinol 195: 1–6.
2. Rhen T, Cidlowski JA (2005) Antiinflammatory action of glucocorticoids—new mechanisms for old drugs. NEnglJMed 353: 1711–1723.
3. Schacke H, Docke WD, Asadullah K (2002) Mechanisms involved in the side effects of glucocorticoids. PharmacolTher 96: 23–43.
4. Schacke H, Berger M, Rehwinkel H, Asadullah K (2007) Selective glucocorticoid receptor agonists (SEGRAs): novel ligands with an improved therapeutic index. MolCell Endocrinol 275: 109–117.
5. van Raalte DH, Ouwens DM, Diamant M (2009) Novel insights into glucocorticoid-mediated diabetogenic effects: towards expansion of therapeutic options? EurJClinInvest 39: 81–93.
6. Dulos J, Vijn P, van Doorn C, Hofstra CL, Veening-Griffioen D, et al. (2010) Suppression of the inflammatory response in experimental arthritis is mediated via estrogen receptor alpha but not estrogen receptor beta. Arthritis ResTher 12: R101.
7. Thompson CS (2008) Animal models of diabetes mellitus: relevance to vascular complications. CurrPharmDes 14: 309–324.
8. Miner JN, Ardecky B, Benbatoul K, Griffiths K, Larson CJ, et al. (2007) Antiinflammatory glucocorticoid receptor ligand with reduced side effects exhibits an altered protein-protein interaction profile. ProcNatlAcadSciUSA 104: 19244–19249.
9. Hwang J, Rodgers K, Oliver JC, Schluep T (2008) Alpha-methylprednisolone conjugated cyclodextrin polymer-based nanoparticles for rheumatoid arthritis therapy. IntJNanomedicine 3: 359–371.
10. Courtenay JS, Dallman MJ, Dayan AD, Martin A, Mosedale B (1980) Immunisation against heterologous type II collagen induces arthritis in mice. Nature 283: 666–668.
11. Stuart JM, Townes AS, Kang AH (1982) Nature and specificity of the immune response to collagen in type II collagen-induced arthritis in mice. JClinInvest 69: 673–683.
12. Monzillo LU, Hamdy O (2003) Evaluation of insulin sensitivity in clinical practice and in research settings. NutrRev 61: 397–412.
13. van Dijk TH, Laskewitz AJ, Grefhorst A, Boer TS, Bloks VW, et al. (2013) A novel approach to monitor glucose metabolism using stable isotopically labelled glucose in longitudinal studies in mice. Lab Anim.
14. Joosten LA, Helsen MM, van de Loo FA, van den Berg WB (2008) Anticytokine treatment of established type II collagen-induced arthritis in DBA/1 mice: a comparative study using anti-TNFalpha, anti-IL-1alpha/beta and IL-1Ra. Arthritis Rheum 58: S110–S122.
15. Dulos J, Verbraak E, Bagchus WM, Boots AM, Kaptein A (2004) Severity of murine collagen-induced arthritis correlates with increased CYP7B activity: enhancement of dehydroepiandrosterone metabolism by interleukin-1beta. Arthritis Rheum 50: 3346–3353.
16. Joosten LA, Helsen MM, Saxne T, van de Loo FA, Heinegard D, et al. (1999) IL-1 alpha beta blockade prevents cartilage and bone destruction in murine type II collagen-induced arthritis, whereas TNF-alpha blockade only ameliorates joint inflammation. JImmunol 163: 5049–5055.
17. van Dijk TH, Boer TS, Havinga R, Stellaard F, Kuipers F, et al. (2003) Quantification of hepatic carbohydrate metabolism in conscious mice using serial blood and urine spots. AnalBiochem 322: 1–13.
18. Lee WN, Byerley LO, Bergner EA, Edmond J (1991) Mass isotopomer analysis: theoretical and practical considerations. BiolMass Spectrom 20: 451–458.
19. Ader M, Ni TC, Bergman RN (1997) Glucose effectiveness assessed under dynamic and steady state conditions. Comparability of uptake versus production components. JClinInvest 99: 1187–1199.
20. Best JD, Kahn SE, Ader M, Watanabe RM, Ni TC, et al. (1996) Role of glucose effectiveness in the determination of glucose tolerance. Diabetes Care 19: 1018–1030.
21. Pacini G, Thomaseth K, Ahren B (2001) Contribution to glucose tolerance of insulin-independent vs. insulin-dependent mechanisms in mice. AmJPhysiol EndocrinolMetab 281: E693–E703.
22. Matthews DR, Hosker JP, Rudenski AS, Naylor BA, Treacher DF, et al. (1985) Homeostasis model assessment: insulin resistance and beta-cell function from fasting plasma glucose and insulin concentrations in man. Diabetologia 28: 412–419.
23. Wallace TM, Levy JC, Matthews DR (2004) Use and abuse of HOMA modeling. Diabetes Care 27: 1487–1495.
24. Kokkola R, Li J, Sundberg E, Aveberger AC, Palmblad K, et al. (2003) Successful treatment of collagen-induced arthritis in mice and rats by targeting extracellular high mobility group box chromosomal protein 1 activity. Arthritis Rheum 48: 2052–2058.

25. Compton MM, Cidlowski JA (1986) Rapid in vivo effects of glucocorticoids on the integrity of rat lymphocyte genomic deoxyribonucleic acid. Endocrinology 118: 38–45.
26. DeFronzo RA, Tobin JD, Andres R (1979) Glucose clamp technique: a method for quantifying insulin secretion and resistance. AmJPhysiol 237: E214–E223.
27. Laskewitz AJ, van Dijk TH, Bloks VW, Reijngoud DJ, van Lierop MJ, et al. (2010) Chronic prednisolone treatment reduces hepatic insulin sensitivity while perturbing the fed-to-fasting transition in mice. Endocrinology 151: 2171–2178.
28. Muniyappa R, Lee S, Chen H, Quon MJ (2008) Current approaches for assessing insulin sensitivity and resistance in vivo: advantages, limitations, and appropriate usage. AmJPhysiol EndocrinolMetab 294: E15–E26.
29. Donath MY, Boni-Schnetzler M, Ellingsgaard H, Ehses JA (2009) Islet inflammation impairs the pancreatic beta-cell in type 2 diabetes. Physiology(-Bethesda) 24: 325–331.
30. Gurzov EN, Germano CM, Cunha DA, Ortis F, Vanderwinden JM, et al. (2010) p53 up-regulated modulator of apoptosis (PUMA) activation contributes to pancreatic beta-cell apoptosis induced by proinflammatory cytokines and endoplasmic reticulum stress. JBiolChem 285: 19910–19920.
31. Thomas CR, Turner SL, Jefferson WH, Bailey CJ (1998) Prevention of dexamethasone-induced insulin resistance by metformin. BiochemPharmacol 56: 1145–1150.
32. Yen TT, Gill AM, Powell JG, Sampson BM (1992) Ciglitazone prevents and reverses dexamethasone-induced hyperglycemia in female viable yellow mice. IntJObesRelat Metab Disord 16: 923–933.
33. Gill AM, Leiter EH, Powell JG, Chapman HD, Yen TT (1994) Dexamethasone-induced hyperglycemia in obese Avy/a (viable yellow) female mice entails preferential induction of a hepatic estrogen sulfotransferase. Diabetes 43: 999–1004.
34. Bernal-Mizrachi C, Weng S, Feng C, Finck BN, Knutsen RH, et al. (2003) Dexamethasone induction of hypertension and diabetes is PPAR-alpha dependent in LDL receptor-null mice. NatMed 9: 1069–1075.
35. Bergman RN, Prager R, Volund A, Olefsky JM (1987) Equivalence of the insulin sensitivity index in man derived by the minimal model method and the euglycemic glucose clamp. JClinInvest 79: 790–800.
36. Gounarides JS, Korach-Andre M, Killary K, Argentieri G, Turner O, et al. (2008) Effect of dexamethasone on glucose tolerance and fat metabolism in a diet-induced obesity mouse model. Endocrinology 149: 758–766.
37. Orland MJ, Permutt MA (1987) Genetic susceptibility to diabetes in inbred strains of mice: measurements of proinsulin mRNA and response to dexamethasone. Diabetologia 30: 934–939.
38. Zhao R, Fuentes-Mattei E, Velazquez-Torres G, Su CH, Chen J, et al. (2011) Exenatide improves glucocorticoid-induced glucose intolerance in mice. Diabetes Metab SyndrObes 4: 61–65.
39. Myers LK, Rosloniec EF, Cremer MA, Kang AH (1997) Collagen-induced arthritis, an animal model of autoimmunity. Life Sci 61: 1861–1878.
40. Clee SM, Attie AD (2007) The genetic landscape of type 2 diabetes in mice. EndocrRev 28: 48–83.
41. van Raalte DH, Nofrate V, Bunck M, van Iersel T, Elassaiss SJ, et al. (2010) Acute and two-week exposure to prednisolone impair different aspects of beta-cell function in healthy men. EurJEndocrinol 162: 729–735.
42. Gulliford MC, Charlton J, Latinovic R (2006) Risk of diabetes associated with prescribed glucocorticoids in a large population. Diabetes Care 29: 2728–2729.
43. Dessein PH, Joffe BI, Stanwix AE, Christian BF, Veller M (2004) Glucocorticoids and insulin sensitivity in rheumatoid arthritis. JRheumatol 31: 867–874.
44. Wolfe F, Michaud K (2004) Severe rheumatoid arthritis (RA), worse outcomes, comorbid illness, and sociodemographic disadvantage characterize ra patients with fibromyalgia. JRheumatol 31: 695–700.
45. van Tuyl LH, Boers M, Lems WF, Landewe RB, Han H, et al. (2010) Survival, comorbidities and joint damage 11 years after the COBRA combination therapy trial in early rheumatoid arthritis. AnnRheumDis 69: 807–812.
46. Svenson KL, Lundqvist G, Wide L, Hallgren R (1987) Impaired glucose handling in active rheumatoid arthritis: effects of corticosteroids and antirheumatic treatment. Metabolism 36: 944–948.
47. Hallgren R, Berne C (1983) Glucose intolerance in patients with chronic inflammatory diseases is normalized by glucocorticoids. Acta MedScand 213: 351–355.
48. den UD, van Raalte DH, Nurmohamed MT, Lems WF, Bijlsma JW, et al. (2012) Metabolic effects of high-dose prednisolone treatment in early rheumatoid arthritis: Balance between diabetogenic effects and inflammation reduction. Arthritis Rheum 64: 639–646.

7

Relationship of Adipocyte Size with Adiposity and Metabolic Risk Factors

Ved Prakash Meena[1], V. Seenu[2], M. C. Sharma[3], Saumya Ranjan Mallick[3], Ashu Seith Bhalla[4], Nandita Gupta[5], Anant Mohan[6], Randeep Guleria[6], Ravindra M. Pandey[7], Kalpana Luthra[8], Naval K. Vikram[1]*

1 Department of Medicine, All India Institute of Medical Sciences, New Delhi, India, **2** Department of Surgical Disciplines, All India Institute of Medical Sciences, New Delhi, India, **3** Department of Pathology, All India Institute of Medical Sciences, New Delhi, India, **4** Department of Radiodiagnosis, All India Institute of Medical Sciences, New Delhi, India, **5** Department of Endocrinology and Metabolism, All India Institute of Medical Sciences, New Delhi, India, **6** Departments of Pulmonary Medicine and Sleep Disorders, All India Institute of Medical Sciences, New Delhi, India, **7** Department of Biostatistics, All India Institute of Medical Sciences, New Delhi, India, **8** Department of Biochemistry, All India Institute of Medical Sciences, New Delhi, India

Abstract

Background: Enlargement of adipocyte is associated with their dysfunction and alterations in metabolic functions.

Objectives: We evaluated the association of adipocyte size of subcutaneous and omental adipose tissue with body composition and cardiovascular risk factors in Asian Indians.

Methodology: Eighty (40 males and 40 females) non-diabetic adult subjects undergoing elective abdominal surgery were included. Pre-surgery evaluation included anthropometric measurements, % body fat by bioimpedance, abdominal fat area at L_{2-3} level (computed tomography) and biochemical investigations (fasting blood glucose and insulin, lipids and hsCRP). During surgery, about 5 grams each of omental and subcutaneous adipose tissue was obtained for adipocyte size determination.

Results: Females had higher BMI, % body fat, skinfold thickness, total and subcutaneous abdominal fat area as compared to males. Overweight was present in 42.5% and 67.5%, and abdominal obesity in 5% and 52.5% males and females, respectively. Subcutaneous adipocyte size was significantly higher than omental adipocyte size. Omental adipocyte size correlated more strongly than subcutaneous adipocyte size with measures of adiposity (BMI, waist circumference, %BF), total and subcutaneous abdominal fat area and biochemical measures (fasting glucose, total cholesterol, triglycerides and HOMA-IR), the correlations being stronger in females. The correlation of adipocyte size with metabolic parameters was attenuated after adjusting for measures of adiposity.

Conclusion: Omental adipocyte size, though smaller than the subcutaneous adipocyte size, was more closely related to measures of adiposity and metabolic parameters. However, the relationship was not independent of measures of adiposity.

Editor: Luísa M. Seoane, Complexo Hospitalario Universitario de Santiago, Spain

Funding: The authors have no support or funding to report.

Competing Interests: The authors have declared that no competing interests exist.

* Email: navalvikram@gmail.com

Introduction

Obesity is a medical condition with accumulation of excess body fat adversely affecting health leading to reduced life expectancy and/or increased health problems. It may be defined as an abnormal growth of the adipose tissue due to an enlargement of fat cell size (hypertrophic obesity) or an increase in fat cell number (hyperplasic obesity) or a combination of both [1]. The prevalence of obesity, particularly abdominal obesity, is increasing rapidly all over the world, including developing countries [2]. Obesity increases the risk of various diseases, including cardiovascular disease, type 2 diabetes, sleep disordered breathing, certain types of cancer, and osteoarthritis [3]. Abdominal obesity is more closely related to insulin resistance, metabolic syndrome and type 2 diabetes [4].

Asian Indians have been shown to be more insulin resistant at any given body mass index (BMI) and are more likely to develop type 2 diabetes and cardiovascular disease as compared to their European counterparts [5,6]. Some unique phenotypic features among Asian Indians, such as increased body fat, abdominal and truncal adiposity may contribute to this increased insulin resistance [4,7]. These features appear to be present from birth as Indian neonates tend to have increased body fat compared to their white Caucasian counterparts despite lower birth weights [8]. These features have been referred to as the "Asian Indian Phenotype or Paradox".

Not all obese subjects develop metabolic abnormalities. Some observations indicate that being moderately overweight may actually be protective against mortality due to non-cancerous and non-cardiovascular cause and have lower mortality from cancer and cardiovascular disease (CVD) [9]. However, a recent systematic review indicates that metabolically healthy overweight and obese individuals may be at increased risk for adverse long-term outcomes [10]. The risk of development of abnormalities may be determined by the number and size of adipocytes (hyperplastic vs. hypertrophic obesity). In the presence of positive calorie balance, the mature adipocytes initially undergo enlargement, which acts as a trigger for recruitment and proliferation of preadipocytes to add more functional adipocytes [11,12,13]. If the process of adipogenesis is impaired after initial hypertrophy, it leads to adipose tissue metabolic and immunologic dysfunction [14,15].

Adipose tissue is not a mere depot for fat storage but is an active endocrine organ and secretes various adipocytokines which include adiponectin, leptin, resistin, and proinflammatory cytokines like tumor necrosis factor alpha (TNF-α) which modulate insulin sensitivity and related metabolic abnormalities. Enlargement of adipocyte is associated with substantial changes in metabolic functions [16]. Several reports have indicated that adipocyte size of the visceral and subcutaneous adipose tissue is associated with insulin resistance. In their study, Weyer *et al.* observed that large subcutaneous adipocytes predicted insulin resistance and type 2 diabetes, independent of obesity in those with normal glucose tolerance (NGT) [17]. Furthermore, In another study involving women, subcutaneous adipocyte size, particularly in the abdominal region, in addition to the amount and distribution of body fat, predicted incidence of type 2 diabetes in later life [18].

Majority of these studies have been conducted on populations other than Asian Indians and a few studies have included migrant Asian Indians. A study involving migrant Asian Indians indicated that subcutaneous fat is a better determinant of insulin resistance than visceral fat [19]. There is paucity of data on Asian Indians from India in this regard. Therefore the present study aimed to evaluate the association of adipocyte size of subcutaneous and omental adipose tissue with body composition, insulin resistance and subclinical inflammation in non-diabetic adult Asian Indian subjects.

Materials and Methods

Study population

This cross-sectional study was undertaken in the Department of Medicine, All India Institute of Medical Sciences, New Delhi, India from 2010 to 2012. The study was approved by the Institutional Ethics Committee of All India Institute of Medical Sciences, New Delhi, and written informed consent was obtained from subjects prior to inclusion in the study. Eighty adult subjects (40 males and 40 females) in the age group of 20–60 years, undergoing elective abdominal surgery in the General Surgery Department of the institute were included in the study. Exclusion criteria included any known malignancy, known seropositivity for HIV, HBV or HCV, any severe acute or chronic medical or surgical illness, pregnancy and lactation.

Measurements

Anthropometry and Biochemical parameters. Subjects underwent detailed clinical evaluation before surgery including detailed clinical history, physical examination and anthropometric measurements (height, weight, body mass index [BMI], waist (WC) and hip (HC) circumferences, waist to hip circumference ratio (WHR) mid-arm and mid-thigh circumferences and skinfold thickness measurements) according to the methods mentioned elsewhere [20]. A venous blood sample was obtained after an overnight fast of at least 10 hours. Biochemical measurements included fasting blood glucose (FBG), total cholesterol (TC), triglycerides (TG), high density lipoprotein cholesterol (HDL-c) and hsCRP levels (using ELISA) performed according to the methods described earlier [20]. Value of low density lipoprotein cholesterol (LDL-c) was calculated using Freidewald's equation [21]. Fasting insulin levels were measured using an eletrochemieluminometric assay on a Roche ELECSYS e411 auto analyser.

Percentage body fat and abdominal fat. Percentage body fat was measured by bioelectrical impedance method (TANITA CORP, JAPAN). Abdominal fat area (cm^2) was determined by computed tomography scan at the level of L_{2-3}. Total (TAF), subcutaneous (SAF) and visceral (VAF) abdominal fat area was measured in L_{2-3} slice by mapping various adipose tissue compartments on the computer screen using a track-ball.

Adipocyte size measurement. In patients who underwent cholecystectomy, subcutaneous (SC) adipose tissue was obtained through a 1 cm transverse incision given about 2 cm below the xiphisternum in the epigastric region to the right of midline. In patients undergoing incisional hernia repair, subcutaneous adipose tissue was obtained through a 1 cm transverse incision given about 2 cm below the umbilicus to the right of midline. Omental (OM) adipose tissue was obtained from the free edge of the greater omentum in all the patients. At the time of surgery, about 5 grams of each OM and SC adipose tissue was obtained and was fixed in 10% neutral buffered formalin. Subsequently, it was routinely processed and 5 μm thick sections were cut and stained with haematoxylin and eosin. Microphotographs were captured at 200 magnification using DP 70 digital camera with Olympus BX51 microscope (M/S –Japan). The images were processed with image pro plus software (image proplus version 7, mediacybernetics USA). Fifty non-overlaping adipocytes were traced in semiautomatic manner. Area and maximum diameter were calculated and the data was transported to Microsoft excel. In about 20% of samples there were less than 100 non-overlapping adipocytes for morphometric analysis, therefore for uniformity, 50 non-overlapping adipocytes were taken for measurements. Furthermore, comparison of adipocyte measurements (mean area and diameter) obtained by analyzing 100 adipocytes versus 50 adipocytes in the same individual did not reveal any significant difference.

Definitions

Overweight was defined as BMI$\geq$23 kg/m^2 [22]. Abdominal obesity was defined as WC>90 cm in males and>80 cm in females [23]. Dyslipidemias were defined as per the criteria of National Cholesterol Education Program, Adult Treatment Panel III (NCEP, ATP III) [24]. The metabolic syndrome was defined as the presence of at least three of the following abnormalities: FBG$\geq$ 100 mg/dL, central obesity (as defined by WC>90 cm in males and>80 cm in females), hypertriglyceridemia (TG$\geq$150 mg/dL), low HDL-c (<40 mg/dL in males and <50 mg/dL in females) and blood pressure $\geq$130/85 mmHg [25]. Impaired fasting glucose (IFG) was defined as FBG 100 to125 mg/dL. High levels of hs-CRP were defined as>3 mg/L [26]. Hyperinsulinemia was defined as levels>10.4 μU/mL. Insulin resistance was determined by the homeostatic model assessment (HOMA-IR) method (fasting glucose [mmol]×fasting insulin [μU/mL]/22.5) [27]. A value of HOMA-IR>2.29 was defined as high indicating insulin resistance [28].

Statistical analysis

Comparison of normally distributed variables among male and female subjects was done by student's 't' test. Comparison of non-normally distributed variables was done by using Wilcoxon ranksum test. Correlations of omental and subcutaneous adipocyte size with body composition and metabolic parameters were evaluated by Spearman's Ranksum correlation coefficient. Multivariate regression analysis was performed to assess whether adipocyte size is correlated with metabolic parameters independent of body composition. Statistical analysis was performed using STATA software (version 9; StataCorp, College Station, TX) and a P value<0.05 was taken as statistically significant.

Results

A total of 132 patients were screened during the time period of June 2010 to May 2012, out of which 80 patients fulfilled the criteria of the study and were included. Out of these, 73 patients were having gall stone disease and 7 patients were having incisional hernia. Fifty two patients were excluded due to malignancy, diabetes mellitus, existing coronary artery disease, liver or kidney disease and 13 patients didn't give consent.

Clinical, anthropometric, body fat and biochemical characteristics (Table 1)

Females were older, had higher BMI, HC and skinfold thickness than males. Mean values of systolic and diastolic blood pressures were comparable among males and females. Mean values of FBG, TC and HDL-c were significantly higher in females as compared to males, whereas serum levels of TG were significantly higher in males. Values of fasting insulin, hsCRP and HOMA-IR were comparable in both males and females (Table 1). Percentage body fat, TAF and SAF were higher in females as compared to males, whereas VAF area was comparable in both genders. The size of adipocytes from SC adipose tissue was greater (59.6 ± 5.10 vs. 54.6 ± 4.4, $p<0.01$) than adipocytes from OM adipose tissue, with no significant difference among the genders.

Prevalence of abnormalities

Overweight was present in 42.5% males and 67.5% females ($p=0.02$) whereas abdominal obesity was present in 5% males and 52.5% females ($p<0.001$). Prevalence of hypertension was comparable in both genders (20% and 25%, p = NS). Among the biochemical abnormalities, IFG was more prevalent in females than males (10% vs. 5%, $p=0.01$). Prevalence of hypercholesterolemia (2.5% and 7.5%), hypertriglyceridemia (32.5 and 20%), low HDL-c (12.5% and 10%), high hsCRP (20% and 27.5%), high HOMA-IR (30% and 35%) and metabolic syndrome (12.5% and 27.5%) were comparable in males and females, respectively.

Correlation of abdominal fat depots with biochemical parameters (Table 2)

Total and subcutaneous abdominal fat area correlated significantly with BMI, WC, WHR and %BF in both males and females, the correlations being stronger in females. Visceral abdominal fat area correlated with BMI, WC, WHR and % BF only in males. Total abdominal fat area correlated significantly with FBG, TC, TG, fasting insulin and HOMA-IR in both genders, with hsCRP and LDL-c only in females, and correlated inversely with HDL-c only in males. Visceral abdominal fat area correlated positively with TG and inversely with HDL-c only in males. Subcutaneous abdominal fat area correlated with FBG, TC, TG, fasting insulin and HOMA-IR in both genders, with hsCRP and LDL-c only in females and inversely with HDL-c only in males.

Correlation of adipocyte size with anthropometric and biochemical parameters

Table 3 is showing the correlation of various anthropometric and biochemical parameters with the diameter of SC and OM adipocytes. In males, BMI and WHR correlated significantly with OM adipocyte size, whereas %BF correlated significantly with both SC and OM adipocyte size. All the skinfold thicknesses correlated significantly with adipocyte size of both depots, but the correlations with OM adipocyte size were stronger. Total, subcutaneous and visceral abdominal fat area showed significant correlations with adipocyte size from both the depots. Among the biochemical parameters, only TG, insulin levels and HOMA-IR correlated significantly with OM adipocyte size.

In females, adipocyte diameters of both adipose depots showed significant correlation with BMI, WC, WHR, %BF, TAF and SAF, the correlations being stronger with OM adipocyte diameter, except for %BF. Among the skinfolds, only biceps skinfold thickness correlated with OM adipocyte diameter. Among the biochemical parameters, levels of FBG, TC, TG, insulin and HOMA-IR correlated significantly with both SC and OM adipocyte diameter (correlations of TC and TG being stronger with OM adipocyte size), whereas LDL-c levels correlated significantly only with OM adipocyte diameter. The size of adipocytes from both the abdominal fat depots was significantly higher in subjects who had metabolic syndrome as compared to those without it.

Regression analysis

Regression analysis was performed to evaluate the influence of increase in adipocyte size of both adipose tissue depots on the biochemical parameters. In females, one unit increase in SC adipocyte size was associated with increase in 1.13 units of FBG ($p=0.007$, 95% CI: 0.33–1.93), 3.34 units of TC ($p=0.001$, 95% CI: 1.38–5.30), 1.90 units of TG ($p=0.01$, 95% CI: 0.35–3.45), 0.13 units of fasting insulin ($p<0.001$, 95% CI: 0.07–0.19) and 0.14 units of HOMA-IR ($p<0.001$, 95% CI: 0.07–0.21). After adjusting for age, BMI, %BF, WC, TAF and SAF, only the relationship with fasting insulin (regression coefficient 0.09, $p=0.03$, 95% CI: 0.008–0.17) and HOMA-IR (regression coefficient 0.10, $p=0.03$, 95% CI: 0.008–0.19) remained significant whereas the relationship with FBG (regression coefficient 0.71), TC (regression coefficient 1.10) and TG (regression coefficient 0.36) became nonsignificant. In males, one unit increase in OM adipocyte size was associated with increase in 2.0 units of TC ($p=0.05$, 95% CI: −0.44–4.02) and 4.0 units of TG ($p<0.001$, 95% CI: 2.10–5.99). This relationship was attenuated after adjusting for age, BMI, %BF, WC, TAF and SAF (TC regression coefficient 0.93, TG regression coefficient 1.73). In females, one unit increase in OM adipocyte size was associated with an increase of 1.3 units of FBG ($p=0.007$, 95% CI: 0.38–2.24), 5.4 units of TC ($p<0.001$, 95% CI: 3.52–7.33), 2.90 units of TG ($p=0.001$, 95% CI: 1.20–4.59), 0.15 units of fasting insulin ($p<0.001$, 95% CI: 0.07–0.22) and 0.16 units of HOMA-IR ($p<0.001$, 95% CI: 0.08–0.24). After adjusting for age, BMI, %BF, WC, TAF and SAF, these relationships were attenuated (FBG regression coefficient −0.26, TC regression coefficient 2.28, TG regression coefficient 0.83, fasting insulin regression coefficient 0.04 and HOMA-IR regression coefficient 0.04).

Table 1. Clinical, anthropometric, body composition and biochemical characteristics.

Parameter	Male (n = 40)	Female (n = 40)	P value
Age (yrs.)	39.1±10.1 (25.9)	43.6±13.1 (30.0)	0.08
Systolic blood pressure (mm Hg)	122.2±5.9 (4.8)	124.7±6.9 (5.6)	0.09
Diastolic blood pressure (mm Hg)	80.9±3.5 (4.4)	80.1±4.7 (5.9)	0.41
Anthropometric and body composition characteristics			
Height (cm)	169.8±5.4 (3.2)	154.1±5.0 (3.2)	<0.001
Weight (kg)	64.1±7.4 (11.6)	60.2±9.7 (16.1)	0.04
Body mass index (kg/m^2)	22.2±2.7 (12.1)	25.6±4.5 (17.6)	<0.001
Waist circumference (cm)	80.2±6.3 (7.9)	82.3±9.2 (11.2)	0.22
Hip circumference (cm)	88.7±5.1 (5.7)	100.2±5.5 (5.6)	<0.001
Waist-to-hip ratio	0.90±.05 (5.9)	0.81±.05 (7.1)	<0.001
Biceps skinfold (mm)	7.7±2.1 (27.3)	11.0±3.2 (29.0)	<0.001
Triceps skinfold (mm)	10.5±2.8 (27.2)	19.0±4 (21.0)	<0.001
Subscapular skinfold (mm)	12.6±4.0 (32.4)	23.6±5.9 (20.9)	<0.001
Suprailiac skinfold (mm)	13.1±3.6 (27.8)	24.5±5.0 (20.5)	<0.001
Fat mass (kg)	11.4±4.7 (40.9)	20.6±5.7 (27.8)	<0.001
% Body fat	17.4±6.0 (34.4)	33.7±4.7 (14.1)	<0.001
Fat free mass (kg)	52.6±4.6 (8.9)	39.4±4.4 (11.2)	<0.001
Total abdominal fat (cm^2)	209±68.6 (32.8)	331.3±56.5 (17.1)	<0.001
Visceral abdominal fat (cm^2)	119.9±37.2 (31.1)	118.3±33.0 (27.9)	0.84
Subcutaneous abdominal fat (cm^2)	72 (56, 117.5)*	197 (167, 261)*	<0.001
Subcutaneous adipocyte size (μm)	59.3±5.08 (8.5)	59.8±5.18 (8.66)	0.66
Omental adipocyte size (μm)	54.8±4.4 (8.0)	54.4±4.46 (8.2)	0.72
Biochemical parameters			
Fasting blood glucose (mg/dL)	82.0±8.2 (10.1)	87.8±13.9 (15.9)	0.02
Total cholesterol (mg/dL)	129.2±28.6 (22.2)	148.4±35.4 (23.9)	0.01
Serum triglycerides (mg/dL)	143.0±31.5 (22.0)	128.9±26.4 (20.5)	0.03
High density lipoprotein cholesterol (mg/dL)	39.1±5.1 (13.1)	49.9±6.3 (12.8)	<0.001
Low density lipoprotein cholesterol (mg/dL)	90.5±29.0 (33.0)	98.8±24.4 (24.7)	0.17
Fasting insulin(μU/mL)*	6.40 (3.59,16.03)	8.12 (3.83, 16.62)	0.36
HOMA-IR*	1.29 (0.68, 3.14)	1.61 (0.75, 3.80)	0.33
hsCRP (mg/L)*	1.0 (0.67, 2.3)	1.55 (0.9, 3.5)	0.11

Values in mean±SD (coefficient of variation);
* mean (interquartile range).
HOMA-IR: Homeostatic model of assessment-insulin resistance; hsCRP: high sensitivity C-reactive protein.

Discussion

The observations of this study involving adult Asian Indians from India indicates that OM adipocyte size correlates more strongly with measures of generalised and abdominal obesity, abdominal fat compartments and metabolic alterations than SC adipocyte size.

A growing body of evidence suggests that variation in adipocyte size occurring in obesity has impact on adipose tissue function [29] [30]. Adipocyte hypertrophy leads to its dysfunction and reduced triglyceride storage which in turn promotes overflow of fatty acids to visceral fat and liver [7]. In addition, adiponectin secretion is reduced with increased pro-inflammatory cytokine secretion [31]. Earlier studies investigating this have included only the influence of SC adipocyte size on metabolic parameters. This may be due to the relative ease of obtaining SC adipose tissue.

There is paucity of data comparing the influence of OM and SC adipocyte size on metabolic alterations, and there are no studies performed in Asian Indians from India, to the best of our knowledge. A comparison of South Asian and Caucasian men showed that abdominal SC adipocyte size was significantly larger in South Asians and it inversely correlated with glucose disposal rate and adiponectin levels. This relationship persisted even after adjusting for SC abdominal fat mass [19]. Observations of another study comparing healthy South Asians and Caucasians revealed that South Asians had relatively higher amount of deep SC and visceral fat compared to Caucasians along with larger adipocytes [32]. Interestingly, the differences in fasting insulin, HDL-c and adiponectin levels among the two ethnic groups were not altered after adjusting for body fat distribution, but were attenuated after adjusting for adipocyte area.

In our study, a clear gender difference in the correlations of adipocyte with anthropometric and biochemical was observed. The correlations of TC, TG and LDL-c were stronger with OM than SC adipocyte size in both genders, the correlations being

Table 2. Spearman correlation analysis of anthropometric and biochemical parameters with abdominal fat depots.

Parameter	Total abdominal fat (Rho)		Visceral abdominal fat (Rho)		Subcutaneous abdominal fat (Rho)	
	Males (n = 40)	Females (n = 40)	Males (n = 40)	Females (n = 40)	Males (n = 40)	Females (n = 40)
Body mass index	0.56[c]	0.85[c]	0.32[a]	0.26	0.55[c]	0.81[c]
Waist circumference	0.70[c]	0.91[c]	0.59[c]	0.25	0.46[b]	0.83[c]
Waist-to-hip ratio	0.65[c]	0.84[c]	0.44[b]	0.21	0.61c	0.80[c]
% Body fat	0.54[c]	0.90[c]	0.40[a]	0.28	0.50[c]	0.81[c]
Fasting blood glucose	0.43[b]	0.50[b]	0.18	−0.01	0.44[b]	0.51[b]
Total cholesterol	0.46[b]	0.56[b]	0.21	−0.12	0.42[b]	0.62[b]
Triglycerides	0.60[c]	0.55[b]	0.38[a]	−0.05	0.62[b]	0.60[b]
High-density lipoprotein cholesterol	−0.52[b]	−0.18	−0.62[b]	−0.09	−0.33[a]	−0.09
Low-density lipoprotein cholesterol	−0.01	0.31[a]	−0.05	−0.24	0.03	0.45[b]
Fasting insulin	0.55[b]	0.59[b]	0.16	0.007	0.65[b]	0.37[b]
hsCRP	0.01	0.38[a]	0.11	0.10	−0.08	0.40[a]
HOMA-IR	0.54[b]	0.58[b]	0.16	−0.01	0.64[b]	0.57[b]

[a]: $p<0.05$;
[b]$p<0.01$;
[c]: $p<0.001$.
hsCRP: high sensitivity C-reactive protein; HOMA-IR: Homeostatic model of assessment-insulin resistance.

stronger in females. These observations are similar to an earlier study which concluded that OM adipose tissue cellularity was important predictor of hypertriglyceridemia in women. An enlargement and increase in number of OM adipocytes by 10% was associated with increased risk of hypertriglyceridemia by four times and 1.5 times, respectively. The association between OM

Table 3. Spearman correlation analysis of anthropometric and biochemical parameters with adipocyte size.

Parameter	Subcutaneous adipocyte diameter		Omental adipocyte diameter	
	Males (n = 40)	Females (n = 40)	Males (n = 40)	Females (n = 40)
Body mass index	0.20	0.48[b]	0.35[a]	0.50[c]
Waist circumference	0.11	0.41[b]	0.22	0.61[c]
Waist-to-hip ratio	0.28	0.42[b]	0.36[a]	0.48[b]
Biceps skinfold	0.35[a]	0.18	0.44[b]	0.50[b]
Triceps skinfold	0.40[a]	−0.01	0.43[b]	0.24
Subscapular skinfold	0.36[a]	0.09	0.50[c]	0.28
Suprailiac skinfold	0.29	0.05	0.46[b]	0.15
% Body fat	0.33[a]	0.66[c]	0.32[a]	0.63[c]
Total abdominal fat	0.52[c]	0.50[c]	0.54[c]	0.56[c]
Subcutaneous abdominal fat	0.44[b]	0.49[b]	0.38[a]	0.62[c]
Visceral abdominal fat	0.43[b]	0.08	0.50[c]	−0.03
Fasting blood glucose	0.14	0.43[c]	0.26	0.44[b]
Total cholesterol	0.21	0.47[b]	0.29	0.67[c]
Serum triglyceride	0.22	0.42[b]	0.50[b]	0.52[c]
High-density lipoprotein cholesterol	−0.18	−0.17	−0.13	−0.11
Low-density lipoprotein cholesterol	−0.01	0.28	0.20	0.41[b]
Fasting insulin	0.21	0.65[c]	0.31[a]	0.62[c]
hsCRP*	−0.12	−0.17	−0.01	0.09
HOMA-IR	0.19	0.62[c]	0.29[a]	0.61[c]

[a]: $p<0.05$;
[b]$p<0.01$;
[c]: $p<0.001$.
HOMA-IR: Homeostatic model of assessment-insulin resistance; hsCRP: high sensitivity C-reactive protein.

adipocyte hypertrophy and lipid profile alterations was observed to be independent of differences in subcutaneous adipose tissue cellularity, body composition, and fat distribution in women [33].

Fasting insulin and HOMA-IR correlated significantly with TAF and SAF but not with VAF in both males and females. This is in line with earlier observations of significant association of truncal subcutaneous adipose tissue with hyperinsulinemia in Asian Indian young adults from India [34] and migrant Asian Indians [19]. However, these observations are contrary to other reports from Indian subcontinent which indicate that VAF is more closely related to insulin resistance [35]. In the present study, the correlations of SC and OM adipocyte size with fasting insulin and HOMA-IR were significantly stronger only in females. After adjusting for age, BMI, WC, %BF, TAF and SAF, only the association of fasting insulin and HOMA-IR remained significant with SC adipocyte size ($p = 0.03$ for both fasting insulin and HOMA-IR). These observations are similar to those reported by Weyer *et al.* in Pima Indians where mean SC abdominal adipocyte size was observed to be 19% and 11% higher in subjects with diabetes and IGT as compared to those with NGT, after adjusting for age, sex and %BF [17]. Enlarged mean SC abdominal adipocyte along with a low insulin sensitivity and acute insulin secretory response independently predicted diabetes in NGT subjects over an average follow up of about nine years. The changes in insulin sensitivity were inversely and independently related to changes in mean SC abdominal adipocyte size and %BF [17]. However, this study did not evaluate the association of OM adipocyte size with insulin sensitivity and risk of development of diabetes mellitus. In another study involving severe obese patients who underwent bariatric surgery, it was observed that OM adipocyte size correlated strongly with insulin resistance, TG/HDL-c ratio and HbA1c. The study subjects were categorised into metabolically healthy and unhealthy groups. Though mean SC adipocyte size was similar in both groups, OM adipocyte size was smaller in metabolically healthy group as compared to metabolically unhealthy group [36]. This may be explained to some extent by their greater metabolic activity and responsiveness to various hormonal alterations.

Whether adipocyte size or body composition in terms of %BF or body fat distribution predicts metabolic complications of obesity is unclear. This was investigated by Mundi *et al.* in a study involving predominantly Caucasian subjects [37]. Serum triglyceride levels were best predicted by visceral fat area in both men and women, whereas fasting insulin levels were best predicted by SC abdominal fat area in women and BMI in men. No independent association of fasting insulin with femoral adipocyte size was noted. In our study, though SC and OM adipocyte size was associated with FBG, TC, TG and insulin levels in females, this relationship was attenuated after adjusting for age, BMI, %BF, WC, TAF and SAF area of abdomen. This may further suggest that body fat distribution may have a greater influence on obesity associated metabolic abnormalities.

The strength of our study consists is that we have evaluated the relationship of adipocyte size from abdominal SC and OM fat depots with measures of generalised and abdominal obesity, abdominal fat distribution, and various biochemical parameters in Asian Indians from India. Some of our observations are similar to those reported earlier such as strong relationship of SC adipocyte size with insulin resistance and that of OM adipocyte size with dyslipidemias, with clear gender differences. This study has some limitations. The relatively small sample size may not be sufficient to draw firm conclusions. Moreover, the prevalence of abdominal obesity was very low in males in this study. This could be related to the sample selection as the subjects were included from individuals undergoing elective surgery and may not be representative of general population. However, this study is first of its kind involving Asian Indians from India and may be helpful in planning further studies involving larger number of subjects. Due to logistic reasons, oral glucose tolerance test could not be performed in the study. We used HOMA-IR as a surrogate marker of insulin resistance instead of clamp study due to limitations of infrastructure. However, HOMA-IR has been used as a valid surrogate marker of insulin resistance by several investigators. Further studies involving larger number of subjects with wide range of BMI, more accurate measures and higher number of parameters are required to draw firm conclusions.

In conclusion, in this study involving Asian Indians from India, the OM adipocyte size, though smaller than SC adipocyte, was more closely related to measures of generalised as well as abdominal obesity and metabolic abnormalities with distinct gender differences. The relationship of adipocyte size with metabolic parameters was attenuated after adjusting for measures of adiposity.

Acknowledgments

The authors are thankful to Dr. Surya Prakash for his assistance in obtaining anthropometric measurements and Mr Punnu Lal for assisting in obtaining and performance of biochemical investigations. The co-operation of subjects who agreed to participate in this study is highly appreciated.

Author Contributions

Conceived and designed the experiments: NKV MCS RG AM. Performed the experiments: VPM SRM MCS ASB NG. Analyzed the data: RMP NKV. Contributed reagents/materials/analysis tools: VS SRM MCS NG KL AM. Wrote the paper: NKV RMP.

References

1. Hager A (1981) Adipose tissue cellularity in childhood in relation to the development of obesity. British medical bulletin 37: 287–290.
2. Misra A, Khurana L (2008) Obesity and the metabolic syndrome in developing countries. The Journal of clinical endocrinology and metabolism 93: S9–30.
3. Haslam DW, James WP (2005) Obesity. Lancet 366: 1197–1209.
4. Misra A, Vikram NK (2003) Clinical and pathophysiological consequences of abdominal adiposity and abdominal adipose tissue depots. Nutrition 19: 457–466.
5. Sanderson JE, Mayosi B, Yusuf S, Reddy S, Hu S, et al. (2007) Global burden of cardiovascular disease. Heart 93: 1175.
6. Razak F, Anand SS, Shannon H, Vuksan V, Davis B, et al. (2007) Defining obesity cut points in a multiethnic population. Circulation 115: 2111–2118.
7. Sniderman AD, Bhopal R, Prabhakaran D, Sarrafzadegan N, Tchernof A (2007) Why might South Asians be so susceptible to central obesity and its atherogenic consequences? The adipose tissue overflow hypothesis. International journal of epidemiology 36: 220–225.
8. Modi N, Thomas EL, Uthaya SN, Umranikar S, Bell JD, et al. (2009) Whole body magnetic resonance imaging of healthy newborn infants demonstrates increased central adiposity in Asian Indians. Pediatric research 65: 584–587.
9. Flegal KM, Graubard BI, Williamson DF, Gail MH (2007) Cause-specific excess deaths associated with underweight, overweight, and obesity. JAMA: the journal of the American Medical Association 298: 2028–2037.

10. Kramer CK, Zinman B, Retnakaran R (2013) Are Metabolically Healthy Overweight and Obesity Benign Conditions? A Systematic Review and Meta-analysis. Annals of internal medicine 159: 758–769.
11. Hausman DB, DiGirolamo M, Bartness TJ, Hausman GJ, Martin RJ (2001) The biology of white adipocyte proliferation. Obesity reviews: an official journal of the International Association for the Study of Obesity 2: 239–254.
12. Marques BG, Hausman DB, Martin RJ (1998) Association of fat cell size and paracrine growth factors in development of hyperplastic obesity. The American journal of physiology 275: R1898–1908.
13. Smas CM, Sul HS (1995) Control of adipocyte differentiation. The Biochemical journal 309 (Pt 3): 697–710.
14. Chandalia M, Abate N (2007) Metabolic complications of obesity: inflated or inflamed? Journal of diabetes and its complications 21: 128–136.
15. Bays H, Blonde L, Rosenson R (2006) Adiposopathy: how do diet, exercise and weight loss drug therapies improve metabolic disease in overweight patients? Expert review of cardiovascular therapy 4: 871–895.
16. Meyer LK, Ciaraldi TP, Henry RR, Wittgrove AC, Phillips SA (2013) Adipose tissue depot and cell size dependency of adiponectin synthesis and secretion in human obesity. Adipocyte 2: 217–226.
17. Weyer C, Foley JE, Bogardus C, Tataranni PA, Pratley RE (2000) Enlarged subcutaneous abdominal adipocyte size, but not obesity itself, predicts type II diabetes independent of insulin resistance. Diabetologia 43: 1498–1506.
18. Lonn M, Mehlig K, Bengtsson C, Lissner L (2010) Adipocyte size predicts incidence of type 2 diabetes in women. FASEB journal: official publication of the Federation of American Societies for Experimental Biology 24: 326–331.
19. Chandalia M, Lin P, Seenivasan T, Livingston EH, Snell PG, et al. (2007) Insulin resistance and body fat distribution in South Asian men compared to Caucasian men. PloS one 2: e812.
20. Vikram NK, Misra A, Pandey RM, Dwivedi M, Luthra K, et al. (2006) Association between subclinical inflammation & fasting insulin in urban young adult north Indian males. The Indian journal of medical research 124: 677–682.
21. Friedewald WT, Levy RI, Fredrickson DS (1972) Estimation of the concentration of low-density lipoprotein cholesterol in plasma, without use of the preparative ultracentrifuge. Clinical chemistry 18: 499–502.
22. Misra A, Chowbey P, Makkar BM, Vikram NK, Wasir JS, et al. (2009) Consensus statement for diagnosis of obesity, abdominal obesity and the metabolic syndrome for Asian Indians and recommendations for physical activity, medical and surgical management. The Journal of the Association of Physicians of India 57: 163–170.
23. Misra A, Vikram NK, Gupta R, Pandey RM, Wasir JS, et al. (2006) Waist circumference cutoff points and action levels for Asian Indians for identification of abdominal obesity. International journal of obesity 30: 106–111.
24. Grundy SM, Cleeman JI, Daniels SR, Donato KA, Eckel RH, et al. (2005) Diagnosis and management of the metabolic syndrome: an American Heart Association/National Heart, Lung, and Blood Institute Scientific Statement. Circulation 112: 2735–2752.
25. Alberti KG, Eckel RH, Grundy SM, Zimmet PZ, Cleeman JI, et al. (2009) Harmonizing the metabolic syndrome: a joint interim statement of the International Diabetes Federation Task Force on Epidemiology and Prevention; National Heart, Lung, and Blood Institute; American Heart Association; World Heart Federation; International Atherosclerosis Society; and International Association for the Study of Obesity. Circulation 120: 1640–1645.
26. Ridker PM (2003) High-sensitivity C-reactive protein and cardiovascular risk: rationale for screening and primary prevention. The American journal of cardiology 92: 17K–22K.
27. Matthews DR, Hosker JP, Rudenski AS, Naylor BA, Treacher DF, et al. (1985) Homeostasis model assessment: insulin resistance and beta-cell function from fasting plasma glucose and insulin concentrations in man. Diabetologia 28: 412–419.
28. Bhatt SP, Misra A, Sharma M, Luthra K, Guleria R, et al. (2012) Ala/Ala genotype of Pro12Ala polymorphism in the peroxisome proliferator-activated receptor-gamma2 gene is associated with obesity and insulin resistance in Asian Indians. Diabetes technology & therapeutics 14: 828–834.
29. Arner E, Westermark PO, Spalding KL, Britton T, Ryden M, et al. (2010) Adipocyte turnover: relevance to human adipose tissue morphology. Diabetes 59: 105–109.
30. van Harmelen V, Skurk T, Rohrig K, Lee YM, Halbleib M, et al. (2003) Effect of BMI and age on adipose tissue cellularity and differentiation capacity in women. International journal of obesity and related metabolic disorders: journal of the International Association for the Study of Obesity 27: 889–895.
31. Skurk T, Alberti-Huber C, Herder C, Hauner H (2007) Relationship between adipocyte size and adipokine expression and secretion. The Journal of clinical endocrinology and metabolism 92: 1023–1033.
32. Anand SS, Tarnopolsky MA, Rashid S, Schulze KM, Desai D, et al. (2011) Adipocyte hypertrophy, fatty liver and metabolic risk factors in South Asians: the Molecular Study of Health and Risk in Ethnic Groups (mol-SHARE). PloS one 6: e22112.
33. Veilleux A, Caron-Jobin M, Noel S, Laberge PY, Tchernof A (2011) Visceral adipocyte hypertrophy is associated with dyslipidemia independent of body composition and fat distribution in women. Diabetes 60: 1504–1511.
34. Misra A, Khurana L (2011) Obesity-related non-communicable diseases: South Asians vs White Caucasians. International journal of obesity 35: 167–187.
35. Indulekha K, Anjana RM, Surendar J, Mohan V (2011) Association of visceral and subcutaneous fat with glucose intolerance, insulin resistance, adipocytokines and inflammatory markers in Asian Indians (CURES-113). Clinical biochemistry 44: 281–287.
36. O'Connell J, Lynch L, Cawood TJ, Kwasnik A, Nolan N, et al. (2010) The relationship of omental and subcutaneous adipocyte size to metabolic disease in severe obesity. PloS one 5: e9997.
37. Mundi MS, Karpyak MV, Koutsari C, Votruba SB, O'Brien PC, et al. (2010) Body fat distribution, adipocyte size, and metabolic characteristics of nondiabetic adults. The Journal of clinical endocrinology and metabolism 95: 67–73.

8

Progression of Cardio-Metabolic Risk Factors in Subjects Born Small and Large for Gestational Age

Valentina Chiavaroli[1,2*], Maria Loredana Marcovecchio[1,2], Tommaso de Giorgis[1,2], Laura Diesse[1], Francesco Chiarelli[1,2], Angelika Mohn[1,2]

1 Department of Paediatrics, University of Chieti, Chieti, Italy, 2 Center of Excellence on Aging, "G. d'Annunzio" University Foundation, University of Chieti, Chieti, Italy

Abstract

Background: Subjects born small (SGA) and large (LGA) for gestational age have an increased risk of cardio-metabolic alterations already during prepuberty. Nevertheless, the progression of their cardio-metabolic profile from childhood to adolescence has not been fully explored. Our aim was to assess potential changes in the cardio-metabolic profile from childhood to adolescence in subjects born SGA and LGA compared to those born appropriate (AGA) for gestational age.

Methods: This longitudinal study included 35 AGA, 24 SGA and 31 LGA subjects evaluated during childhood (mean age (±SD) 8.4±1.4 yr) and then re-assessed during adolescence (mean age 13.3±1.8 yr). BMI, blood pressure, insulin resistance (fasting insulin, HOMA-IR) and lipids were assessed. A cardio-metabolic risk z-score was applied and this consisted in calculating the sum of sex-specific z-scores for BMI, blood pressure, HOMA-IR, triglycerides and triglycerides:high-density lipoprotein cholesterol ratio.

Results: Fasting insulin and HOMA-IR were higher in SGA and LGA than AGA subjects both during childhood (all $P<0.01$) and adolescence (all $P<0.01$). Similarly, the clustered cardio-metabolic risk score was higher in SGA and LGA than AGA children (both $P<0.05$), and these differences among groups increased during adolescence (both $P<0.05$). Of note, a progression of the clustered cardio-metabolic risk score was observed from childhood to adolescence within SGA and within LGA subjects (both $P<0.05$).

Conclusions: SGA and LGA subjects showed an adverse cardio-metabolic profile during childhood when compared to AGA peers, with a worsening of this profile during adolescence. These findings indicate an overtime progression of insulin resistance and overall estimated cardiovascular risk from childhood to adolescence in SGA and LGA populations.

Editor: Marta Letizia Hribal, University of Catanzaro Magna Graecia, Italy

Funding: The authors have no support or funding to report.

Competing Interests: The authors have declared that no competing interests exist.

* Email: valentinachiavaroli@hotmail.it

Introduction

Birth weight is now recognized to have important implications for cardio-metabolic health in adulthood. Children born small (SGA) and large (LGA) for gestational age are at greater risk of developing type 2 diabetes and cardiovascular disease as they age [1–6]. These groups have been shown to have metabolic alterations in childhood and adolescence, suggesting a phenotype of metabolic dysfunction in early life, finally leading to the emergence of disease in adulthood [2,6–10].

The determinants of birth weight are multifactorial including genetics, ethnicity, maternal nutrition, obesity, smoking and diabetes [11,12]. Birth weight is a marker of intrauterine nutrition, hence it is likely that the mechanisms mediating the increased metabolic risk of those born SGA are different to those born LGA. Nevertheless, decreased insulin sensitivity has a key role linking birth weight to the development of chronic disease in both these groups [6,7]. Metabolic risk is further modulated by the post-natal growth pattern, and infants born SGA who show early catch-up growth are at increased risk [13–15]. Reduced insulin sensitivity and increased fat accumulation have also been detected in LGA subjects [15–17].

Most studies investigating the relationship between birth weight and metabolic risk have been cross-sectional [13–15,17]. It is important to reassess cohorts of children prospectively to investigate whether markers of metabolic risk are stable or progress overtime.

We have previously shown in a cohort of prepubertal children that those born SGA or LGA were more insulin resistant and had greater oxidative stress than those born appropriate (AGA) for gestational age [15]. Further, these factors were greater in those who were obese.

Therefore, in the present study we have reassessed a group of adolescents born AGA, SGA and LGA, most of whom belonged to the previous cohort of prepubertal children, to describe how markers of metabolic risk change after puberty.

Materials and Methods

Ethics Statement

This study was approved by the Ethical Committee of the University of Chieti. Written informed parental consent, oral assent from children and written consent from adolescents were obtained.

Recruitment

We recruited 115 Caucasian children, living in the district of Chieti (Abruzzo, Central Italy). These children were admitted to the Department of Pediatrics of the University of Chieti, for minor illness or cranio-facial trauma. During hospitalization, parents were informed about the study and children were invited to participate.

Children were eligible for the study if they were born at term (37–41 weeks of gestation) from singleton pregnancies. Children were excluded if they had a first degree relative or grandparent with type 2 diabetes, or were born to a mother with gestational diabetes mellitus [18], obesity or hypertension. In addition, potential participants were excluded if they had congenital anomalies, developmental delay, chronic diseases, took regular medication or if they were involved in regular programmed physical activity or dietary programs.

Participants were divided into three groups according to birth weight: AGA children, defined on a birth weight between the 10th to 90th percentile for gestational age; SGA children, defined on a birth weight less than or equal to −2 SD, with evidence of catch-up growth [actual height SD score (SDS) within 1.3 SD of the target height SDS] to investigate those with the characteristic SGA growth pattern [19]; and LGA children, defined on a birth weight above the 90th percentile for gestational age. Information regarding birth weight and maternal-perinatal history was obtained by parents and ascertained throughout delivery records and health booklets.

Assessment of the study population during childhood

Anthropometric measurements and blood samples were taken after complete recovery from the illness for which children were admitted to hospital. All children had a physical examination including anthropometric measurements, blood pressure (BP) and pubertal staging (all participants were prepubertal corresponding to Tanner stage 1). Fasting blood samples were obtained to measure glucose, insulin and lipid profile [including total cholesterol, high-density lipoprotein (HDL) cholesterol, low-density lipoprotein (LDL) cholesterol, triglycerides, and triglycerides-to-HDL cholesterol (triglycerides:HDL) ratio]. Fasting glucose and insulin concentrations were used to calculate the homeostasis model assessment of insulin resistance (HOMA-IR).

Assessment of the study population during adolescence

The whole study cohort was invited for reevaluation at least 2 years from the first visit. Participants had a repeated physical examination including anthropometric measurement, BP and pubertal staging. Fasting blood samples were obtained to assess fasting glucose, insulin and lipid profile. Thus, the anthropometric and laboratory measurements were consistent between the childhood and adolescent assessments. In this second evaluation, all subjects had pubertal characteristics, corresponding to stage ≥3 (3 = mid-puberty, 4 = late puberty, 5 = post-puberty, respectively).

Anthropometric measurements

Body weight was determined to the nearest 0.1 kg, and height was measured with a Harpenden stadiometer to the nearest 0.1 cm. Body mass index (BMI) was calculated as weight/height^2 and expressed as kg/m^2. Subjects with BMI >95th percentile for the age and sex were defined as obese. Height and BMI SDS were calculated based on the age and sex reference values for Italian children using the LMS method [20]. Maternal and paternal heights were recorded for all participants. Target height (cm) was calculated using Tanner's formula: (the sum of both parents' heights−13)/2 for girls and (the sum of both parents' heights+13)/2 for boys, respectively [21].

Blood pressure

All BP measurements were obtained by the same researcher properly trained in the techniques of BP assessment. Systolic BP and diastolic BP were measured three times at intervals of at least 1 minute from the non-dominant arm, after five minutes of rest in the supine position using the same calibrated and accurately maintained sphygmomanometer, and then averaged [22].

Biochemical analysis

Plasma glucose level was determined by the glucose oxidase method, and plasma insulin was measured with a 2-site immunoenzymometric assay (AIAPACK IRI; Tosoh, Tokyo, Japan). The limit of detection was 0.5 μU/mL with intraassay and interassay coefficients of variation of <7%. HOMA-IR was calculated with the formula: fasting insulin (μU/mL) x fasting glucose (mmol/L)/22.5 [23].

Lipid analysis

Serum total cholesterol, HDL cholesterol, and triglycerides concentrations were determined by the calorimetric enzymatic method. LDL cholesterol was calculated according to the Friedewald formula (LDL cholesterol = total cholesterol−HDL cholesterol−triglycerides/5).

Score of cardio-metabolic risk

The cardio-metabolic risk was assessed on the basis of the following clinical characteristics and biochemical parameters: BMI, systolic BP, HOMA-IR, triglycerides, and triglycerides:HDL ratio. The sex-specific z-score [z = (value−mean)/SD] for each component was calculated based on the mean and the SD of the whole study population (AGA, SGA, and LGA). The sex-specific z-score for each variable was then summed to obtain the clustered cardio-metabolic score for each of the three birth weight groups during childhood and adolescence, respectively. The rationale for selecting this cardio-metabolic score and its components was based on previous studies, in which similar risk score and factors were used [24–26].

Statistical analysis

According to birth weight all children were divided into three groups (AGA, SGA, LGA). Only subjects for whom data for both visits (childhood and adolescence) were available were included in the statistical analysis. All values were expressed as means ± SD unless otherwise stated. Variables of interest non-normally distributed were logarithmically transformed for analyses (insulin, HOMA-IR, and triglycerides). Differences in variables among the three groups were analyzed by general linear model with Bonferroni's test for post hoc comparison of means between each pair of groups. Adjustments for important confounders have been made: BP assessments have been adjusted for subject's height, height has been adjusted for target height, anthropometric measurements (height, weight, BMI) and biochemical parameters (lipid profile) prior to and during puberty have been adjusted for sex, and glucose homeostasis (glucose, insulin, HOMA-IR) has been adjusted for BMI SDS and age. Differences in sex ratio were compared by Fisher's exact test. Paired-Samples T test was performed for evaluating intragroup differences for the clustered risk score and its components between childhood and adolescence. A multiple linear regression analysis was performed to evaluate the independent contribution of birth weight on the clustered risk z-scores obtained during childhood and during adolescence. In addition, a multiple linear regression analysis was performed to evaluate the independent contribution of birth weight and the clustered risk z-score obtained during childhood on the clustered risk z-score obtained during adolescence. In the models, data have been adjusted for age and sex (included as a continuous variable and as a categorical variable, respectively). The birth weight categories have been included as predictors in the regression model. As the use of more than two categorical variables as predictors is not allowed in the multiple regression analysis, dummy coding was used to categorize birth weight, and in the models the birth weight categories were included as dummy variables (AGA *versus* SGA, and AGA *versus* LGA, respectively). P values <0.05 were considered statistically significant. SPSS program version 16.0 for Windows was used.

For the purpose of the sample estimation, changes in insulin resistance between childhood and adolescence were based on data from the literature [27]. A sample size of 30 for each group would provide a power of roughly 90% to detect a 1.51 difference in HOMA-IR among groups, with a SD of 0.68, and a 5% significance level.

Results

The whole study population was recalled for a longitudinal evaluation after at least 2 years from the first visit (mean time interval (±SD) 5.0±2.0 yr). Invitation letters together with an information leaflet about the study were send to the study participants. From the initial 115 participants, 90 adolescents (35 AGA, 24 SGA, 31 LGA; girls:boys ratio approximately 2:1) agreed to participate in this part of the study and were re-assessed. The remaining 25 subjects from the original study population were not recruited either due to lack of interest in the study, and inability to make contact or failing to meet the inclusion criteria (involvement in regular and programmed physical activity and/or dietary intervention). The primary reasons for losing boys to the longitudinal part of the study were involvement in physical activity programs and a follow-up time not long enough to reach adolescence.

Childhood assessment

Clinical characteristics and laboratory investigations of the study population during childhood are reported in Table 1.

The AGA, SGA and LGA groups were similar for gestational weeks, age and sex, whereas a difference was found in birth weight ($P<0.01$). No difference was observed among AGA, SGA and LGA children in height SDS, BMI SDS, BP, and lipid profile.

Fasting insulin and HOMA-IR values were higher in the SGA group compared to AGA subjects (both $P<0.01$). Similarly, LGA children showed higher fasting insulin and HOMA-IR values compared to the AGA group (both $P<0.01$).

Adolescence assessment

Clinical characteristics and laboratory investigations of the study population during adolescence are reported in Table 1.

The AGA, SGA and LGA groups were similar for age. No difference was found in height SDS, BMI SDS, BP, and lipid profile.

Fasting insulin and HOMA-IR values were higher in SGA adolescents compared to AGA peers (both $P<0.01$). Similarly, LGA adolescents showed higher fasting insulin and HOMA-IR values than the AGA group (both $P<0.01$).

Intragroup differences in cardio-metabolic markers between childhood and adolescence

An increase in systolic BP and HOMA-IR was found from childhood to adolescence within each birth weight group (all $P<0.01$). A reduction was detected in BMI SDS within LGA and AGA subjects (both $P<0.05$), without considerable difference in the SGA group. Triglycerides remained stable over time in LGA and AGA subjects, while a trend to an increase was observed in the SGA group ($P=0.058$). No intragroup difference was found in triglycerides:HDL ratio.

Cardio-metabolic risk score from childhood to adolescence

The clustered risk z-scores of AGA, SGA and LGA subjects during childhood and adolescence are shown in Figure 1.

The clustered risk scores were higher in SGA and LGA children than those born AGA (both $P<0.05$). During adolescence, both SGA and LGA subjects showed higher cardio-metabolic risk scores than AGA peers ($P=0.01$ and $P<0.01$, respectively).

Of note, a progression of the clustered risk score from childhood to adolescence was observed within the SGA group ($P<0.05$) and within the LGA group ($P<0.05$), while no difference was detected in the AGA group.

Associations between birth weight and the clustered risk z-scores

A multiple linear regression analysis was performed to evaluate the potential associations between birth weight categories and the clustered z-scores during childhood and during adolescence (Table 2). A positive and significant association was found between SGA and LGA categories and the clustered risk z-scores during childhood and adolescence.

In addition, a multiple linear regression analysis was performed to evaluate the potential role of birth weight categories and the childhood risk score as independent predictors for the risk score obtained during adolescence (Table 3). In this model, both the SGA and LGA groups and the childhood clustered z-score were significantly and independently related to the clustered z-score during adolescence.

Discussion

In this longitudinal study children born SGA and LGA had greater insulin resistance than those born AGA, which was shown to increase from childhood to adolescence. Similarly, the clustered risk score was higher in SGA and LGA children than AGA peers, and these differences among groups increased during adolescence. Notably, a global increase in the risk score was observed within the SGA and the LGA group, suggesting an overtime progression of their cardio-metabolic risk.

A large body of evidence has highlighted that SGA and LGA children are at increased risk of cardio-metabolic diseases at a young age [2,6,16]. The first metabolic abnormality seems to be insulin resistance, which can be observed during the first years of life in SGA and LGA children through adolescence [13–17,28]. In

Table 1. Longitudinal evaluation of clinical characteristics and biochemical evaluation of the study population during childhood and adolescence.

	CHILDHOOD (*n*=90)			ADOLESCENCE (*n*=90)		
	AGA	**SGA**	**LGA**	**AGA**	**SGA**	**LGA**
Clinical characteristics						
Number	35	24	31	35	24	31
Age (years)	8.7±1.0	8.6±1.4	8.0±1.7	13.5±1.7	13.4±1.9	13.0±2.0
Sex ratio	11M/24F	8M/16F	10M/21F			
Birth weight (g)	3364±283	2514±136**	4141±223**			
Gestational weeks	39.6±1.2	39.4±1.4	39.7±1.4			
Height SDS	0.5±1.1	0.4±1.0	0.7±0.7	0.3±0.9	0.0±0.9	0.5±0.6
BMI SDS	1.35±1.10	1.59±1.06	1.71±1.04	0.82±1.25	1.36±0.68	1.34±1.01
Obese subjects (%)	34	41	45	14	23	25
Pubertal stage (%)	100	100	100	20/34/46	25/33/42	26/29/45
Systolic BP (mmHg)	103±6	102±5	103±8	115±8	117±6	117±7
Diastolic BP (mmHg)	62±5	62±4	63±5	69±4	71±7	71±5
Lipid profile						
Total cholesterol (mg/dl)	160.8±17.6	160.9±11.8	166.9±19.3	163.8±22.4	169.3±18.5	176.2±28.8
HDL cholesterol (mg/dl)	56.4±7.0	55.9±7.4	52.2±6.2	53.6±8.1	52.7±7.3	50.4±3.3
LDL cholesterol (mg/dl)	92.0±17.3	90.8±10.5	98.1±20.1	96.8±24.9	96.3±16.7	108.6±27.4
Triglycerides (mg/dl)	71.1±18.6	72.3±28.1	83.1±25.4	83.7±31.4	87.3±17.0	93.9±26.9
Triglycerides:HDL ratio	1.29±0.44	1.33±0.57	1.53±0.50	1.57±0.67	1.62±0.31	1.58±0.38
Glucose metabolism						
Fasting glucose (mg/dl)	78.8±6.1	84.5±8.0**	86.6±6.0**	82.9±4.7	86.6±5.1**	86.4±3.2*
Fasting insulin (μU/ml)	7.7±3.2	12.0±4.8**	13.1±5.4**	13.2±5.8	20.3±6.6**	18.9±4.7**
HOMA-IR	1.55±0.72	2.57±1.20**	2.85±1.24**	2.94±1.18	4.59±1.56**	4.04±0.91**

Values are means (± SD). **P*<0.05 and ***P*<0.01, for comparisons to AGA group by *post hoc* analysis.
Pubertal stage is presented as % in phase 1 during childhood, and as % in phase 3, 4 and 5, respectively, during adolescence.
AGA = Appropriate for Gestational Age; SGA = Small for Gestational Age; LGA = Large for Gestational Age; M = Male; F = Female; SDS = Standard Deviation Score; BP = Blood Pressure; HDL = High-Density Lipoprotein; LDL = Low-Density Lipoprotein; HOMA-IR = Homeostasis Model Assessment of Insulin Resistance.

a longitudinal analysis performed retrospectively on data collected from the Bogalusa Heart Study, Frontini et al. reported that low birth weight is associated with adverse metabolic outcomes, including altered glucose homeostasis, from childhood to adolescence [29]. In line with these observations, the present study showed greater insulin resistance in the same group of SGA and LGA subjects from childhood to early adolescence. No detectable differences have been found in adiposity, BP and lipid profile among the three birth weight groups. Thus, insulin resistance in itself seems to be a persisting characteristic of both SGA and LGA population. Although the exact mechanisms remain to be determined, prenatal exposure to an adverse metabolic environment and rapid post-natal catch-up growth might play a major role in influencing insulin sensitivity [7,8,11,12].

Interestingly, an emerging concept of clustering cardiovascular and metabolic risk factors has been introduced by several authors to assess subjects at major risk for future diseases [24,26,30]. According to this concept, several scores have been proposed combining both cardiovascular and metabolic criteria in adults [24,30] and children [26,31], allowing estimation of the individual risk level.

We decided to use a risk score combining both clinical characteristics and biochemical parameters, including adiposity, BP, insulin resistance and lipids, as they can easily be collected in clinical practice and, even more importantly, all of them have been recognized as major predictors of cardiovascular disease [2,32–34]. In addition, in line with previous studies a clustered risk z-score was used to compensate for daily variations in each factor [27,35,36]. Of interest, our data suggest a global increase in cardiovascular risk as calculated by the composite risk Z-score from childhood to adolescence in SGA and LGA categories. These findings suggest that early interventions to improve long-term cardiovascular outcomes in those born SGA and LGA may be warranted. Hence, clustering of risk factors in SGA and LGA subjects could be useful in assessing the cardio-metabolic risk and its overtime progression.

Our data support an independent effect of birth weight categories on later metabolic disturbances. Moreover, a rising attractive question is whether childhood cardio-metabolic profile could be associated to the later cardio-metabolic risk score. In this respect, we found a significant association between the childhood score and that one obtained during adolescence, suggesting that the cardio-metabolic profile showed during infancy seems to be predictive of future abnormalities. These findings are in accordance with other studies where infancy and childhood have been recognized as critical time periods for subsequent development of cardiovascular and metabolic alterations [37,38]. Therefore, childhood may represent an important window of opportunity to optimize risk factors in SGA and LGA populations.

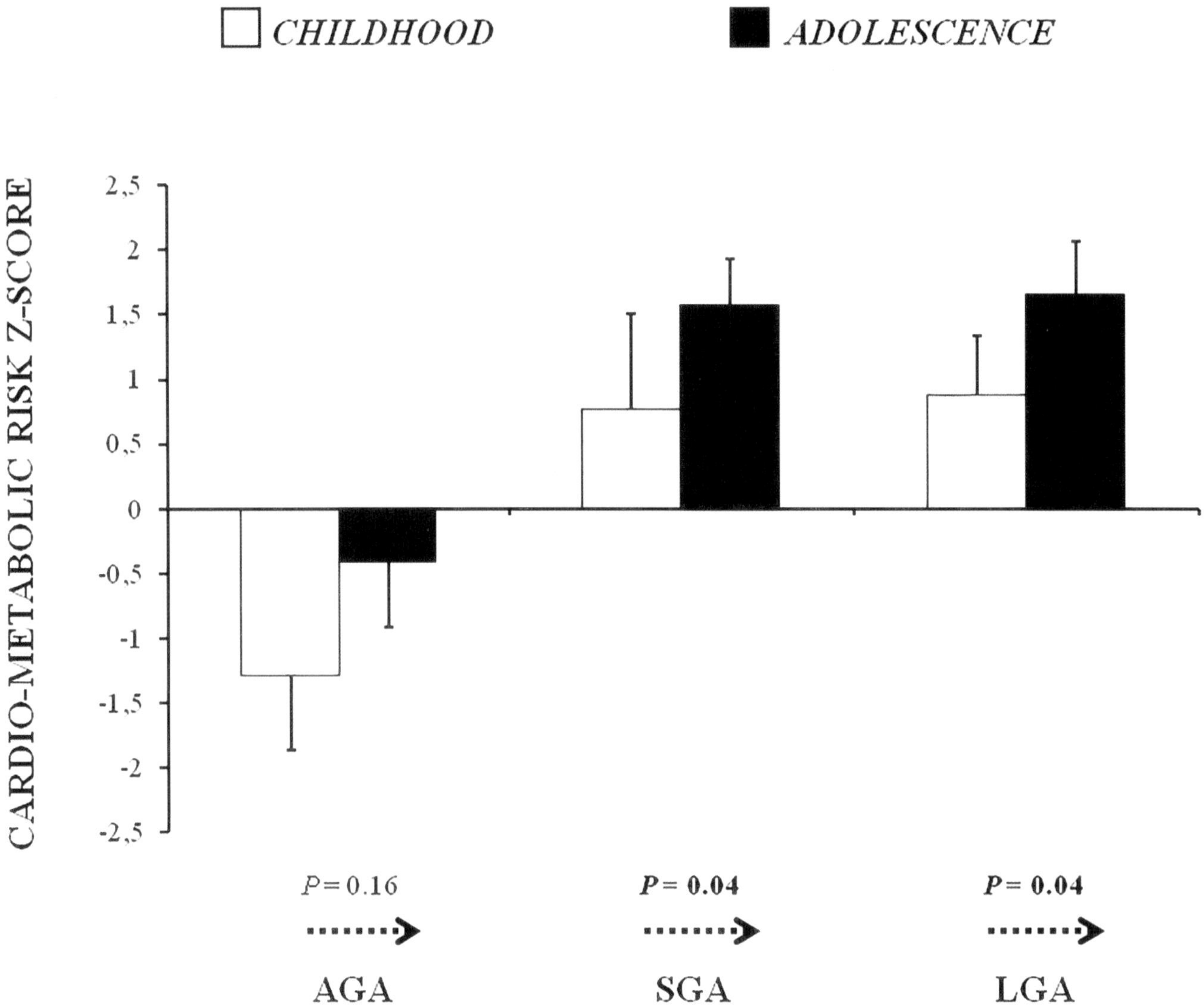

Figure 1. Cardio-metabolic risk z-scores of AGA, SGA and LGA subjects during childhood and adolescence. Values are means (± SE). *P* values by Paired-Samples T test for temporal change (arrows) in the cardio-metabolic risk score from childhood to adolescence within each group. AGA = Appropriate for Gestational Age; SGA = Small for Gestational Age; LGA = Large for Gestational Age.

It needs to be acknowledged that, although several scores have been proposed to identify adults and youths at potential high risk for future diseases [24–26,30], defining accurate clusters of risk factors still remains a challenge. Thus, using a composite risk score may represent a limitation in terms of overfitting and validation as risk scores must be validated with actual cardiovascular and diabetes outcomes to find out if the composite score is more predictive than individual components. In addition, we used risk z-scores based on a relatively small cohort and not on population norms.

Table 2. Association between birth weight categories and cardio-metabolic risk z-scores during childhood and adolescence.

	Cardio-metabolic risk z-score			
	Childhood		*Adolescence*	
	β Coefficient	*P*	**β Coefficient**	*P*
AGA *vs* SGA	0.334	0.008	0.344	0.003
AGA *vs* LGA	0.330	0.01	0.409	0.001

Dependent variable: cardio-metabolic risk z-score. R^2 during childhood = 0.14. R^2 during adolescence = 0.17. Data were adjusted for age and sex.
AGA = Appropriate for Gestational Age; SGA = Small for Gestational Age; LGA = Large for Gestational Age.

Table 3. Association between birth weight categories, the cardio-metabolic risk z-score during childhood and the cardio-metabolic risk z-score during adolescence.

	Cardio-metabolic risk z-score during adolescence	
	β Coefficient	**P**
AGA vs SGA	0.328	0.004
AGA vs LGA	0.336	0.005
Cardio-metabolic risk z-score during childhood	0.395	<0.001

Dependent variable: cardio-metabolic risk z-score during adolescence. $R^2 = 0.37$. Data were adjusted for age and sex.
AGA = Appropriate for Gestational Age; SGA = Small for Gestational Age; LGA = Large for Gestational Age.

A further limitation is the exclusion of children following exercise and dietary programs, which may represent an important bias due to the potential missing of subjects with the highest cardiovascular risk. Although this exclusion criterion may limit generalizability of our finding to the wider population, we chose children who did not regularly exercise to increase the ability to detect a difference between groups. In addition, this ensured that physical activity was similar between groups as exercise has insulin sensitizing effects, which may have obscured differences in insulin resistance between birth weight categories.

Conclusions

SGA and LGA populations are known to have increased cardio-metabolic risk factors in childhood and adulthood. Our study adds to this literature showing that there is progression of these risk factors as children enter early adolescence. Further longer longitudinal studies are needed to elucidate the mechanisms responsible for progression of cardio-metabolic risk factors from infancy to adolescence in SGA and LGA subjects.

Acknowledgments

We thank all nurses of the Department of Paediatrics, University of Chieti, in particular Sabbion P, Di Domenica S, Finamore C, for their daily support in clinical research and care of children.

Author Contributions

Conceived and designed the experiments: VC MLM TDG LD FC AM. Performed the experiments: VC MLM TDG AM. Analyzed the data: VC MLM TDG LD FC AM. Contributed reagents/materials/analysis tools: VC MLM TDG AM. Wrote the paper: VC MLM TDG LD FC AM. Drafted the article and revised it critically: VC MLM TDG LD FC AM. Final approval of the version to be published: VC MLM TDG LD FC AM.

References

1. Johnson RC, Schoeni RF (2011) Early-life origins of adult disease: national longitudinal population-based study of the United States. Am J Public Health 101(12): 2317–2324. doi: 10.2105/AJPH.2011.300252.
2. Efstathiou SP, Skeva II, Zorbala E, Georgiou E, Mountokalakis TD (2012) Metabolic syndrome in adolescence: can it be predicted from natal and parental profile? The Prediction of Metabolic Syndrome in Adolescence (PREMA) study. Circulation 125(7): 902–910. doi: 10.1161/CIRCULATIONAHA.111.034546.
3. Dyer JS, Rosenfeld CR, Rice J, Rice M, Hardin DS (2007) Insulin resistance in Hispanic large-for-gestational-age neonates at birth. J Clin Endocrinol Metab 92(10): 3836–3843.
4. Boney CM, Verma A, Tucker R, Vohr BR (2005) Metabolic syndrome in childhood: association with birth weight, maternal obesity, and GD mellitus. Pediatrics 115(3): 290–296.
5. Barker DJ, Hales CN, Fall CH, Osmond C, Phipps K, et al. (1993) Type 2 (non-insulin-dependent) diabetes mellitus, hypertension and hyperlipidaemia (syndrome X): relation to reduced fetal growth. Diabetologia 36(1): 62–67.
6. Norris SA, Osmond C, Gigante D, Kuzawa CW, Ramakrishnan L, et al. (2012) Size at birth, weight gain in infancy and childhood, and adult diabetes risk in five low- or middle-income country birth cohorts. Diabetes Care 35(1): 72–79. doi: 10.2337/dc11-0456.
7. Evagelidou EN, Kiortsis DN, Bairaktari ET, Giapros VI, Cholevas VK, et al. (2006) Lipid profile, glucose homeostasis, blood pressure, and obesity-anthropometric markers in macrosomic offspring of nondiabetic mothers. Diabetes Care 29(6): 1197–1201.
8. Taal HR, Vd Heijden AJ, Steegers EA, Hofman A, Jaddoe VW (2013) Small and large size for gestational age at birth, infant growth, and childhood overweight. Obesity (Silver Spring) 21(6): 1261–1268. doi: 10.1002/oby.20116.
9. Brufani C, Grossi A, Fintini D, Tozzi A, Nocerino V, et al. (2009) Obese children with low birth weight demonstrate impaired beta-cell function during oral glucose tolerance test. J Clin Endocrinol Metab 94(11): 4448–4452. doi: 10.1210/jc.2009-1079.
10. Bueno AC, Espineira AR, Fernandes-Rosa FL, de Souza RM, de Castro M, et al. (2010) Adiponectin: serum levels, promoter polymorphism, and associations with birth size and cardiometabolic outcome in young adults born large for gestational age. Eur J Endocrinol 162: 53–60. doi: 10.1530/EJE-09-0697.
11. Langer O (2000) Fetal macrosomia: etiologic factors. Clin Obstet Gynecol 43: 283–297.
12. Campbell MK, Cartier S, Xie B, Kouniakis G, Huang W, et al. (2012) Determinants of small for gestational age birth at term. Paediatr Perinat Epidemiol 26(6): 525–533. doi: 10.1111/j.1365-3016.2012.01319.x.
13. Deng HZ, Deng H, Su Z, Li YH, Ma HM, et al. (2012) Insulin resistance and adiponectin levels are associated with height catch-up growth in pre-pubertal Chinese individuals born small for gestational age. Nutr Metab (Lond) 9(1): 107. doi: 10.1186/1743-7075-9-107.
14. Mohn A, Chiavaroli V, Cerruto M, Blasetti A, Giannini C, et al. (2007) Increased oxidative stress in prepubertal children born small for gestational age. J Clin Endocrinol Metab 92(4): 1372–1378.
15. Chiavaroli V, Giannini C, D'Adamo E, de Giorgis T, Chiarelli F, et al. (2009) Insulin resistance and oxidative stress in children born small and large for gestational age. Pediatrics 124(2): 695–702. doi: 10.1542/peds.2008-3056.
16. Renom Espineira A, Fernandes-Rosa FL, Bueno AC, de Souza RM, Moreira AC, et al. (2011) Postnatal growth and cardiometabolic profile in young adults born large for gestational age. Clin Endocrinol (Oxf) 75(3): 335–341. doi: 10.1111/j.1365-2265.2011.04054.x.
17. Evagelidou EN, Giapros VI, Challa AS, Cholevas VK, Vartholomatos GA, et al. (2010) Prothrombotic state, cardiovascular, and metabolic syndrome risk factors in prepubertal children born large for gestational age. Diabetes Care 33(11): 2468–2470. doi: 10.2337/dc10-1190.
18. International Association Of Diabetes And Pregnancy Study Groups Consensus Panel. (2010) International Association of Diabetes and Pregnancy Study Groups recommendations on the diagnosis and classification of hyperglycemia in pregnancy. Diabetes Care 33(3): 676–682. doi: 10.2337/dc09-1848.
19. Boukes FS, Merkx JAM, Rikken B, Huisman J (1998) Tracing, tracking, and diagnostics in general practice and criteria for referral. In: De Muinch Ueizer-Schrama SMPF, editors. Diagnostics short stature in childhood. Alphen aen den Rijn, The Netherlands. Van Zuiden Communications.
20. Cacciari E, Milani S, Balsamo A, Spada E, Bona G, et al. (2006) Italian cross-sectional growth charts for height, weight and BMI (2 to 20 yr). J Endocrinol Invest 29: 581–593.
21. Tanner JM, Goldstein H, Whitehouse RH (1970) Standards for children's height at ages 2–9 years allowing for heights of parents. Arch Dis Child 45: 755–762.
22. National High Blood Pressure Education Program Working Group on High Blood Pressure in Children and Adolescents (2004) The fourth report on the diagnosis, evaluation and treatment of high blood pressure in children and adolescents. Pediatrics 114(2): 555–576.

23. Heinze E, Holl RW (2003) Tests of beta-cell function in childhood and adolescence. In: Ranke MB, editors. Diagnostics of Endocrine Function in Children and Adolescents. Basel, Switzerland: Karger.
24. Thorn LM, Forsblom C, Fagerudd J, Pettersson-Fernholm K, Kilpikari R, et al. (2007) Clustering of risk factors in parents of patients with type 1 diabetes and nephropathy. Diabetes Care 30(5): 1162–1167.
25. Brage S, Wedderkopp N, Ekelund U, Franks PW, Wareham NJ, et al. (2004) Features of the metabolic syndrome are associated with objectively measured physical activity and fitness in Danish children: the European Youth Heart Study (EYHS). Diabetes Care 27(9): 2141–2148.
26. Andersen LB, Sardinha LB, Froberg K, Riddoch CJ, Page AS, et al. (2008) Fitness, fatness and clustering of cardiovascular risk factors in children from Denmark, Estonia and Portugal: the European Youth Heart Study. Int J Pediatr Obes 3(1): 58–66. doi: 10.1080/17477160801896366.
27. Bugge A, El-Naaman B, McMurray RG, Froberg K, Andersen LB (2013) Tracking of clustered cardiovascular disease risk factors from childhood to adolescence. Pediatr Res 73(2): 245–249. doi: 10.1038/pr.2012.158.
28. Fabricius-Bjerre S, Jensen RB, Færch K, Larsen T, Mølgaard C, et al. (2011) Impact of birth weight and early infant weight gain on insulin resistance and associated cardiovascular risk factors in adolescence. PLoS One 6(6): e20595. doi: 10.1371/journal.pone.0020595.
29. Frontini MG, Srinivasan SR, Xu J, Berenson GS (2004) Low birth weight and longitudinal trends of cardiovascular risk factor variables from childhood to adolescence: the bogalusa heart study. BMC Pediatr 4(1): 22.
30. Setayeshgar S, Whiting SJ, Vatanparast H (2013) Prevalence of 10-year risk of cardiovascular diseases and associated risks in canadian adults: the contribution of cardiometabolic risk assessment introduction. Int J Hypertens 2013: 276564. doi: 10.1155/2013/276564.
31. Camhi SM, Katzmarzyk PT (2010) Tracking of cardiometabolic risk factor clustering from childhood to adulthood. Int J Pediatr Obes 5(2): 122–129. doi: 10.3109/17477160903111763.
32. Kassi E, Pervanidou P, Kaltsas G, Chrousos G (2011) Metabolic syndrome: definitions and controversies. BMC Medicine 9: 48. doi: 10.1186/1741-7015-9-48.
33. Giannini C, Santoro N, Caprio S, Kim G, Lartaud D, et al. (2011) The triglyceride-to-HDL cholesterol ratio: association with insulin resistance in obese youths of different ethnic backgrounds. Diabetes Care 34(8): 1869–1874. doi: 10.2337/dc10-2234.
34. de Giorgis T, Marcovecchio ML, Di Giovanni I, Giannini C, Chiavaroli V, et al. (2013) Triglycerides-to-HDL ratio as a new marker of endothelial dysfunction in obese prepubertal children. Eur J Endocrinol 170(2): 173–180. doi: 10.1530/EJE-13-0452.
35. Andersen LB, Harro M, Sardinha LB, Froberg K, Ekelund U, et al. (2006) Physical activity and clustered cardiovascular risk in children: a cross-sectional study (The European Youth Heart Study). Lancet 368(9532): 299–304.
36. Brouwer SI, Stolk RP, Liem ET, Lemmink KA, Corpeleijn E (2013) The role of fitness in the association between fatness and cardiometabolic risk from childhood to adolescence. Pediatr Diabetes 14(1): 57–65. doi: 10.1111/j.1399-5448.2012.00893.x.
37. Baird J, Fisher D, Lucas P, Kleijnen J, Roberts H, et al. (2005) Being big or growing fast: systematic review of size and growth in infancy and later obesity. BMJ 331(7522): 929.
38. Liem ET, van Buuren S, Sauer PJ, Jaspers M, Stolk RP, et al. (2013) Growth during infancy and childhood, and adiposity at age 16 years: ages 2 to 7 years are pivotal. J Pediatr 162(2): 287–292. doi: 10.1016/j.jpeds.2012.07.053.

Insulin Resistance Induced by Hyperinsulinemia Coincides with a Persistent Alteration at the Insulin Receptor Tyrosine Kinase Domain

Karyn J. Catalano[1], Betty A. Maddux[1,2], Jaroslaw Szary[1], Jack F. Youngren[2], Ira D. Goldfine[2], Fred Schaufele[1]*

1 Department of Obstetrics and Gynecology and the Diabetes Center, University of California San Francisco, San Francisco, California, United States of America, **2** Division of Endocrinology and Metabolism, University of California San Francisco, San Francisco, California, United States of America

Abstract

Insulin resistance, the diminished response of target tissues to insulin, is associated with the metabolic syndrome and a predisposition towards diabetes in a growing proportion of the worldwide population. Under insulin resistant states, the cellular response of the insulin signaling pathway is diminished and the body typically responds by increasing serum insulin concentrations to maintain insulin signaling. Some evidence indicates that the increased insulin concentration may itself further dampen insulin response. If so, insulin resistance would worsen as the level of circulating insulin increases during compensation, which could contribute to the transition of insulin resistance to more severe disease. Here, we investigated the consequences of excess insulin exposure to insulin receptor (IR) activity. Cells chronically exposed to insulin show a diminished the level of IR tyrosine and serine autophosphorylation below that observed after short-term insulin exposure. The diminished IR response did not originate with IR internalization since IR amounts at the cell membrane were similar after short- and long-term insulin incubation. Förster resonance energy transfer between fluorophores attached to the IR tyrosine kinase (TK) domain showed that a change in the TK domain occurred upon prolonged, but not short-term, insulin exposure. Even though the altered 'insulin refractory' IR TK FRET and IR autophosphorylation levels returned to baseline (non-stimulated) levels after wash-out of the original insulin stimulus, subsequent short-term exposure to insulin caused immediate re-establishment of the insulin-refractory levels. This suggests that some cell-based 'memory' of chronic hyperinsulinemic exposure acts directly at the IR. An improved understanding of that memory may help define interventions to reset the IR to full insulin responsiveness and impede the progression of insulin resistance to more severe disease states.

Editor: Makoto Kanzaki, Tohoku University, Japan

Funding: This work was supported by an Early Exploration award from the NovoNordisk Diabetes Innovation Award Program, a Pilot and Feasibility award and support for the Diabetes Center Microscopy Core from the NIH-funded, UCSF Diabetes and Endocrine Research Center (P30 DK063270) and a Strategic Opportunities Support award from the NIH-funded UCSF Clinical and Translational Science Institute (UL1 RR024131). The funders had no role in study design, data collection and analysis, decision to publish, or preparation of the manuscript.

Competing Interests: The work was funded by an unrestricted grant from the NovoNordisk Diabetes Innovation Award Program.

* Email: freds@diabetes.ucsf.edu

Introduction

Insulin resistance, or the impaired ability of insulin to mediate glucose disposal, is a risk factor for several disorders including the metabolic syndrome, type 2 diabetes mellitus, gestational diabetes, cardiovascular disease and several forms of cancer [1]. Modifications in insulin signaling, often associated with imbalances in energy homeostasis such as obesity, have been linked to a predisposition towards the development of insulin resistance [2]. Once insulin resistance develops, the body responds through compensatory mechanisms designed to maintain insulin signaling. Here we examine how one of those compensatory alterations, an elevation in the concentration of circulating insulin, may itself cause a further decline in insulin signaling.

Insulin mediates its physiological effects by acting through a multimeric, transmembrane insulin receptor (IR) present at the surface of responsive cells. Once insulin is bound, the IR's intracellular tyrosine kinase domain becomes activated and phosphorylates specific tyrosines on the β-subunits of the IR dimer partners. This autophosphorylation initiates several signaling cascades that lead to insulin's downstream effects [3–7]. Insulin resistance could originate with a decreased amount of IR available to effect signaling. However, decreased overall IR levels are not typically observed in insulin-resistant patients with type 2 diabetes [8]. Furthermore, deficiencies in insulin signaling downstream of the IR have been heavily studied as a cause of insulin resistance in humans [9].

Insulin signaling also can be directly inhibited at the IR itself [2] as serine/threonine phosphorylation of the IR β-subunit, possibly through the protein kinase C pathway [10–13], inhibits IR tyrosine kinase activity [4,14]. A direct inhibition of IR signaling also has been observed in mouse models in which insulin resistance is associated with a loss of IR phosphorylation upon elevation of protein tyrosine phosphatase 1B (PTP1B) [15–16]. Still further, an

IR-interacting membrane glycoprotein, PC-1 (also called ENPP-1), has been implicated in insulin resistance and type 2 diabetes [17–21]; PC-1 seems to impair IR tyrosine kinase activity through a direct interaction of PC-1 with IR that does not affect insulin binding [22–23]. Thus, there is some evidence to suggest that some alterations at the IR itself may contribute to insulin resistance.

In individuals with functioning beta-cells, insulin resistance is often compensated for by increased beta-cell secretion of insulin. However, an elevated insulin concentration itself can induce or exacerbate insulin resistance [24]. For example, transgenic mice expressing multiple copies of the insulin gene, although lean and normoglycemic, exhibited marked insulin resistance [25]. Patients with primary insulinomas and no medical history of metabolic syndrome also have been observed to acquire insulin resistance, possibly as a result of their tumor-induced insulinemia [24]. Furthermore, diabetic patients receiving pulsatile, rather than continuous insulin infusion display better glucose control, suggesting that chronic insulin stimulation is best avoided for optimal insulin response [24]. While it might be tempting to suspect that an insulin-initiated turnover in IR could decrease the amount of IR available for signaling, most insulin resistant patients do not exhibit reduced skeletal muscle IR expression [26]. The mechanism by which an elevated or prolonged exposure to insulin (referred to here as hyperinsulinemia, regardless of origin) exerts its deleterious effects on insulin signaling remains unclear.

We examined whether prolonged insulin exposure induces a change in IR activity, membrane localization or structure that may render the IR less capable of being re-activated upon re-stimulation. Since the origins by which an individual may become hyperinsulinemic are variable, the studies presented here were conducted in cell culture models in which the amount and duration of insulin exposure could be carefully regulated independent of any other physiologic responses to hyperinsulinemia. The changes in IR structure and autophosphorylation detected in this study make it possible that the level and duration of insulin stimulation may act partially at the IR to initiate or progressively worsen insulin resistance.

Materials and Methods

Cell Culture

Rat hepatoma cells (HTCs) and Chinese Hamster Ovary (CHO) cells, obtained originally from the UCSF Cell Culture facility, were modified and maintained as described below. All cells were grown in Dulbecco's modified Eagle's medium containing 1 g/l glucose supplemented with 10% fetal bovine serum (Hyclone, Thermo Scientific, Waltham, MA, USA), 100 units/ml penicillin and streptomycin, and 1 mM glutamine at 37°C in 5% CO_2.

HTC cells were genetically modified to express the cDNA for the B-isoform of the human IR (HTC-IR) [27], or the human IR fused at its C-terminus in frame with the yellow fluorescent protein (IR-YFP). The IR expression cassettes were co-integrated into the genome with a linked expression cassette conferring resistance to the antibiotic G418. The culture media for HTC-IR or HTC-IR-YFP stable cell lines was supplemented with 500 μg/ml G418 (Axenia Biologix, Dixon, CA, USA). The CHO cells were modified with either a PC-1 expression cassette linked to the G418-resistance expression cassette (CHO-PC1) or with the G418-resistance cassette only (CHO). Both CHO cell lines were maintained with 800 μg/ml G418.

Insulin Treatments and Lysate Collection

For IR phosphorylation studies in HTC cells, extracts were prepared from cells grown in 10 cm plates to ~80% confluence. On the day of the study, cells were washed twice with 'starvation media' containing no fetal calf serum or selection drugs but supplemented with 1% bovine serum albumin. Cells were serum starved for 4 hrs and then treated with recombinant human insulin (Sigma-Aldrich, St. Louis, MO, USA) at the indicated doses and times. At the conclusion of treatment, cells were rapidly washed with ice-cold PBS 3 times and solubilized in 0.5–1.0 ml of lysis buffer containing 50 mM HEPES (pH 7.6), 150 mM sodium chloride, 1% Triton X-100, 1 mM phenylmethylsulfonyl fluoride (PMSF), and 2 mM sodium orthovanadate at 4°C for 60 min. To remove cellular debris, lysates were spun at 14,000 g for 20 min at 4°C. Protein content was determined in each sample using the Pierce BCA protein assay kit (Thermo Scientific) per manufacturer's instructions.

Determination of Total Insulin Receptor Tyrosine and Serine Phosphorylation

Total IR phosphorylation was determined using an enzyme-linked immunosorbent assay (ELISA) as previously described [28]. Equal amounts of cell lysates (20 μg protein) were loaded onto a 96-well plate coated with monoclonal anti-human IR antibody (MA-20, prepared in-house), that does not cross-react with the related receptor for insulin-like growth factor 1 [29]. Lysates were incubated with the IR-specific antibody for 18 hr at 4°C. Next, plates were washed with Tris-buffered saline containing 150 mM sodium chloride, 0.05% Tween-20, and 20 mM Tris (pH 7.4). Horse radish peroxidase (HRP)-conjugated mouse monoclonal anti-phosphotyrosine pY-20 (Santa Cruz Biotechnology, Santa Cruz, CA, USA) or rabbit polyclonal anti-phosphoserine (Abcam, Cambridge, England) antibodies were then added and allowed to incubate for 2 hr at 22°C; wells treated with the anti-phosphotyrosine antibody were subsequently incubated with horseradish peroxidase-linked streptavidin. Binding was measured upon the addition of the peroxidase substrate, 3,3′,5,5′-tetramethylbenzidine (TMB). The amount of tyrosine or serine phosphorylation was determined by reading the optical density (absorption at 451 nm) of the converted substrate. Measurements were conducted in triplicate and averaged. The means +/− standard deviation of the measurements from multiple independent studies are shown in the figures (see figure legend for numbers of studies). As absolute numbers vary from study to study, the data in the figures are shown normalized to a standard treatment condition common to all studies (see Fig. 1 legend).

Western Blotting

Lysates (10 μg), prepared as described above, were diluted with an equal volume of 2× loading buffer and subjected to SDS-PAGE on a gradient gel (8–16%), followed by transfer onto a 0.45 μm nitrocellulose membrane. Membranes were blocked for 1–2 hr at room temperature in Odyssey Blocking Buffer (LI-COR Biosciences, Lincoln, NE, USA) and incubated overnight at 4°C with the following primary antibodies in blocking buffer containing 0.1% Tween-20: mouse monoclonal anti-IR (MA-20, 0.17 μg/ml final concentration), rabbit polyclonal anti-pY972 (Abcam, ab-5678, 1:4000), rabbit polyclonal anti-pY1162,1163 (Santa Cruz, sc-25103, 1:500), mouse monoclonal anti-ERK (Cell Signaling Technology, 1:4000, Beverly, MA, USA), rabbit polyclonal anti-pERK (Cell Signaling Technology, 1:2000), rabbit polyclonal anti-AKT (Cell Signaling Technology, 1:2000), rabbit polyclonal anti-pAKT (Cell Signaling Technology, 1:1000), rabbit polyclonal anti-

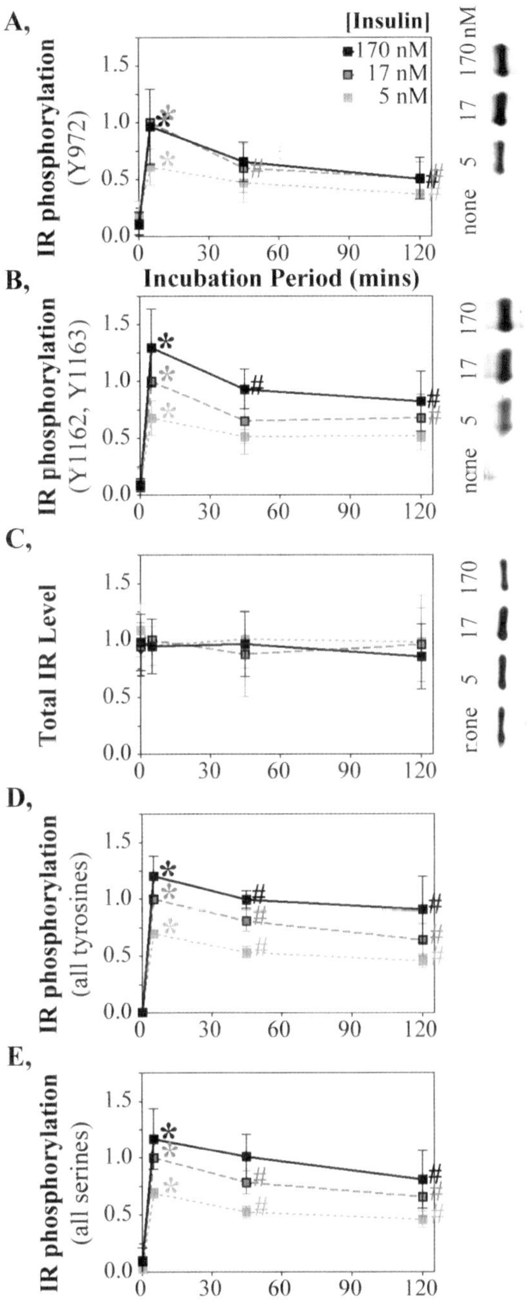

Figure 1. Chronic insulin exposure down-regulates IR activity. Timecourse and insulin dose response of IR phosphorylation at (**A**) pY IR^{972} and (**B**) pY $IR^{1162,1163}$ detected by western blot with phospho-specific rabbit polyclonal antibodies. Detection and quantification was by infrared immunofluorescence linked to the anti-rabbit secondary antibody. Representative westerns shown for a dose response (right panels; only shown for the shortest insulin incubation period). (**C**) Total IR protein quantified on the same western blots with an anti-IR mouse monoclonal antibody conjugated with an anti-mouse secondary antibody linked to a distinct infrared fluorophore. Total (**D**) tyrosine and (**E**) serine phosphorylation, over all sites on the IR determined by ELISA, in response to insulin stimulation. Data are presented as mean ± sd from 3, 10 and 9 independent studies for the 5 nm, 17 nM and 170 nM doses. The intermediate 45 mins time point was included in a subset of those studies (3, 4 and 4 studies for the 5 nm, 17 nM and 170 nM doses). Since the absolute 'light unit' values quantified differ from experiment to experiment, the data were normalized to a treatment condition common amongst all experimental conditions. The earliest time point of induction (2–10′) with 17 nM insulin was set as 1.0 and all other data points within each study were normalized to that. *, increased IR phosphorylation ($p<0.05$) at the 2–10′ time point relative to the no insulin control. #, diminished IR phosphorylation at longer insulin incubation periods ($p<0.05$) relative to the 2–10′ time point. The data normalization and statistical symbols are applied similarly to the data presented in the remaining figures.

GSK (Cell Signaling Technology, 1:1000), and mouse monoclonal anti-pGSK (Cell Signaling Technology, 1:1000). Membranes were then washed and incubated for 30 min at room temperature with 1:10,000 dilutions of species-specific secondary antibodies (LI-COR Biosciences) conjugated with either 680 nm or 800 nm fluorophores. The secondary antibodies were removed by two washes of washing buffer and the fluorescence from each band was detected on the Odyssey Infrared Imaging System (LI-COR Biosciences). Fluorescence levels were quantified using Image Studio Software Version 2.1.10 (LI-COR Biosciences) with an in-lane background region used to subtract fluorescence values originating from noise. The means +/− standard deviation of those measurements from multiple independent studies (see figure legend for numbers of studies) are shown in the figures.

Insulin Receptor Localization

Two days after seeding HTC-IR-YFP cells at 2,000 cells per well in 384-well tissue-culture-treated imaging plates (Greiner BioOne; Frickenhausen, Germany), wells were washed twice with starvation media and incubated in 30 µl starvation media for four hours prior to insulin addition. To each well was added 10 µl starvation media containing insulin diluted so that the final concentration was 17 nM insulin in 40 µl media. For control wells, 10 µl of starvation media without insulin was added. Images of the YFP-tagged IR were collected over a 6 minute period+/− 3 minutes to the time points indicated in the figures. 30 minutes prior to image collection was added the membrane staining dye CellMask Orange and the nuclear staining dye Hoechst 33342 (Invitrogen, Carlsbad, CA, USA) to 2.5 µg/ml and 5.0 µg/ml final concentrations, respectively.

Images were captured with a 40×, 0.95 NA objective on an Olympus IX-70 microscope using a triple band-pass dichroic mirror and filter sets (Chroma Corp.; Brattleboro, VT) that distinguish, in order of image collection, the fluorescence of the YFP-tagged IR (excite 480–495 nm, collect 500–530 nm) from the CellMask Orange-stained membrane (excite 550–560 nm, collect 580–630 nm) and from the Hoechst 33342-stained nucleus (excite 365–395 nm, collect 435–465 nm). Image collection times were 1000, 25 and 50 ms, respectively. Filter wheels (Sutter Corp., Novato, CA, USA) rapidly move filters to collect sequential images within <200 ms of the end of the prior collection. Images were captured at 14-bit depth on a CCD camera (Andor Technology, Belfast, Northern Ireland) set at gain 1.5. Image collection was controlled by Metamorph 7.1 software (Molecular Device Corp., Downingtown, PA, USA).

Images were analyzed with Metamorph 7.1's multi-wavelength cell scoring module. Individual cells were identified by the nuclear marker, from which the cellular margins of each cell was established by the location of the membrane marker. The image analysis alogarithms best define membranes using a 'negative' of the CellMask Orange image (i.e., that image subtracted at each pixel from the maximal 14-bit values). Visual inspection shows that the cell margins defined by that alogarithm parallel a user's perception of the location of the stained membrane in the images although perhaps 50% of membrane segments show folds that do not precisely track with the alogarithm-defined cell margins. All membranes are included if the membrane margin is expanded

400 nm towards the interior of the cell. The IR-YFP intensities within that expanded membrane mask are shown in the figure. The IR-YFP intensities reported for the cytoplasm cover a cellular area that starts a further 600 nm interior to the membrane mask and do not include the cell nucleus defined by the nuclear marker.

Förster Resonance Emission Transfer (FRET)

HTC or CHO cells were transiently transfected with a vector expressing a tandem repeat of cyan fluorescent protein (CFP) and YFP appended to the C-terminus of the IR (IR-CFP-YFP). Control transfections expressed either IR-CFP or IR-YFP. Cells first were plated into 6-well dishes containing sterile 22×22 mm Number 1 borosilicate coverglasses. Cells were grown an additional two days, then transfected using a total of 1.875 µg of each plasmid and 10 µl Lipofectamine LTC (Invitrogen) per well. Transfected cells were grown overnight following which cells were subjected to 4 hour insulin starvation prior to the initiation of insulin incubation (100 nM), as described in the prior sections. The cover slips were removed for imaging following insulin incubation for the times indicated in the figures. For some CHO studies, the remaining cells were collected for extract preparation and measurement of IR auto-phosphorylation by ELISA, as described above. Only in CHO cells was the transfection efficiency great enough to permit those autophosphorylation studies.

The 'acceptor' YFP (excite 490–510 nm, collect 520–550 nm), 'donor' CFP (excite 431–441 nm, collect 455–485 nm) and FRET (excite 431–441 nm, collect 520–550 nm) channels were collected on Hamamatsu (Tokyo, Japan) ORCA camera on an Olympus IX-70 microscope. Exposure times were 200, 400 and 100 ms, respectively, at camera gain 5. Excitation was with a 200 W Hg/Xe light source (OptiQuip; Highland Mills, NY, USA) that possesses a strong 436 nm peak optimal for exciting CFP.

FRET was calculated as previously described [30–31]. Briefly, when energy is transferred from the donor fluorophore (CFP) to the acceptor fluorophore (YFP), CFP intensities become dimmer whereas the amount of yellow light emitted upon CFP excitation (the FRET channel) increases. Because CFP and YFP both are independently excited by, and emit in, the FRET channel, the amounts of that 'donor bleedthrough' and 'acceptor bleedthrough' are determined from control cells transfected with only the CFP or YFP expression vectors. The background-subtracted and bleed-through-corrected intensities in the donor and FRET channels are used to establish the percentage of donor energy transferred to the acceptor (E), on a microscope calibrated to define constants for that conversion. In the figures, E represents the mean +/− sd of multiple independent studies in which an average of 47 CHO cells or 27 HTC cells were collected for each measurement point in each independent study.

Statistical Analysis

All Data were reported as mean ± sd from multiple independent studies. All studies were compared using a One-Way ANOVA with Tukey's post-hoc tests for individual comparisons. Statistical significance was set at $p<0.05$.

Results

Down-Regulation of Insulin Response Upon Chronic Insulin Exposure

To establish how the length of duration of insulin stimulation affects IR signaling, HTC-IR cells, in which the human insulin receptor is expressed and readily measured [22] were incubated with insulin at various doses and periods of time. Insulin responsiveness was measured first by the most proximal IR function activated by insulin following four hours growth of the cells in insulin-deprived media. Almost immediately upon insulin addition, activation of the IR tyrosine kinase results in tyrosine autophosphorylation of the IR at all insulin doses (5, 17 and 170 nM) examined (Fig. 1; *, $p<0.01$).

pY^{972} and $pY^{1162,1163}$ are important sites for receptor activation that leads to further IR autophosphorylation and the binding/phosphorylation of IR interacting factors within the insulin signaling cascade. At all insulin doses, IR autophosphorylation at Y^{972} (Fig. 1A) and $Y^{1162,1163}$ (Fig. 1B), measured by quantitative western blot with phospho-specific anti-IR antibodies, was induced within ten minutes of insulin stimulation and declined below that activated level at later time points (#, $p<0.05$). The changes in IR autophosphorylation were not accompanied by any changes in total IR amount (Fig. 1C). The progressive loss of IR autophosphorylation over time therefore was not a consequence of any diminution of the total IR pool.

The stimulation and down-regulation of IR global autophosphorylation also was evident by ELISA measurement of all anti-phospho-tyrosine antibody bound to insulin captured by an anti-insulin antibody (Fig. 1D). This suggests a bulk down-regulation in tyrosine phosphorylation scattered, across all 13 known IR autophosphorylation sites. ELISA studies of pan-serine phosphorylation of the IR showed a similar down-regulation (Fig. 1E). Thus, a general diminution of IR phosphorylation occurs upon chronic insulin stimulation.

There are similarities in tyrosine phosphorylation sites in the IR and the insulin-like growth factor-1 receptor (IGF1R). Some cross-reactivity has been reported for binding of the phosphotyrosine-specific IR antibodies used in figures 1A and 1B to both phospho-IR and phospho-IGF1R. The ELISA assay (Fig. 1D) is specific for the IR [29] and shows an insulin response pattern similar to that of the two phospho-IR/IGF1R-targeted antibodies. The apparent down-regulation of tyrosine phosphorylation upon chronic insulin exposure therefore seems to occur at multiple sites throughout the IR. With no change in IR level (Fig. 1C), the reduction in IR phosphorylation upon prolonged insulin exposure reflects an average loss of phosphorylation per IR, not a net loss in the amounts of IR present.

Divergent Downstream Signaling Responses to Chronic Insulin Exposure

The activation of IR autophosphorylation by insulin initiates a number of divergent signaling pathways, some of which were measured to define the consequences of phospho-IR down-regulation to downstream signaling. Phosphorylation of Erk1/2 at Thr202/Tyr204 was used as a read-out of insulin activation of the MAPK/ERK pathway. ERK showed a very strong and transient phosphorylation at 5 mins for all doses followed by a very rapid decline by 45 mins of insulin exposure (Fig. 2A). The changes in total ERK phosphorylation were not accompanied by any changes in total ERK protein (Fig. 2B). The activation of other insulin-regulated signaling pathways, measured by AKT phosphorylation at Ser473 and GSK3α/β phosphorylation at Ser21/Ser9, also reached maximum by 10 min at all insulin doses (Figs. 2C, E). Total AKT and total GSK3 protein levels similarly were unchanged by time or dose (Fig. 2D, F). No declines in AKT or GSK3 autophosphorylation were detected even 120 minutes after insulin addition (Fig. 2C, E). This does not necessarily mean that those signaling pathways are chronically activated as they may be down-regulated by other modifications at other sites.

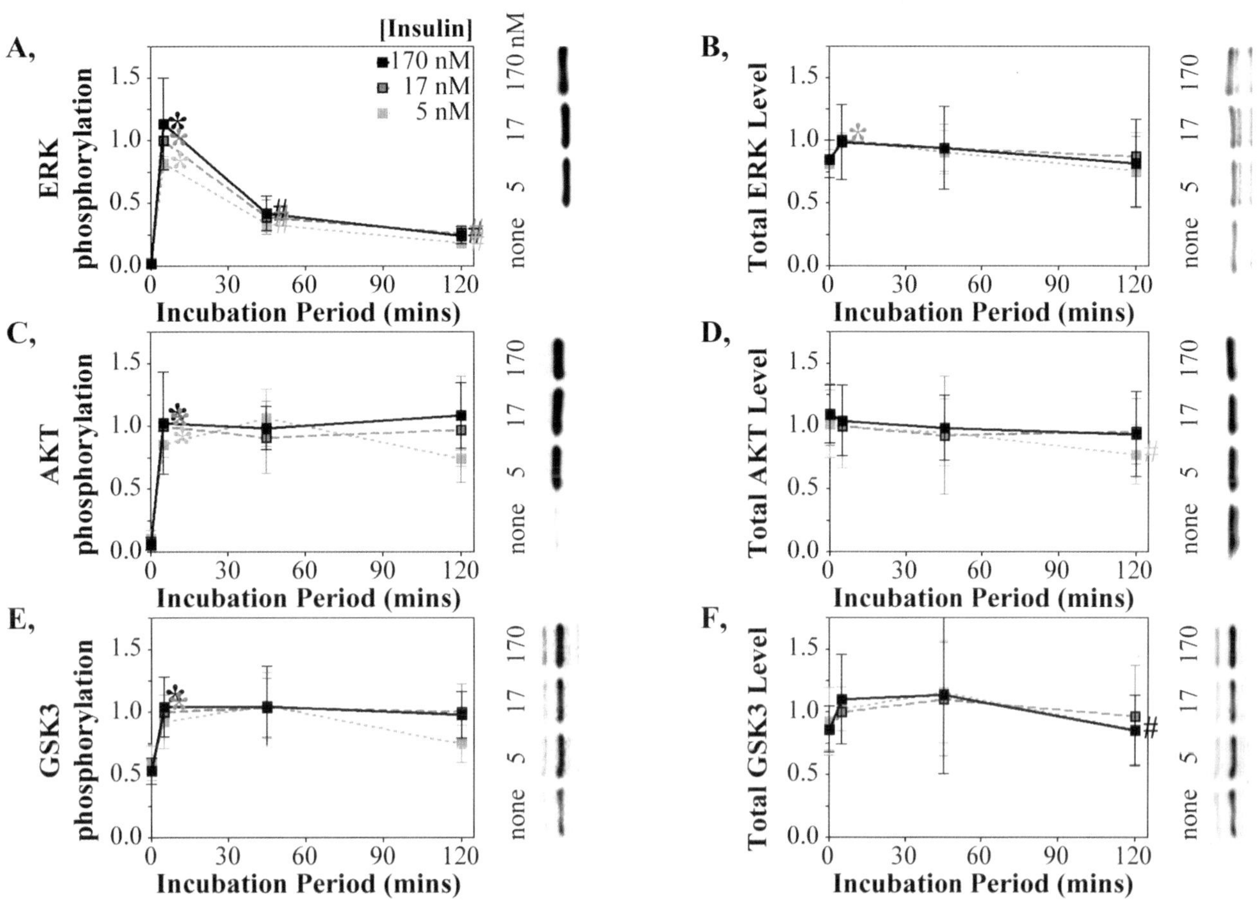

Figure 2. Differential down-regulation of downstream signaling pathways following chronic insulin stimulation. (**A**) phospho-ERK, (**B**) total ERK (**C**) phospho-AKT, (**D**) total AKT, (**E**) phospho-GSKβ, and (**F**) total GSKβ proteins quantified by western blot using the same extracts analyzed in figure 1. The fluorescence intensities of pERK and ERK, or pGSK and GSK, were quantified on the same blot with the phospho-specific and total protein antibodies (of rabbit and mouse origin) conjugated to specific-specific secondary antibodies with distinguishable fluorophores. The pAKT and total AKT antibodies both originated from rabbits and were probed in separate blots. Data normalization, number of studies, symbols and representative westerns are as described in figure 1.

Insulin Refractory Response

The diminution of IR autophosphorylation following insulin stimulation may be a natural response that enables the IR to avoid an over-reaction to a lingering insulin stimulus. Once the remnants of that prior stimulation are erased, the expectation may be that the previously down-regulated IR will regain a full response to subsequent insulin stimulation. We therefore examined how chronic insulin stimulation affects the IR's ability to respond to subsequent insulin stimulation (Fig. 3).

HTC-IR cells were exposed for short (2 mins) or prolonged (120 mins) periods of 170 nM insulin (Figs. 3A–C, left panels) or 17 nM insulin (right panels), followed by removal of the insulin and a subsequent 2 min re-stimulation with the same insulin concentration. As in the earlier studies (Fig. 1), IR Y^{972} (Fig. 3A, black bars) and $pY^{1162,1163}$ (Fig. 3B, black bars) phosphorylation was strongly elevated 2 minutes after insulin addition (*, $p<0.05$) and diminished by 120 minutes of insulin incubation (#, $p<0.05$). Following the primary 2 or 120 minute stimulation, the insulin was removed and the cells were incubated for only ten minutes with no insulin (gray bars). That washout of insulin was sufficient to erase most of the IR autophosphorylation. This rapid decrease in IR phosphorylation suggests that IR tyrosine phosphorylation is rapidly removed unless insulin remains present. Therefore, even at 120 minutes of chronic insulin stimulation, IR phosphorylation likely remains ongoing but is shifted to a lower level.

The critical question is whether, after wash-out of the insulin, the cell resets the IR so that the IR now responds to a second 2 minute stimulus (Fig. 3, checkered bars) equivalently to the initial 2 minute stimulus (black bars). Secondary insulin stimulation following 120 mins insulin exposure permitted the IR to regain only the diminished autophosphorylation level characteristic of the 120 mins time point. Thus, the conditions at the IR that caused it to have a diminished insulin response following 120 mins of chronic insulin exposure persisted after the wash. There was no change in the amount of IR present within the cell (Fig. 3C) that could account for that diminished response. By contrast, an initial exposure to only 2 mins of insulin was insufficient to diminish the second IR stimulation (Figs. 3A, B). This shows that the 'insulin refractory state' must first be achieved for the memory of that state to persist. As discussed later, even removing insulin for up to 180 minutes was insufficient to overcome the persistently diminished IR state.

For the 17 nM insulin studies, extracts also were collected 30 minutes following the initial insulin stimulation. Following 30 mins insulin exposure, IR phosphorylation at $Y^{1162,1163}$ was already diminished and remained diminished upon insulin wash-

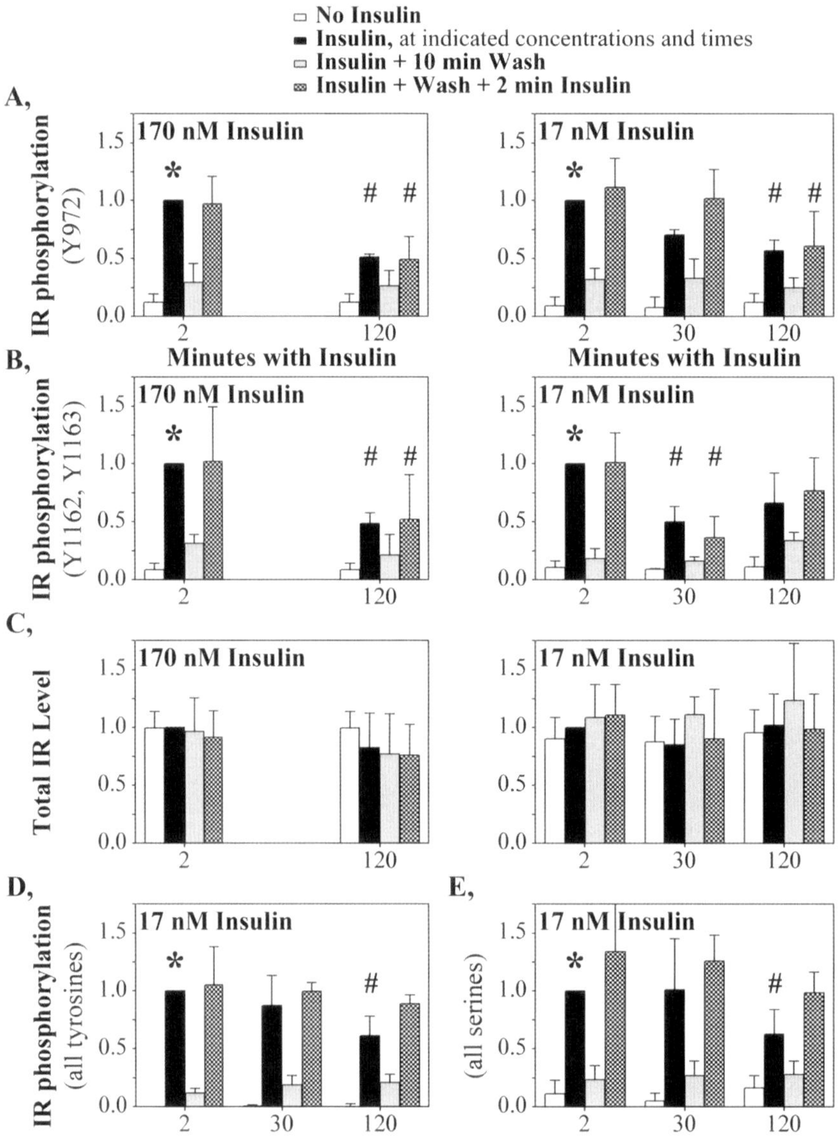

Figure 3. Chronically stimulated IR is refractory to subsequent re-stimulation following removal of insulin. Insulin receptor tyrosine phosphorylation at (**A**) pY IR^{972} (170 nM: n = 4 independent studies; 17 nM: n = 5) and (**B**) pY $IR^{1162,1163}$ (170 nM: n = 4; 17 nM: n = 3) quantified by western blot in response to repeated insulin stimulation. (**C**) total IR protein quantified on the same blots. (**D**) Total tyrosine (n = 5) and (**E**) total serine (n = 5) phosphorylation, measured by ELISA (17 nM treatments). Data normalization and symbols are as described in figure 1.

out and re-stimulation (Fig. 3B). For Y^{972}, the reduction in IR phosphorylation at 30 minutes of insulin exposure did not achieve statistical significance and the subsequent 2 mins insulin exposure was able to restimulate IR autophosphorylation to the level of the primary 2 mins stimulus.

Some differences in other phosphorylation responses were noted in the re-stimulation studies. Autophosphorylation across all IR tyrosines (Fig. 3D) or serines (Fig. 3E) was mostly or completely recovered by the ten minute wash-out of insulin. Thus, pY^{972} and $pY^{1162,1163}$ are unusual amongst the insulin-induced phosphorylation sites in not rapidly recovering. Because pY^{972} and $pY^{1162,1163}$ represent key sites in the initiation of the insulin signaling cascade, the refractory nature of re-stimulation at these sites may have an outsized effect on some aspects on a deadened insulin response when the IR is exposed to insulin for prolonged times.

The markers of downstream insulin signaling similarly were assessed for complete or partial recovery of the secondary insulin response following chronic insulin stimulation (Fig. 4). Erk phosphorylation could not be re-stimulated after a second 2 min stimulation following initial short- or long-term exposures (Figs. 4A, B; 2 mins or 120 mins). Thus, once stimulated by insulin, even for 2 minutes, Erk seems to be unable to respond to any secondary stimulation. Erk therefore appears to have rigidly controlled mechanisms of preventing secondary phosphorylation responses that are likely distinct from the more modest changes in IR pY^{972} and $pY^{1162,1163}$ response to secondary stimulus following prolonged activation. Neither Akt nor Gsk3β phosphorylation was reduced by removing insulin (Figs. 4C–E) which is consistent either with sustained activity or a mechanism of down-regulation that does not involve removal of the activating phosphorylation.

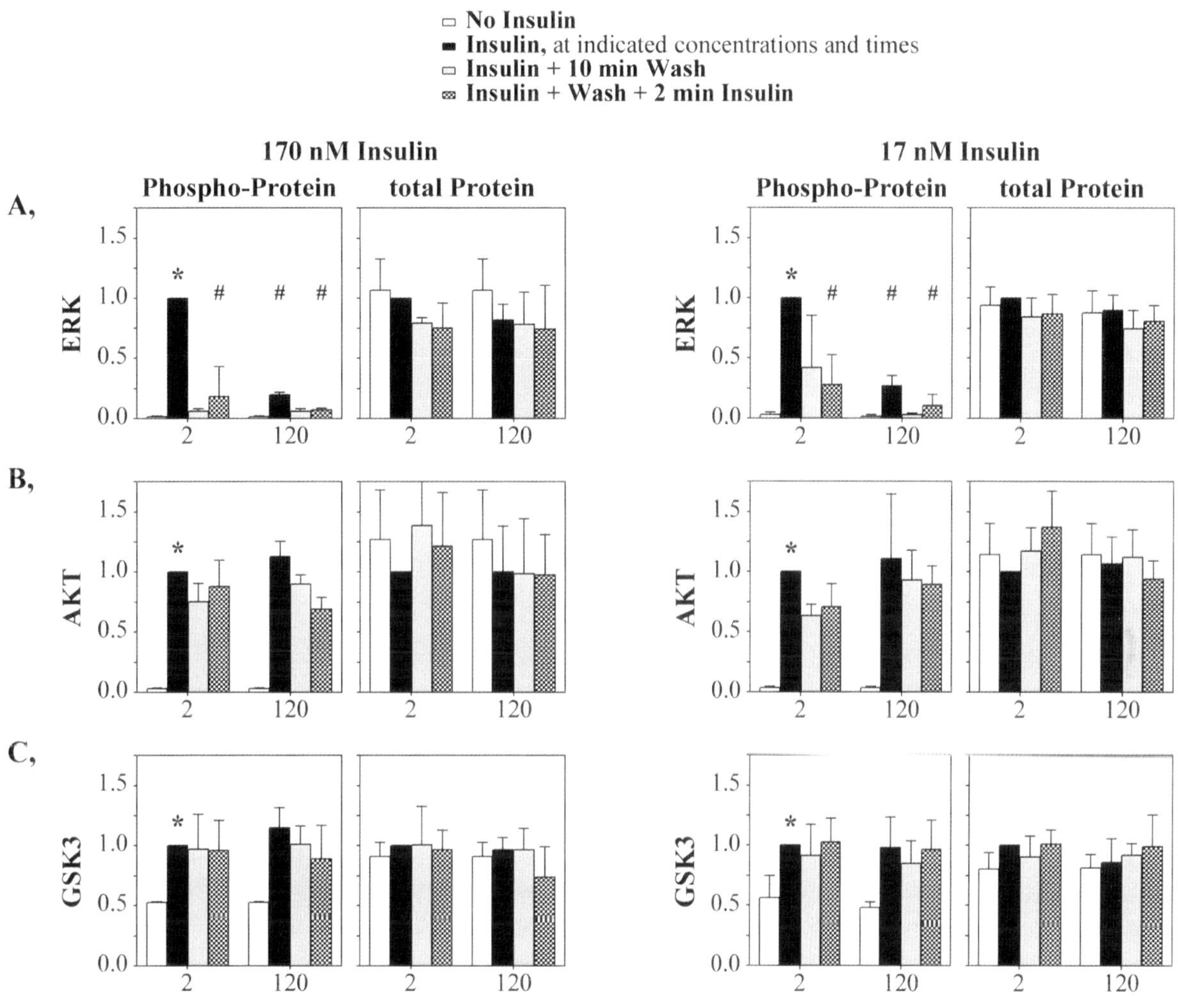

Figure 4. Differential impact of re-stimulation on pathways downstream of the IR. (**A**) pERK, (**B**) total ERK, (**C**) pAKT, (**D**) total AKT (**E**) pGSKβ and (**F**) total GSKβ proteins quantified by western blot in response to repeated insulin stimulation. See Fig. 2 for measurement details. Data are represented as mean ± SD from three (170 nM) and four (17 nM) independent studies. Data normalization and symbols are as described in figure 1.

IR Internalization Does Not Account for the Refractory Response

The studies of total insulin receptor level (Figs. 1C, 3C) showed no change in IR levels that could account for the diminished IR phosphorylation. However, long-term exposure to insulin could increase internalization of IR and sequester IR from the membrane to blunt insulin response. To test this possibility, HTC cells were created that stably expressed the cDNA for the human IR fused in frame at the C-terminus of the β-subunit with the cDNA for the yellow fluorescent protein (YFP). Fluorescence microscopy of these HTC-IR-YFP cells (Fig. 5A) showed that IR-YFP fluorescence coincided predominantly with cell membranes stained by the CellMask Orange membrane-specific dye. IR tyrosine autophosphorylation studies showed that the YFP-tagged IR responded to insulin dose and time-course studies (Fig. 5B) similarly to that measured for the untagged IR (see Fig. 1D). This HTC-IR-YFP cell line therefore was competent for comparing diminished IR autophosphorylation upon chronic insulin exposure with IR distribution in cellular membranes and cytoplasm.

Quantification of the amounts of IR-YFP at the cell membrane (marked by the membrane marker) and within the cytoplasm (Fig. 5C) showed that diminished IR phosphorylation induced by 17 nM insulin was not accompanied by any reduction in IR amount at the cell membrane. Similar measurements of the membrane marker (Fig. 5D) serve as a control for quantification accuracy and similarly did not change with insulin doses or incubation period. Less than 10% of the total YFP signal was detected in the cytosol, likely representing background, as quantification of the membrane stain showed a similar result. These findings make it unlikely that the strong reduction in IR phosphorylation after long-term insulin exposure arose exclusively from a reduction in IR availability to insulin at the cell membrane.

The IR Tyrosine Kinase Domain Acquires an Altered State Upon Chronic Insulin Exposure

The above studies showed that the insulin refractory response was not linked to changes in IR level or localization. We next investigated if it could be associated with any persistently altered tyrosine kinase (TK) state induced by prolonged insulin exposure. Changes in the structure of, or environment around, the IR TK domain were investigated by Förster resonance energy transfer (FRET). A human IR was tagged at the C-terminal TK domain with a fused CFP-YFP fluorophore and expressed in cells (Fig. 6A). Any insulin-induced conformational change, modifica-

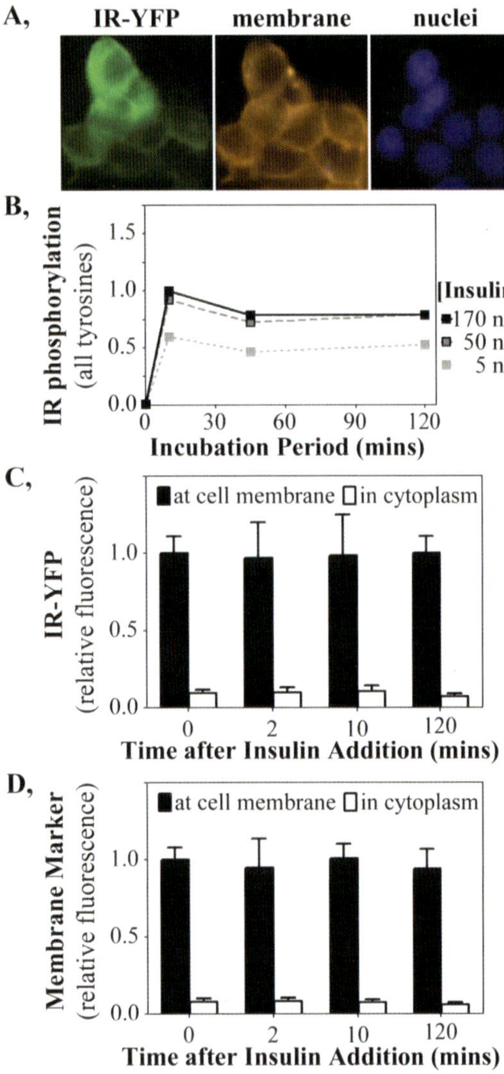

Figure 5. The IR remains membrane localized following chronic insulin stimulation of HTC-IR-YFP cells. (**A**) YFP fused to the IR fluoresces green and co-localizes with the membrane-specific stain (orange) and not with nuclei (blue). (**B**) Total IR tyrosine phosphorylation in HTC-IR-YFP cells, detected by ELISA, mirrors that of the unfused similar to HTC-IR in response to insulin stimulation (see Fig. 1D). The fluorescence intensity of (**C**) YFP (IR) and (**D**) the membrane marker were quantified at the membrane and in the cytosol of HTC-IR-YFP cells.

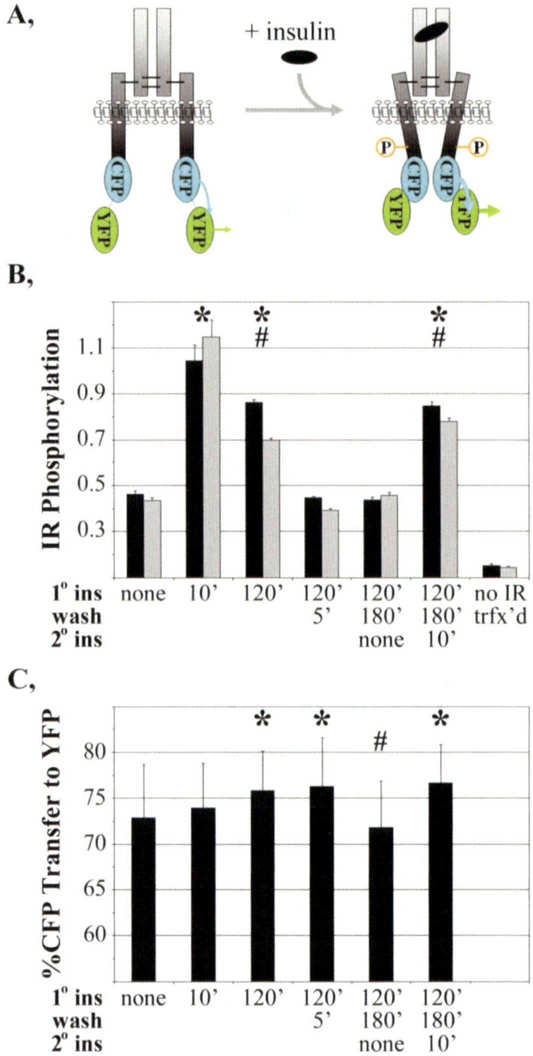

Figure 6. FRET measurement of altered IR structure or environment associated with insulin resistance in CHO cells. (**A**) Schematic representation of the IR-CFP-YFP probe and alterations in (**B**) total IR tyrosine phosphorylation or (**C**) energy transfer in that probe under acute or chronic insulin stimulation and after re-stimulation following insulin removal. The probe was transiently expressed in CHO cells. Symbols are as described in figure 1. Gray bars (Fig. 6B) represent IR phosphorylation levels normalized to IR expression levels determined by IR-CFP-YFP fluorescence.

tion, or interaction with other factors, near the IR TK domain would shift CFP and YFP relative to each other. Such a shift would alter the percentage of CFP (donor) fluorophore energy transferred to the nearby YFP (acceptor) fluorophore.

Autophosphorylation studies were first conducted to assess if the IR-CFP-YFP probe remained functional. The autophosphorylation studies were conducted in CHO cells which were more readily transfected than HTC cells. Upon transient expression in CHO cells, IR-CFP-YFP was maximally phosphorylated within 10 min of insulin incubation (Fig. 6B, 10′); the level of autophosphorylation is presented per amount of extract (black bars) or adjusted for minor variations in transfection level (Fig. 6B, gray bars; normalized to YFP fluorescence from the IR). Both measurements showed that, as in the earlier studies in HTC cells stably expressing the untagged or YFP-tagged IR (Figs. 1, 3, 5), autophosphorylation of the transiently expressed IR-CFP-YFP probe became diminished after 120 mins of insulin exposure. Subsequent secondary insulin stimulation also permitted IR-CFP-YFP autophosphorylation only to the diminished 'insulin-refractory' level, even after washing away the insulin for 180 minutes. The IR-CFP-YFP probe thus retained the insulin refractory response characteristic of the non-tagged IR.

The availability of a functional IR-CFP-YFP probe allowed FRET investigation of alterations in the IR TK domain that might occur upon acute or chronic insulin exposure. The percentage of donor (CFP) energy transferred to acceptor (YFP) within the IR-CFP-YFP probe expressed in CHO cells was high (>70%) in the absence of insulin stimulation (Fig. 6C, none). This reflects the close proximity of the CFP and YFP attached in tandem to the most C-terminal amino acid within the IR. 10 minutes incubation with insulin did not alter that level of energy transfer ($p>0.05$). Thus, no gross change in the environment surrounding the IR TK domain was associated with the rapid induction of IR autophosphorylation.

By contrast, prolonged insulin stimulation increased ($p<0.05$) the amount of energy transfer (Fig. 6C, 120′). That suggested that the positions of the CFP and YFP tagged to the IR TK domain shifted upon prolonged insulin exposure. FRET changes may occur experimentally, as a consequence of the photobleaching of a fluorophore over repetitive excitation. That was avoided by measuring, for each time point, naïve cells grown on a separate slide and never exposed to light until a one-time, rapid automated image collection at the specific time-point. Thus, the data collection procedures minimized the potential for photobleaching artifacts. Furthermore, FRET increased at the 120′ insulin exposure time whereas photobleaching would have decreased FRET as a consequence of preferential photobleaching of the YFP 'FRET acceptor' that is more photolabile than the CFP 'FRET donor' [32].

A short wash-out of insulin was sufficient to permit the rapid loss of IR-CFP-YFP autophosphorylation (Fig. 6B, 5′ wash). However, that de-phosphorylated IR still maintained the 'insulin refractory' FRET level (Fig. 6C, 5′ wash) indicating that the altered fluorophore positions acquired upon chronic insulin stimulation was not linked to continued IR phosphorylation. It is possible that the persistence of insulin-refractory IR-CFP-YFP FRET may reflect an altered IR TK structure that constitutes a 'memory' state responsible for the reduced level of phosphorylation upon subsequent re-stimulation. However, that particular IR TK structure does not confer the memory state itself as the altered FRET state was expunged with a prolonged wash-out of insulin (Fig. 6C, 180′ wash) but still rapidly re-acquired with the subsequent 10′ re-stimulation.

The insulin refractory FRET state also was observed when the IR-CFP-YFP probe was transiently expressed in HTC cells (Fig. 7, black bars). The baseline level of IR-CFP-YFP FRET in HTC cells was slightly lower than that in CHO cells. However, as in CHO cells, prolonged incubation of HTC cells with insulin increased the amount of energy transfer within IR-CFP-YFP (120′), whereas short insulin incubation did not (10′). As a negative FRET measurement control, the amounts of energy transfer also are shown for a probe in which CFP and YFP were attached to the amino- and carboxy-termini of the IR-interacting factor, IRS-1 (gray bars). That positioned the fluorescent proteins too far apart for efficient FRET which was accurately measured in the current studies.

The Insulin-Refractory State Also is Acquired upon PC-1 Expression

Our prior studies also showed that insulin response, measured by IR autophosphorylation, was decreased upon the expression of PC-1 [33]. PC-1 is a membrane glycoprotein associated with insulin resistance in humans and in transgenic mice modified to over-express PC-1 [17,19–21]. We therefore examined whether the shift in IR TK conformation, measured by IR-CFP-YFP FRET, occurred in the presence of PC-1.

The IR-CFP-YFP probe was transiently expressed in CHO cell lines that stably expressed PC-1 linked to a G418-resistance cassette, or just the G418 cassette only (Fig. 8). Expression of the IR-CFP-YFP probe in PC-1-expressing cells resulted, even in the absence of chronic insulin exposure, in an elevated FRET signal reminiscent of that which occurs following chronic (120′) insulin exposure of cells not overexpressing PC-1. Statistical significance was not achieved in this study set, but the general trend is towards an elevated FRET level upon chronic insulin exposure ($p=0.068$) or PC-1 overexpression ($p=0.066$). The IR TK alteration detected by FRET thus may be a general marker of insulin resistance initiated by divergent mechanisms, including PC-1 expression or hyperinsulinemia.

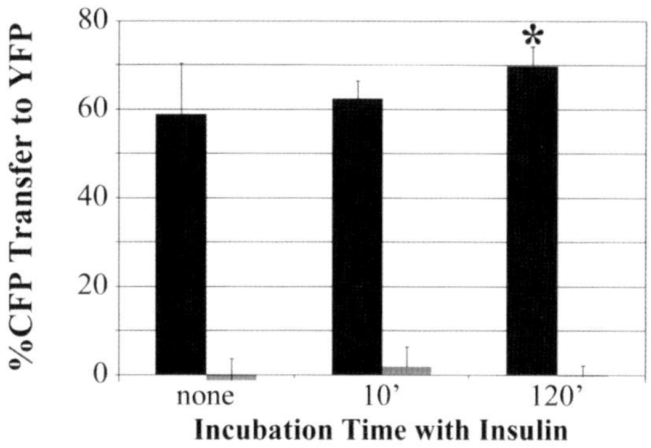

Figure 7. Insulin refractory IR structure in HTC cells. Energy transfer of IR-CFP-YFP probe transiently expressed in HTC cells subjected to acute (10′) and chronic (120′) insulin exposure. Gray bars, minimal energy transfer of CFP and YFP attached to the amino and carboxy termini of IRS1 (too far apart for energy transfer) demonstrates FRET measurement accuracy. Data represent the mean ± sd of the average FRET measurements of an average of 44 cells per point in each of three independent studies.

Discussion

That long-term or continuous insulin exposure could lead to insulin resistance is not a new concept. Insulin is normally released in low-amplitude pulses and rapidly cleared from the circulation [34–35] possibly so that the body avoids chronic insulin exposure. Indeed, a pulsatile delivery of exogenous insulin also appears to confer improved glucose control compared to continuous infusion of insulin [24,36–41]. Given that insulin signaling must be exquisitely controlled to maintain metabolic control, it is logical that the body would possess mechanisms to prevent insulin signaling under conditions of insulin excess. Thus, in transgenic

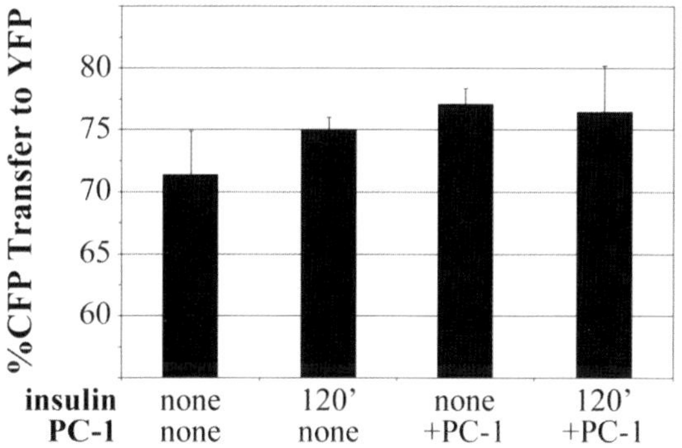

Figure 8. IR-CFP-YFP structure induced by chronic insulin exposure is similar to that induced by expression of PC-1. FRET levels of the IR-CFP-YFP probe transiently expressed in CHO cells or in CHO cells stably overexpressing PC-1. Measurements are conducted prior to insulin treatment or after chronic (120′) insulin exposure (n = 3 independent studies). Data represent the mean ± sd of the average FRET measurements of an average of 27 cells per point in each of three independent studies.

mice over-expressing insulin [25] or in patients with insulinomas [42–45], the resulting hyperinsulinemia is counteracted by a diminished insulin response. While such studies reveal a clear negative effect of hyperinsulinemia on insulin action, they do not elucidate the mechanism by which this process occurs so that it may be avoided.

We hypothesized that some deficit in IR activity may contribute to insulin resistance conferred by hyperinsulinemia. Once pre-incubated with insulin for prolonged times, the ability of IR to autophosphorylate in response to insulin became curtailed (Fig. 3). The deficit in IR phosphorylation following long-term insulin stimulation appeared to occur in the absence of any changes in either IR amount or membrane localization (Fig. 5). Notably, the refractory phosphorylation state occurred in concert with a distinct change, measured by FRET, in the position of FPs attached to the IR tyrosine kinase domain (Figs. 6, 7). The detection of the IR structural alteration in two cell lines and its parallel to the pronounced decrease in IR autophosphorylation upon prolonged insulin exposure suggests that the subtle FRET change measured may be affiliated with the down-regulation of IR signaling. The similar, subtle change in IR structure upon the induction of insulin resistance by another means (Fig. 8) further supports the structural/functional association although, as described below, this particular structure does not constitute the physical 'memory' that causes the retention of a diminished IR response characteristic of chronic insulin stimulation.

It has long been recognized that the kinetics of insulin binding to the IR are complex [46], possibly originating with alternative insulin binding sites within the IR [47–48] that may become more available with prolonged exposure. A lag time between insulin binding and an IR conformational change [49] similarly may constitute a component of a diminished IR autophosphorylation capacity upon prolonged insulin exposure. At the IR itself, insulin resistance has been associated with binding of PC-1 to the IR through a site in the IR [22] implicated in structural studies to act as a hinge that moves upon insulin binding [23,50]. However, the relationship of the change in IR conformation measured here (Figs. 6, 7) to any of those events remains unknown. We also found that the altered insulin structure reported here and the lowered capacity for IR autophosphorylation were erased by a 180 min washout of insulin, but rapidly reformed thereafter. This suggests that the IR retained a memory of the insulin resistant state even after the phosphorylation mark and FRET structure were erased by long-term insulin removal. The physical origin of that memory thus remains unknown although it may be informative that the altered IR structure and impaired IR autophosphorylation may be similar to that observed upon overexpression of PC-1 (Fig. 8). Overall, the study suggested that persistent hyperinsulinemia induces a still poorly understood change in the IR or in factors binding to the IR that render it less efficacious following repeated stimulation.

Other studies showed that insulin resistance induced by inflammation is associated with insulin signaling events downstream of the IR. The development of insulin resistance is therefore expected to be complex and may occur at many levels. In the current studies of resistance induced by chronic insulin stimulation, we detected no dysregulation of the downstream effectors Akt or GSK3. Other studies at the IR itself suggest that insulin resistance may involve alterations in IR serine phosphorylation [4,14] or in tyrosine phosphatase activities, possibly at Y^{972} [39–41], whose phosphorylation is critical for interaction with IRS-1 [51]. Indeed, in our studies of insulin resistance initiated by chronic insulin exposure, Y^{972} and $Y^{1162,\ 1163}$ were refractory for re-stimulation by insulin (Fig. 3).

Overall, our data demonstrate an effect of long-term insulin stimulation that leads to a down-regulation of IR phosphorylation. That down-regulation appears to be associated with some change within the IR TK domain or in proteins interacting with the domain that persists after the insulin stimulus is removed. The prolonged wash-out studies in which the apparent insulin-refractory IR conformation was restored to its native state but was rapidly recovered upon re-stimulation, indicate that there is more to the mechanism than has been uncovered here. Our current hypothesis is that a molecular memory of prior chronic insulin exposure must consist of some lingering environment or transient interaction that remains primed, even after the insulin has been removed for 180 minutes, to rapidly affect IR conformation and phosphorylation. The persistence of this memory for so long has significant repercussions to the influence of our lifestyles and eating patterns on the development of insulin resistance. It also impacts discussions about optimal insulin delivery protocols for diabetic patients.

Acknowledgments

We thank Dr. Fusheng Li for Ms. Rachel Jaffe for the construction and characterization of fluorescent protein-tagged expression vectors and for helpful discussion.

Author Contributions

Conceived and designed the experiments: KJC BAM JFY IDG FS. Performed the experiments: KJC BAM JS FS. Analyzed the data: KJC BAM FS. Contributed reagents/materials/analysis tools: KJC BAM JS JFY IDG FS. Wrote the paper: KJC FS.

References

1. Reaven GM (1988) Banting lecture 1988. Role of insulin resistance in human disease. Diabetes 37: 1595–1607.
2. Youngren JF (2007) Regulation of insulin receptor function. Cell Mol Life Sci 64: 873–891.
3. Backer JM, Shoelson SE, Weiss MA, Hua QX, Cheatham RB, et al. (1992) The insulin receptor juxtamembrane region contains two independent tyrosine/beta-turn internalization signals. J Cell Biol 118: 831–839.
4. Cherqui G, Reynet C, Caron M, Melin B, Wicek D, et al. (1990) Insulin receptor tyrosine residues 1162 and 1163 control insulin stimulation of myristoyl-diacylglycerol generation and subsequent activation of glucose transport. J Biol Chem 265: 21254–21261.
5. White MF, Shoelson SE, Keutmann H, Kahn CR (1988) A cascade of tyrosine autophosphorylation in the beta-subunit activates the phosphotransferase of the insulin receptor. J Biol Chem 263: 2969–2980.
6. Dickens M, Tavare JM (1992) Analysis of the order of autophosphorylation of human insulin receptor tyrosines 1158, 1162 and 1163. Biochem Biophys Res Commun 186: 244–250.
7. Ellis L, Clauser E, Morgan DO, Edery M, Roth RA, et al. (1986) Replacement of insulin receptor tyrosine residues 1162 and 1163 compromises insulin-stimulated kinase activity and uptake of 2-deoxyglucose. Cell 45: 721–732.
8. Biddinger SB, Kahn CR (2006) From mice to men: insights into the insulin resistance syndromes. Annu Rev Physiol 68: 123–158.
9. Samuel VT, Shulman GI (2012) Mechanisms for insulin resistance: common threads and missing links. Cell 148: 852–871.
10. Considine RV, Nyce MR, Allen LE, Morales LM, Triester S, et al. (1995) Protein kinase C is increased in the liver of humans and rats with non-insulin-dependent diabetes mellitus: an alteration not due to hyperglycemia. J Clin Invest 95: 2938–2944.
11. Avignon A, Yamada K, Zhou X, Spencer B, Cardona O, et al. (1996) Chronic activation of protein kinase C in soleus muscles and other tissues of insulin-resistant type II diabetic Goto-Kakizaki (GK), obese/aged, and obese/Zucker rats. A mechanism for inhibiting glycogen synthesis. Diabetes 45: 1396–1404.
12. Donnelly R, Qu X (1998) Mechanisms of insulin resistance and new pharmacological approaches to metabolism and diabetic complications. Clin Exp Pharmacol Physiol 25: 79–87.

13. Ishizuka T, Miura A, Kajita K, Yamada K, Wada H, et al. (1998) Alterations in insulin-induced postreceptor signaling in adipocytes of the Otsuka Long-Evans Tokushima fatty rat strain. J Endocrinol 156: 1–13.
14. Caron M, Reynet C, Wicek D, Picard J, Cherqui G, et al. (1994) Insulin receptor mutation at tyrosines 1162 and 1163 alters both receptor serine phosphorylation and desensitization. Metabolism 43: 757–765.
15. Delibegovic M, Bence KK, Mody N, Hong EG, Ko HJ, et al. (2007) Improved glucose homeostasis in mice with muscle-specific deletion of protein-tyrosine phosphatase 1B. Mol Cell Biol 27: 7727–7734.
16. Galic S, Hauser C, Kahn BB, Haj FG, Neel BG, et al. (2005) Coordinated regulation of insulin signaling by the protein tyrosine phosphatases PTP1B and TCPTP. Mol Cell Biol 25: 819–829.
17. Costanzo BV, Trischitta V, Di Paola R, Spampinato D, Pizzuti A, et al. (2001) The Q allele variant (GLN121) of membrane glycoprotein PC-1 interacts with the insulin receptor and inhibits insulin signaling more effectively than the common K allele variant (LYS121). Diabetes 50: 831–836.
18. Dong H, Maddux BA, Altomonte J, Meseck M, Accili D, et al. (2005) Increased hepatic levels of the insulin receptor inhibitor, PC-1/NPP1, induce insulin resistance and glucose intolerance. Diabetes 54: 367–372.
19. Goldfine ID, Maddux BA, Youngren JF, Reaven G, Accili D, et al. (2008) The role of membrane glycoprotein plasma cell antigen 1/ectonucleotide pyrophosphatase phosphodiesterase 1 in the pathogenesis of insulin resistance and related abnormalities. Endocr Rev 29: 62–75.
20. Maddux BA, Chang YN, Accili D, McGuinness OP, Youngren JF, et al. (2006) Overexpression of the insulin receptor inhibitor PC-1/ENPP1 induces insulin resistance and hyperglycemia. Am J Physiol Endocrinol Metab 290: E746–749.
21. Maddux BA, Sbraccia P, Kumakura S, Sasson S, Youngren J, et al. (1995) Membrane glycoprotein PC-1 and insulin resistance in non-insulin-dependent diabetes mellitus. Nature 373: 448–451.
22. Maddux BA, Goldfine ID (2000) Membrane glycoprotein PC-1 inhibition of insulin receptor function occurs via direct interaction with the receptor alpha-subunit. Diabetes 49: 13–19.
23. Yip CC, Ottensmeyer P (2003) Three-dimensional structural interactions of insulin and its receptor. J Biol Chem 278: 27329–27332.
24. Shanik MH, Xu Y, Skrha J, Dankner R, Zick Y, et al. (2008) Insulin resistance and hyperinsulinemia: is hyperinsulinemia the cart or the horse? Diabetes Care 31 Suppl 2: S262–268.
25. Marban SL, Roth J, editors(1996) Transgenic hyperinsulinemia: a mouse model of insulin resistance and glucose intolerance without obesity. Boston: Birkhauser. 201–224 p.
26. Gavin JR, 3rd, Roth J, Neville DM, Jr., de Meyts P, Buell DN (1974) Insulin-dependent regulation of insulin receptor concentrations: a direct demonstration in cell culture. Proc Natl Acad Sci U S A 71: 84–88.
27. Hawley DM, Maddux BA, Patel RG, Wong KY, Mamula PW, et al. (1989) Insulin receptor monoclonal antibodies that mimic insulin action without activating tyrosine kinase. J Biol Chem 264: 2438–2444.
28. Youngren JF, Goldfine ID, Pratley RE (1999) Insulin receptor autophosphorylation in cultured myoblasts correlates to glucose disposal in Pima Indians. Am J Physiol 276: E990–994.
29. Forsayeth JR, Montemurro A, Maddux BA, DePirro R, Goldfine ID (1981) Effect of monoclonal antibodies on human insulin receptor autophosphorylation, negative cooperativity, and down-regulation. J Biol Chem 262: 4134–4140.
30. Kofoed E, Guerbadot M, Schaufele F (2008) Dimerization between aequorea fluorescent proteins does not affect interaction between tagged estrogen receptors in living cells. J Biomed Opt 13: 031207.
31. Koushik SV, Chen H, Thaler C, Puhl HL, Vogel SS (2006) Cerulean, Venus, and VenusY67C FRET reference standards. Biophys J 91: L99–L101.
32. Day RN, Periasamy A, Schaufele F (2001) Fluorescence Resonance Energy Transfer Microscopy of Localized Protein Interactions in the Living Cell Nucleus. Methods 25: 4–18.
33. Li M, Youngren JF, Manchem VP, Kozlowski M, Zhang BB, et al. (2001) Small molecule insulin receptor activators potentiate insulin action in insulin-resistant cells. Diabetes 50: 2323–2328.
34. Hansen BC, Jen KC, Belbez Pek S, Wolfe RA (1982) Rapid oscillations in plasma insulin, glucagon, and glucose in obese and normal weight humans. J Clin Endocrinol Metab 54: 785–792.
35. Lang DA, Matthews DR, Peto J, Turner RC (1979) Cyclic oscillations of basal plasma glucose and insulin concentrations in human beings. N Engl J Med 301: 1023–1027.
36. Matthews DR, Naylor BA, Jones RG, Ward GM, Turner RC (1983) Pulsatile insulin has greater hypoglycemic effect than continuous delivery. Diabetes 32: 617–621.
37. Paolisso G, Sgambato S, Torella R, Varricchio M, Scheen A, et al. (1988) Pulsatile insulin delivery is more efficient than continuous infusion in modulating islet cell function in normal subjects and patients with type 1 diabetes. J Clin Endocrinol Metab 66: 1220–1226.
38. Schmitz O, Arnfred J, Nielsen OH, Beck-Nielsen H, Orskov H (1986) Glucose uptake and pulsatile insulin infusion: euglycaemic clamp and [3-3H]glucose studies in healthy subjects. Acta Endocrinol (Copenh) 113: 559–563.
39. Bratusch-Marrain PR, Komjati M, Waldhausl WK (1986) Efficacy of pulsatile versus continuous insulin administration on hepatic glucose production and glucose utilization in type I diabetic humans. Diabetes 35: 922–926.
40. Paolisso G, Sgambato S, Passariello N, Scheen A, D'Onofrio F, et al. (1987) Greater efficacy of pulsatile insulin in type I diabetics critically depends on plasma glucagon levels. Diabetes 36: 566–570.
41. Koopmans SJ, Sips HC, Krans HM, Radder JK (1996) Pulsatile intravenous insulin replacement in streptozotocin diabetic rats is more efficient than continuous delivery: effects on glycaemic control, insulin-mediated glucose metabolism and lipolysis. Diabetologia 39: 391–400.
42. Bar RS, Gorden P, Roth J, Siebert CW (1977) Insulin receptors in patients with insulinomas: changes in receptor affinity and concentration. J Clin Endocrinol Metab 44: 1210–1213.
43. Del Prato S, Riccio A, Vigili de Kreutzenberg S, Dorella M, Avogaro A, et al. (1993) Mechanisms of fasting hypoglycemia and concomitant insulin resistance in insulinoma patients. Metabolism 42: 24–29.
44. Nankervis A, Proietto J, Aitken P, Alford F (1985) Hyperinsulinaemia and insulin insensitivity: studies in subjects with insulinoma. Diabetologia 28: 427–431.
45. Skrha J, Sindelka G, Haas T, Hilgertova J, Justova V (1996) Comparison of insulin sensitivity in patients with insulinoma and obese Type 2 diabetes mellitus. Horm Metab Res 28: 595–598.
46. de Meyts P, Roth J, Neville Jr DM, Gavin 3rd JR, Lesniak MA (1973) Insulin interactions with its receptors: experimental evidence for negative cooperativity. Biochem Biophys Res Commun 55: 154–161.
47. De Meyts P (1994) The structural basis of insulin and insulin-like growth factor-I receptor binding and negative co-operativity, and its relevance to mitogenic versus metabolic signalling. Diabetologia 37: S135–S148.
48. Schäffer L (1994) A model for insulin binding to the insulin receptor. Eur J Biochem: 1127–1132.
49. Schlein M, Havelund S, Kristensen C, Dunn MF, Kaarsholm NC (2000) Ligand-induced conformational change in the minimized insulin receptor. J Mol Biol 303: 161–169.
50. Luo RZ, Beniac DR, Fernandes A, Yip CC, Ottensmeyer FP (1999) Quaternary structure of the insulin-insulin receptor complex. Science 285: 1077–1080.
51. Combettes-Souverain M, Issad T (1998) Molecular basis of insulin action. Diabetes Metab 24: 477–489.

10

Endothelial Function and Insulin Resistance in Early Postmenopausal Women with Cardiovascular Risk Factors: Importance of *ESR1* and *NOS3* Polymorphisms

Ruth Clapauch[1,2]*, André Felipe Mourão[3], Anete S. Mecenas[1], Priscila A. Maranhão[1], Ana Rossini[3], Eliete Bouskela[1]

1 Laboratory for Clinical and Experimental Research on Vascular Biology (BioVasc), Biomedical Center, State University of Rio de Janeiro, Rio de Janeiro, Brazil, **2** Hospital da Lagoa, Endocrinology Sector, Health Ministry, Rio de Janeiro, Brazil, **3** Departamento de Bioquímica, IBRAG, State University of Rio de Janeiro, Rio de Janeiro, Brazil

Abstract

Cardiovascular benefits from estradiol activation of nitric oxide endothelial production may depend on vascular wall and on estrogen receptor alpha (*ESR1*) and nitric oxide synthase (*NOS3*) polymorphisms. We have evaluated the microcirculation *in vivo* through nailfold videocapillaroscopy, before and after acute nasal estradiol administration at baseline and after increased sheer stress (postocclusive reactive hyperemia response) in 100 postmenopausal women, being 70 controls (healthy) and 30 simultaneously hypertensive and diabetic (HD), correlating their responses to *PvuII* and *XbaI ESR1* polymorphisms and to *VNTR*, *T-786C* and *G894T NOS3* variants. In HD women, C variant allele of *ESR1 PvuII* was associated to higher vasodilatation after estradiol (1.72 *vs* 1.64 mm/s, p = 0.01 compared to TT homozygotes) while *G894T and T-786C NOS3* polymorphisms were connected to lower increment after shear stress (15% among wild type and 10% among variant alleles, p = 0.02 and 0.04). The G variant allele of *ESR1 XbaI* polymorphism was associated to higher HOMA-IR (3.54 *vs.* 1.64, p = 0.01) in HD and higher glucose levels in healthy women (91.8 vs. 87.1 mg/dl, p = 0.01), in which increased waist and HOMA-IR were also related to the G allele in *NOS3 G894T* (waist 93.5 *vs* 88.2 cm, p = 0.02; HOMA-IR 2.89 *vs* 1.48, p = 0.05). *ESR1 PvuII, NOS3 G894T* and *T-786C* polymorphism analysis may be considered in HD postmenopausal women for endothelial response prediction following estrogen therapy but were not discriminatory for endothelial response in healthy women. *ESR1 XbaI* and *G894T NOS3* polymorphisms may be useful in accessing insulin resistance and type 2 diabetes risks in all women, even before menopause and occurrence of metabolic disease.

Editor: Antimo Migliaccio, II Università di Napoli, Italy

Funding: This work was supported by grant 474116/2008-5 from the National Research Council of Brazil (CNPq- htpp://www.cnpq.br) and grant E-26/110.318/2007 from the State of Rio de Janeiro Research Supporting Agency (FAPERJ - htpp://www.faperj.br). The funders had no role in study design, data collection and analysis, decision to publish, or preparation of the manuscript.

Competing Interests: The authors have declared that no competing interests exist.

* Email: rclapauch@uol.com.br

Introduction

Cardiovascular (CV) disease remains the leading cause of female mortality [1]. Women's CV risk increases steadily after 60 years [2], i.e., ten years after menopause, potentially due to loss of estrogen cardio protective effects. However, studies examining hormone therapy (HT) in relation to CV events are contradictory, probably due to different vascular wall conditions, which can be affected by HT timing and also by co-morbidities [3]. Nowadays 28% of 45–64 years old American women present 2–3 chronic conditions, hypertension/diabetes (HD) being the second most prevalent dyad, representing 23.6% of the couplets [4]. Early postmenopausal simultaneously HD women would likely present a more advanced-for-age vascular impairment. Predicting HT CV effects in HD women would be particularly important, since their baseline CV risk may be higher than that of healthy early postmenopausal ones.

The central target of estrogen anti-atherosclerotic action is the endothelium, a monolayer of cells covering internally the vascular wall. It functions as a barrier, but, most importantly, produces nitric oxide (NO) by converting L-arginine to L-citrulline upon activation of endothelial nitric oxide synthase (eNOS) [5]. Other stimuli like sheer-stress after exercise physiologically activate eNOS genomic production, resulting in hyperemia due to NO vasodilatatory effect. NO modulates blood flow and pressure and has important anti-atherogenic effects on platelets and vascular smooth muscle cells. Endothelial dysfunction, i.e., the inability of the endothelium to liberate NO properly, is considered the first step of the atherosclerotic process and a predictor of CV disease; moreover, the lack of endothelial-derived NO is associated to vasospasm and vascular infarction [6], [7]. Estradiol (E2) has a major impact on the vasculature, enhancing the release of dilating factors such as NO, prostacyclin, and endothelium-derived hyperpolarizing factor (EDHF), and decreasing the vasoconstricting ones like endothelin and angiotensin II [8]. Both destruction of the endothelial layer and administration of NO inhibitors were shown to prevent estrogen vascular effects in rats [9]. Later on, a sequence of non-classical, non-genomic, E2 receptor membrane actions involving rapid signal-transduction pathways was detailed, including activation of phosphatidylinositol 3-kinase, protein kinase B (Akt) cascade generation and, by Gαi-protein interaction, long lasting estrogen-mediated eNOS phosphorylation and genomic NO production [10], [11], [12].

Estradiol actions are manifest through estrogen nuclear receptors alpha (ERα) and beta (ERβ), encoded by *ESR1* and *ESR2* genes, respectively [13], and one G-protein coupled receptor [8]. Most reports consolidated ERα as the main responsible for E2 endothelial effects [14]: eliminating ERα from endothelial cells resulted in abolishment of E2-induced NO release [15]; likewise, NO bioavailability and the consequent vasodilatation induced by E2 were abolished in ERα KO mice [11]. *ESR1* is located in chromosome 6p25.1 and encodes a 6.8-kilobase mRNA containing eight exons [16]. *PvuII* (rs2234693) and *XbaI* (rs9340799), mapped in intron 1, are the two most studied polymorphisms of *ESR1* associated to CV risk factors, such as dyslipidemia, insulin resistance, hypertension, central obesity and type 2 diabetes [17], [18], [19]. The *PvuII* polymorphism, caused by a C>T transition is located ≈0.4 kb upstream from exon 2 and the *XbaI* polymorphism, caused by a G>A transition, is located approximately 50 bp apart from the *PvuII* polymorphic site [20], [21]. Genetic influences on E2 vasodilatatory effect involve also the *NOS3* gene, located on chromosome 7q35–36 [22], from which few polymorphisms have proven functional importance. In this study, we focused in three *NOS3* variants: *VNTR* (27 bp TR), *T-786C* (rs2070744), and *G894T* (rs1799983). *VNTR* is characterized by variable tandem repeats of 27 bp in intron 4 (4a/b) and has been associated with variations in NO, nitrite, and nitrate plasma levels that may reflect eNOS activity [23]. *T-786C*, a T> C transition in the promoter region of the gene reduces its activity and affects eNOS protein expression and function [24], [25]. *G894T*, a G>T substitution at nucleotide 894 in exon 7, causes structural change of eNOS protein that down regulates eNOS activity [26], [27].

Microvascular endothelial function can be studied through nailfold videocapillaroscopy (NVC), a well-validated technique which measures vasodilatation (reactive hyperemia response) as an evidence of NO liberation after ischemia/reperfusion, provoked by an occlusion distal to the examined area, with subsequent release and consequent sheer-stress endothelial stimulation. In this study we have used this technique to assess endothelial function before and after acute estradiol administration in HD and healthy postmenopausal women and analyzed the responses in each group in relation to *ESR1* and *NOS3* polymorphisms, in order to identify genetic benefit/risk determinants of HT endothelial effects, both in healthy and CV risk patients.

Patients and Methods

Ethics Statement

This study was conducted according to principles expressed in the Declaration of Helsinki and was approved by Hospital da Lagoa Ethics Committee (Research protocol no. 02/2005). The participants were informed about the design of the study and possible risks and discomforts related to the experiment, and all of them signed a written informed consent, approved by the Ethics Committee.

Patients

One hundred postmenopausal women were selected from the Gynecological Endocrinology Clinic (Hospital da Lagoa, Rio de Janeiro, RJ, Brazil). Patients were divided into 2 groups: HD (n = 30), defined as simultaneously hypertensive (blood pressure [BP] >140×90 mmHg in at least 3 occasions or known hypertension controlled with medication) coupled with altered fasting plasma glucose (>110 mg% in at least 2 occasions) or diabetes mellitus using oral hypoglycemic agents; and healthy (n = 70), normotensive (BP <140×90 mmHg) and normoglycemic (fasting plasma glucose <100 mg%). In addition, HD women should be <60 years old and have <10 years of hormone deprivation (defined as time since menopause *minus* years of HT). Points for age, previous total and HDL cholesterol, smoking status and systolic blood pressure through the Framingham Risk Score were used to select HD patients with a 10-year risk for coronary heart disease <1% [28]. In most postmenopausal women composing the control group, mean age and time since menopause were similar to HD, although a larger limit for age (above 60 up to 70 years in 13 patients) and years of hormone deprivation >10 years (in 3 women) were tolerated for inclusion, as long as these women remained healthy.

Exclusion criteria were BP >160/100 mmHg, previous CV event, thyroid dysfunction, use of Ca^{++}-channel or β-blockers, sulfonylureas, corticosteroids, tranquilizers and soy isoflavones, evidence or suspicion of hormone dependent cancer and past venous thromboembolism. The procedure was fully explained to each patient. Women on current HT (n = 10 in HD group and n = 17 in C group) withhold it one month before NVC evaluation, scheduled at the Laboratory for Clinical and Experimental Research on Vascular Biology (BioVasc).

Methods

On the day of the experiment, each patient arrived in the morning, after 12 hours fasting, had the blood sample collected and waited for 30 min, acclimatized at 24±1°C, during which she answered clinical questions and had her blood pressure and waist assessed by the same observer. From the same blood sample, hormone and inflammatory markers determinations were performed at Laboratório Diagnósticos da América; biochemical determinations at Hospital da Lagoa, according to methodology and reference values given below. Genetic determinations were performed in part of the total blood collected, maintained in EDTA tubes without heparin and stored in a −70°C freezer until DNA extraction.

Glucose and insulin were measured by enzymatic colorimetric method (reference value <99 mg/dl) and chemiluminescence kit (reference values 3–16 mcUI/ml), respectively. HOMA- IR index [29], an estimation of insulin resistance, was calculated as fasting insulin (mU/l) x fasting glucose/22.5 (reference value 2.1±0.7). Estradiol was measured by chemiluminescence using an automated XP kit (Siemens Diagnostics; reference values for postmenopausal women without HT were <44 pg/ml). TSH (for exclusion of thyroid dysfunction) was measured by chemiluminescence using an automated Advia Centaur XP kit (Siemens Diagnostics; reference values 0.350–5.900 mcU/ml). High sensitivity C-reactive protein was measured by nefelometry, being considered indicative of low if≤0.099 mg/dl; intermediate if between 0.1 to 0.3 mg/dl and high cardiovascular risk if >0.3 mg/dl. Oxidated LDL was determined by espectofotometry (reference value < 0,5 nM/mg ApoPt). Triglycerides, total and HDL cholesterol were determined by enzymatic colorimetric kits (reference values <150 mg/dl, <200 mg/dl and >40 mg/dl, respectively). LDL cholesterol was calculated from previous dosages (reference values <130 mg/dl).

Nailfold videocapillaroscopy (NVC)

This technique is a non-invasive, accurate and reproducible exam derived from capillaroscopy [30] fully described previously [31]. Briefly, the patient was comfortably seated in a chair with her 4th finger of the left hand positioned at the heart level under the view of a microscope (DM/LM, Leica, Wetzlar, Germany) connected to a CD recorder. Capillaries, microvessels with only the endothelial layer, and red blood cells passing through them were directly visualized and images stored to be further analyzed by another observer, with the help of specific computer assisted-software. Red blood cell velocity (RBCV, mm/s) at rest was used to quantify blood flow and tissue perfusion. A maneuver to elicit NO production was performed, namely 1 min ischemia and subsequent reactive hyperemia response upon occlusion release, eliciting red blood cell velocity to reach a peak ($RBCV_{max}$, mm/s). The time to reach the peak ($TRBCV_{max}$, s) was used to infer the elasticity of the vascular wall. NVC was performed twice in each patient: at baseline (NVC_1) and, in continuity, 1 hour after acute nasal 17β-estradiol application (NVC_2). This approved drug for menopause treatment in Brazil acts in a pulsed fashion, with plasma estradiol levels reaching 1,200–1,500 pg/dl up to 30 min after administration, saturating estrogen receptors and returning to postmenopausal values after 2 hours. Succeeding NVC_2, the patient received breakfast and was discharged.

DNA extraction and genotyping analysis

Genomic DNA was extracted from peripheral blood leukocytes using a QIAamp DNA Blood Mini Kit following manufacturer's protocol (Qiagen). All DNA samples were assayed using polymerase chain reaction (PCR) for detection of polymorphisms in *ESR1* (*PvuII* and *XbaI*) and *NOS3 genes* (*VNTR*, *T-786C* and *G894T*). PCR reactions were performed in a final volume of 25 μl, containing approximately 50 ng of genomic DNA, 1 μmol/l of each primer, 0.2 mmol/l dNTPs, and 1.25 U of DNA Polymerase (Life Technologies).

Genotyping of *ESR1* polymorphism was performed using PCR–restriction fragment-length polymorphism (PCR–RFLP) analysis [32]. Genotyping of *PvuII* and *XbaI* polymorphisms was performed using the following oligonucleotide primers: 5′CTG CCA CCC TAT CTGTAT CTT TTC CTATTC TCC3′ (sense) and 5′TCT TTC TCT GCC ACC CTG GCG TCG ATT ATC TGA3′ (antisense). To differentiate *PvuII* and *XbaI* polymorphisms, PCR product of 1,372 bp was digested for 3 h with *PvuII* and *XbaI* restriction enzymes, separately. Digestion products were electrophoresed on 2.5% agarose gel stained with GelRed (Biotium). After *PvuII* digestion, wild-type TT produced fragments of 982, and 390 bp, while mutated homozygous variant CC exhibited one fragment of 1,372 bp. Fragments for *XbaI* digestion were: mutated homozygous variant AA produced fragments of 936, and 436 bp, and the wild-type GG exhibited one fragment of 1,327 bp.

The *VNTR* region of *NOS3* was amplified using the primers 5′AGG CCC TAT GGT AGT GCC TTT3′ (sense) and 5′TCT CTT AGT GCT GTG GTC AC3′ (antisense), as described elsewhere [33]. PCR products were visualized in 4% agarose gels stained with GelRed (Biotium). Alleles obtained when this region was amplified were classified according to number of repeating units. Alleles *c*, *a*, *b*, and *y* were found, consisting of 3, 4, 5, 6 or 7 repeating units. For analysis, only alleles with four or five repeating units were included. For T-*786C* polymorphism of *NOS3*, 282 bp fragment was amplified using primers 5′TGG AGA GTG CTG GTG TAC CCC A3′ (sense) and 5′GCC TCC ACC CCC ACC CTG TC3′ (anti-sense) as described elsewhere [34]. PCR products were then digested for 3 hours by *MspI* and visualized in 4% agarose gels stained with GelRed (Biotium). TT homozygotes had two fragments (140 bp and 40 bp), TC heterozygotes had four DNA bands (194 bp, 149 bp, 88 bp and 45 bp), and CC homozygotes showed three fragments (90 bp, 50 bp, and 40 bp). For *NOS3 G894T* polymorphism, PCR primers were generated to amplify a 248 bp fragment encompassing the missense mutation: 5′AAG GCA GGA GAC AGT GGA TGG A3′ (sense) and 5′CCC AGT CAA TCC CTT TGG TGC TCA3′ (antisense). PCR products were then digested for 16 hours with *BanII* and visualized in 3% agarose gels stained with GelRed (Biotium). As described previously [34], GG homozygotes had two fragments (163 bp and 85 bp), GT heterozygotes had three DNA bands (248 bp, 163 bp and 85 bp), and TT homozygotes showed only one fragment (248 bp).

Hardy-Weinberg equilibrium was determined with use of a χ^2 goodness-of-fit test on the basis of expected frequencies, calculated using the assumption of Hardy-Weinberg equilibrium. Statistical analysis was performed on each group separately using the Windows software SPSS version 14.0. Failure of data to confirm the normality hypothesis meant that ANOVA or t-tests could not be performed and nonparametric tests, U-Mann Whitney to contrast two samples, and Kruskal-Wallis (with Dunn's multiple comparison test) to contrast more than two samples were therefore applied. Results were considered significantly different for $p<0.05$.

Results

Clinical, videocapillaroscopy and laboratorial data from 100 postmenopausal women, divided into HD ($n = 30$) and healthy ($n = 70$) groups, are presented in Table 1. Although many results do not follow a Gaussian distribution, mean and median values were very close. Mean age, time since menopause, intensity of vasomotor symptoms, estradiol levels, previous smoking or oral contraceptive use, and inflammatory markers were similar. As expected, most anthropometric and metabolic analyzed parameters differed between groups. Videocapillaroscopy results were similar between groups, except for time to reach maximal red blood cell velocity before estradiol ($TRBCV_{max1}$), which was shorter in HD women. Estradiol increased at rest and peak RBCV both in HD and healthy women.

The frequency of *ESR1* (*PvuII* and *XbaI*) and *NOS3* (*VNTR*, *T-786C* and *G894T*) polymorphisms in HD and healthy women are shown in Table 2. Few variants were not successfully genotyped in every sample, thus numbers reported for specific polymorphism may vary. In most instances, polymorphic homozygotes and heterozygotes were grouped because some variant alleles were underrepresented among groups, hindering statistical analysis. All polymorphisms analyzed did not deviate significantly from Hardy–Weinberg equilibrium in both groups. We found similar distribution of polymorphisms in white and non-white individuals (data not shown), as well as in HD and healthy women, except for *NOS3 VNTR*: the frequency of *aa* genotype was higher among HD women (17.2%) than in the healthy group (3.1%, $p = 0.02$).

ESR1 polymorphisms associated outcomes

When the vasodilatatory response to estradiol was correlated to *ESR1* polymorphisms, we found that HD women who had at least one variant (C) allele of *ESR1 Pvull* polymorphism exhibited higher $RBCV_2$ (1.72 *vs* 1.64 mm/s, $p = 0.01$ compared to TT group, Figure 1A). After estradiol this subgroup of HD women's RBCV was close to the absolute median value reached by healthy women (1.71 mm/s). In the healthy group, RBCV response after estradiol did not differ in relation to *ESR1 Pvull* polymorphisms.

Table 1. Clinical and laboratory data in HD and healthy women.

	HD			HEALTHY			
Variable	**N**	**Mean ± S.D.**	**Median (min–max)**	**N**	**Mean ± S.D.**	**Median (min–max)**	
Age (years)	30	52.7±4.4	54 (42–59)	70	53.4±7.7	54 (34–70)	0.70
BMI (kg/m^2)	30	2.9±4.9	26.7 (20–38)	70	25.9±3.7	25.7 (18.8–36.6)	0.070
Time since menopause (years)	30	6.0±4.1	5.5 (1–20)	70	7.0±5.8	6.0 (0.42–24)	0.78
Intensity of vasomotor symptoms (0–10)	30	6.3±3.6	7.0 (0–10)	68	5.8±3.2	6.5 (0–10)	0.36
Oral contraceptives use duration (years)	30	7.3±6.5	7.0 (0–24)	70	6.9±6.5	5.5 (0–21)	0.81
Number of smoked cigarettes in the lifetime	30	203.0±377.6	0 (0–1200)	70	121.4±385.1	0 (0–3000)	0.47
Waist circumference (cm)	30	93.1±11.9	93.5 (70–111)	70	85.9±9.2	85 (69–107)	**0.004**
Systolic blood pressure (SBP, mmHg)	30	144.7±22.1	140 (100–200)	70	121.9±13.8	120 (80–160)	**0.0001**
Diastolic blood pressure (DBP, mmHg)	30	85.7±11.0	85 (60–110)	70	76.1±8.8	80 (50–93)	**0.0001**
$RBCV_1$ (mm/s)	29	1.46±0,09	1.46 (1.25–1.68)	70	1.49±0.10	1.49 (1.20–1.74)	0.13
$RBCV_{max1}$ (mm/s)	30	1.66±0.10	1.63 (1.50–1.95)	69	1.69±0.11	1.68 (1.48–2.0)	0.11
$RBCV_1$ increment (%)	29	13.5±6.60	12.3 (1.62–31.6)	69	13.2±7.1	11.2 (−1.90–41.7)	0.65
$TRBCV_{max1}$ (s)	30	7.9±1.5	8.0 (4–12)	69	8.7±1.8	9 (4–13)	**0.019**
$RBCV_2$ (mm/s)	30	1.69±0.08	1.67 (1.54–1.88)	69	1.69±0.12	1.71 (1.28–2.08)	0.47
$RBCV_{max2}$ (mm/s)	30	1.84±0.08	1.85 (1.69–1.99)	68	1.84±0.12	1.83 (1.63–2.40)	0.78
$RBCV_2$ increment (%)	30	9.3±4.4	8.5 (2.8–18.3)	68	9.1±5.7	8.2 (−1.74–29,0)	0.80
$TRBCV_{max2}$ (s)	30	5.9±1.2	6 (4–9)	68	6.1±1.4	6 (2–10)	0.25
Glucose (mg/dl)	30	145.2±66.2	118.5 (82–327)	69	89.4±10.4	90 (69–125)	**0.0001**
HOMA-IR	28	2.59±1,83	2.21 (0.38–7.68)	68	1.31±0.77	1.19 (0.36–3.98)	**0.0002**
Triglycerides, mg/dl	30	168.1±98.2	146.5 (46–406)	68	112.0±51.3	103.5 (40–277)	**0.006**
HDL cholesterol, mg/dl	30	51.8±13.1	51.5 (29–84)	68	57.0±13.8	55.5 (24–95)	0.089
hs C-reactive protein, mg/dl	30	0,42±0,47	0,21 (0,07–1,78)	67	0,29±0,26	0,22 (0,07–1,51)	0,38
Estradiol, pg/ml	30	18.0±11.4	15 (6–56)	67	17.2±11.1	15 (6–75)	0.76
Oxidized LDL, nmol/mg ApoPt	30	0.22±0.08	0.2 (0.1–0.4)	68	0.23±0.08	0.2 (0.1–0.4)	0.99

Reference values: HOMA-IR, 2.1 T 0.7; Triglycerides, <150 mg/dl; HDL cholesterol, >50 mg/dl; hS C-reactive protein, <0.3 mg/dl; Estradiol, <44 pg/ml (post menopause without HT); Oxidized LDL, <0.5 nmol/mg ApoPt.

BMI, body mass index; HOMA-IR, homeostasis model assessment of insulin resistance; $RBCV_1$: red blood cell velocity before estradiol: $RBCV_{max1}$: peak red blood cell velocity before estradiol: $RBCV_1$ increment: % of $RBCV_{max1}$ increase in relation to $RBCV_1$; $TRBCV_{max1}$: time to reach peak red blood cell velocity before estradiol; $RBCV_2$: red blood cell velocity after estradiol: $RBCV_{max2}$: peak red blood cell velocity after estradiol: $RBCV_2$ increment: % of $RBCV_{max2}$ increase in relation to $RBCV_2$: $TRBCV_{max2}$: time to reach peak red blood cell velocity after estradiol Comparison between groups was performed by Mann Whitney test.

Table 2. Frequencies of *ESR1* and *NOS3* polymorphisms in HD and healthy women.

	HD	HEALTHY	
ESR1	**n (%)**	**n (%)**	**P value**
PvuII			
TT	11 (36.7)	24 (34.3)	reference
TC	18 (60.0)	36 (51.4)	1.00
CC	1 (3.3)	10 (14.3)	0.242
TC + CC	19 (63.3)	46 (65.7)	0.823
Total	30	70	
XbaI			
AA	15 (50.0)	37 (52.9)	reference
AG	14 (46.7)	30 (42.8)	0.825
GG	1 (3.3)	3 (4.3)	1.00
AG + GG	15 (50.0)	33 (47.1)	0.830
Total	30	70	
NOS3	**n (%)**	**n (%)**	**P value**
VNTR			
aa	5 (17.2)	2 (3.1)	reference
ab	8 (27.6)	17 (26.2)	0.091
bb	16 (55.2)	46 (70.7)	**0.024**
ab + bb	24 (82.8)	63 (96.9)	**0.027**
Total	29	65	
T-786C			
TT	19 (63.3)	33 (47.1)	reference
TC	11 (36.7)	32 (45.7)	0.276
CC	0	5 (7.2)	0.158
TC + CC	11 (36.7)	37 (52.9)	0.190
Total	30	70	
G894T			
GG	19 (63.3)	38 (55.1)	reference
GT	11 (36.7)	28 (40.6)	0.658
TT	0	3 (4.3)	0.545
GT + TT	11 (36.7)	31 (44.9)	0.512
Total	30	69	

Comparison between genotypes was performed by Fisher's exact test.

ESR1 XbaI polymorphisms did not influence videocapillaroscopy responses to estradiol in the healthy group (1.69 mm/s for AA and AG/GG groups). $RBCV_2$ tended to be higher in HD women harboring at least one G allele, but the results were not statistically significant (1.71 for AG or GG *vs* 1.67 mm/s for AA genotype, $p=0.10$, Figure 1C). HD women who had at least one variant allele of the *XbaI* polymorphism (AG or GG genotypes) showed higher HOMA-IR (3.54) than the wild-type homozygous ones (1.64, $p=0.01$); healthy women with at least one G allele showed higher glucose levels than the AA subgroup (91.8 vs. 87.1 mg/dl, $p=0.01$, Table 3).

NOS3 polymorphisms associated outcomes

VNTR NOS3 polymorphisms, which showed different frequencies between HD and healthy women, did not correlate with any studied variables. On the other hand, *NOS3 T-786C* C and *G894T* T alleles were associated with lower $RBCV_1$ increments after the reactive hyperemia response in HD women, being these increments of about 15% among wild type and about 10% among those harboring variant alleles ($p=0.02$ and 0.04, respectively, Figures 2D and F).

An association with lower HOMA-IR tended to occur in healthy women in relation to T allele in *NOS3 G894T* polymorphism, although this result could be due to a narrower waist circumference in this subgroup (Table 3).

In summary, *ESR1 PvuII*, *NOS3 T-786C* and *G894T* polymorphisms influenced endothelial-mediated vasodilatatory responses to estradiol and sheer stress, respectively, in early HD postmenopausal women, while these genetic differences seemed not to affect microvascular responses in healthy women.

The presence of G allele in *ESR1 XbaI* was associated with increased insulin resistance in HD patients and higher glucose

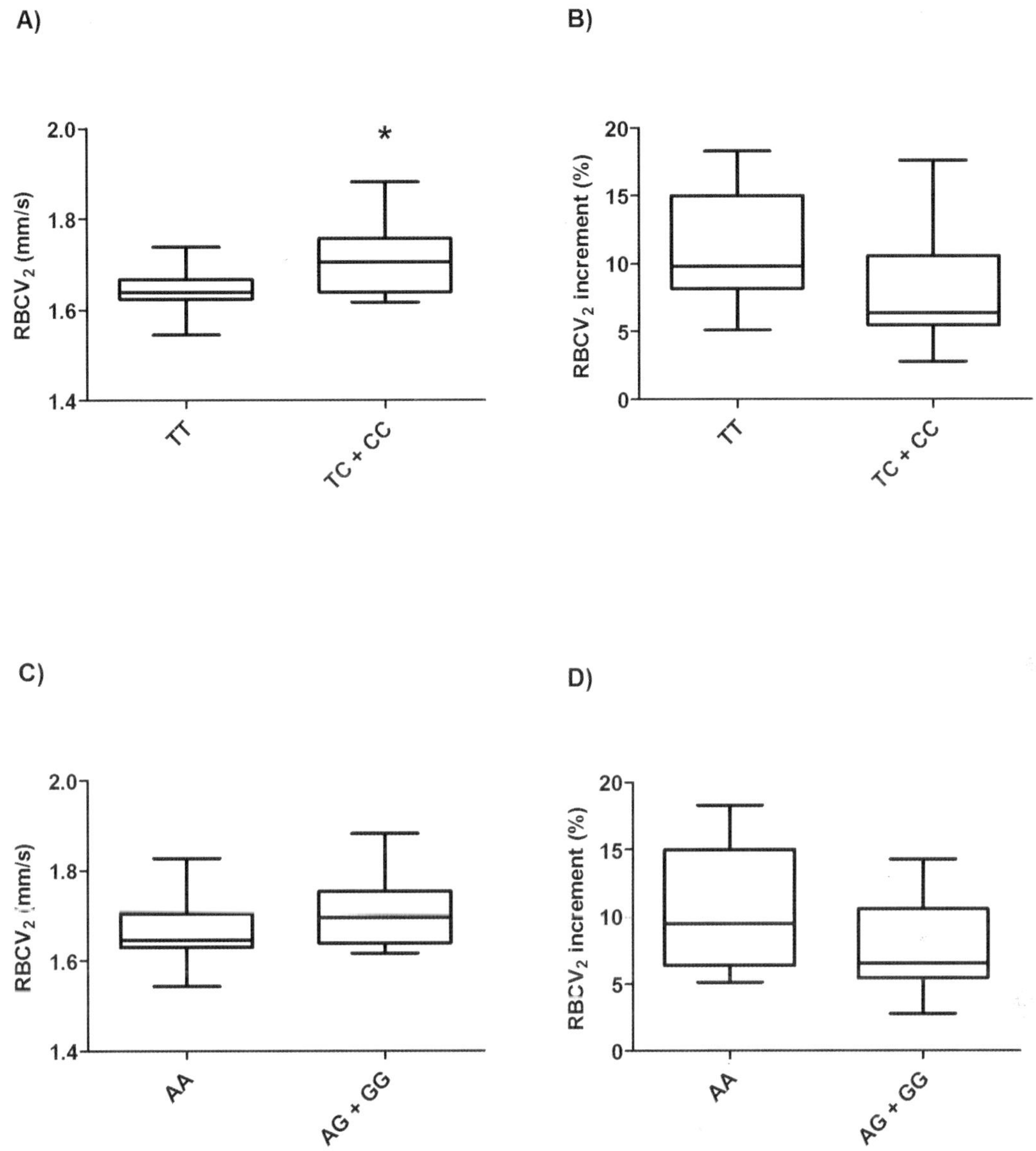

Figure 1. $RBCV_2$ and $RBCV_2$ increment in HD women according to *ESR1 PvuII* and *XbaI* genotypes. Data are presented as Whiskers plot. Comparison between groups was made by Mann Whitney test. $RBCV_2$: Red blood cells velocity (mm/s) after estrogen administration. $RBCV_2$ increment: Red blood cells velocity increment (%) after 1 min ischemia and subsequent reactive hyperemia response upon occlusion release after estrogen administration. A and C, $RBCV_2$ and *PvuII* and *XbaI* genotypes, respectively. B and D, $RBCV_2$ increment and *PvuII* and *XbaI* genotypes, respectively.

levels in healthy women. *NOS3 G894T* T allele in healthy women was associated with narrower waist and tendency to lower HOMA-IR.

Discussion

Endothelial function can be studied through well-validated techniques such as videocapillaroscopy, plethysmograhy and flow mediated dilatation, which assess baselne flow and vasodilatation during the reactive hyperemia response as evidence of NO liberation, upon sheer-stress stimuli obtained after release from induced ischemia. Acute nasal estradiol administration was based on findings that, on cultured human endothelial cells, high transient estradiol levels for one hour were shown to trigger eNOS expression and activity by the same amount observed with 24 h continuous exposure [35]. To know which polymorphisms influence endothelial NO generation following estrogen could help to understand an important endogenous mechanism against initial atherosclerosis progression. Moreover, screening for specific polymorphisms could be useful in predicting how early postmenopausal women with CV risk factors would react in response to estradiol replacement therapy in terms of endothelial function activation and *NO* release as a surrogate marker of future cardiovascular benefits or risks.

Videocapillaroscopy results were similar between HD and healthy women, except for time to reach maximum red blood cell velocity before estradiol ($TRBCV_{max1}$), which was shorter in HD women, as previously described [36], probably due to higher vascular wall stiffness, denoting some degree of atherosclerotic infiltration. Nevertheless, women with CV risk factors in early postmenopausal years showed to retain an endothelial function

Table 3. Association of *ESR1* polymorphism (*XbaI*), *NOS3* polymorphism (*G894T*), waist circumference and HOMA-IR in HD and healthy women.

	HD					HEALTHY				
ESR1 polymorphism (Xbal)	**AA**		**AG + GG**			**AA**		**AG + GG**		
	n	**Mean ± SD**	**n**	**Mean ± SD**	**P value**	**n**	**Mean ± SD**	**n**	**Mean ± SD**	**P value**
Waist circumference (cm)	15	91.1±11.8	15	95.1±12.0	0.42	37	85.8±8.7	33	86.0±9.7	0.85
BMI (kg/m^2)	15	27.5±5.5	15	28.3±4.5	0.48	37	26.1±3.8	37	25.5±3.7	0.69
Glucose	15	134±72.6	15	156±59.2	0.11	36	87.1±12.1	33	91.8±7.7	**0.01**
HOMA-IR	14	1.64±0.91	14	3.54±2.05	**0.01**	35	1.25±0.69	33	1.36±0.86	0.70
Triglycerides, mg/dL	15	177.6±95.2	15	158.5±103.5	0.38	35	111.7±47.0	33	112.5±56.2	0.72
HDL cholesterol, mg/dL	15	53.5±13.0	15	50.1±13.4	0.52	35	56.9±14.4	33	57.2±13.2	0.99
Estradiol, pg/mL	15	18.3±12.1	15	17.7±11.1	0.97	35	19.2±13.5	32	15.0±7.0	0.30
	HD					HEALTHY				
NOS3 polymorphism (G894T)	**GG**		**GT + TT**			**GG**		**GT + TT**		
	n	**Mean ± SD**	**n**	**Mean ± SD**	**P value**	**n**	**Mean ± SD**	**n**	**Mean ± SD**	**P value**
Waist circumference (cm)	19	93.5±13.2	11	92.4±9.7	0.76	38	88.2±8.9	31	83.0±8.9	**0.02**
BMI (kg/m^2)	19	27.9±5.6	11	27.8±3.7	0.93	38	26.6±4.0	31	24.9±3.2	0.10
Glucose	19	142.1±65.6	11	150.6±70.0	0.67	37	91.0±12.0	31	87.5±8.2	0.28
HOMA-IR	17	2.89±1.56	11	2.13±2.19	0.10	36	1.48±0.87	31	1.09±0.60	**0.05**
Triglycerides, mg/dL	19	178.8±102.4	11	149.5±92.0	0.40	36	116.2±43.6	31	105.3±58.9	0.085
HDL cholesterol, mg/dL	19	50.9±14.0	11	53.2±11.9	0.49	36	57.5±14.8	31	57.0±12.7	0.78
Estradiol, pg/mL	19	15.5±6.2	11	22.4±16.6	0.50	35	19.2±13.3	31	14.9±7.6	0.15

Reference values: HOMA-IR, 2.1 T 0.7; Triglycerides, <150 mg/dl; HDL cholesterol, >50 mg/dl; Estradiol, <44 pg/ml (post menopause without HT).
BMI, body mass index; HOMA-IR, homeostasis model assessment of insulin resistance. Comparison between groups was performed by Mann Whitney test.

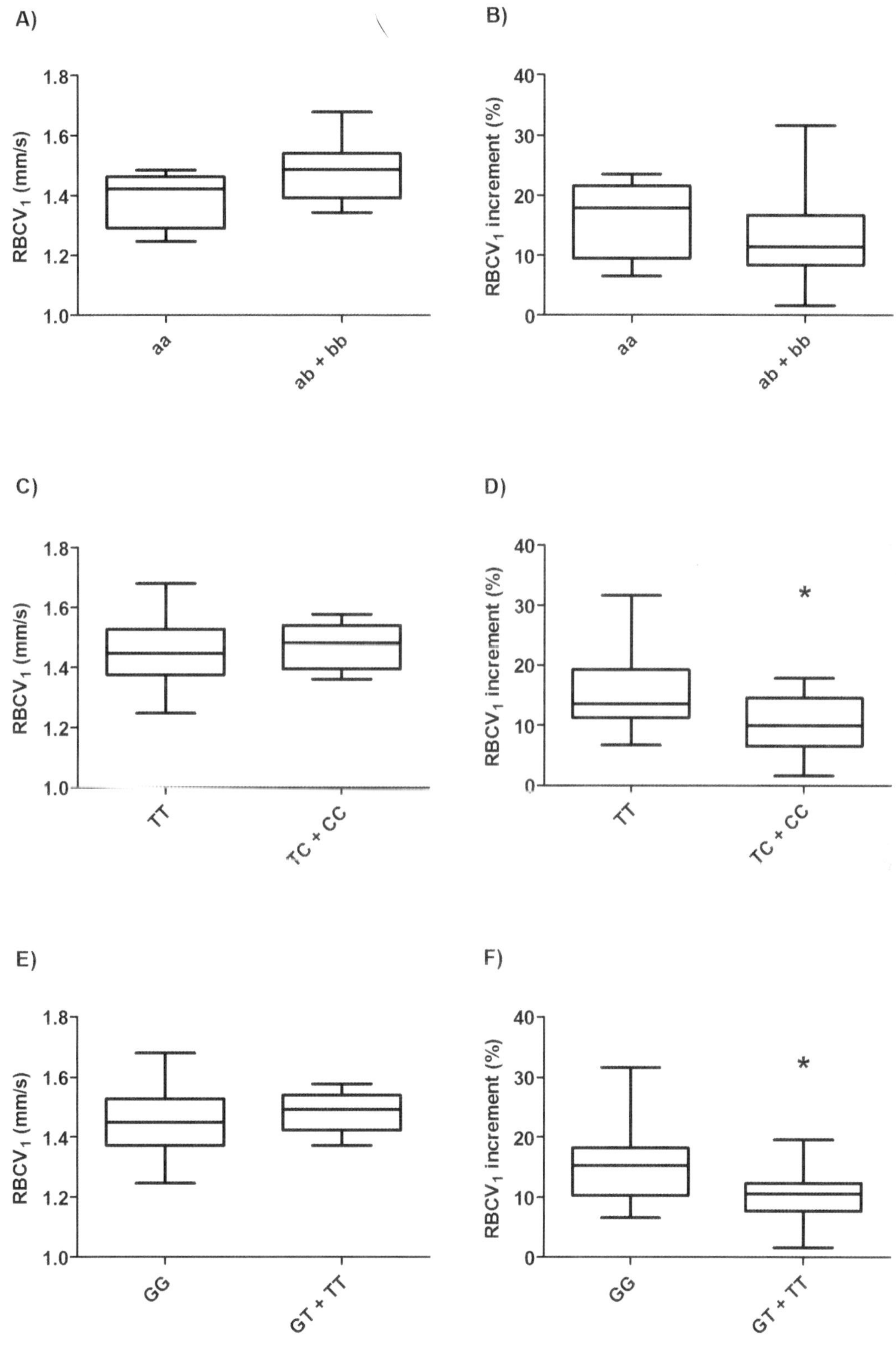

Figure 2. $RBCV_1$ and $RBCV_1$ increment in HD women according to *NOS3 T-786C and G894T* genotypes. Data are presented as Whiskers plot. Comparison between groups was made by Mann Whitney test. $RBCV_1$: Red blood cells velocity (mm/s). $RBCV_1$ increment: Red blood cells velocity increment (%) after 1 min ischemia and subsequent reactive hyperemia response upon occlusion release. A, C, and E, $RBCV_1$ and *VNTR*, *-786C*, and *G894T* genotypes, respectively. B, D, and F, $RBCV_1$ increment and *VNTR*, *-786C*, and *G894T* genotypes, respectively.

comparable to healthy ones. Timing of initiation, or window of opportunity, ultimately considered to be between 50–59 years or <10 years after menopause [37], may reflect a critical period of estrogen deficiency not long enough to impair receptor responsiveness by allowing methylation upon disuse. We have to emphasize that all HD women here studied were <60 years old and had a Framingham Score estimating a 10-year risk for coronary heart disease of less than 1%, with low inflammatory markers, supporting that, in initial endothelial dysfunction, microvascular responses to estradiol and sheer-stress may be preserved and enhanced to further halter atherosclerosis injury and progression. In this sense, recent symptomatic postmenopausal women with CV risk factors may benefit from HT vascular and quality of life climacteric symptoms.

HD women who had at least one C allele of *ESR1 PvuII* polymorphism exhibited higher $RBCV_2$. *ESR1 PvuII* is one of the most studied polymorphisms described to alter CV risk, yet the mechanisms through which this risk is mediated are not completely understood [38]. Most studies, performed in older male samples, showed that C allele confers more CV risk. When the offspring cohort of the Framingham Heart Study was genetically studied, 1739 unrelated mean age 60 years subjects were followed during 16 years for incident CV events [39]. After adjusting for covariates, the wild, although less common, *ESR1 PvuII CC* genotype was associated with an OR = 2.0 (1.32–3.2, p = 0.004) for major atherosclerotic CVD and an OR = 3.0 (1.7–5.2; p<0.001) for myocardial infarction, while having T allele (*CT* or *TT* genotypes) conferred CV protection. Later on, *ESR1 PvuII* CC genotype was found to be associated with myocardial infarction in different studies in older (>60 years old) men [40], older southern Brazilian subjects [41] and over 1,000 Chinese men [42]. However, estradiol cardiovascular effects may perform differently according to the extent of vascular atherosclerotic disease. Estrogen levels were shown to modulate endothelial ER expression throughout the menstrual cycle [43], so postmenopausal women subjected to HT could present distinct outcomes in relation to their *ESR1* receptor polymorphisms enhancement or down regulation. A Greek team compared the same *ESR1* polymorphisms we have studied in relation to the extent of coronary artery disease (CAD) in 173 older women with various CV risk factors referred to angiography [19]. They found a significant correlation for CC *PvuII* genotype and CAD severity, as well as for the G allele in *XbaI* polymorphismsm, which in our study was linked to insulin resistance but not to NO induced vasodilatation. We have studied early postmenopausal women and a significantly higher vascular response to estradiol was present in around 65% of our HD group, who had at least one C allele of *PvuII*. Our findings provide further evidence that NO bioavailability may be the main mechanism linked to *PvuII* C allele CV protection or hazard, depending on the stage of the atherosclerotic process. A larger NO bioavailability brought by CC or CT *PvuII* genotypes can be translated into interaction of NO with superoxide anions, present in aged microvessels, producing peroxynitrite, a reactive oxygen species (ROS), which causes vasoconstriction instead of vasodilatation [44]. Previous findings that *ESR1 PvuII* CC was associated with increased systolic blood pressure in men and coronary intima thickness in women [38] reinforce NO estrogen-mediated release as an impaired physiological mechanism determined by this genotype.

In HD women *G894T* T and *T-786C* C alleles in *NOS3* polymorphisms were associated with lower $RBCV_1$ increments after reactive hyperemia. The first study showing the impact of *NOS3 G894T* T was published in 2007 [45], where human umbilical vein endothelial cells were subjected to shear stress and eNOS protein levels, phosphorylation, and enzyme function were evaluated. Variant T genotypes had lower NO production pre- and post-shear stress due to an altered localization of the variant protein at the caveolae, leading to diminished shear-dependent responses and impaired coordination of eNOS regulatory cycle. Many other studies then aimed to correlate endothelial function and *NOS3* alleles. The Prospective Investigation of the Vasculature in Uppsala Seniors (PIVUS), a population-based cohort study, analyzed 25 SNPs distributed over a region of about 5 kb upstream and 2 kb downstream from the *NOS3* gene [46] while endothelial function was evaluated with brachial artery ultrasound to assess flow-mediated vasodilatation. In this older population *NOS3 G894T* T allele was associated to higher endothelium-dependent vasodilatation in conduit arteries while another study in 230 normotensive male and female Malay individuals between 18 and 40 years [47] found that heterozygotes for the *NOS3 G894T* polymorphism had lower baseline skin perfusion when compared with wild type homozygous (p = 0.029), like in our study. Another Brazilian study [48] is also in accordance with our findings, as in 110 healthy volunteers the polymorphic group presented lower vascular reactivity 120 min after maximal cardiopulmonary exercise. Regarding *NOS3 T-786C* polymorphism, a German proteomic study in human primary cultured endothelial cells compared fluid shear stress (FSS)-induced protein expression. Cells with CC genotype exhibited a greatly reduced FSS-induced eNOS expression as well as diminished NO synthesis capacity when compared to TT cells [49]. Again, results seem to point to caution when interpreting results related to polymorphisms and vascular reactivity, since they are subjected to many variables, like experimental design, biochemical parameters, ethnic differences, but especially age and pre-existing diseases determining baseline degree of vascular damage.

The presence of the G allele in *ESR1 XbaI* was associated to increased insulin resistance in HD patients and higher glucose levels in healthy women. These are important findings, since the use of estrogen alone and estrogen plus progestin in the prospective randomized double blind trial Women's Health Initiative were associated with decreased risk for type 2 diabetes [37]. To know which woman is at risk for diabetes mellitus type 2, by anthropometrical, laboratorial and now genetic data could help to identify further HT individualized benefits. Estrogen receptors are expressed in non-reproductive tissues, including skeletal and smooth muscle, adipose tissue and pancreas, supporting their involvement with multiple systems [38]. *ESR1* was described to be important for proper glucose homeostasis: female and male αERKO obese mice show adipocyte hyperplasia and insulin resistance, while ERα resistant men present impaired glucose metabolism, insulin resistance, hyperinsulinemia, elevated glycosylated hemoglobin level, and acanthosis nigricans [50]. In male and female mice, estradiol was shown to protect against glucose intolerance induced by high fat diet [51] and also to promote β-pancreatic cell survival by preventing apoptosis through non-classical ER mediated extra-nuclear mechanisms, with predominant ERα effect [52]. Recent papers emphasize non-hepatic actions [53] in adipose tissue or skeletal muscle. Membrane effects are the most implicated mechanisms for estrogen-mediated insulin sensitivity, because estrogen binding to its membrane receptor could influence mitogen-activated protein kinase (MAPK), located on phosphorylated aminoacid residues, signaling the insulin pathway and influencing insulin receptor expression especially on adipocytes [38]. *ESR1 XbaI* G alelle was associated to insulin sensitivity and metabolic syndrome in the Study of Women's Health Across the Nation [54], but only in Asian ones. Furthermore, *ESR1 XbaI* polymorphism was associated to metabolic syndrome in 548 individuals from 42 African-American families from the Insulin Resistance Atherosclerosis Family Study (OR = 1.53; 1.05–2.27, p = 0.029) [55]. Other studies related *ESR1 XbaI* G allele to lower insulin secretory capacity, suggesting a role on diabetes type 2 installation [38]. However, these findings are not universal, G polymorphisms frequencies may vary across populations, and most importantly, have different consequences depending on age, gender and hormonal status, not allowing for extrapolations. For example, in 500 normoglycemic controls and type 2 diabetic patients *ESR1 XbaI* genotypes were not associated to diabetes or fasting glucose levels in Iranian females, but rather in males ($p = 0.02$) [56]. Insulin resistance is a complex pathophysiological feature with different organs and targets in the carbohydrate metabolism that can be genetically influenced; in this setting our study reinforces *ESR1 XbaI* polymorphism as a piece in insulin sensitivity.

One of our study strengths was to analyze genetic determinants of estrogen action in early postmenopausal women, since they are the ones who most benefit from HT. Also, we have examined the whole chain involved in endothelial NO generation, namely two *ESR1* and three *NOS3* polymorphisms most implicated in CV disease. Another important point was to include, along with healthy ones, a group of recent postmenopausal women with CV risk factors, in which initial endothelial dysfunction was already installed, and in fact we could see that in their slightly impaired endothelial function the polymorphisms influence was more evident.

The finding that in our HD women, with Framingham Risk Score <1%, the C allele of *PvuII ESR1* was associated to increased endothelial response after estrogen is consistent to the thoughts that later on, in a more damaged endothelium with atherosclerotic infiltration and unstable plaques, this observed beneficial activation could lead to an increase in cardiovascular risk, as seen in older male populations. This phenomenon was described by Vanhoutte in a review article "Endothelium-dependent contractions: when a good guy turns bad!" (57). In brief, Vanhoutte describes the constant balance within the endothelium between the production of relaxing factors (NO being the major one) and of cyclooxygenase-derived vasoconstrictor substances (EDCF, especially prostanoids such as COX). This balance is decisive for blood flow regulation according to physiological necessities like temperature and exercise changes. However, in a model of spontaneous hypertension, a progressively dysfunctional endothelium develops. At an advanced setting, in response to acetylcholine (a known NO synthesis stimulator, through M3 muscarinic endothelial receptors), a concomitant endothelial release of EDCF occurs, impairing or reversing the expected vasodilator response. Endothelium-dependent relaxations in response to acetylcholine are also blunted in diabetes, where high glucose levels result in increased oxidative stress and over- expression of EDCFs such as COX-1 and COX-2. This evidence let us conclude that the mentioned C allele of *PvuII ERS1* is linked to endothelial activation: however, depending on endothelial status, this activation may lead to a predominant vasodilator, neutral or vasoconstrictor effect, a beautiful example of genetic-acquired interaction. These opposite effects may explain why HT cardiovascular outcomes are so conflicting. Women already presenting CV risk factors in early menopause undergoing estrogen therapy must be followed for atherosclerotic progression with care.

The small number of HD patients could be a limitation but in fact we found significant results in this group and even associations between insulin resistance and genetic polymorphisms, which was not our main goal. The small number of individuals was limiting for more sophisticated studies, such as haplotype analysis. Some haplotypes would be so rare that statistical analysis would be impossible. However, the study was designed to have a robust group of clinical and laboratorial data, consisting of women showing similar time since menopause and hormonal profiles. Moreover, this group of women was included in other studies of the group and their vascular responses before and after administration of estradiol were already well established. The Brazilian population is mixed and that could represent a limitation, although we did not find different polymorphism distributions between white and non-white women. Polymorphism frequencies vary between populations and their distribution must be taken into account in each specific community. Compared to previous studies, enhancement of endothelial response to estradiol may represent a benefit or risk, depending on vascular atherosclerotic stage.

Conclusions

ESR1 and NOS3 polymorphisms influenced vasodilatatory baseline and after estradiol responses in HD but not in healthy early postmenopausal women. The C variant allele of *ESR1 PvuII* polymorphism was associated to higher RBCV values after estradiol while *G894T and T-786C NOS3* polymorphisms were associated to lower $RBCV_1$ reactive hyperemia increment.

In relation to metabolic outcomes, G variant allele of *ESR1 XbaI* polymorphism was associated to higher HOMA-IR in HD women. In healthy women increased waist and HOMA-IR were found in association with G alelle in *NOS3 G894T* polymorphism.

Different estrogen receptors polymorphisms may play a role in CV risk related to different outcomes. When balancing HT risks and benefits in early postmenopausal women with CV risk factors such as diabetes and hypertension, *ESR1 PvuII, NOS3 G894T* and *T-786C* polymorphism analysis may be considered in relation to endothelial-mediated benefits, fundamental in atherosclerosis progression process. Atherosclerotic stage may determine whether endothelial increase NO production after estrogen will produce favorable or unfavorable outcomes. *ESR1 XbaI* and *G894T NOS3* polymorphisms may be useful in accessing insulin resistance and type 2 diabetes risks, even before menopause and occurrence of metabolic disease.

Acknowledgments

Laboratórios Servier do Brasil for the gift of a sufficient amount of nasal estradiol samples to perform the experiments; Hospital da Lagoa and Diagnósticos da América for performing laboratorial determinations; Rosangela Aparecida Martins Noe , MSc in Statistics, from the Federal University of Rio de Janeiro for statistical analysis.

Author Contributions

Conceived and designed the experiments: RC AR EB. Performed the experiments: RC AFM ASM PAM AR. Analyzed the data: RC AR. Contributed reagents/materials/analysis tools: AR EB. Contributed to the writing of the manuscript: RC AR EB.

References

1. Go AS, Mozaffarian D, Roger VL, Benjamin EJ, Berry JD, et al American Heart Association Statistics Committee and Stroke Statistics Subcommittee (2013) Executive summary: heart disease and stroke statistics-2013 update: a report from the American Heart Association. Circulation 127: 143 152.
2. Mikkola TS, Gissler M, Merikukka M, Tuomikoski P, Ylikorkala O (2013) Sex differences in age-related cardiovascular mortality. PLoS One 8: e63347.
3. Nofer JR (2012) Estrogens and atherosclerosis: insights from animal models and cell systems. Journal of Molecular Endocrinology 48: R13 29.

4. Ward BW, Schiller JS (2013) Prevalence of Multiple Chronic Conditions Among US Adults: Estimates From the National Health Interview Survey, 2010. Preventing chronic disease 10: E65.
5. Moncada S, Higgs A (1993) The L-arginine-nitric oxide pathway. New England Journal of Medicine 329: 2002-2012.
6. Channon KM, Guzik TJ (2002) Mechanisms of Superoxide Production in Human Blood Vessels: Relationship to Endothelial Dysfunction, Clinical and Genetic Risk Factors. Journal of Physiology and Pharmacology 53: 515-524.
7. Gilchrist M, Shore AC, Benjamin N (2011) Inorganic nitrate and nitrite and control of blood pressure. Cardiovascular Research 15: 492-498.
8. Masood D, Roach EC, Beauregard KG, Khalil RA (2010) Impact of Sex Hormone Metabolism on the Vascular Effects of Menopausal Hormone Therapy in Cardiovascular Disease. Current Drug Metabolism 11: 693-714.
9. Holm P, Korsgaard N, Shalmi M, Andersen HL, Hougaard P, et al. (1997) Significant reduction of the antiatherogenic effect of estrogen by long-term inhibition of nitric oxide synthesis in cholesterol-clamped rabbits. Journal of Clinical Investigation 100: 821-828.
10. Kim KH, Bender JR (2009) Membrane-initiated actions of estrogen on the endothelium. Molecular and Cellular Endocrinol 308: 3-8.
11. Arnal JF, Fontaine C, Billon-Galés A, Favre J, Laurell H, et al. (2010) Estrogens receptors and endothelium. Arteriosclerosis, Thrombosis, and Vascular Biology 30: 1506-1512.
12. Chow RW, Handelsman DJ, Ng MK (2010) Minireview: rapid actions of sex steroids in the endothelium. Endocrinology 151: 2411-2422.
13. Speroff L (2000) A clinical understanding of the estrogen receptor. Annals of the New York Academy of Sciences 900: 26-39.
14. Knowlton AA, Lee AR (2012) Estrogen and the cardiovascular system. Pharmacology & Therapeutics 135: 54-70.
15. Billon-Galés A, Fontaine C, Douin-Echinard V, Delpy L, Berges H, et al. (2009) Endothelial estrogen receptor-α plays a crucial role in the atheroprotective action of 17β-estradiol in low-density lipoprotein receptor-deficient mice. Circulation 120: 2567-2576.
16. Bollig A, Miksicek RJ (2000) An estrogen receptor-α splicing variant mediates both positive and negative effects on gene transcription. Molecular Endocrinology 14: 634-649.
17. Lu H, Higashikata T, Inazu A, Nohara A, Yu W, et al. (2002) Association of estrogen receptor-alpha gene polymorphisms with coronary artery disease in patients with familial hypercholesterolemia. Arteriosclerosis, Thrombosis, and Vascular Biology 1: 817-823.
18. Kjaergaard AD, Ellervik C, Tybjaerg-Hansen A, Axelsson CK, Gronholdt ML, et al. (2007) Estrogen receptor alpha polymorphism and risk of cardiovascular disease, cancer and hip fracture: Cross sectional, cohort, and case-control studies and a meta-analysis. Circulation 115: 861-871.
19. Alevizaki M, Saltiki K, Cimponeriu A, Kanakakis I, Xita N, et al. (2007) Severity of cardiovascular disease in postmenopausal women: Associations with common estrogen receptor alpha polymorphic variants. European Journal of Endocrinology 156: 489-496.
20. Yaich L, Dupont WD, Cavener DR, Parl FF (1992) Analysis of the PvuII restriction fragment-length polymorphism and exon structure of the estrogen receptor gene in the breast cancer and peripheral blood. Cancer Research 52: 77-83.
21. Andersen TI, Heimdal KR, Skrede M, Tveit K, Berg K, et al. (1994) Oestrogen receptor (ESR) polymorphisms and breast cancer susceptibility. Human Genetics 94: 665-670.
22. Marsden PA, Heng HH, Scherer SW, Stewart RJ, Hall AV, et al. (1993) Structure and chromosomal localization of the human constitutive endothelial nitric oxide synthase gene. The Journal of Biological Chemistry 268: 17478-17488.
23. Li R, Lyn D, Lapu-Bula R, Oduwole A, Igho-Pemu P, et al. (2004) Relation of endothelial nitric oxide synthase gene to plasma nitric oxide level, endothelial function, and blood pressure in African Americans. Am J Hypertens 17: 560-567.
24. Nakayama M, Yasue H, Yoshimura M, Shimasaki Y, Kugiyama K, et al. (1999) T-786 >C mutation in the 5′-flanking region of the endothelial nitric oxide synthase gene is associated with coronary spasm. Circulation 99: 2864-2870.
25. Doshi AA, Ziolo MT, Wang H, Burke E, Lesinski A, et al. (2010) Promoter polymorphism of the endothelial nitric oxide synthase gene is associated with reduced mRNA and protein expression in failing human myocardium. Journal of Cardiac Failure 16: 314-319.
26. Tesauro M, Thompson WC, Rogliani P, Qi L, Chaudhary PP, et al. (2000) Intracellular processing of endothelial nitric oxide synthase isoforms associated with differences in severity of cardiopulmonary diseases: cleavage of proteins with aspartate vs. glutamate at position 298. Proceedings of the National Academy of Sciences of the United States of America 97: 2832-2835.
27. Leeson CP, Hingorani AD, Mullen MJ, Jeerooburkhan N, Kattenhorn M, et al. (2002) Glu298Asp endothelial nitric oxide synthase gene polymorphism interacts with environmental and dietary factors to influence endothelial function. Circulation Research 90: 1153-1158.
28. Wilson PWF, D'Agostino RB, Levy D, Belanger AM, Silbershatz H, et al. (1998) Prediction of coronary heart disease using risk factor categories. Circulation 97: 1837-1847.
29. Matthews DR, Hosker JP, Rudenski AS, Naylor BA, Treacher DF, et al. (1985) Homeostasis Model Assessment: Insulin Resistance And Beta-Cell Function From Fasting Plasma Glucose And Insulin Concentrations In Man. Diabetologia 28: 412-419.
30. Ostergren J, Fagrell B (1986) Skin capillary blood cell velocity in man. Characteristics and reproducibility of the reactive hyperemia response. International Journal of Microcirculation Clinical and Experimental 5: 37-51.
31. Clapauch R, Mecenas AS, Maranhão PA, Bouskela E (2009) Microcirculatory function in postmenopausal women: role of aging, hormonal exposure and metabolic syndrome. Microvascular Research 78: 405-412.
32. Safarinejad MR, Shafiei N, Safarinejad S (2010) Association of polymorphisms in the estrogen receptors alpha, and beta (ESR1, ESR2) with the occurrence of male infertility and semen parameters. The Journal of Steroid Biochemistry and Molecular Biology 122: 193-203.
33. Tanus-Santos JE, Desai M, Deak LR, Pezzullo JC, Abernethy DR, et al. (2002) Effects of endothelial nitric oxide synthase gene polymorphisms on platelet function, nitric oxide release, and interactions with estradiol. Pharmacogenetics 12: 407-413.
34. Safarinejad MR, Safarinejad S, Shafiei N, Safarinejad S (2013) Effects of the T-786C, G894T, and Intron 4 VNTR (4a/b) polymorphisms of the endothelial nitric oxide synthase gene on the risk of prostate cancer. Urologic Oncology 31(7): 1132-1140.
35. Simoncini T, Fornari L, Mannella P, Varone G, Caruso A, et al. (2005) Differential estrogen signaling in endothelial cells upon pulsed or continuous administration. Maturitas 50: 247-258.
36. Clapauch R, Mecenas AS, Maranhão PA & Bouskela E (2012) Early postmenopausal women with cardiovascular risk factors improve microvascular dysfunction after acute estradiol administration. Menopause 19: 672-679.
37. Santen RJ, Allred DC, Ardoin SP, Archer DF, Boyd N, et al Endocrine Society (2010) Postmenopausal hormone therapy: an Endocrine Society scientific statement. The Journal of Clinical Endocrinology and Metabolism 95: s1-s66.
38. Casazza K, Page GP, Fernandez JR (2010) The association between the rs2234693 and rs9340799 estrogen receptor alpha gene polymorphisms and risk factors for cardiovascular disease: a review. Biological Research for Nursing 12: 84-97.
39. Shearman AM, Cupples L, Demissie S, Peter I, Schmid CH, et al. (2003) Association Between Estrogen Receptor α Gene Variation and Cardiovascular Disease. JAMA 290: 2263-2270.
40. Shearman AM, Cooper JA, Kotwinski PJ, Miller GJ, Humphries SE, et al. (2006) Estrogen receptor alpha gene variation is associated with risk of myocardial infarction in more than seven thousand men from five cohorts. Circulation Research 98: 590-592.
41. Almeida S, Hutz MH (2006) Estrogen receptor 1 gene polymorphisms and coronary artery disease in the Brazilian population. Brazilian Journal of Medical and Biological Research 39: 447-454.
42. Shen C, Chen J, Fan S, Li Z, Hu Y, et al. (2012) Association between the polymorphism of estrogen receptor α and coronary artery disease in a Chinese population. European Journal of Internal Medicine 23: 175-178.
43. Gavin KM, Seals DR, Silver AE, Moreau KL (2009) Vascular Endothelial Estrogen Receptor Is Modulated by Estrogen Status and Related to Endothelial Function and Endothelial Nitric Oxide Synthase in Healthy Women. Journal of Clinical Endocrinology and Metabolism 94: 3513-3520.
44. Rodriguez-Mañas L, El-Assar M, Vallejo S, López-Dóriga P, Solis J, et al. (2009) Endothelial dysfunction in aged humans is related with oxidative stress and vascular inflammation. Aging Cell 8(3): 226-238.
45. Joshi MS, Mineo C, Shaul PW, Bauer JA (2007) Biochemical consequences of the NOS3 Glu298Asp variation in human endothelium: altered caveolar localization and impaired response to shear. The FASEB Journal 21: 2655-2663.
46. Ingelsson E, Syvanen AC, Lind L (2008) Endothelium-dependent vasodilation in conduit and resistance vessels in relation to the endothelial nitric oxide synthase gene. Journal of Human Hypertension 22: 569-578.
47. Rasool AIG, Ghazali DM, Abdullah H, Halim AS, Wong AR (2009) Endothelial nitric oxide synthase G894T gene polymorphism and response to skin reactive hyperemia Microvascular Research 78: 230-234.
48. Neves FJ, Silva BM, Rocha NG, Salesa ARK, Ribeiro GS, et al. (2010) Effect of the 894G>T polymorphism of the endothelial nitric oxide synthase on vascular reactivity following maximal dynamic exercise Journal of Hypertension 28: 764-770.
49. Asif AR, Oellerich M, Armstrong VW, Hecker M, Cattaruzza M (2009) T-786C Polymorphism of the nos-3 Gene and the Endothelial Cell Response to Fluid Shear Stress - A Proteome Analysis. Journal of Proteome Research 8: 3161-3168.
50. Nilsson S, Gustafsson JA (2011) Estrogen Receptors: Therapies Targeted to Receptor Subtypes. Clinical Pharmacology and Therapeutics 89: 44-55.
51. Riant E, Waget A, Cogo H, Arnal JF, Burcelin R, et al. (2009) Estrogens protect against high-fat diet-induced insulin resistance and glucose intolerance in mice. Endocrinology 150: 2109-2117.
52. Liu S, Mauvais-Jarvis F (2009) Rapid, nongenomic estrogen actions protect pancreatic islet survival. Islets 1: 273-275.
53. Matic M, Bryzgalova G, Gao H, Antonson P, Humire P, et al. (2013) Estrogen signalling and the metabolic syndrome: targeting the hepatic estrogen receptor alpha action. PLoS One 8: e57458.
54. Lo JC, Zhao X, Scuteri A, Brockwell S, Sowers MR (2006) The association of genetic polymorphisms in sex hormone biosynthesis and action with insulin

sensitivity and diabetes mellitus in women at midlife. American Journal of Medicine 119: S69–S78.

55. Gallagher CJ, Langefeld CD, Gordon CJ, Campbell JK, Mychaleckyj JC, et al. (2007) Association of the estrogen receptor-alpha gene with the metabolic syndrome and its component traits in African-American families: the Insulin Resistance Atherosclerosis Family Study. Diabetes 56: 2135–2141.

56. Meshkani R, Saberi H, MohammadTaghvaei N, Tabatabaiefar MA (2012) Estrogen receptor alpha gene polymorphisms are associated with type 2 diabetes and fasting glucose in male subjects. Molecular and Cellular Biochemistry 359: 225–233.

57. Vanhoutte PM, Tang EH (2008) Endothelium-dependent contractions: when a good guy turns bad! J Physiol 586(Pt22): 5295–5304.

11

Go-6976 Reverses Hyperglycemia-Induced Insulin Resistance Independently of cPKC Inhibition in Adipocytes

Katherine A. Robinson[2], Krisztina Hegyi[1], Yusuf A. Hannun[3], Maria G. Buse[2], Jaswinder K. Sethi[1]*

1 The Department of Clinical Biochemistry, University of Cambridge Metabolic Research Laboratories, Institute of Metabolic Science, Addenbrooke's Hospital, Cambridge, United Kingdom, **2** The Departments of Biochemistry and Molecular Biology and Medicine, Division Diabetes, Endocrinology and Medical Genetics, Medical University of South Carolina, Charleston, South Carolina, United States of America, **3** The Department of Medicine and the Stony Brook Cancer Center, Stony Brook University, Stony Brook, New York, United States of America

Abstract

Chronic hyperglycemia induces insulin resistance by mechanisms that are incompletely understood. One model of hyperglycemia-induced insulin resistance involves chronic preincubation of adipocytes in the presence of high glucose and low insulin concentrations. We have previously shown that the mTOR complex 1 (mTORC1) plays a partial role in the development of insulin resistance in this model. Here, we demonstrate that treatment with Go-6976, a widely used "specific" inhibitor of cPKCs, alleviates hyperglycemia-induced insulin resistance. However, the effects of mTOR inhibitor, rapamycin and Go-6976 were not additive and only rapamycin restored impaired insulin-stimulated AKT activation. Although, PKCα, (but not –β) was abundantly expressed in these adipocytes, our studies indicate cPKCs do not play a major role in causing insulin-resistance in this model. There was no evidence of changes in the expression or phosphorylation of PKCα, and PKCα knock-down did not prevent the reduction of insulin-stimulated glucose transport. This was also consistent with lack of IRS-1 phosphorylation on Ser-24 in hyperglycemia-induced insulin-resistant adipocytes. Treatment with Go-6976 did inhibit a component of the mTORC1 pathway, as evidenced by decreased phosphorylation of S6 ribosomal protein. Raptor knock-down enhanced the effect of insulin on glucose transport in insulin resistant adipocytes. Go-6976 had the same effect in control cells, but was ineffective in cells with Raptor knock-down. Taken together these findings suggest that Go-6976 exerts its effect in alleviating hyperglycemia-induced insulin-resistance independently of cPKC inhibition and may target components of the mTORC1 signaling pathway.

Editor: Juergen Eckel, GDC, Germany

Funding: This work was supported by grants from the Biotechnology and Biological Sciences Research Council (David Phillips Fellowship, JF16994), Diabetes UK (BDA:RD06/0003237) and British Heart Foundation (PG/10/38/28359) to J.K. Sethi and also from National Institute of Diabetes and Digestive and Kidney Diseases (DK-02001) to M.G. Buse. The funders had no role in study design, data collection and analysis, decision to publish, or preparation of the manuscript.

Competing Interests: The authors have declared that no competing interests exist.

* Email: j.sethi@oxon.org

Introduction

Insulin resistance is a common pathological condition defined as the reduced ability of insulin to produce its biological effects. Clinically, it refers to the reduced effectiveness of insulin to lower plasma glucose. Insulin resistance is a major feature of Type 2 diabetes and is commonly associated with numerous other conditions, *e.g.* obesity, the metabolic syndrome, polycystic ovary syndrome, glucocorticoid excess, *etc.* The molecular basis of insulin resistance is currently incompletely understood, but in each of these conditions is likely to be multi-factorial, being induced by glucotoxicity, lipotoxicity, and hormones. In contrast, the insulin resistance that accompanies uncontrolled Type 1 diabetes is primarily attributed to glucotoxicity and is reversible with insulin therapy *in vivo* [1,2]. However, the mechanistic basis of hypergylcemia-induced insulin resistance is controversial. Its expression appears to be tissue/cell-type specific and may differ from that caused by lipotoxicity.

We have studied the mechanism(s) of insulin resistance in an *in vitro* model of glucotoxicity in 3T3-L1 adipocytes in some detail [3,4]. This represents a model of 'fasting hyperglycemia-induced insulin resistance' as is observed in diabetes. Under control conditions (*i.e.* after incubation in 5 mM glucose), adipocytes are exquisitely insulin responsive - as assessed by the insulin stimulated glucose uptake. Chronic preincubation in either high glucose (25 mM) or in the presence of a relatively low dose of insulin (0.6 nM) alone does not alter the insulin-stimulated response. However, chronic preincubation with both high glucose and low insulin causes a 40–60% impairment of subsequent insulin-stimulated glucose transport. This state of insulin resistance is not accompanied by changes in the expression of the glucose transporters, GLUT1 and GLUT4 and the proximal insulin signaling cascade appears to be intact, as judged by the insulin response of insulin receptor substrate-1 (IRS-1)-bound phosphatidylinositol (PI) 3-kinase activity [3]. However, in this model there is a block downstream of PI3-kinase activation, which is manifested by markedly impaired activation of protein kinase B/Akt [5].

Since we had evidence that flux through the hexosamine synthesis pathway was increased by exposure to high glucose, we explored the possibility that the insulin resistance reflected enhanced O-GlcNAc modification of some regulatory proteins. However, increased expression of the enzyme which removes O-GlcNAc from proteins or >90% knock-down of O-GlcNAc transferase did not affect the development of insulin resistance in our model, suggesting that other pathways certainly played a role [6]. Similarly, we found no evidence to suggest that enhanced superoxide production caused the insulin resistance in this model [7].

We discovered that basal PtdIns(3,4,5)P_3 was unaltered in control and insulin resistant cells, however, following insulin stimulation, the response was diminished by 34% in the latter. Concomitantly, the amount of PTEN protein, a lipid phosphatase, which dephosphorylates PtdIns(3,4,5)P_3 in the 3-position was significantly and specifically increased in the insulin resistant cells. Treatment with rapamycin, a specific inhibitor of mTORC1, inhibited increased PTEN expression and partially restored insulin-stimulated glucose transport and Akt activation to the insulin resistant cells. Thus, we have evidence that at least one mechanism, which causes insulin resistance in our model, involves the mTOR pathway [7].

Given that blocking mTORC1 restored the insulin resistance only partially, we continued the search for other pathways, which may be involved. Protein kinase C (PKC) seemed to be a logical candidate, particularly because it is known to be activated under some conditions by exposure to high glucose [8]. This hypothesis was supported by initial experiments, which showed that treating cells with Go-6976 partially prevented the development of insulin resistance in cells, which had been pretreated with high glucose and low dose insulin. Go-6976 is a widely used inhibitor of PKC, which is relatively selective for the conventional PKC isoforms, (cPKC α and β) and has much less affinity for the novel and atypical PKC-s. PKCβ is not expressed in NIH/hIR cells (mouse fibroblasts overexpressing the human insulin receptor) [9], and we were unable to detect it by immunoblotting in murine 3T3-L1 adipocytes, which are also fibroblast derived. PKCα was abundantly expressed in our cells, suggesting that we may have identified a candidate, which would be partially responsible for the development of glucose/insulin mediated insulin resistance. However, Go-6976 can also inhibit other enzymes including S6-kinase 1 [10], a substrate of mTORC1. It is also a potent *in vivo* inhibitor of protein kinase D (PKD) [11,12]. The experiments described here led us to the conclusion that PKCα may not be involved in causing hyperglycemia-induced insulin resistance in adipocytes, and that at least some of the effects caused by Go-6976 may have been mediated via its inhibition of the mTORC1 pathway.

Research Design and Methods

Cell culture and glucose transport assay

3T3-L1 fibroblasts (ATCC 2001; cat #CL-173) were differentiated into adipocytes as previously described [3]. Cells were studied on days 8–12 from the initiation of the differentiation protocol, when >95% of the cells exhibited the adipocyte phenotype. They were maintained in Dulbecco's modified Eagle's medium (DMEM) containing 25 mM glucose and 10% fetal bovine serum (FBS). Before experiments the cells were exposed for 18 h to DMEM containing 1% FBS and either 5 mM or 25 mM glucose, with or without 0.6 nM insulin, as indicated. They were then serum and insulin deprived for 2 h, and after washing placed into Krebs Ringer bicarbonate/HEPES (KRBH) buffer without glucose for 10 min and then incubated with or without a maximally stimulating insulin dose (100 nM) for 15 min [3]. Glucose transport was assessed as the uptake of 2-deoxy-D-glucose (2-DOG) for 3 min as described [3] and normalized to protein concentration assessed using the Coomassie Protein Reagent (Pierce). In some experiments activators and/or inhibitors of PKC were added to the media before assay. The activator used was phorbol 12-myristate 13-acetate (PMA) (Calbiochem), the inhibitors used were Go-6976, a cell permeable inhibitor of PKC, which selectively inhibits PKCα and β1 isozymes, at nM concentrations, but does not affect the kinase activities of Ca2+ independent isozymes, δ, ε and ζ, even at μM concentrations (Cat. No. 365250), and bisindolylmaleimide I, Go-6850, which is a broader PKC inhibitor (Cat. No. 203290, both from Calbiochem). We also tested Ruboxistaurin (LY379196), kindly provided by Lilly Research Laboratories, which at the doses used (300 nM) is a highly selective inhibitor of PKCβ [8,13].

RNAi

To test the role of PKCα, PKCλ and mTORC1 pathway in our model of insulin resistance we investigated the effect of reducing their expression via transfection of mouse specific small interfering siRNA-s. We purchased SMARTpool reagents from Dharmacon against PKCα, PKCλ and against Raptor, each consist of a mixture of 4 unique siRNA-s developed against the targeted gene and are guaranteed to silence the RNA by >75%. For cells treated with non-targeting siRNA, we used Dharmacon's non-targeting siRNA pool of 4.

3T3-L1 adipocytes are notoriously difficult to transfect and until recently their successful siRNA transfection usually involved electroporation [14]. Recently, a technology using virus derived amphipatic peptides has been developed, that directly interact with nucleic acid cargos to form nanoparticles, which diffuse through plasma membranes and release their cargos inside the cell [15]. The technology has been adapted by the manufacturer (Panomics, Fremont, CA) to several cell lines, including 3T3-L1 adipocytes. We adopted the following protocol for transfection of the latter [6]. On day 6 after initiation of the differentiation protocol, cells were subcultured to a density of 2.5×10^4 cells/cm^2 and incubated overnight in DME containing 25 mM glucose and 10% FBS. Then FBS was removed and cells were washed with PBS and transfected with a final concentration of 40 nM non-targeting or targeting siRNA using the DeliverX Plus Kit (Panomics). Following 4 h incubation with the siRNA, FBS was added to a concentration of 10% and cells were incubated for an additional 18 h. Media was replaced with fresh DME containing 25 mM glucose and 10% FBS for 24 h. Cells were then incubated for 18 h in DME containing 1% FBS and 5 mM glucose or 25 mM glucose+0.6 nM insulin, with or without Go-6976 or rapamycin, then serum- and insulin-deprived for 2 h and glucose transport measured as described. The degree of knock-down was assessed by Western blotting for the respective protein.

Western blots

Total post-nuclear cell lysates were prepared in lysis buffer as previously described [3,6]. Cell extracts were separated on 7% or 12% SDS-PAGE and transferred to nitrocellulose. They were blocked for 1 h and then incubated overnight in blocking buffer containing one of the following: rabbit P-PKC α/β (Thr 638/641) antibody, P-Akt (Ser473) antibody, rabbit P-p70 S6kinase (Thr 389) antibody, rabbit P-S6 ribosomal protein (Ser 240/244) antibody or rabbit anti-Raptor antibody (all 1:1000, each from

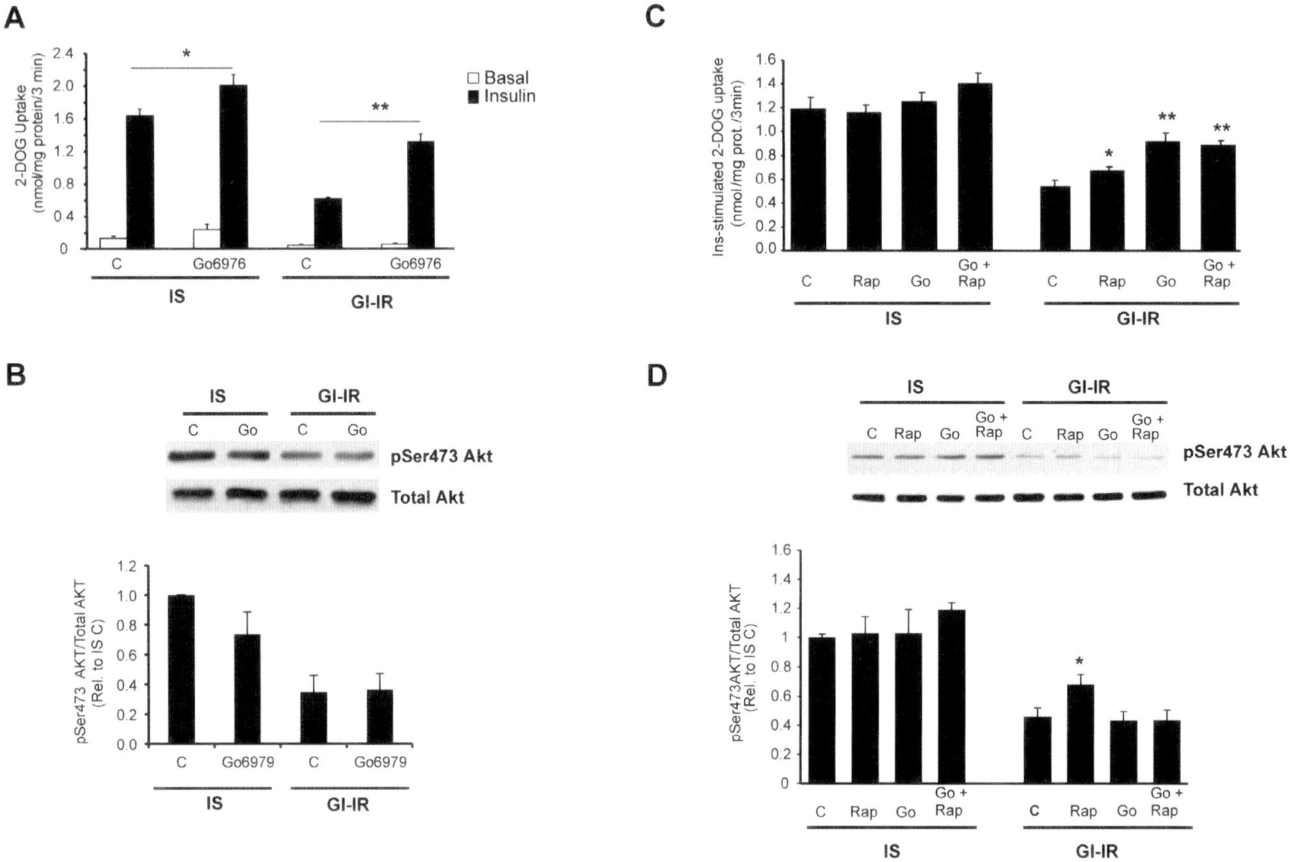

Figure 1. Treatment with Go-6976, reverses hyperglycemia-induced insulin resistance in adipocytes. A. Effect of Go-6976 on Glucose transport. Insulin sensitive (IS) Adipocytes were preincubated in 5 mM glucose while Glucose-induced insulin resistant, (GI-IR) were generated by preincubation in 25 mM glucose+0.6 nM insulin for 18 h. During serum and insulin deprivation for 2 h, adipocytes were received 0.3 mM Go-6976 or vehicle control during the last hour of incubation. Glucose (2DOG) uptake was determined in unstimulated (open bars, basal) or in insulin-stimulated (100 nM for 15 min; filled bars, Insulin) cells. **B.** Effect of Go-6976 on insulin-stimulated Akt phosphorylation. Adipocytes were treated as in A, following acute insulin stimulation, cell lysates were collected and both phospho-Akt and total AKT was measured. Quantification represents ratios of phosphoAKT/Total AKT protein expressed relative to ratios obtained in from control insulin sensitive (IS) adipocytes. **C.** The effects of rapamycin and Go-6976 on insulin-stimulated glucose transport. Adipocytes were treated as in A, except that only cells, which have been acutely stimulated with insulin, are shown. Go-6976 (0.3 mM) and rapamycin (100 nM) are added during the last hour of incubation. **D.** The effects of rapamycin and Go-6976 on insulin-stimulated Akt phosphorylation. Adipocytes were treated as in C, following acute insulin stimulation, cell lysates were collected and both phospho-Akt and total AKT was measured. Quantification represents ratios of phosphoAKT/Total AKT protein expressed relative to ratios obtained in from control insulin sensitive (IS) adipocytes. Statistical significance is indicated by *$p<0.05$, and ** = $p<0.005$ compared to controls with the same preincubation.

Cell Signaling). Following washing, membranes were incubated in goat anti-rabbit IgG (1:10,000, Jackson Immunoresearch) for 1 h, washed, developed with West Pico ECL Reagent (Pierce), exposed to film, and quantified by laser densitometry using a National Institute of Health Image Analyzer Program. Membranes that had been exposed to P-PKC α/β_2 antibody were stripped and reanalyzed with an antibody to PKCα (1:1000, Cell Signaling); while blots developed with anti-phospho- p70 S6kinase or with anti-phospho S6 ribosomal protein antibody were stripped and analyzed with mouse p70 S6kinase antibody (1:200, Santa Cruz) or with rabbit anti-S6 ribosomal protein antibody (1:1000, Cell Signaling), respectively. Finally, most gels were stripped and analyzed with rabbit β-tubulin antibody (1:200, Santa Cruz) to document equal loading of the gel.

In some experiments the phosphorylation of Ser 24 of IRS-1 was tested, because this site is directly responsive to stimulation by PKCα [9]. The preparation of this antibody has been described [9]. Total post-nuclear cell lysates (1 mg protein) were immunoprecipitated with 2 µg of rabbit anti-IRS-1 antibody (Upstate/Chemicon) overnight at 4°C. Immunocomplexes were collected for 2 h with protein G Sepharose, washed and eluted with Laemmli's sample buffer for 10 min at 95°C. The eluates were separated by SDS-PAGE and exposed to P-IRS-1 (Ser 24) rabbit antibody, at a dilution of 1:100 overnight at 4°C. Subsequent development with goat anti-rabbit IgG was as described above.

Results and Discussion

Go-6976 treatment enhances insulin-sensitivity in cultured adipocytes

To generate hyperglycemia- and insulin-induced insulin resistant (GI-IR) adipocytes, 3T3-L1 adipocytes were preincubated for 18 h in culture media containing 25 mM glucose and supplemented with 0.6 nM insulin. In contrast, control 'insulin-sensitive' adipocytes (IS) were generated by preincubation with 5 mM glucose without insulin supplementation. Insulin-stimulated glucose uptake was then determined in materials and methods. As previously reported, preincubation in high glucose

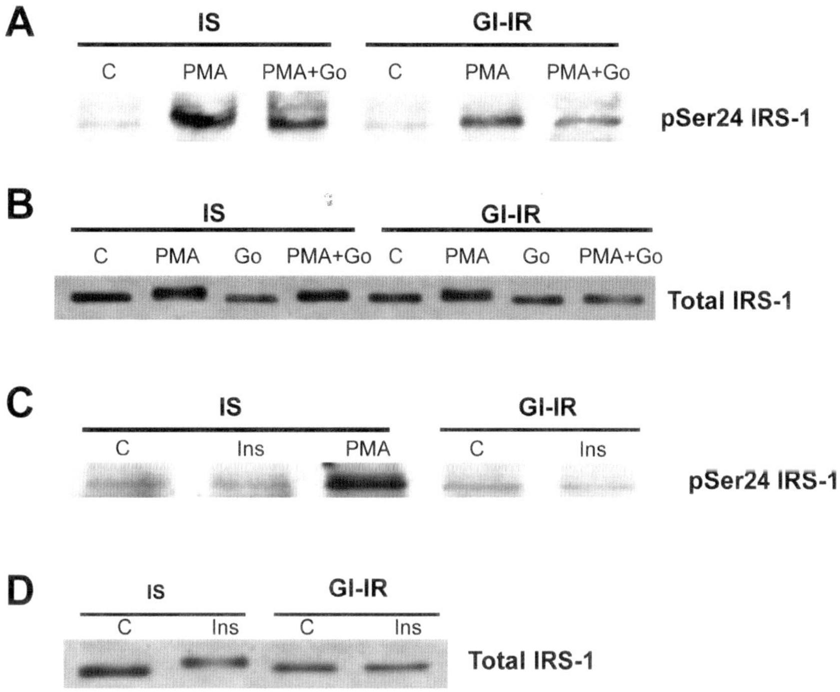

Figure 2. Hyperglycemia-induced insulin resistance does not promote pSer24 IRS-1, a target of cPKC. Adipocytes were preincubated for 18 h in 5 mM glucose (IS) or in 25 mM glucose+0.6 nM insulin (GI-IR). **A and B.** During the last hour, cells were exposed to either vehicle control (C), PMA (1 mM), Go-6976 (1 mM) or both. IRS-1 was immunoprecipitated from subsequent cell extracts and following gel separation western blotted with an anti-pSer 24 IRS1 (**A**) or anti-IRS1 (**B**), as described in Methods. **C.** pSer 24 IRS1 levels are unaffected by preincubation treatment and acute insulin stimulation. **D.** Total IRS1 protein exhibit a mobility shift following acute stimulation with 100 nM insulin for 15 min. All gels are representative of 3 similar experiments.

together with low dose insulin inhibited insulin-stimulated ($p < 0.001$) glucose transport (**Fig. 1A**) confirming that these GI-IR adipocytes were indeed insulin resistant. To identify potential serine kinases that may be involved in mediating this insulin resistance and amenable to pharmacological intervention, we screened a number of kinase inhibitors. Amongst these, Go-6976 was identified as an inhibitor of cPKC isoforms [9] that significantly enhanced insulin-stimulated glucose transport both in the GI-IR adipocytes (by 114%, $p<0.001$) as well in IS adipocytes (by 23%, $p<0.05$). Although Go-6976 did not completely restore insulin stimulated glucose transport to control levels ($p<0.04$), the effects only required incubation with 0.3 µM inhibitor for 1 h immediately following the pretreatment and preceding determination of insulin sensitivity.

We have previously shown that the insulin resistance that develops in this model is associated with a marked inhibition of insulin-stimulated Akt activation [5,7] and this was again observed in these experiments (**Fig. 1B**). However, Go-6976 treatment did not restore insulin-stimulated Akt activation, suggesting that the target of Go-6976 action is either downstream of, or occurs parallel to, Akt activation. This observation contrasts with our previous study in which exposure of GI-IR adipocytes for one hour to the mTOR inhibitor, rapamycin, partially restored the insulin resistant glucose transport, and simultaneously corrected the impaired activation of Akt [7]. To establish whether the effects of both serine kinase inhibitors (Go-6976 and rapamycin) on glucose transport were of equal magnitude, additive and/or synergistic, we performed additional parallel experiments. In this study there were no significant effects in control insulin sensitive (IS) adipocytes (**Fig. 1C**). However, in GI-IR adipocytes, insulin-stimulated glucose transport was decreased by ~60%. This was significantly reversed both by rapamycin and Go-6976 treatments when used individually, however, there was no evidence of any additive effect when these inhibitors were combined (**Fig. 1C**) suggesting that they may target the same pathway. Notably, insulin resistance was again not completely restored and insulin-stimulated AKT phosphorylation was also not restored with Go-6976 alone or combination with rapamycin (**Fig. 1D**).

GI-IR adipocytes do not exhibit enhanced IRS-1 phosphorylation on Ser-24

We recently reported that protein kinase C activators such as phorbol esters can promote insulin resistance through phosphorylation of Serine-24 on IRS-1 and that this was also inhibited by Go-6976 [9]. We therefore next investigated whether IRS-1 phosphorylation on Ser-24 was enhanced in GI-IR adipocytes. **Figure 2A** shows that 1 µM PMA can induce phosphorylation of IRS-1 on Ser-24 in IS adipocytes and this coincided with a mobility shift in total IRS-1 (**Fig. 2B**). Inclusion of Go-6976 (1 µM) with the PMA reduced both Ser-24 phosphorylation of IRS1 and the reduction in total IRS-1 mobility (**Fig. 2A and 2B**). This is consistent with similar findings reported for NIH3T3 cells [9]. However, in GI-IR adipocytes, basal IRS-1 Ser-24 phosphorylation was unaltered and the response to PMA with or without Go-6976 was similar to IS adipocytes. **Figure 2C** also shows that acute stimulation with insulin alone (100 nM, 15 min) also did not induce Ser-24 phosphorylation in the control (IS) or in the insulin resistant (GI-IR) adipocytes. However, acute insulin was sufficient to induce a mobility shift in total IRS-1 at least in IS adipocytes (**Fig. 2D**). These data suggest that PKCα-mediated phosphoryla-

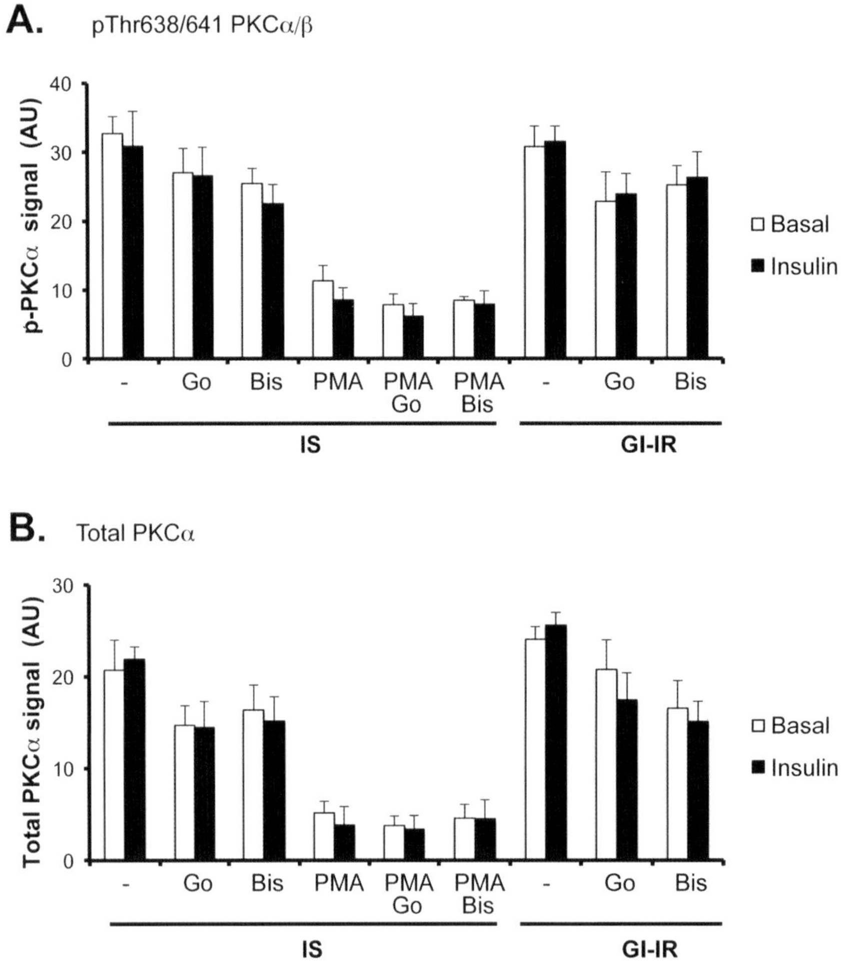

Figure 3. Phosphorylated PKCalpha and total PKCalpha are not altered by hyperglycemia-induced insulin resistance. Adipocytes were preincubated for 18 h in 5 mM glucose (IS) or in 25 mM glucose+0.6 nM insulin (GI-IR). During the last 2 hours cells were exposed to either vehicle control or PMA (1 mM), or during the last hour with Go-6976 (1 mM, Go) or bis-indolylmaleimide (1 mM, Bis). Acute insulin stimulation (black bars) or non-stimulation (white bars) were performed for 15 min with or without 100 nM insulin. Cells were lysed, proteins extracted and subjected to western blotting with antibodies to either phosphorylated pThr638/641 PKCalpha/beta (**A**) or to Total PKCalpha (**B**). Quantification was determined as described in Methods. The graph data represents means +/− SE of 6 observations.

tion of Ser24 on IRS-1 is not involved in hyperglycemia-induced insulin resistance.

GI-IR adipocytes do not exhibit altered PKCα expression or activating phosphorylation

Since Go-6976 is widely reported to be an inhibitor of cPKCs (PKCα/β), and cPKCs have themselves been implicated in other models of insulin resistance, we next investigated their presence and putative regulation in GI-IR adipocytes. We were unable to detect PKCβ expression in our cells (data not shown). However, PKCα protein was detected, as was pThr638/641- PKCα, an indicator of active PKCα levels (**Fig. 3 and Fig. S1**). Importantly, neither the preincubation conditions (low glucose versus high glucose plus low dose insulin) nor acute stimulation with high dose insulin affected either the total amount or the phosphorylation of PKCα significantly (**Fig. 3 and Fig. S1**), suggesting that PKCα is not involved in this model of insulin-resistance. However, the addition of Go-6976 significantly reduced the expression of PKCα (**Fig. 3B**, $p<0.001$). Nonetheless, there was no difference in the effect of Go-6976 between IS adipocytes (preincubated in 5 mM glucose) and GI-IR adipocytes. The effect of Go-6976 on the phosphorylation of PKCα showed the same trend as that of total PKCα expression. Although the effect was less pronounced, it was significant by analysis of variance ($p<0.01$). In contrast, incubation of adipocytes for two hours with 1 μM PMA markedly reduced the expression and phosphorylation of PKCα (**Fig. 3**, $p<0.001$). The ratio of phospho-PKC:Total PKCα was not significantly affected suggesting that PMA-stimulated effects involved primarily PKCα degradation. Indeed it is well known that sustained exposure to PMA promotes activation followed by degradation of cPKC [9]. Addition of Go-6976 or bisindolylmaleimide I for 1 hour to PMA pretreated cells did not change the PMA effect. The surprising lack of effect of the PKC inhibitors likely reflects the fact that adipocytes were first treated with PMA for 1 hr followed by a further 1 hr with inhibitors (Go-6976 or of bisindolylmaleimide I) together with PMA. An alternative commonly used albeit preventative approach, would have been to pretreat adipocytes with these inhibitors prior to and during PMA exposure. This approach may have yielded different results with respect to the effects of PMA.

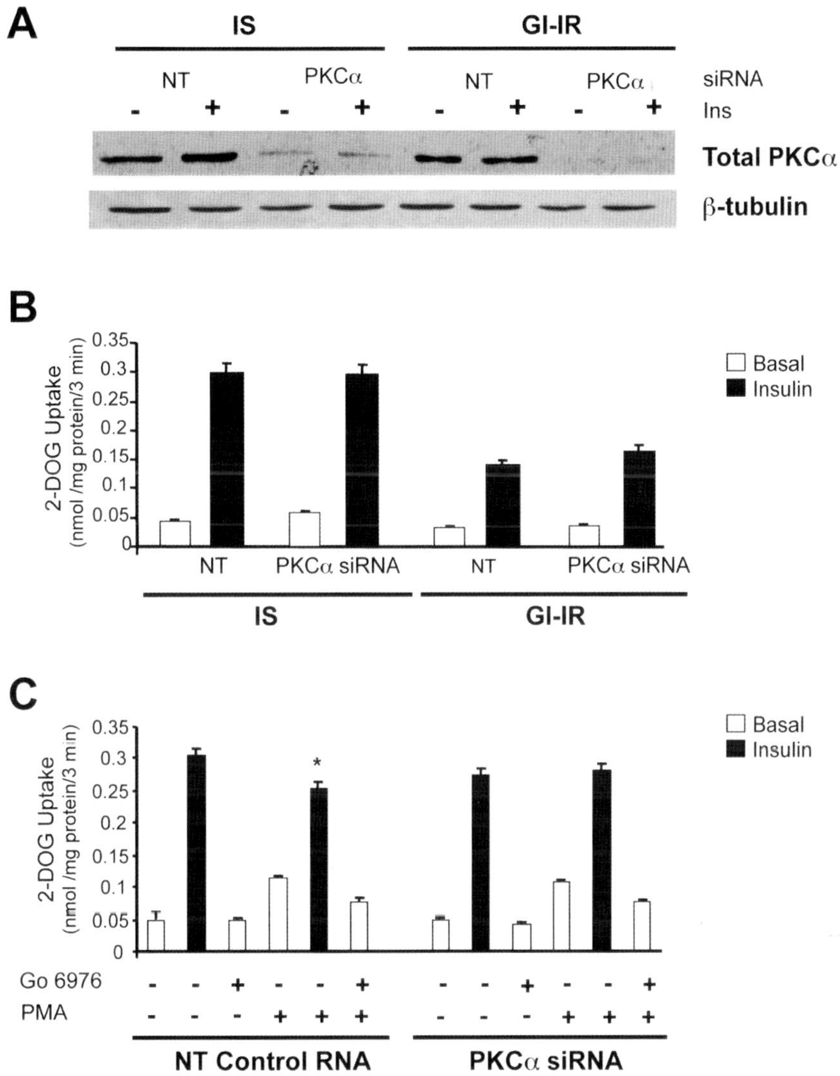

Figure 4. PKCalpha knock-down does not prevent the development of hyperglycemia-induced insulin resistance. A. The expression of PKCαlpha is reduced (by 75–78%) in adipocytes treated with anti-PKCαlpha siRNA compared with cells infected with non-targeting (NT) siRNA. **B.** Experiment designed was as described for Fig. 1 except cells were treated with indicated siRNA prior to glucose uptake determination. **C.** PMA-induced insulin resistance is lost in cells infected with anti-PKCαlpha siRNA. Adipocytes were infected with non-targeting or with anti-PKCalpha siRNA, then treated with or without PMA (1 μM, 1 h) followed by acute insulin stimulation and glucose uptake determined. Statistical significance is indicated by *$p<0.005$ vs. no PMA.

PKCα knock-down does not alter insulin resistance in GI-IR adipocytes

To further assess the role of PKCα, we tested the effect of its knock-down on the development of insulin resistance in our model. Cells transfected with siRNA against PKCα were compared to cells transfected with non-targeting RNA and tested 72 h after transfection. PKCα expression at this time was reduced by 75–78% as judged by Western blots (**Fig. 4A**). As shown in **Fig. 4B**, glucose transport and the development of insulin resistance were not affected by the PKCα knock-down in either IS or GI-IR adipocytes. To further assess whether PKCα knock-down had any effect on insulin-stimulated glucose transport, we compared the effects of PMA and Go-6976, in the presence or absence of insulin on glucose transport in IS adipocytes (**Fig. 4C**). PMA (1 μM, 1 h) stimulated glucose transport (>2-fold over basal) in both the PKCα knock-down and the non-targeted controls and the addition of Go-6976 to PMA partially blocked this effect. The only significant difference between the PKCα knock-down and the non-targeting controls was that in the latter PMA inhibited maximally insulin-stimulated glucose transport by ~17% ($p<0.005$) while this did not occur in the PKCα knock-down cells. The data suggests that while PKCα does play a role in the effect of PMA on glucose transport in these cells, confirming previous observations [16], it does not seem to participate, in the development of hyperglycemia-induced insulin resistance in GI-IR adipocytes.

PKCβ inhibition does not reverse insulin resistance in GI-IR adipocytes

Although we had no evidence that PKCβ is expressed in our 3T3-L1 adipocytes, we also tested whether incubation with a specific inhibitor of this isoform would alter the insulin resistant glucose transport in our experiments. Ruboxistaurin had no effect on glucose transport under any of the conditions tested and failed

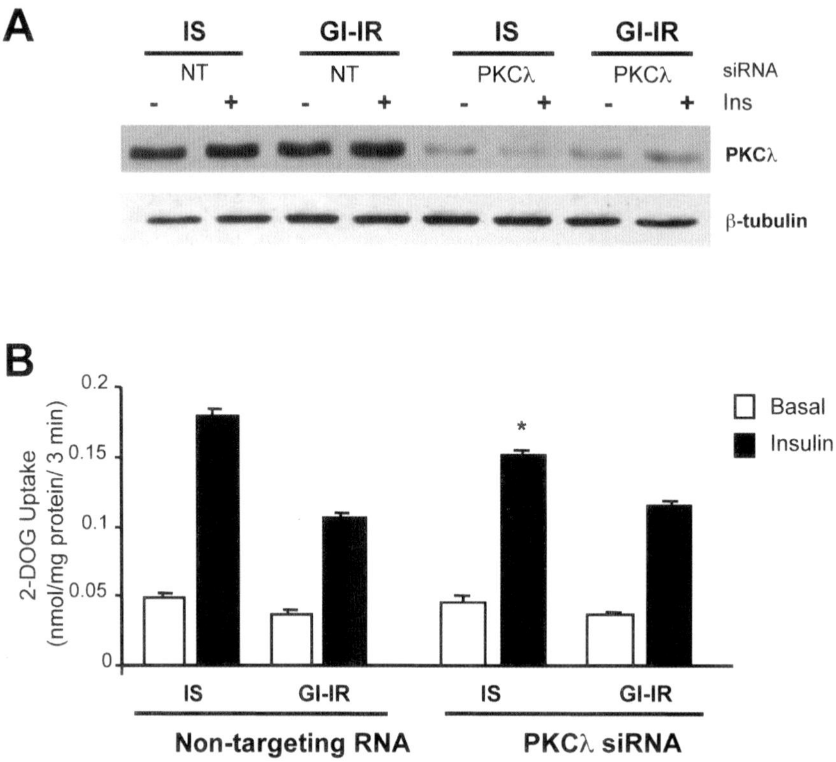

Figure 5. The effect of PKCλ knock-down on hyperglycemia-induced insulin resistance. A. Western blot showing depletion (by 84%) of PKCλ in cells treated with anti-PKCλ siRNA as compared to cells treated with NT control RNA. **B.** cells preincubated in 5 mM glucose (IS) vs. 25 mM glucose+0.6 nM insulin (GI-IR) and then stimulated (the black bars) or not (basal) with acute, 100 nM insulin. Knock-down of PKCλ mRNA decreased the insulin-stimulation of glucose transport by ~20%, in IS adipocytes, but had no additional effect in GI-IR adipocytes. (*$p<0.001$, $n=15$).

to affect the insulin response of glucose transport ($n=5$, from two experiments, **Fig. S2**).

Effect of PKCλ knock-down on insulin-stimulated glucose transport

In view of the elegant demonstration that atypical PKC's are required for insulin-stimulated glucose transport in 3T3-L1 adipocytes [17] we also investigated the role of PKCλ (the a-PKC expressed in adipocytes) in our model. PKCλ expression was decreased by 84% in cells transfected with mouse specific small interfering si-RNA against PKCλ (**Fig. 5A**). In cells incubated in 5 mM glucose the insulin effect on glucose transport was decreased by 20% in RNAi treated adipocytes (**Fig. 5B**, $p<0.001$) compared to cells treated with a non-targeting RNA. Our data qualitatively reproduces previously published observations [17]. However, it is of interest, that in GI-IR adipocytes, knock-down of PKCλ had no additional inhibitory effect.

Go-6976 affects the phosphorylation of S6 ribosomal protein

In view of the above findings we next investigated whether Go-6976 may reverse the development of insulin resistance by inhibiting enzyme(s) other than cPKC but downstream of AKT. Indeed, *In vitro* studies using recombinant peptides have suggested that Go-6976 can interact with additional kinases, including p70 S6 kinase-1 [10], which we previously reported to be involved in our model of insulin resistance [7]. We therefore next measured the insulin-stimulated activation of S6 kinase-1 (i.e. pThr389-S6K:Total S6K ratio) and the phosphorylation of its substrate, S6 ribosomal protein (on Ser 240/244). As reported previously [7], acute insulin treatment of IS adipocytes markedly stimulated the activation of S6 kinase (8–10-fold) and increased the expression of phosphorylated S6 ribosomal protein (3–5-fold, **Fig. 6A**). In GI-IR adipocytes, basal levels of active S6 kinase-1 and S6 ribosomal protein phosphorylation was significantly elevated (**Fig. 6B**) and Go-6976 treatment prevented direct correlation between active S6K and phosphorylated S6 ribosomal protein (**Fig. 6B**). However, insulin-stimulated activation of this pathway was reduced in GI-IR adipocytes, and Go-6976 treatment further reduced both active S6K and S6 ribosomal protein phosphorylation (**Fig. 6C**). These data suggest that p70 S6 kinase-1 is a candidate target for Go-6976 action in adipocytes.

Raptor knock-down enhances insulin-stimulated glucose transport in GI-IR adipocytes but is additive with Go-6976

Since S6K-1 is a downstream target of mTOR-associated proteins such as raptor we next investigated whether insulin-stimulated glucose transport was altered in our model when Raptor was knocked-down. Raptor expression decreased by 76% in the cells treated with siRNA for Raptor (**Fig. 7A**). In IS adipocytes, insulin stimulated glucose transport was not significantly different in the Raptor knock-down cells as compared to the non-targeted controls (**Fig. 7B**). However, in GI-IR adipocytes, insulin-stimulated glucose transport increased by 40% in the Raptor-deficient cells, a significant effect (**Fig. 7B**, $p<0.04$). We next compared the response to Go-6976 of glucose transport between non-targeted and knock-down cells (**Fig. 7C**). In IS adipocytes, there was no difference either in basal or acute insulin stimulated glucose transport between control and Raptor deficient

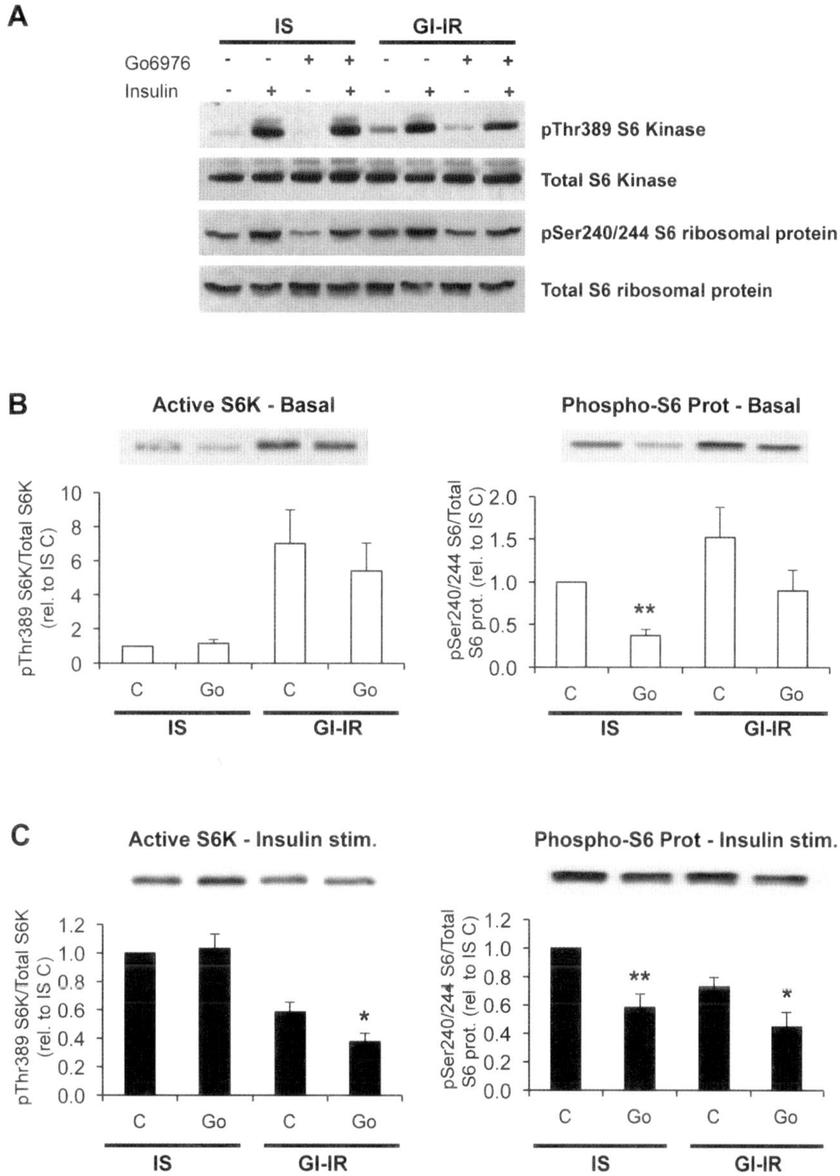

Figure 6. Effect of Go-6976 on S6 Kinase activity. Adipocytes were preincubated for 18 h in 5 mM glucose (IS) or in 25 mM glucose+0.6 nM insulin (GI-IR). **A.** Acute insulin treatment (100 nM for 15 min) stimulated activating phosphorylation of S-6 kinase (8–10-fold) and of its substrate S-6 ribosomal protein (4–5-fold). Under basal conditions, GI-IR adipocytes exhibited enhanced S6K phosphorylation. For quantification purposes, unstimulated (**B**) and acute insulin-stimulated (**C**) samples were also analysed on separate gels with exposure to times adjusted to within linear ranges. Under these conditions it is evident that the acute insulin stimulated S6K activity was decreased in the GI-IR cells. This was further reduced by treatment with Go-6976 (1 mM for 1 h). Statistical significance is indicated by $^*p<0.05$ vs. control without Go-6976, $^{**}p<0.001$. n = 9.

cells and the addition of 1 µM Go-6976 also had no effect. However, in GI-IR adipocytes, Go-6976 significantly increased insulin-stimulated glucose transport in the non-targeted cells ($p<0.03$) but was unable to further improve glucose transport in Raptor knock-down cells (**Fig. 7C**). Again, without Go-6976 treatment the insulin-stimulated glucose transport was greater ($p<0.005$) in the Raptor knock-down cells than in the non-targeted controls (**Fig. 7C**). These data suggest that the mTORC1 pathway indeed plays an important role in GI-IR adipocytes and that Go-6976 alleviates this by targeting inhibition of mTORC1 dependent pathway(s).

In summary, the major message of this paper is that the mTORC1 pathway does play a role in eliciting high glucose/low dose insulin mediated insulin resistance (GI-IR) in cultured adipocytes, while we were unable to detect any significant role of cPKC with the methods used here. This is important, because cPKCs are thought to be important mediators of hyperglycemia-associated pathology and experiments with the widely used cPKC inhibitor Go-6976 initially suggested that cPKC-s might play a major role in high glucose-induced insulin resistance in adipocytes. However, our data clearly indicate that Go-6976 exerts its major effects by inhibiting mTORC1 dependent pathways in the GI-IR adipocytes. It is worth noting that this study has focused on one *in vitro* model of hyperglycemia-induced insulin resistance in murine adipocytes. As such, our findings do not rule out the possibility that other PKC's, novel or atypical, may play a role in the development

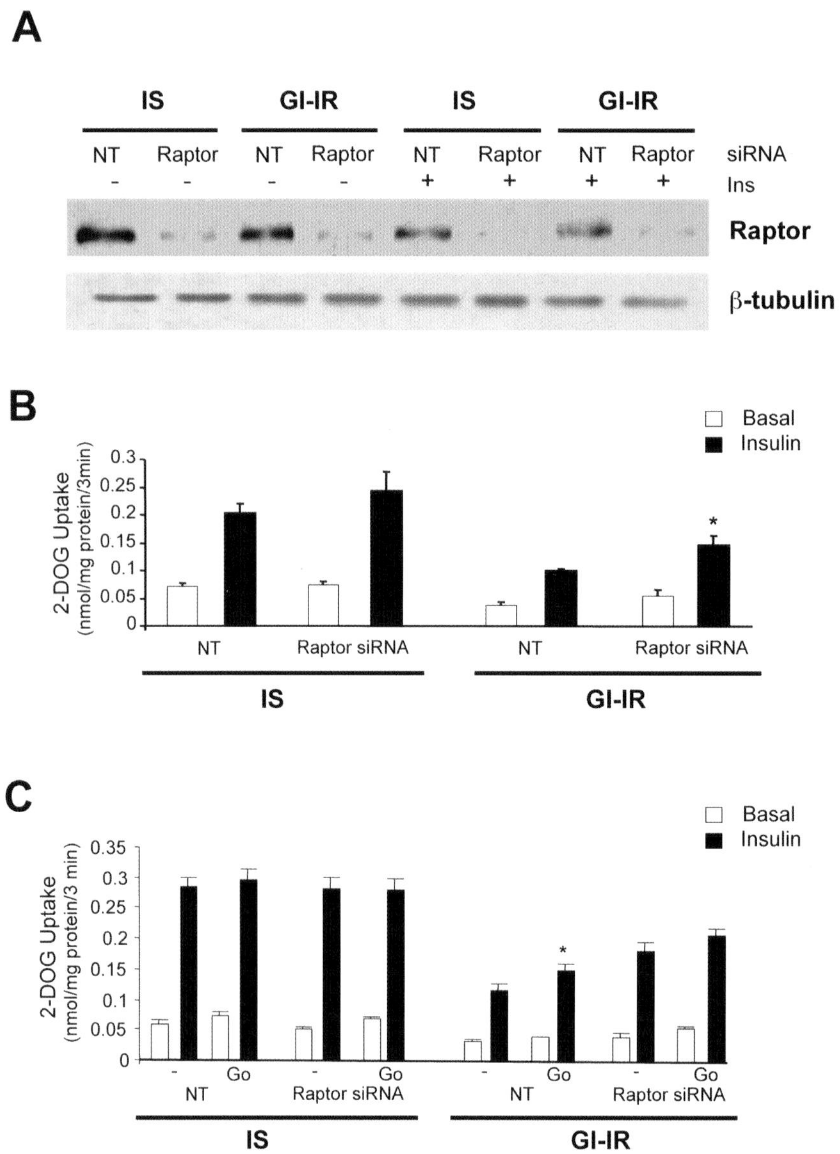

Figure 7. Raptor knock-down enhances the effect of insulin on glucose transport in insulin resistant cells. **A** Raptor expression was decreased by 76% in adipocytes treated with anti-Raptor siRNA compared to cells treated with NT RNA. **B** Insulin-stimulated glucose transport is enhanced by ~40% in hyperglycemia-induced insulin resistant (GI-IR) Raptor knock-down cells (* = $p < 0.005$ vs. NT). **C** Go-6976 enhances insulin stimulated glucose transport only in the insulin resistant NT cells (* = $p < 0.03$), but not in the Raptor knock-down cells.

of insulin resistance induced by other mediators on in other cellular systems. Indeed, there is ample evidence that lipid/FFA-induced insulin resistance is associated with activation of PKCθin rodent skeletal muscle and PKCδ and -β in human muscle. Furthermore, in liver lipid-induced insulin resistance has been linked to PKCε activity (reviewed in [18]). Hence, additional studies are warranted before a significant clinical impact can be assigned to our findings. Such studies should elucidate the molecular target of Go-6976 action and confirm that similar therapeutic effects also occur in human adipocytes and other insulin target tissues. Such mechanistic insights will be crucial in informing future targeted therapeutics aimed at treating patients with hyperglycemia and IR while avoiding unanticipated side effects.

Nonetheless, our findings highlight the fact that caution should be exercised when interpreting mechanistic data from pharmacological studies alone because potentially misleading conclusions can be drawn from use of very modest doses a 'specific' pharmacological inhibitor in cultured cells. That Go-6976 may not be as specific as advertised has been reported previously, where its inhibition of recombinant S6 kinase 1 has been demonstrated [10]. By combining both targeted pharmaceuticals with specific gene modulation we have demonstrated that a more reliable and powerful approach can be taken to dissect complex signaling pathways.

Supporting Information

Figure S1 Phosphorylated PKCalpha and total PKCalpha are not altered by hyperglycemia-induced insulin resistance. Adipocytes were treated as described for Figure 3.

Representative western blots are shown for basal (A) and Insulin stimulated (B) samples. Quantification is shown in Figure 3.

Figure S2 The PKCbeta inhibitor, Ruboxistaurin does not affect insulin resistance in 3T3-L1 adipocytes. Cells were preincubated in 5 mM glucose (IS) or in 25 M glucose+ 0.6 nM insulin (GI-IR) and then acutely stimulated with (the black bars) or without (the white bars) 100 nM insulin for 15 min. Some samples were also supplemented with 300 nM Ruboxistaurin (Rbxn) for 18 h or for 2 h, before insulin stimulation. Ruboxistaurin did not affect insulin stimulation of glucose transport under any of the conditions tested (n = 6).

Author Contributions

Conceived and designed the experiments: JKS MGB. Performed the experiments: KAR KH. Analyzed the data: KAR KH YAH MGB JKS. Contributed reagents/materials/analysis tools: MGB JKS. Wrote the paper: KAR KH YAH MGB JKS.

References

1. Rossetti L, Giaccari A, DeFronzo RA (1990) Glucose toxicity. Diabetes Care 13: 610–630.
2. Yki-Jarvinen H, Helve E, Koivisto VA (1987) Hyperglycemia decreases glucose uptake in type I diabetes. Diabetes 36: 892–896.
3. Nelson BA, Robinson KA, Buse MG (2000) High glucose and glucosamine induce insulin resistance via different mechanisms in 3T3-L1 adipocytes. Diabetes 49: 981–991.
4. Nelson BA, Robinson KA, Buse MG (2002) Insulin acutely regulates Munc18-c subcellular trafficking: altered response in insulin-resistant 3T3-L1 adipocytes. J Biol Chem 277: 3809–3812.
5. Nelson BA, Robinson KA, Buse MG (2002) Defective Akt activation is associated with glucose- but not glucosamine-induced insulin resistance. Am J Physiol Endocrinol Metab 282: E497–506.
6. Robinson KA, Ball LE, Buse MG (2007) Reduction of O-GlcNAc protein modification does not prevent insulin resistance in 3T3-L1 adipocytes. Am J Physiol Endocrinol Metab 292: E884–890.
7. Robinson KA, Buse MG (2008) Mechanisms of high-glucose/insulin-mediated desensitization of acute insulin-stimulated glucose transport and Akt activation. Am J Physiol Endocrinol Metab 294: E870–881.
8. Idris I, Gray S, Donnelly R (2001) Protein kinase C activation: isozyme-specific effects on metabolism and cardiovascular complications in diabetes. Diabetologia 44: 659–673.
9. Nawaratne R, Gray A, Jorgensen CH, Downes CP, Siddle K, et al. (2006) Regulation of insulin receptor substrate 1 pleckstrin homology domain by protein kinase C: role of serine 24 phosphorylation. Mol Endocrinol 20: 1838–1852.
10. Davies SP, Reddy H, Caivano M, Cohen P (2000) Specificity and mechanism of action of some commonly used protein kinase inhibitors. Biochem J 351: 95–105.
11. Haxhinasto SA, Bishop GA (2003) A novel interaction between protein kinase D and TNF receptor-associated factor molecules regulates B cell receptor-CD40 synergy. J Immunol 171: 4655–4662.
12. Sumara G, Formentini I, Collins S, Sumara I, Windak R, et al. (2009) Regulation of PKD by the MAPK p38delta in insulin secretion and glucose homeostasis. Cell 136: 235–248.
13. Mehta NN, Sheetz M, Price K, Comiskey L, Amrutia S, et al. (2009) Selective PKC beta inhibition with ruboxistaurin and endothelial function in type-2 diabetes mellitus. Cardiovasc Drugs Ther 23: 17–24.
14. Mitra P, Zheng X, Czech MP (2004) RNAi-based analysis of CAP, Cbl, and CrkII function in the regulation of GLUT4 by insulin. J Biol Chem 279: 37431–37435.
15. Deshayes S, Gerbal-Chaloin S, Morris MC, Aldrian-Herrada G, Charnet P, et al. (2004) On the mechanism of non-endosomial peptide-mediated cellular delivery of nucleic acids. Biochim Biophys Acta 1667: 141–147.
16. Bandyopadhyay G, Standaert ML, Galloway L, Moscat J, Farese RV (1997) Evidence for involvement of protein kinase C (PKC)-zeta and noninvolvement of diacylglycerol-sensitive PKCs in insulin-stimulated glucose transport in L6 myotubes. Endocrinology 138: 4721–4731.
17. Sajan MP, Rivas J, Li P, Standaert ML, Farese RV (2006) Repletion of atypical protein kinase C following RNA interference-mediated depletion restores insulin-stimulated glucose transport. J Biol Chem 281: 17466–17473.
18. Morino K, Petersen KF, Shulman GI (2006) Molecular mechanisms of insulin resistance in humans and their potential links with mitochondrial dysfunction. Diabetes 55 Suppl 2: S9–S15.

The rs225017 Polymorphism in the 3′UTR of the Human *DIO2* Gene Is Associated with Increased Insulin Resistance

Leonardo B. Leiria, José M. Dora, Simone M. Wajner, Aline A. F. Estivalet, Daisy Crispim*, Ana Luiza Maia

Thyroid Section, Endocrine Division, Hospital de Clínicas de Porto Alegre, Universidade Federal do Rio Grande do Sul, Porto Alegre, RS, Brazil

Abstract

The Thr92Ala (rs225014) polymorphism in the type 2 deiodinase (*DIO2*) gene has been associated with insulin resistance (IR) and decreased enzyme activity in human tissues but kinetic studies failed to detect changes in the mutant enzyme, suggesting that this variant might be a marker of abnormal *DIO2* expression. Thus, we aimed to investigate whether other *DIO2* polymorphisms, individually or in combination with the Thr92Ala, may contribute to IR. The entire coding-region of *DIO2* gene was sequenced in 12 patients with type 2 diabetes mellitus (T2DM). Potentially informative variants were evaluated in 1077 T2DM patients and 516 nondiabetic subjects. IR was evaluated using the homeostasis model assessment (HOMA-IR) index. *DIO2* gene sequencing revealed no new mutation but 5 previously described single nucleotide polymorphisms (SNPs). We observed that all T2DM patients displaying high HOMA-IR index (n = 6) were homozygous for the rs225017 (T/A) polymorphism. Further analysis showed that the median fasting plasma insulin and HOMA-IR of T2DM patients carrying the T/T genotype were higher than in patients carrying the A allele ($P = 0.013$ and $P = 0.002$, respectively). These associations were magnified in the presence of the Ala92Ala genotype of the Thr92Ala polymorphism. Moreover, the rs225017 and the Thr92Ala polymorphisms were in partial linkage disequilibrium ($|D'| = 0.811$; $r^2 = 0.365$). In conclusion, the rs225017 polymorphism is associated with greater IR in T2DM and it seems to interact with the Thr92Ala polymorphism in the modulation of IR.

Editor: Qingyang Huang, Central China Normal University, China

Funding: This study was supported by grants from Conselho Nacional de Desenvolvimento Científico e Tecnológico (CNPq), Coordenação de Aperfeiçoamento de Pessoal de Nivel Superior (CAPES) and Fundo de Incentivo a Pesquisa (FIPE), Brazil. The funders had no role in study design, data collection and analysis, decision to publish, or preparation of the manuscript.

Competing Interests: The authors have declared that no competing interests exist.

* Email: dcmoreira@hcpa.ufrgs.br

Introduction

Thyroid hormones are critical to the development, growth and metabolism of virtually all tissues [1,2]. The iodothyronine deiodinases types 1 (D1), 2 (D2) and 3 (D3) are selenoenzymes of the oxidoreductase family which catalyze iodine removal from the outer (D1 and D2) or inner (D1 and D3) ring of thyroid hormones. While D1 and D2 convert T4 to the metabolically active hormone T3, D3 inactivates both T4 and T3 [2]. In humans, D2 is the most important deiodinase for intracellular T3 generation in target tissues [1,2] and, together with D1, contributes for 80% of peripheral T3 [3]. The gene that encodes D2 (*DIO2*) is expressed in the thyroid, pituitary, brain, heart, placenta, skeletal muscle and adipocytes [4,5,6,7,8,9]. D2 activity is tightly regulated at transcriptional, post-transcriptional and post-translational levels [10,11], which thereby supports the hypothesis that this enzyme plays an important homeostatic role in metabolism.

Type 2 diabetes mellitus (T2DM) is a heterogeneous group of disorders usually characterized by varying degrees of insulin insufficiency and insulin resistance (IR), which result in increased blood glucose concentrations. Ultimately, IR results either from inappropriately increased hepatic gluconeogenesis or decreased glucose disposal rate in tissues such as skeletal muscle, adipose tissue and liver [12].

Glucose homeostasis may be affected by thyroid status [13,14]. Thyroid hormone affects insulin action in skeletal muscle and adipose tissue in part by upregulating the expression of the glucose transporter 4 (GLUT4) and, therefore, increasing glucose uptake [15,16]. An increase in both hepatic endogenous glucose disposal and insulin mediated-glucose uptake is observed in patients with hyperthyroidism when compared with euthyroid subjects [17,18,19]. In contrast, studies showed that, in hypothyroidism, there is a decrease in both glucose disposal [19] and insulin mediated-glucose uptake in muscle, and also an impaired ability of insulin to stimulate glucose disposal related to insulinaemia [19,20]. In animal models, experimental induction or spontaneous forms of thyroid dysfunction are also associated with impaired glucose tolerance [20]. Mice with targeted disruption of the *dio2* gene have higher insulin levels during glucose tolerance tests and reduced glucose uptake during insulin tolerance tests, consistent with the occurrence of IR [21]. According to these findings, it is plausible to postulate that a lower intracellular D2-generated T3 in skeletal muscle might create a state of relative intracellular hypothyroidism, decreasing the expression of genes involved in energy use, such as GLUT4, and thus resulting in increased IR.

Previous studies have demonstrated that polymorphisms in the *DIO2* gene might interfere in the phenotypic expression of D2 [7,22]. The *DIO2* single-nucleotide polymorphism (SNP), in which a threonine (Thr) changes to alanine (Ala) at codon 92 (Thr92Ala, rs225014, A/G), was associated with IR in obese white women and with a 20% lower glucose disposal rate in white non-diabetic women [23]. The Ala92Ala genotype was also associated with a more pronounced IR in patients with T2DM and the frequency of this variant allele was found to be increased in some ethnic groups, such as Pima Indians and Mexican-Americans, who have a higher prevalence of IR [23]. Even though some studies have failed to demonstrate an association between the Thr92Ala polymorphism and glycemic traits or T2DM [24,25,26], the association between this polymorphism and T2DM is supported by data reported in a recent systematic review and meta-analysis [27]. However, the mechanism by which this occurs is still not clear. Decreased D2 activity has been observed in human tissue biopsy samples [7,27] but studies failed to identify any changes in the *ex vivo* biochemical properties of the mutant enzyme [7,28], suggesting that this variant might be only a marker for abnormal *DIO2* expression. Here, we aimed to determine whether other SNPs in the *DIO2* gene, individually or in combination with the Thr92Ala polymorphism, contribute to the IR phenotype.

Materials and Methods

Ethics statement

The information obtained during the study did not affect the patients' diagnosis or treatment. The protocol was approved by the Committee on Research Ethics from Hospital de Clínicas de Porto Alegre, and all subjects signed an informed consent term. Clinical investigation was conducted according to the principles expressed in the Declaration of Helsinki.

Study population

In the first phase of this study, we used direct automated sequencing of the *DIO2* gene to search for SNPs in 12 T2DM patients with different degrees of IR. These 12 patients were selected from two subgroups in our T2DM population: 6 patients with a low HOMA-IR index (ranging from 0.32 to 1.3) and 6 patients with a high HOMA-IR index (6.2–23.4). The results generated by sequencing the *DIO2* gene in T2DM patients were compared with the sequences of the human *DIO2* gene available in GenBank (http://www.ncbi.nlm.nih.gov/genbank/).

In the second phase of the study, allele and genotype frequencies of a potentially informative *DIO2* variants found by sequencing were compared between 1077 patients with T2DM and 516 nondiabetic subjects. The criteria used to select the variant for further analysis were: 1) the polymorphism was not known to be a neutral variation; 2) it involved change between chemically different amino acids or was localized at regulatory regions, such as the promoter or 3′- untranslated region (3′UTR); 3) its frequency was not low (minor allele frequency less than 5% in the literature or GenBank); and 4) the frequency of the variant was different in the groups under analysis (in this case, low and high HOMA-IR groups) [29,30]. Additionally, haplotypes constructed from the combination of this polymorphism with the Thr92Ala polymorphism were analyzed regarding their effect on IR in T2DM patients.

The 1077 patients with T2DM were selected from a multicenter study that started recruiting patients in southern Brazil in 2002 and whose purpose was to investigate risk factors for T2DM and its complications. Initially, it included 4 tertiary-teaching hospitals in the Brazilian state of Rio Grande do Sul, namely Grupo Hospitalar Conceição, Hospital São Vicente de Paula, Hospital Universitário de Rio Grande and Hospital de Clínicas de Porto Alegre. The detailed description of that study can be found elsewhere [31]. The group of subjects without diabetes was composed of 516 healthy volunteers who came to Hospital de Clínicas de Porto Alegre to donate blood.

Clinical and anthropometric profiles and laboratory analyses

A standard questionnaire was used to collect information from all patients about age, age at T2DM diagnosis and drug treatment. All patients with T2DM were white. The ethnic group was defined on the basis of self-classification and subjective classification (skin color, nose and lip shapes, hair texture and family history).

All T2DM patients underwent physical and laboratory evaluations. They were weighed (barefoot and wearing light outdoor clothing) and had their height measured. Body mass index (BMI) was calculated as weight (kg) divided by height squared (m^2). Blood pressure (BP) was measured twice, in the sitting position, with a 5-min rest between measurements, using a mercury sphygmomanometer (Korotkoff phases I and V). The mean of the two measurements was used to record systolic and diastolic BP. Arterial hypertension was defined as BP≥140/90 mmHg or use of antihypertensive drugs regardless of BP at the time of assessment.

Serum samples for laboratory tests were collected after a 12-h fast from all patients with T2DM. Glucose levels were determined by a glucose oxidase method; creatinine by the Jaffé reaction; glycated haemoglobin (A1C) by an ion-exchange HPLC procedure (Merck-Hitachi L-9100 glycated haemoglobin analyzer, Merck, Darmstadt, Germany; reference range: 2.7–6.0%); and total plasma cholesterol, HDL-cholesterol, and triglycerides, by enzymatic methods. LDL-cholesterol was calculated using the Friedewald equation. Serum insulin was measured by radioassay (Elecsys Systems 1010/2010/modular analytics E170, Roche Diagnostics, Indianapolis, IN). Insulin sensitivity was estimated by the HOMA-IR index [fasting insulin (milliunits per millilitre) x fasting glucose (millimoles per litre)/22.5] [32]. The mean HOMA-IR index of control subjects in our laboratory was 1.84±1.02 [33].

Molecular analysis

DNA was extracted from peripheral blood leukocytes by a standardized salting-out procedure. A search for variants of the *DIO2* gene was performed in 12 patients with T2DM by direct sequencing of all exons, partial intron sequences (500 bp of exon-intron junctions), and 5′UTR and 3′UTR sequences (1000 bp each, including the selenocysteine insertion sequence element - ESECIS - in the 3′UTR). Screening of this limited number of individuals may fail to detect some rarer polymorphisms; however, this number seems to be adequate to identify representative variants which are sufficiently polymorphic to warrant association studies. Direct sequencing in an automated ABI 3100 *Avant Genetic Analyzer* (Life Technologies, Foster City, CA, USA) was performed using ABI Prism Big Dye Terminator Cycle Sequence Ready reaction kit (Life Technologies) according to the manufacturers' recommendations, and using primers described in **Table S1**.

Potentially informative variants identified through the sequencing of the *DIO2* gene were selected for subsequent genotyping in all patients with T2DM and nondiabetic subjects. These SNPs, together with the rs225014 (Thr92Ala) polymorphism, were determined using primers and probes contained in Human

Custom TaqMan Genotyping Assays 40x (Assays-By-Design Service, Life Technologies). Sequences of primers and probes used for genotyping are shown in **Table S1**. Reactions were conducted in 96-well plates, at a total reaction volume of 5 µL and using 2 ng of genomic DNA, TaqMan Genotyping Master Mix 1x (Life Technologies), and Custom TaqMan Genotyping Assay 1x. Plates were then placed in a real-time PCR thermal cycler (7500 Fast Real-Time PCR System, Life Technologies) and heated for 10 minutes at 95°C, followed by 45 cycles of 95°C for 15 seconds and 62°C for 1 minute. Fluorescence data files of each plate were analyzed using automated allele-calling software (SDS 2.1, Life Technologies).

Statistical analyses

Results are expressed as mean ± SD, % or median (minimum-maximum values). Allelic frequencies were determined by gene counting, and departures from the Hardy-Weinberg equilibrium (HWE) were investigated using chi-squared test. Linkage disequilibrium (LD) between the candidate polymorphism and the Thr92Ala polymorphism was examined using Lewontin's D′ |D′| and r^2 measures [34,35]. Haplotypes constructed from the combination of these *DIO2* polymorphisms and their frequencies were inferred using the Phase 2.1 program, which uses a Bayesian statistical method [35,36]. We also used this program to compare the distributions of *DIO2* haplotypes between patients with T2DM and nondiabetic subjects by permutation analyses of 1,000 random replicates [35].

Clinical and laboratory characteristics were compared using ANOVA, unpaired Student *t* test or chi-squared test, as appropriate. Variables with a skewed distribution were logarithmically transformed before analyses. To check if the candidate polymorphism was independently associated with T2DM, a multiple logistic regression analysis was performed with T2DM as the dependent variable and age, sex, and the possible informative polymorphism as independent variables. A linear regression analysis was performed to evaluate the independent association between the candidate polymorphism and IR parameters after adjusting for covariates (age, sex, BMI and use of T2DM medication). Haplotype interaction between the candidate polymorphism and the Thr92Ala polymorphism in modulating fasting insulin and HOMA-IR index was tested by general linear model univariate analyses (GLM), after adjusting for covariates (age, sex, BMI and use of T2DM medication). In these interaction analyses, each of the polymorphisms was modeled as a dichotomous variable.

All analyses were performed using the SPSS 18.0 (SPSS, Chicago, IL, USA). The level of statistical significance was set at P less than 0.05. Power calculations for the case-control study were done using the software PEPI, version 4.0, and showed that this study has a power of approximately 80% at a significance level of 0.05 to detect an OR of 1.35 or higher (for a 40% frequency of the minor allele).

Results

DIO2 screening and identification of candidate polymorphisms for association with insulin resistance

An interim study comprising samples of 12 patients with T2DM was used to search for polymorphisms in the *DIO2* gene. This first phase study identified 448 amplicons (data not shown). Although no new mutation was detected in the data set, 5 previously described SNPs were identified (**Figure 1**). These SNPs included two polymorphisms in the 5′ flanking region (rs199598135,

A

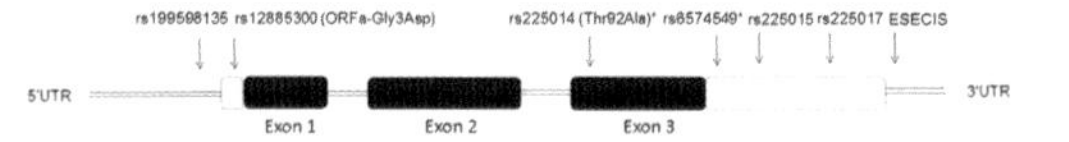

B

Patients	Sex	Age	Candidate Polymorphisms					HOMA-IR index
			rs199598135 (-/T)	rs12885300 (Gly/Asp)*	rs225014 (Thr/Ala)	rs225015 (A/G)	rs225017 (A/T)	
High HOMA-IR index								
#1	M	55	T	Gly	Ala	A	T	23.40
#2	M	78	-	Gly	Ala	A	T	20.09
#3	M	45	-	Gly	Ala	G	T	19.07
#4	F	52	-	Asp	Ala	A	T	7.78
#5	M	38	-	Gly	Thr	A	T	7.54
#6	F	66	-	Gly	Ala	G	T	6.20
Frequency (%)	-	-	1/6 (16)	5/6 (83)	5/6 (83)	4/6 (67)	6/6 (100)	-
Low HOMA-IR index								
#7	F	48	-	Gly	Ala	A	T	1.33
#8	M	64	-	Asp	Thr	A	A	1.22
#9	M	64	-	Gly	Ala	G	T	0.88
#10	M	59	-	Asp	Thr	G	A	0.48
#11	F	67	-	Gly	Thr	A	A	0.46
#12	M	49	-	Asp	Thr	A	A	0.32
Frequency (%)	-	-	0/6 (0)	3/6 (50)	2/6 (33)	4/6 (67)	2/6 (33)	-

Figure 1. Candidate polymorphisms identified by sequencing of the *DIO2* gene. A. The vertical arrows show the five candidate variants in human *DIO2* gene identified through sequencing. Black boxes are coding regions. *polymorphisms associated with T2DM/IR/fasting insulin. ESECIS, Selenocysteine Insertion Sequence Element; 3′UTR = 3′-untranslated region. **B.** The characteristics of the 12 patients with T2DM selected for the screening of the *DIO2* gene. These patients had extreme HOMA-IR indexes and were selected from two subgroups according low or high HOMA-IR values.

rs12885300), one polymorphism in exon 3 (rs225014 - Thr92Ala), and two in the 3′UTR (rs225015, rs225017).

The characteristics of the 12 patients with T2DM selected for the screening of the *DIO2* gene, as well as the occurrence of the 5 *DIO2* polymorphisms identified in these patients are shown in **Figure 1**. We observed that the T/T genotype of the rs225017 (A/T) polymorphism was more frequent in patients with a high HOMA-IR index (6 in 6) than in patients with a low HOMA-IR index (2 in 6). Moreover, the relative frequency of this polymorphism for white subjects in GenBank was 0.36 whereas in our sample was 0.66 (P = 0.129). This polymorphism also fills the criteria for selecting an informative polymorphism (see Material and Methods Section) and was then selected for further analysis in an association study. The Thr92Ala polymorphism also fulfilled the above criteria; however, this polymorphism was already reported in our sample population as being associated with both T2DM risk [27] and increased IR and insulin levels [37]. Thus, in the present study, we aimed to evaluate whether haplotypes constructed from the combination of Thr92Ala polymorphism with the rs225017 polymorphism are associated with IR in T2DM patients.

The rs225017 variant and T2DM development in a case-control study

The baseline characteristics of the 1077 patients with T2DM and the 516 nondiabetic subjects included in the study were as follows: mean age was 59.2±10.1 years *vs.* 46.2±10.3 years (P< 0.001), and males comprised 47% and 63% of the sample (P< 0.001).

The T allele frequency of the rs225017 polymorphism did not differ significantly between patients with T2DM and nondiabetic subjects (0.51 *vs.* 0.48, P = 0.196). In addition, genotypes frequencies of this polymorphism were similar between T2DM patients and nondiabetic subjects (25.9% A/A, 47.2% A/T, 26.9% T/T vs. 28.5% A/A, 46.9% A/T, 24.6% T/T; P = 0.452). These findings did not change after logistic regression analysis adjusting for age and sex (OR = 1.15, 95% CI = 0.86–1.55; P = 0.354). Genotype frequencies of the rs225017 polymorphism were in HWE in patients with T2DM and nondiabetic subjects (P>0.05).

Table 1. Clinical and laboratory characteristics of patients with T2DM broken down according to *DIO2* rs225017 (T/A) polymorphism.

		Genotypes		
	Total (n = 1077)	**A/A or A/T (n = 798)**	**T/T (n = 279)**	**P**
Age (Years)	59.2±10.1	59.6±9.8	58.2±10.3	0.051
Duration of diabetes (Years)	11.7±8.8	12.1±9.0	10.5±7.9	0.009
Sex (% males)	47.0	49.0	42.0	0.038
BMI (kg/m^2)	28.9±4.9	28.8±4.8	29.3±5.3	0.117
Total cholesterol (mmol/l)	5.4±1.2	5.4±1.2	5.5±1.2	0.419
Systolic BP (mm Hg)	141.9±23.2	141.9±23.7	141.8±21.8	0.953
Diastolic BP (mm Hg)	85.0±12.8	84.8±12.7	85.6±13.1	0.823
HDL cholesterol (mmol/l)	1.17±0.3	1.17±0.3	1.16±0,3	0.753
LDL cholesterol (mmol/l)	1.29±1.1	1.29±1.1	1.31±1.1	0.533
Serum creatinine (μmol/l)[a]	102.8 (35.4–937)	81.4 (26.5–937)	79.6 (35.4–540)	0.127
Triglycerides (mmol/l)[a]	2.00 (0.3–13.2)	2.00 (0.3–13.2)	1.99 (0.5–8.7)	0.821
Fasting plasma glucose (mmol/l)	9.4 (2.9–21.9)	9.3 (2.9–21.9)	9.8 (3.3–20.5)	0.144
SU/Met/SU + Met (%)	32.5/38.5/16.5	31.1/36.0/14.3	34.8/45.9/22.9	0.249/0.027/0.015
A1C (%)	7.2±2.0	7.1±2.0	7.3±1.8	0.343
Fasting insulin (UI/ml)[a,b]	13.9 (1–46.1)	10.6 (1–44.9)	15.7 (3.2–46.1)	0.005
HOMA–IR index[a,b]	3.8 (0.3–20.1)	3.5 (0.3–19.5)	5.2 (0.6–20.1)	0.005

Data are mean ± SD, median (minimum - maximum values) or %. A1C, glycated haemoglobin; BMI, body mass index; HOMA-IR, homeostasis model assessment - insulin resistance; Met, metformin; SU, sulfonylureas; WHR, waist-to-hip ratio; P values were estimated by χ^2 or ANOVA, as appropriate.
[a]Variables which were logarithmically transformed before analyses.
[b]For comparisons of fasting insulin levels and HOMA-IR index among rs225017 genotypes, we analyzed only 227 individuals (162 individuals harboring the A/A or A/T genotypes and 65 individuals harboring the T/T genotype).

The rs225017 DIO2 polymorphism is associated with insulin resistance in patients with T2DM

Table 1 summarizes the clinical and laboratory characteristics of patients with T2DM grouped according to the different genotypes of the rs225017 polymorphism. Assuming a recessive model of inheritance, patients with A/A or A/T genotypes were grouped and compared with patients carrying the T/T genotype. T2DM duration (P = 0.009), sex proportion (P = 0.038) and use of metformin alone (P = 0.027) or metformin + sulfonylurea (P = 0.015) for treatment of T2DM were differentially distributed between patients with the T/T genotype and A allele carriers. It is worth mentioning that none of the variables showed in **Table 1** attained statistical significance when assuming dominant (A/A *vs.* A/T-T/T) or additive (A/A *vs.* T/T) models of inheritance (data not shown).

A subgroup of 227 patients with T2DM who were not receiving insulin was further analyzed for IR measurements. This subgroup was representative of the whole sample: mean age was 59.3±9.3 years (P = 0.803 for the comparison with the whole sample), mean T2DM duration was 11.2±8.2 years (P = 0.580), mean A1C was 7.3±1.7% (P = 0.12), and mean BMI was 28.9±4.7 kg/m^2 (P = 0.89). Males comprised 45.3% (n = 103) of the sample (P = 0.45).

In this subgroup of patients, median fasting plasma insulin levels were higher in patients with the T/T genotype than in patients carrying the A allele [15.71 (3.2–46.1) *vs.* 10.57 (1–44.9), P = 0.005], whereas fasting plasma glucose levels did not differ significantly between groups (P = 0.144). Moreover, T/T genotype patients showed a higher HOMA-IR index than patients carrying the A allele [5.20 (0.6–20.1) *vs.* 3.50 (0.3–19.5), P = 0.005]. Because insulin sensitivity is known to be affected by multiple independent factors, multiple linear regression analyses were performed with HOMA-IR index ($\log_{10}$ HOMA-IR) or insulin level ($\log_{10}$ fasting insulin) as dependent variables. The T/T genotype of the rs225017 polymorphism remained significantly associated with HOMA-IR [standardized coefficient B for T/T genotype = −0.366, 95% CI (−0.654 −0.078); P = 0.013] and insulin levels [standardized coefficient B for T/T genotype = −0.268, 95% CI (−0.441 −0.096); P = 0.002], after adjusting for age, sex, BMI and use of medication for T2DM (mainly metformin or sulfonylureas).

Association of the DIO2 rs225017 and Thr92Ala variants with insulin resistance

We used a Bayesian statistical method to estimate the frequencies of different haplotypes produced by the combination of the rs225017 and Thr92Ala polymorphisms in patients with T2DM. The first letter of the haplotypes refers to the Thr92Ala polymorphism, and the second, to the rs225017 polymorphism. The wild type haplotype (Thr/A) was observed in 49.0% of the sample, the Thr/T haplotype was observed in 18.0%, the Ala/A haplotype in 4.0%, and the Ala/T haplotype (double mutated) in 29.0% of the sample.

Taking these results into account, we tested whether any haplotype constituted by the rs225017 and Thr92Ala polymorphisms might affect fasting plasma insulin levels or HOMA-IR index differently as compared with the effect of each polymorphism analyzed separately. To test this hypothesis, we performed GLM analyses using fasting insulin levels or the HOMA-IR index as the dependent variable, and age, sex, BMI, use of medication for T2DM and the polymorphic combinations of the two *DIO2* variants as independent variables. These interaction analyses are

Table 2. Interaction analyses between the *DIO2* rs225017 (T/A) and rs225014 (Thr92Ala) polymorphisms according to fasting plasma insulin and HOMA-IR index.

	rs225017						
	A/X			T/T			
Thr92Ala	Thr/X (n = 138)	Ala/Ala (n = 14)	P[a]	Thr/X (n = 35)	Ala/Ala (n = 30)	P[a]	F; P[b]
Age (years)	59.7±9.9	57.2±10.5	0.177	58.2±10.6	58.1±10.0	0.941	-
Sex (% males)	49.0	42.0	0.439	39.0	49.0	0.417	-
BMI (kg/m^2)	28.8±4.9	28.6±4.5	0.865	29.4±5.5	29.3±5.1	0.959	-
SU/Met/SU + Met (%)	31.3/35.6/14.0	28.6/50.0/14.0	0.830/0.270/0.997	35.3/51.5/22.0	34.3/40.3/24.0	0.907/0.196/0.803	-
Fasting insulin (UI/ml)[c,d]	10.8 (1–44.9)	8.6 (4.0–39.0)	0.794	11.9 (4.5–44.6)	16.8 (3.2–46.1)	0.011	11.072; 0.001
HOMA-IR index[c,e]	3.5 (0.3–19.5)	2.8 (1.6–13.6)	0.916	3.9 (0.6–13.5)	6.1 (0.9–20.1)	0.034	4.740; 0.010

Data are mean ± SD, median (minimum - maximum values) or %. BMI, body mass index; HOMA-IR, homeostasis model assessment - insulin resistance; Met, metformin; SU, sulfonylureas.
[a]Data were analyzed using the Student *t* test or χ^2, as appropriate.
[b]F and P values obtained from the general linear model-interaction analyses, after adjusting for age, sex, BMI and use of medication for T2DM.
[c]Variables which were logarithmically transformed before analyses.
[d]Adjusted R squared for fasting plasma insulin = 0.135.
[e]Adjusted R squared for HOMA-IR = 0.111.

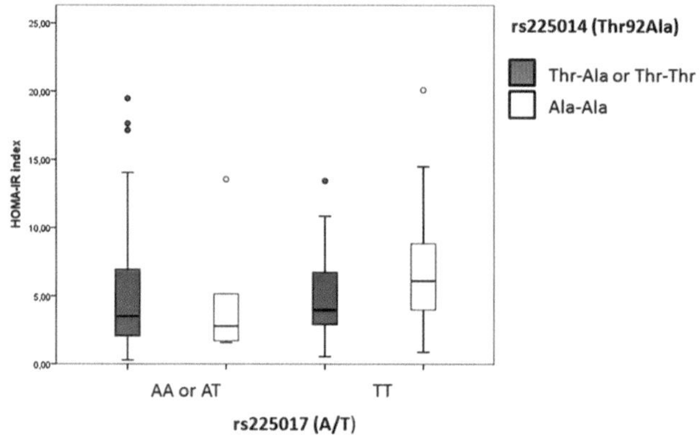

Figure 2. Possible interaction between rs225017 and Thr92Ala variants in modulation of insulin resistance. HOMA-IR indexes in T2DM patients according to different genotypes of *DIO2* rs225017 (A/T) and rs225014 (Thr92Ala) polymorphisms. Results are expressed as median (percentiles 25% and 75%). Circles represent outlier values. Interaction P value = 0.010, adjusted for age, sex, BMI, and use of medication for T2DM.

shown in **Table 2**. Patients carrying the Ala/Ala – T/T haplotype showed higher fasting insulin values than patients with other genotype combinations, adjusting for covariables (F = 11.072, P = 0.001). Likewise, patients carrying the Ala/Ala – T/T haplotype showed a higher HOMA-IR index than patients with other genotype combinations (F = 4.740; P = 0.010) (**Figure 2**).

To determine whether the rs225017 (A/T) and rs225014 (Thr92Ala) polymorphisms were in LD in T2DM patients, we used Lewontin's |D′| and r^2 measures. The analysis showed that the rs225017 polymorphism was in partial LD with the rs225014 polymorphism (|D′| = 0.811; r^2 = 0.365). These results were confirmed in the HAPMAP Project (http://hapmap.ncbi.nlm.nih.gov/).

Discussion

Insulin resistance is a heterogeneous disorder influenced by multiple environmental and genetic factors [38,39,40]. Previous studies indicate that the Thr92Ala polymorphism in the *DIO2* gene is involved in IR pathogenesis [7,23,37]. Even though the Ala/Ala genotype was associated with lower D2 activity in thyroid biopsy samples, *in vitro* studies did not show any change in the biochemical properties of the mutated enzyme, suggesting that this SNP might be only a polymorphic marker [7]. Therefore, here we searched for other informative SNPs in the *DIO2* gene which might be associated with IR or T2DM. We report a new *DIO2* polymorphism associated with increased IR in T2DM patients. Homozygosis for the allele T of the rs225017 (A/T) polymorphism was associated with IR in patients with T2DM, whereas patients carrying a combination of the T/T genotype of the rs225017 polymorphism and the Ala/Ala genotype of the Thr92Ala polymorphism showed an increased HOMA-IR index as compared with patients with other genotype combinations, suggesting that they might interact in the modulation of IR.

The rs205017 (A/T) polymorphism is located at the 3′UTR of the *DIO2* gene. In selenoenzymes, the 3′UTR contains the selenocysteine insertion sequence (SECIS), which is very important for looping formation in the mechanism of cis-acting mRNA structure of selenocysteine insertion [41,42]. The 3′UTR is also the main site for ligation of microRNAs (miRNAs) that can function as translational repressors or triggers of transcript degradation by partially pairing to this region in target mRNAs [43]. Currently, it is universally recognized that miRNAs are major regulators of gene expression and key controllers of several biologic and pathologic processes, as such those involved in the T2DM pathogenesis [44]. Hence, it is reasonable to speculate that the rs205017 polymorphism could be involved in a ligation site for a given miRNA, decreasing the *DIO2* expression. Therefore, we used the TargetScan software to look for potential miRNA targets in the *DIO2* gene [45]. Six predicted interaction regions with miRNA families were found in the *DIO2* sequence: miR-9, miR-29abcd, miR-30abcdef, miR-193, miR-203 and miR-216a. Interestingly, miR-9, miR-29 and miR-30 seem to have a role in insulin resistance [44,46]. Although the rs225017 SNP is not located at any of these miRNA regions, it is close to some of them and, therefore, we could not rule out a potential effect of this SNP on *DIO2* gene expression. Alternatively, it could be obstructing the mechanism of selenocysteine insertion and, thereby, reducing the amount of D2 available for the activation of T3. In this context, polymorphic D2, generated from the Ala/T haplotype sequence, might generate less T3 in skeletal muscle and adipocytes, which, consequently, may create a local state of intracellular hypothyroidism, decreasing the expression of genes involved in metabolism, such as GLUT4, and leading to IR.

Recently, the *DIO2* rs6574549 polymorphism, also located at the 3′UTR, was associated with elevated fasting insulin levels and higher insulin action, but not with T2DM in Pima Indians [47]. This polymorphism may also be a candidate for the functional variant associated with IR. The rs6574549 polymorphism is in strong LD with the Thr92Ala [47] and rs205017 [48] polymorphisms (LD>0.8; HAPMAP Project, http://hapmap.ncbi.nlm.nih.gov/). Therefore, further studies are necessary to determine: 1) which polymorphism is the functional variant interacting with the Thr92Ala polymorphism in the modulation of IR; 2) whether there is another functional polymorphism in the *DIO2* gene yet to be identified; and 3) whether these polymorphisms have combined effects on D2 function. The results presented here add to the understanding of the molecular interactions controlling IR and might partially explain the association with the Thr92Ala polymorphism.

Some factors unrelated to the rs205017 and Thr92Ala polymorphisms may have interfered with the findings of the present study. First, medications for T2DM treatment may have played a role because some are known to affect insulin sensitivity. However, we minimized such possibility by excluding insulin-treated patients from the group of 227 patients analyzed for IR. Furthermore, the rs205017 variant and the Ala/Ala-T/T haplotype remained independently associated with the HOMA-IR index and plasma insulin levels after adjusting for medications for T2DM, including metformin and sulfonylurea. In addition, none of the patients were using thiazolidinediones, agents that change insulin sensitivity. Second, IR was assessed by calculation of the HOMA-IR index rather than by the reference method, the euglycaemic-hyperinsulinemic clamp [32,49,50]. Although the HOMA-IR index is only an approximate estimate of IR, it is simple to calculate and shows a good correlation with the reference method [32,49]; therefore, it is a good approach for cohort and epidemiological studies [50]. Third, we cannot rule out the possibility of stratification bias in our sample, although we studied only self-defined white subjects and thus reduced the risk of false positive or false negative associations due to this bias. In addition, the 227 patients with T2DM analyzed for IR were representative of the whole sample (n = 1077) with respect to age, T2DM duration, A1c, sex, BMI and presence of arterial hypertension. The frequencies of the rs205017 and Thr92Ala polymorphisms were also similar between these 227 patients and the whole T2DM sample (data not shown). Fourth, screening only 12 patients with T2DM for the occurrence of *DIO2* polymorphisms might have failed to detect rare polymorphisms [49]; however, this number was enough to detect most representative variants, which are sufficiently polymorphic to warrant association studies. Finally, our results might represent a type 1 error, but the scientific plausibility of the reported association provides evidence against it.

In summary, the *DIO2* rs225017 (A/T) polymorphism is a new polymorphism associated with IR in white patients with T2DM, and it seems to interact with the Thr92Ala polymorphism in the modulation of this characteristic. Further studies are needed to evaluate the functional and epidemiological importance of the rs205017 polymorphism in IR and T2DM.

Author Contributions

Conceived and designed the experiments: LBL AAFE DC ALM. Performed the experiments: LBL AAFE SMW. Analyzed the data: LBL JMD SMW AAFE DC ALM. Contributed reagents/materials/analysis tools: DC ALM. Wrote the paper: LBL DC ALM.

References

1. Yen PM (2001) Physiological and molecular basis of thyroid hormone action. Physiol Rev 81: 1097–1142.
2. Maia AL, Goemann IM, Meyer EL, Wajner SM (2011) Deiodinases: the balance of thyroid hormone: type 1 iodothyronine deiodinase in human physiology and disease. J Endocrinol 209: 283–297.
3. Maia AL, Kim BW, Huang SA, Harney JW, Larsen PR (2005) Type 2 iodothyronine deiodinase is the major source of plasma T3 in euthyroid humans. J Clin Invest 115: 2524–2533.
4. Croteau W, Davey JC, Galton VA, St Germain DL (1996) Cloning of the mammalian type II iodothyronine deiodinase. A selenoprotein differentially expressed and regulated in human and rat brain and other tissues. J Clin Invest 98: 405–417.
5. Itagaki Y, Yoshida K, Ikeda H, Kaise K, Kaise N, et al. (1990) Thyroxine 5′-deiodinase in human anterior pituitary tumors. J Clin Endocrinol Metab 71: 340–344.
6. Salvatore D, Tu H, Harney JW, Larsen PR (1996) Type 2 iodothyronine deiodinase is highly expressed in human thyroid. J Clin Invest 98: 962–968.
7. Canani LH, Capp C, Dora JM, Meyer EL, Wagner MS, et al. (2005) The type 2 deiodinase A/G (Thr92Ala) polymorphism is associated with decreased enzyme velocity and increased insulin resistance in patients with type 2 diabetes mellitus. J Clin Endocrinol Metab 90: 3472–3478.
8. Grozovsky R, Ribich S, Rosene ML, Mulcahey MA, Huang SA, et al. (2009) Type 2 deiodinase expression is induced by peroxisomal proliferator-activated receptor-gamma agonists in skeletal myocytes. Endocrinology 150: 1976–1983.
9. Heemstra KA, Soeters MR, Fliers E, Serlie MJ, Burggraaf J, et al. (2009) Type 2 iodothyronine deiodinase in skeletal muscle: effects of hypothyroidism and fasting. J Clin Endocrinol Metab 94: 2144–2150.
10. Steinsapir J, Bianco AC, Buettner C, Harney J, Larsen PR (2000) Substrate-induced down-regulation of human type 2 deiodinase (hD2) is mediated through proteasomal degradation and requires interaction with the enzyme's active center. Endocrinology 141: 1127–1135.
11. Gereben B, Goncalves C, Harney JW, Larsen PR, Bianco AC (2000) Selective proteolysis of human type 2 deiodinase: a novel ubiquitin-proteasomal mediated mechanism for regulation of hormone activation. Mol Endocrinol 14: 1697–1708.
12. Frojdo S, Vidal H, Pirola L (2009) Alterations of insulin signaling in type 2 diabetes: a review of the current evidence from humans. Biochim Biophys Acta 1792: 83–92.

13. Chidakel A, Mentuccia D, Celi FS (2005) Peripheral metabolism of thyroid hormone and glucose homeostasis. Thyroid 15: 899–903.
14. Kim SR, Tull ES, Talbott EO, Vogt MT, Kuller LH (2002) A hypothesis of synergism: the interrelationship of T3 and insulin to disturbances in metabolic homeostasis. Med Hypotheses 59: 660–666.
15. Weinstein SP, O'Boyle E, Haber RS (1994) Thyroid hormone increases basal and insulin-stimulated glucose transport in skeletal muscle. The role of GLUT4 glucose transporter expression. Diabetes 43: 1185–1189.
16. Torrance CJ, Devente JE, Jones JP, Dohm GL (1997) Effects of thyroid hormone on GLUT4 glucose transporter gene expression and NIDDM in rats. Endocrinology 138: 1204–1214.
17. Dimitriadis G, Baker B, Marsh H, Mandarino L, Rizza R, et al. (1985) Effect of thyroid hormone excess on action, secretion, and metabolism of insulin in humans. Am J Physiol 248: E593–601.
18. Dimitriadis G, Maratou E, Alevizaki M, Boutati E, Psara K, et al. (2005) Thyroid hormone excess increases basal and insulin-stimulated recruitment of GLUT3 glucose transporters on cell surface. Horm Metab Res 37: 15–20.
19. Rochon C, Tauveron I, Dejax C, Benoit P, Capitan P, et al. (2003) Response of glucose disposal to hyperinsulinaemia in human hypothyroidism and hyperthyroidism. Clin Sci (Lond) 104: 7–15.
20. Dubaniewicz A, Kaciuba-Uscilko H, Nazar K, Budohoski L (1989) Sensitivity of the soleus muscle to insulin in resting and exercising rats with experimental hypo- and hyper-thyroidism. Biochem J 263: 243–247.
21. Marsili A, Aguayo-Mazzucato C, Chen T, Kumar A, Chung M, et al. (2011) Mice with a targeted deletion of the type 2 deiodinase are insulin resistant and susceptible to diet induced obesity. PLoS One 6: e20832.
22. Coppotelli G, Summers A, Chidakel A, Ross JM, Celi FS (2006) Functional characterization of the 258 A/G (D2-ORFa-Gly3Asp) human type-2 deiodinase polymorphism: a naturally occurring variant increases the enzymatic activity by removing a putative repressor site in the 5′ UTR of the gene. Thyroid 16: 625–632.
23. Mentuccia D, Proietti-Pannunzi L, Tanner K, Bacci V, Pollin TI, et al. (2002) Association between a novel variant of the human type 2 deiodinase gene Thr92Ala and insulin resistance: evidence of interaction with the Trp64Arg variant of the beta-3-adrenergic receptor. Diabetes 51: 880–883.
24. Maia AL, Dupuis J, Manning A, Liu C, Meigs JB, et al. (2007) The type 2 deiodinase (DIO2) A/G polymorphism is not associated with glycemic traits: the Framingham Heart Study. Thyroid 17: 199–202.
25. Mentuccia D, Thomas MJ, Coppotelli G, Reinhart LJ, Mitchell BD, et al. (2005) The Thr92Ala deiodinase type 2 (DIO2) variant is not associated with type 2 diabetes or indices of insulin resistance in the old order of Amish. Thyroid 15: 1223–1227.
26. Grarup N, Andersen MK, Andreasen CH, Albrechtsen A, Borch-Johnsen K, et al. (2007) Studies of the common DIO2 Thr92Ala polymorphism and metabolic phenotypes in 7342 Danish white subjects. J Clin Endocrinol Metab 92: 363–366.
27. Dora JM, Machado WE, Rheinheimer J, Crispim D, Maia AL (2010) Association of the type 2 deiodinase Thr92Ala polymorphism with type 2 diabetes: case-control study and meta-analysis. Eur J Endocrinol 163: 427–434.
28. Peeters RP, van Toor H, Klootwijk W, de Rijke YB, Kuiper GG, et al. (2003) Polymorphisms in thyroid hormone pathway genes are associated with plasma TSH and iodothyronine levels in healthy subjects. J Clin Endocrinol Metab 88: 2880–2888.
29. Adams DR, Sincan M, Fuentes Fajardo K, Mullikin JC, Pierson TM, et al. (2011) Analysis of DNA sequence variants detected by high-throughput sequencing. Hum Mutat 33: 599–608.
30. Cooper DN, Chen JM, Ball EV, Howells K, Mort M, et al. (2010) Genes, mutations, and human inherited disease at the dawn of the age of personalized genomics. Hum Mutat 31: 631–655.
31. Canani LH, Costa LA, Crispim D, Goncalves Dos Santos K, Roisenberg I, et al. (2005) The presence of allele D of angiotensin-converting enzyme polymorphism is associated with diabetic nephropathy in patients with less than 10 years duration of Type 2 diabetes. Diabet Med 22: 1167–1172.
32. Bonora E, Targher G, Alberiche M, Bonadonna RC, Saggiani F, et al. (2000) Homeostasis model assessment closely mirrors the glucose clamp technique in the assessment of insulin sensitivity: studies in subjects with various degrees of glucose tolerance and insulin sensitivity. Diabetes Care 23: 57–63.
33. Seligman BG, Biolo A, Polanczyk CA, Gross JL, Clausell N (2000) Increased plasma levels of endothelin 1 and von Willebrand factor in patients with type 2 diabetes and dyslipidemia. Diabetes Care 23: 1395–1400.
34. Hedrick PW (1987) Gametic disequilibrium measures: proceed with caution. Genetics 117: 331–341.
35. Barrett JC, Fry B, Maller J, Daly MJ (2005) Haploview: analysis and visualization of LD and haplotype maps. Bioinformatics 21: 263–265.
36. Stephens M, Smith NJ, Donnelly P (2001) A new statistical method for haplotype reconstruction from population data. Am J Hum Genet 68: 978–989.
37. Estivalet AA, Leiria LB, Dora JM, Rheinheimer J, Boucas AP, et al. (2010) D2 Thr92Ala and PPARgamma2 Pro12Ala polymorphisms interact in the modulation of insulin resistance in type 2 diabetic patients. Obesity (Silver Spring) 19: 825–832.
38. Irvin MR, Wineinger NE, Rice TK, Pajewski NM, Kabagambe EK, et al. (2011) Genome-wide detection of allele specific copy number variation associated with insulin resistance in African Americans from the HyperGEN study. PLoS One 6: e24052.
39. North KE, Williams K, Williams JT, Best LG, Lee ET, et al. (2003) Evidence for genetic factors underlying the insulin resistance syndrome in american indians. Obes Res 11: 1444–1448.
40. North KE, Almasy L, Goring HH, Cole SA, Diego VP, et al. (2005) Linkage analysis of factors underlying insulin resistance: Strong Heart Family Study. Obes Res 13: 1877–1884.
41. Mix H, Lobanov AV, Gladyshev VN (2007) SECIS elements in the coding regions of selenoprotein transcripts are functional in higher eukaryotes. Nucleic Acids Res 35: 414–423.
42. Ryan K, Bauer DL (2008) Finishing touches: post-translational modification of protein factors involved in mammalian pre-mRNA 3′ end formation. Int J Biochem Cell Biol 40: 2384–2396.
43. Ambros V (2004) The functions of animal microRNAs. Nature 431: 350–355.
44. Guay C, Regazzi R (2013) Circulating microRNAs as novel biomarkers for diabetes mellitus. Nat Rev Endocrinol 9: 513–521.
45. Lewis BP, Burge CB, Bartel DP (2005) Conserved seed pairing, often flanked by adenosines, indicates that thousands of human genes are microRNA targets. Cell 120: 15–20.
46. Guay C, Roggli E, Nesca V, Jacovetti C, Regazzi R (2011) Diabetes mellitus, a microRNA-related disease? Transl Res 157: 253–264.
47. Nair S, Muller YL, Ortega E, Kobes S, Bogardus C, et al. (2012) Association analyses of variants in the DIO2 gene with early-onset type 2 diabetes mellitus in Pima Indians. Thyroid 22: 80–87.
48. Altshuler DM, Gibbs RA, Peltonen L, Altshuler DM, Gibbs RA, et al. (2010) Integrating common and rare genetic variation in diverse human populations. Nature 467: 52–58.
49. Emoto M, Nishizawa Y, Maekawa K, Hiura Y, Kanda H, et al. (1999) Homeostasis model assessment as a clinical index of insulin resistance in type 2 diabetic patients treated with sulfonylureas. Diabetes Care 22: 818–822.
50. Wallace TM, Levy JC, Matthews DR (2004) Use and abuse of HOMA modeling. Diabetes Care 27: 1487–1495.

13

Characterising the Inhibitory Actions of Ceramide upon Insulin Signaling in Different Skeletal Muscle Cell Models

Rana Mahfouz[1,2,3], Rhéa Khoury[1,2,3], Agnieszka Blachnio-Zabielska[4], Sophie Turban[5], Nicolas Loiseau[6], Christopher Lipina[5], Clare Stretton[5], Olivier Bourron[1,2,3,7], Pascal Ferré[1,2,3], Fabienne Foufelle[1,2,3], Harinder S. Hundal[5], Eric Hajduch[1,2,3]*

1 INSERM, UMR-S 1138, Centre de Recherche des Cordeliers, Paris, France, **2** Université Pierre et Marie Curie – Paris 6, UMR-S 1138, Paris, France, **3** Université Paris Descartes, UMR-S 1138, Paris, France, **4** Department of Physiology, Medical University of Bialystok, Bialystok, Poland, **5** Division of Cell Signalling and Immunology, College of Life Sciences, University of Dundee, Dundee, United Kingdom, **6** INRA, UMR1331 Toxalim, Research Centre in Food Toxicology, Toulouse, France, **7** Département de Diabétologie et Maladies métaboliques, AP-HP, Hôpital Pitié-Salpêtrière, Paris, France

Abstract

Ceramides are known to promote insulin resistance in a number of metabolically important tissues including skeletal muscle, the predominant site of insulin-stimulated glucose disposal. Depending on cell type, these lipid intermediates have been shown to inhibit protein kinase B (PKB/Akt), a key mediator of the metabolic actions of insulin, via two distinct pathways: one involving the action of atypical protein kinase C (aPKC) isoforms, and the second dependent on protein phosphatase-2A (PP2A). The main aim of this study was to explore the mechanisms by which ceramide inhibits PKB/Akt in three different skeletal muscle-derived cell culture models; rat L6 myotubes, mouse C2C12 myotubes and primary human skeletal muscle cells. Our findings indicate that the mechanism by which ceramide acts to repress PKB/Akt is related to the myocellular abundance of caveolin-enriched domains (CEM) present at the plasma membrane. Here, we show that ceramide-enriched-CEMs are markedly more abundant in L6 myotubes compared to C2C12 myotubes, consistent with their previously reported role in coordinating aPKC-directed repression of PKB/Akt in L6 muscle cells. In contrast, a PP2A-dependent pathway predominantly mediates ceramide-induced inhibition of PKB/Akt in C2C12 myotubes. In addition, we demonstrate for the first time that ceramide engages an aPKC-dependent pathway to suppress insulin-induced PKB/Akt activation in palmitate-treated cultured human muscle cells as well as in muscle cells from diabetic patients. Collectively, this work identifies key mechanistic differences, which may be linked to variations in plasma membrane composition, underlying the insulin-desensitising effects of ceramide in different skeletal muscle cell models that are extensively used in signal transduction and metabolic studies.

Editor: Cedric Moro, INSERM/UMR 1048, France

Funding: This work was supported by INSERM, the Société Francophone du Diabète (ANTADIR grant), from an Agence Nationale de la Recherche (ANR) project (ANR 11 BSV1 03101-Crisalis), and from the Fondation pour Recherche Médicale (Equipe FRM DEQ20140329504). The funders had no role in study design, data collection and analysis, decision to publish, or preparation of the manuscript.

Competing Interests: The authors have declared that no competing interests exist.

* Email: eric.hajduch@crc.jussieu.fr

Introduction

Once bound to its receptor, insulin stimulates a signalling network that functions to regulate whole-body glucose homeostasis by coordinating numerous physiological processes. Defects in the activation of insulin-induced signalling cascades are often associated with insulin resistance, a characteristic feature of obesity and type 2 diabetes [1]. The mechanisms by which insulin resistance develops are not yet fully understood but recent work has shown that forcing cells to accumulate fatty acids beyond their storage capacity may lead to insulin desensitisation through the generation of toxic lipid intermediates such as ceramide [2,3].

Skeletal muscle is the major tissue responsible for insulin-stimulated glucose disposal and therefore considered as a primary target in the onset of insulin resistance. Various studies have suggested that ectopic accumulation of ceramide in response to oversupply of saturated fatty acids including palmitate may underlie the development of insulin resistance in this tissue [4–6].

Indeed, we and others have demonstrated that ceramide can impair insulin action through inhibition of protein kinase B (PKB/Akt), a key signal transduction intermediate that plays a pivotal role in coordinating the insulin-dependent uptake and utilization of glucose [7,8]. Two skeletal muscle cell lines that have been extensively used to study the deleterious effects of ceramide upon insulin action are rat L6 and mouse C2C12 muscle cells. In differentiated rat L6 myotubes, treatment with palmitate or exogenous ceramide leads to the activation of the atypical protein kinase C isoform PKCζ which in turn directly interacts with and phosphorylates the pleckstrin homolog (PH) domain of PKB/Akt at Thr34. As a result of this interaction, PKB/Akt becomes sequestered into specialized domains of the plasma membrane known as caveolin-enriched microdomains (CEM) thereby preventing its recruitment to PIP3-enriched regions where it is normally activated in response to insulin [9–11]. In contrast, whilst exposure of C2C12 myotubes to palmitate has also been shown to result in the activation of aPKCζ, PKB/Akt becomes repressed primarily through its dephosphorylation by protein phosphatase 2A (PP2A) [12].

In this study, we set out to explore this differential mode of inhibition by ceramide upon insulin signalling in L6 and C2C12 myotubes. Importantly, we previously reported that in cells which lack CEM (e.g. fibroblasts), ceramide does not inhibit PKB/Akt through the "PKCζ-CEM" pathway, but rather through activation of PP2A [11]. This is in contrast to cells with abundant CEM (e.g. 3T3-L1 adipocytes) wherein ceramide acts to repress PKB/Akt via the PKCζ-CEM pathway [11]. We therefore hypothesised that variations in CEM content between these different muscle cell lines may account for the distinct signalling pathways utilised by ceramide to impair insulin action. Herein, we demonstrate that whilst ceramide impairs insulin-stimulated PKB/Akt activation *via* the 'PKCζ-CEM' pathway in L6 myotubes, this same lipid intermediate does so *via* a PP2A-dependent mechanism in C2C12 myotubes which exhibit a lower CEM content relative to L6 myotubes.

In addition, little is known about the functional mechanism(s) responsible for conveying the insulin desensitising effects of ceramide in human skeletal muscle. Therefore, we explored the potential involvement of the 'PKCζ-CEM' and PP2A pathways in primary cultured human muscle cells, which represent a good model for studying human skeletal muscle function [13] and can be modulated *ex vivo* [13]. We show that similar to L6 myotubes, it is the "PKCζ-CEM" pathway which predominantly mediates the repressive effects of ceramide upon PKB/Akt in human muscle cells.

Methods

Materials

All reagent-grade chemicals, insulin, palmitate, and BSA were purchased from Sigma-Aldrich. C_2-ceramide was obtained from Cayman Chemical Company. Complete protein phosphatase inhibitor tablets were obtained from Boehringer-Roche Diagnostics. Antibodies against native PKB/Akt, Ser473-PKB/Akt and $^{21/9}$Ser GSK3α/β were from Cell Signalling (New England Biolabs), caveolin-3, PKCζ, PP2A and hemagglutinin from Santa Cruz Biotechnology and β-actin from Sigma-Aldrich. Horseradish peroxidase anti-rabbit, -mouse and -sheep/goat IgGs were from Jackson ImmunoResearch Laboratories and the enhanced chemiluminescent substrate was from Pierce-Perbio Biotechnology.

Cell culture

L6 muscle cells were grown as a monolayer as described previously [14] to the stage of myotubes in α-minimum essential medium containing 2% fetal calf serum and 1% antimicotic/antibiotic solution. C2C12 myoblasts were maintained in Dulbecco's modified Eagle's medium (Gibco) containing 10%(v/v) fetal bovine serum. For differentiation into myotubes, the myoblasts were grown to confluence and the media were replaced with DMEM containing 2% horse serum. Both cell lines were maintained at 37°C in a humidified atmosphere of 5% CO_2, 95% air. Myotubes were used for experiments 4 days following differentiation.

Human skeletal muscle cells

Biopsies from healthy adult lean volunteers were obtained in the context of approved preclinical and clinical trials [15], and *via* the Tissue Bank for Research (Myobank) of the French Association against Myopathies (AFM), in agreement with the French bioethical law (law no 94–654 of 29 July 1994, modified 22 January 2002) on informed consent. Muscle samples from three adult type 2 diabetic patients were obtained from healthy tissue after leg amputation. Donors had no clinical signs of muscular disease and sampled tissues had no bacterial contamination. No clinical and biological infection has been observed (ultra-sensitive C reactive protein at 6.6+/−2.6 mg/L). At baseline, HbA1c and fasting glycaemia of type 2 diabetic patients were respectively 7.9+/−0.31% and 7.59+/−0.44 mmoles/L. Fresh muscle samples were minced and enzymatically dissociated with collagenase. Myoblasts were purified, grown and differentiated as myotubes as previously described [16].

Preparation of whole cell lysates

Cells were lysed following experimental manipulation (see figure legends) in an appropriate volume of lysis buffer [14].

Preparation of detergent-resistant membranes (DRM)

DRM were prepared as described previously [10]. Cells were homogenized into 25 mM MES (2-[N-Morpholino]ethanesulfonic acid), pH 6.0, 150 mM NaCl, 1% (w/v) Triton X-100, complete inhibitor tablet and lysate ran on a sucrose gradient. The gradient was centrifuged at 120,000 *g* for 20 h at 4°C. DRM fractions were then collected and frozen at −20°C until required.

DRM-containing ceramide quantification

700 μL of each DRM fraction were freeze-dried and subsequently extracted once with chloroform/methanol (C/M) (2:1), once with C/M (1:1) and once with C/M (1:2). The combined C/M extracts were freeze dried and solubilized in 2 mL of C/M (1:1) with 3M of potassium hydroxide. The solution is incubated overnight at 50°C. 800 μL of distilled water (W) is added. The solution is neutralized using hydrochloric acid 1N. Organic extract was washed twice with C/M/W (3:48:47), dried under nitrogen and dissolved in 50 μL of C/M (1:1) before analysis. High Performance Thin Layer Chromatography (HPTLC) analyses were performed with a multistep development. A first development was realized with the solvent system Hexane/diethyl ether/acetic acid (30:15:0.5) until a developing distance of 80 mm (from the lower edge of the plate). The second and third development was realized with the solvent system C/M/W (40:10:1) until the respective developing distance of 30 mm and 50 mm. The fourth development was realized with the solvent system C/M/acetic acid (47:2:0.5) until a developing distance of 80 mm. And the last development was realized with the solvent system Hexane/diethyl ether/acetic acid (30:15:0.5) until a developing distance of 80 mm. After each development the plate was dried 5 minutes. Bands were detected after immersion in a charring solution and drying at 250°C during 1 minute. Quantification was realized by densitometry with CAMAG TLC scanner 4 and winCATS software in absorption mode at 560 nm using a tungsten lamp.

Analysis of sphingolipid content

Sphingolipids were extracted an assessed as described previously [17].

Glucose transport

Human myotubes were washed rapidly with HEPES-buffered saline (HBS; 20 mM HEPES-Na (pH 7.4), 140 mM NaCl, 2.5 mM $MgSO_4$, 5 mM KCl, 1 mM $CaCl_2$), and glucose uptake was assayed by incubating cells with 10 μM 2-deoxy-[3H]-D-glucose (1 μCi/ml, 26.2 Ci/mmol) for 15 min in HBS. Carrier-mediated uptake was determined by quantitating cell-associated radioactivity in the presence of 10 mM cytochalasin B (an inhibitor of facilitative glucose transport). Radioactive medium was aspirated rapidly followed by three cell washes in ice-cold isotonic saline solution (0.9% NaCl, w/v) prior to lysis in 0.05 M NaOH [18]. Cell-associated radioactivity was determined by liquid scintillation counting and protein determined by the method of Bradford [19].

Immunoblotting

Cell lysates were subjected to SDS/PAGE and immunoblotted as previously reported [14]. Nitrocellulose membranes were probed with various antibodies as described in the figure legends. Detection of primary antibodies were performed using appropriate peroxidase-conjugated IgGs and protein signals were visualized using enhanced chemiluminescence (Thermo Scientific Pierce) by exposure to Kodak autoradiographic film.

Statistical analysis

Statistical analysis was carried out using a Student's t test. Data were considered statistically significant at p values <0.05 and notified by *.

Results

In an initial attempt to identify factors underpinning the distinct mechanisms involved in mediating the repressive effects of ceramide upon PKB/Akt in L6 and C2C12 myotubes through PKCζ and PP2A respectively, we hypothesised that differences in CEM abundance and/or composition may account for these differential modes of action. This was based on our previous published work demonstrating the key role that CEM abundance plays in determining ceramide-induced pathways leading to PKB/Akt inhibition in non-muscle cell types [11]. We selected caveolin-3 as a CEM marker since this protein is the predominant caveolin isoform expressed in muscle cells and is known to play a crucial role in maintaining CEM structure [20]. Immunoblot analysis of caveolin-3 revealed no significant difference in total caveolin-3 protein content in whole cell lysates of fully differentiated L6 and C2C12 muscle cells (around 3 ng caveolin-3 per μg total protein lysate), as shown in figure 1A. We next examined caveolin-3 protein abundance in CEM structures by isolating detergent resistant membranes (DRM) on discontinuous sucrose density gradients [10], and immunoblotting the resulting DRM fractions for caveolin-3. Interestingly, Figure 1B shows that caveolin-3 protein expression in DRM (fractions 3 to 5) obtained from L6 myotubes was approximately 3-fold greater compared to those isolated from C2C12 myotubes. This suggests higher CEM abundance in L6 versus C2C12 plasma membranes. Because ceramide is known to accumulate within CEMs [21], we assessed whether ceramide concentration would correlate with CEM caveolin-3 content in DRM fractions isolated from these two muscle cell lines. To investigate this, we treated L6 and C2C12 myotubes with 100 μM short-chain C2-ceramide for two hours prior to isolation of DRM fractions that were subsequently used for quantitative determination of ceramide content. Figure 1 C shows that ceramide accumulates in DRM fractions 3 to 6 of both cell lines but to a far lesser extent (10 times less in terms of abundance) in C2C12 compared to L6 myotubes. Therefore, lower CEM abundance in C2C12 myotubes may account for the reduced capacity of these cells to retain ceramide in active membrane microdomains. This may also help to explain why inhibition of PKB/Akt by ceramide occurs outside these membrane domains and is mainly dependent upon PP2A activation in C2C12 myotubes [8–10].

To test this possibility, we examined whether the "PKCζ-CEM" pathway which inhibits PKB/Akt in L6 myotubes may also be functional in C2C12 myotubes. As predicted based on comparative CEM analysis, whilst C2-ceramide promotes the recruitment of PKCζ into L6 CEM domains, no PKCζ was detected in CEMs (fractions 3–5) isolated from C2C12 myotubes challenged with C2-ceramide (figure 2A). Furthermore, PP2A was not detected in ceramide-treated CEM from either muscle cell lines (figure 2A) in accordance with previous work showing that ceramide-activated PP2A acts outside the CEM environment [11].

Having established that PKCζ is not recruited to CEM in response to ceramide in C2C12 myotubes, we next assessed whether the presence of CEM was dispensable for ceramide to repress PKB/Akt in these cells. Figure 2B shows that in L6 myotubes, ceramide-mediated inhibition of PKB/AktSer473 phosphorylation in response to insulin was prevented by methyl β-cyclodextrin (MβCD), a cholesterol depleting agent that has been shown to disrupt CEM integrity without affecting insulin signalling capacity [10]. This demonstrates the importance of CEM in supporting ceramide action in these cells. Moreover, we used either okadaic acid (OKA), a potent inhibitor of protein phosphatase 2A (PP2A), and the pharmacological Protein Kinase C (PKC) inhibitor Ro 31.8220 to determine which ceramide-activated pathway (aPKCζ or PP2A) mediates the repressive effect of ceramide on PKB/Akt. The bisindolemaleimide Ro 31.8220 potently inhibits conventional and novel PKCs in an ATP-competitive manner with IC50 values in the submicromolar range, as well as atypical PKCs in the micromolar range [9]. Figure 2C shows that whilst applying OKA (500 nM) displays no significant effect, Ro 31.8220 (at 5 μM, optimal final concentration to counteract the activation of aPKCζ by ceramide in L6 myotubes, figure S1A) is able to largely prevent the negative action of ceramide upon the insulin-induced phosphorylation of PKB/Akt, thereby confirming the importance of the "CEM- PKCζ" pathway in mediating this insulin desensitising effect in L6 myotubes.

In contrast, in C2C12 myotubes, treatment with MβCD did not prevent the repressive action of either palmitate (ceramide precursor) or C2-ceramide upon insulin-stimulated PKB/Akt Ser473 phosphorylation, or upon phosphorylation of one of its physiological downstream targets, GSK3α/β (figure 2D). The lack of CEM involvement in ceramide action in C2C12 myotubes was further confirmed by overexpressing an inactive dominant negative PKCζ mutant (KD- PKCζ) in these cells. Figure 2D shows that, in contrast to what has previously been reported in L6 myotubes [9], prevention of PKCζ activation does not counteract either palmitate nor ceramide mediated repression of insulin-induced PKB/Akt and GSK3α/β phosphorylation. Furthermore, inhibition of PP2A using OKA (at 500nM, optimal final concentration to counteract the activation of PP2A by ceramide in C2C12 myotubes, figure S1B) was found to completely prevent palmitate and ceramide mediated suppression of PKB/Akt and GSK3α/β phosphorylation in insulin treated C2C12 myotubes (figure 2D). Together, these observations suggest that, depending on cellular CEM abundance, fatty acid overload can inhibit insulin induced PKB signalling through at least one of two distinct mechanisms.

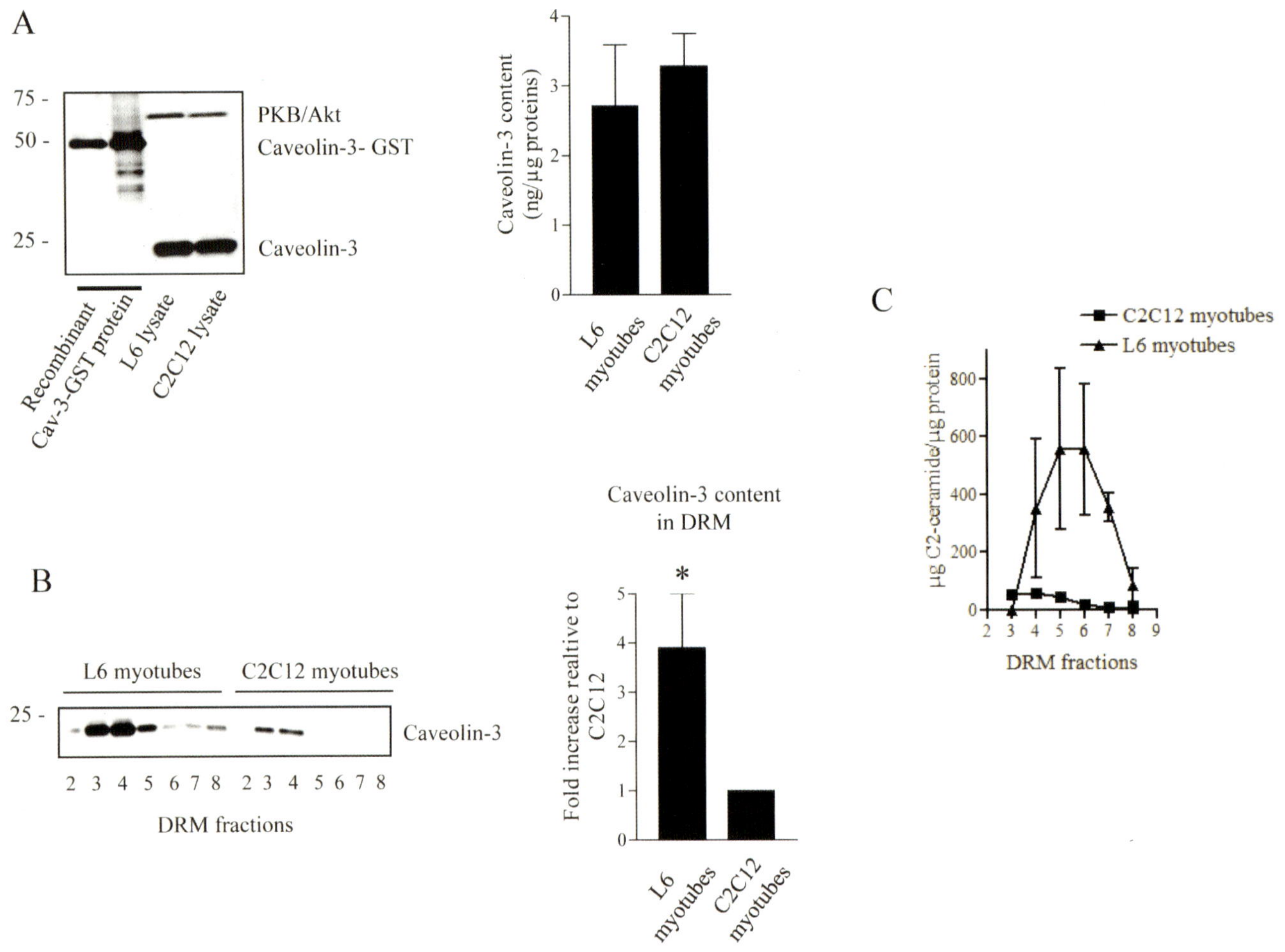

Figure 1. Levels of caveolin expression and ceramide content in both L6 and C2C12 myotubes. A. 15 µg of L6 and C2C12 lysates were immunoblotted alongside 65 ng and 130 ng of recombinant caveolin-3-GST (cav-3-GST) protein with an antibody against caveolin-3 (left panel). Bands were quantified and compared to known quantities of recombinant cav-3 proteins. Results were expressed as ng of cav-3 protein per µg of L6 or C2C12 protein lysat (right panel). B. L6 and C2C12 myotubes were solubilized in 1% Triton X-100 at 4°C and fractionated on sucrose gradients to isolate detergent resistant membranes (DRM) as described in the Methods section. Resulting fractions were collected from top to bottom of the gradient. Equal amounts of protein (1 µg) from fractions 2 to 8 of the sucrose gradient were then immunoblotted using an anti-caveolin-3 antibody. Bands were quantified and caveolin-3 content in L6 cells was expressed as fold increase relative to caveolin-3 content in C2C12 cells. * Significant change $p<0.05$ relative to C2C12 cells. These are representative of at least three independent experiments. C. Total ceramide content was quantified in DRM-containing fractions (3–8 of the sucrose gradient) from both L6 and C2C12 myotubes. These are representative of three independent experiments.

We next explored which of these mechanisms is likely to predominate in human muscle cells.

To investigate this, we used primary cultures of muscle cells derived from human biopsies. These cells have been shown to differentiate into myotubes in culture and are insulin responsive [16]. First, we wanted to establish whether our primary human muscle cells responded to palmitate treatment through assessing their ability to generate ceramide. Figure 3A shows that incubation of cultured human myotubes with 0.75 mM palmitate for 24 h led to significant increases in the cellular content of three distinct ceramide species (i.e. C16-, C18-, and C20 ceramides). Importantly, the ability of palmitate to promote these elevations in intracellular ceramide was attenuated in the presence of myriocin, a pharmacological inhibitor of the enzyme serine palmitoyl transferase (SPT) which catalyses the initial rate limiting step of *de novo* ceramide synthesis [22].

Subsequently, we assessed whether endogenous ceramide production from palmitate would impair insulin action in human muscle cells. Figure 3B shows that prolonged (24 h) incubation of human myotubes with palmitate completely abrogated insulin-induced PKB/Akt Ser473 phosphorylation. However, when human myotubes were pre-incubated with myriocin, the insulin desensitising effect of palmitate was completely prevented, thereby highlighting the important role that ceramide accumulation plays in mediating palmitate induced insulin resistance in human muscle cells (figure 3B).

Next, we explored the mechanism by which ceramide inhibits insulin signalling in human muscle cells. To do this, we treated human myotubes with C2-ceramide for 2 h prior isolating CEM domains. As observed in L6 myotubes (figure 2A), C2-ceramide treatment induced recruitment of PKCζ into CEM domains of human myotubes (figure 4A). Then, to determine whether the ceramide-activated PKCζ pathway was involved in repressing PKB/Akt activity in human muscle cells, we suppressed ceramide induced activation of PKCζ using either Ro 31.8220 (5 µM), or by overexpressing the inactive kinase-dead (KD)-PKCζ mutant in

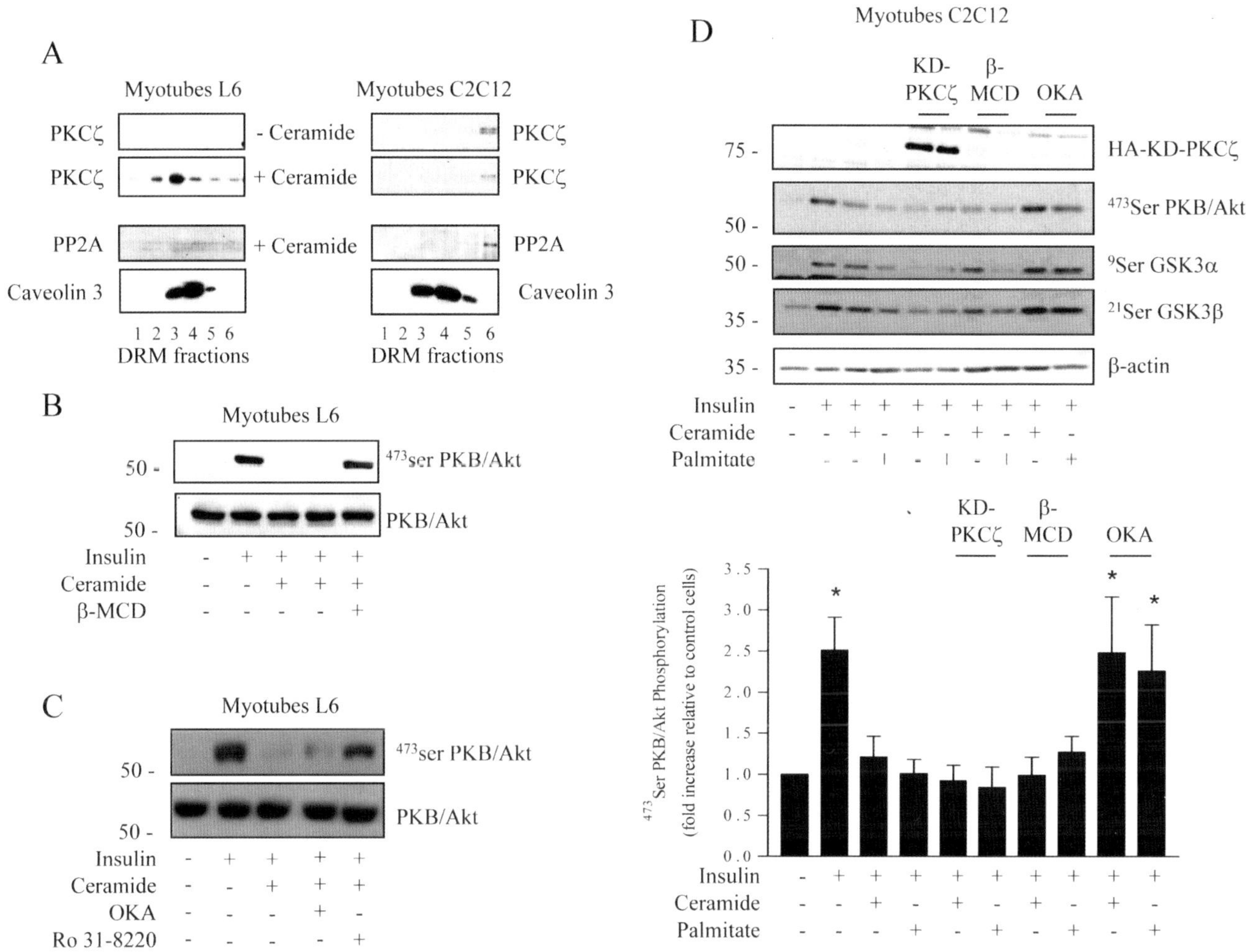

Figure 2. Mechanism of ceramide action on the insulin signalling pathway in both L6 and C2C12 myotubes. A. L6 and C2C12 myotubes were treated with 100 μM C2-ceramide for 2 h before isolation of DRMs. Equal amounts of protein (1 μg) of each fraction were then immunoblotted for the presence of PKCζ, PP2A and caveolin-3. These are representative immunoblots from three independent experiments. B. L6 myotubes were pre-incubated with 100 μM C2-ceramide for 2 h and with 5 mM MβCD for the last 30 min. Cells were then stimulated with 100 nM insulin for 10 min before being lysed and immunoblotted using either a phospho-specific antibody directed against Ser^{473}PKB/Akt or a pan PKB antibody. C. Control C2C12 myotubes or KD-PKCζ-infected C2C12 myotubes were incubated with 100 μM C2-ceramide for 2 h or with 0.75 mM palmitate for 16 h. Control C2C12 myotubes were then treated with 500 nM okadaic acid (OKA) or with 5 mM MβCD the last 30 min. All cells were treated with 100 nM insulin for the last 10 min before being lysed. Cell lysates were immunoblotted with antibodies against native PKB/Akt, Ser^{473}PKB/Akt, $Ser^{21/9}$GSK3 α/β, β-actin and hemagglutinin (HA). Scanning densitometry was performed to quantify changes in Ser^{473}PKB/Akt abundance in cell lysates. Bars represent mean +/− SEM. * Significant change $p<0.05$ relative to the untreated control. Blots shown represent at least three separate experiments.

these cells. Figure 4B shows that application of Ro 31.8220 or expression of the KD- PKCζ mutant were able to prevent the ability of palmitate to reduce insulin-stimulated phosphorylation of PKB/Akt in human cells. In contrast, the PP2A inhibitor okadaic acid did not counteract the repressive action of palmitate towards PKB/Akt (figure 4B). In accordance with its ability to induce PKB/Akt activation, insulin stimulated glucose uptake by over 2-fold in control human myotubes (figure 4C). Importantly, whilst palmitate provision led to a profound reduction in insulin-induced glucose transport, this inhibition was completely prevented in human muscle cells cotreated with Ro 31.8220 (figure 4C). These findings indicate that, in human muscle cells, ceramide acts to impair PKB/Akt predominantly through activation of the PKCζ pathway.

Several studies have previously demonstrated that myotubes derived from type 2 diabetic patients conserve important characteristics of the diabetic phenotype [23–25]. For example, insulin stimulated PKB/Akt phosphorylation in cultured human diabetic myotubes is reduced compared to that observed in non-diabetic human myotubes (figure 5A). Interestingly, pre-incubation with Ro 31.8220, but not OKA, markedly improved insulin responsiveness in diabetic myotubes (figure 5B). In contrast, neither Ro 31.8220 nor OKA significantly altered insulin stimulated PKB/Akt phosphorylation in human control myotubes (figure 5C).

Collectively these observations indicate that it is the PKCζ pathway which prevails in conveying the inhibition of PKB/Akt signalling by excess of lipids in the context of type 2 diabetes.

Discussion

The findings presented in the current study indicate that the inhibitory effects of ceramide on insulin-induced PKB/Akt signalling can be mediated through two distinct mechanisms

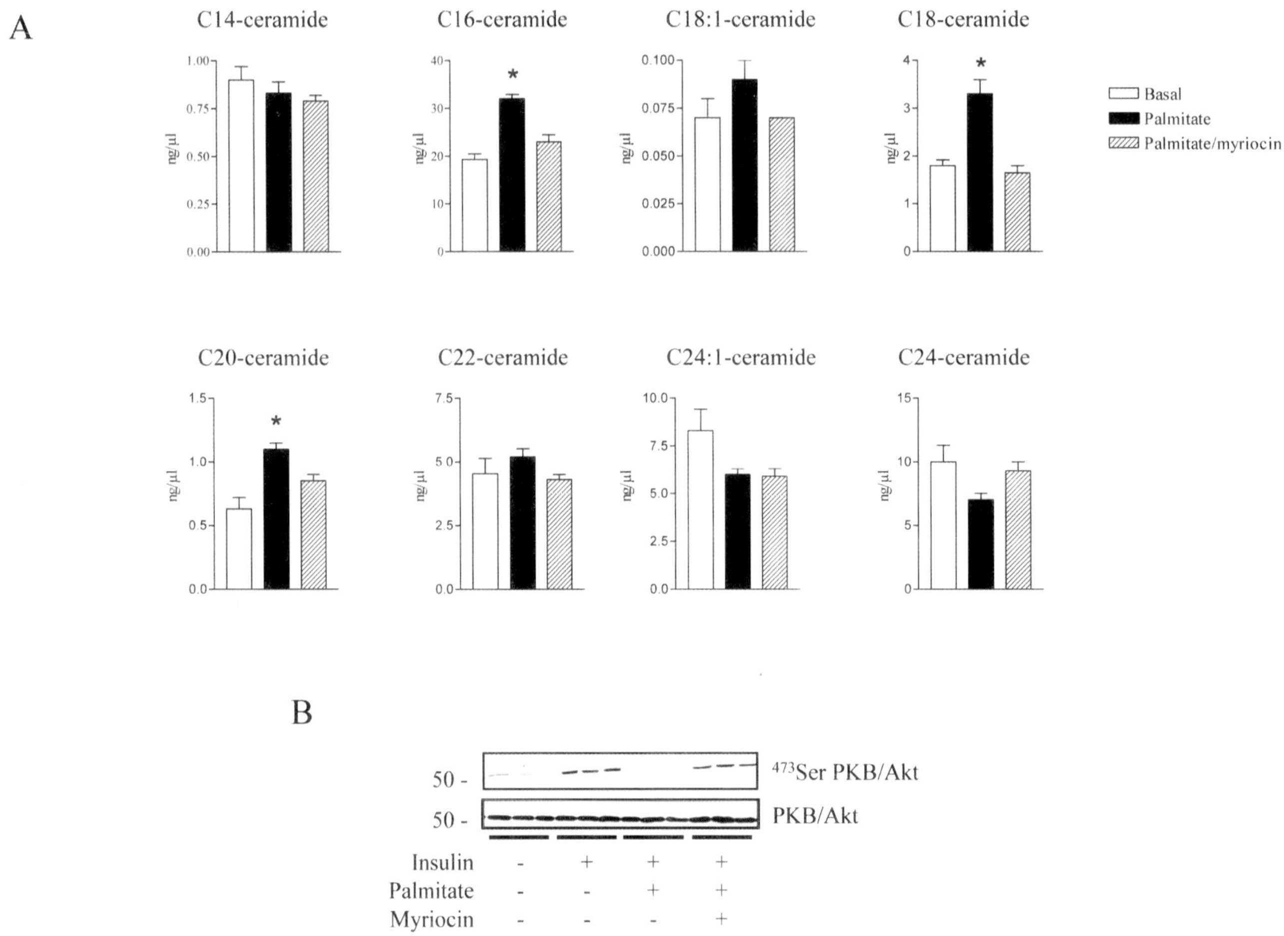

Figure 3. Effect of Palmitate on ceramide production and insulin sensitivity in human muscle cells. Human myotubes were incubated with 0.75 mM palmitate for 48 h in the presence or absence of 10 µM myriocin. A. Following this incubation, muscle cells were harvested in ice-cold PBS and lipids extracted to assess ceramide species content as described in the Methods section. Bars represent mean ± SEM from 3 separate experiments and * denote a significant difference from the untreated control values ($P<0.05$). B. Cells were then stimulated with 100 nM insulin for the last 10 min before being lysed and immunoblotted using either a phospho-specific antibody directed against Ser^{473}PKB/Akt or a pan PKB antibody.

depending on muscle cell type. In rat L6 myotubes, ceramide acts by promoting the activation of PKCζ and its subsequent recruitment to plasma membrane CEMs. In contrast, in mouse C2C12 myotubes, ceramide represses PKB/Akt activity through stimulation of cytoplasmic phosphatase PP2A. Importantly, we show that differences in CEM abundance may be an important factor in determining which mechanism is prominent within any particular cell type.

One possible explanation for the observed differences in CEM abundance and distinct modes of ceramide action in these two muscle cell lines, may be partly due to their contrasting abilities to differentiate from myoblasts into mature myotubes. Both L6 and C2C12 myoblasts exhibit characteristic features of muscle myogenesis, including migration and proliferation in medium containing 10% (v/v) foetal calf serum, followed by elongation and fusion to form myotubes following serum reduction. Interestingly, previous studies have shown that L6 cells differentiate readily into myotubes when maintained in medium containing 2% (v/v) serum, whereas C2C12 differentiation is more pronounced in serum-free medium compared to a serum-containing system [26,27]. Thus, under standard conditions used to differentiate both cell lines (i.e. 2% (w/w) serum), it is possible that L6 myotubes mature more rapidly and/or more efficiently than C2C12 myotubes. However, since caveolins are late differentiation markers [28] and we see similar levels of caveolin-3 content in both differentiated cell types (figure 1A), this is unlikely to account for any mechanistic differences, and rather suggest that these two muscle cell models display different membrane characteristics, reinforcing the importance of our study.

Another key finding from this work concerns the identification of the process by which ceramide mediates insulin desensitisation in human muscle cells. To investigate this, we utilised human muscle satellite cells obtained from either insulin sensitive or diabetic donors that we differentiated *in vitro* into mature myotubes. There are several advantages using this cell model, including its morphological, biochemical and metabolic similarity to adult skeletal muscle cells [13]. Importantly, these cultured myotubes have been shown to maintain metabolic properties of the donor [13]. Similar to what we observed in L6 and C2C12 myotubes, we found that treatment of cultured insulin sensitive human myotubes with palmitate led to both an increase in the biosynthesis of three ceramide species (C16-, C18- and C20-ceramides) and an associated reduction in insulin stimulated PKB/Akt activation. Interestingly, the levels of similar ceramide species

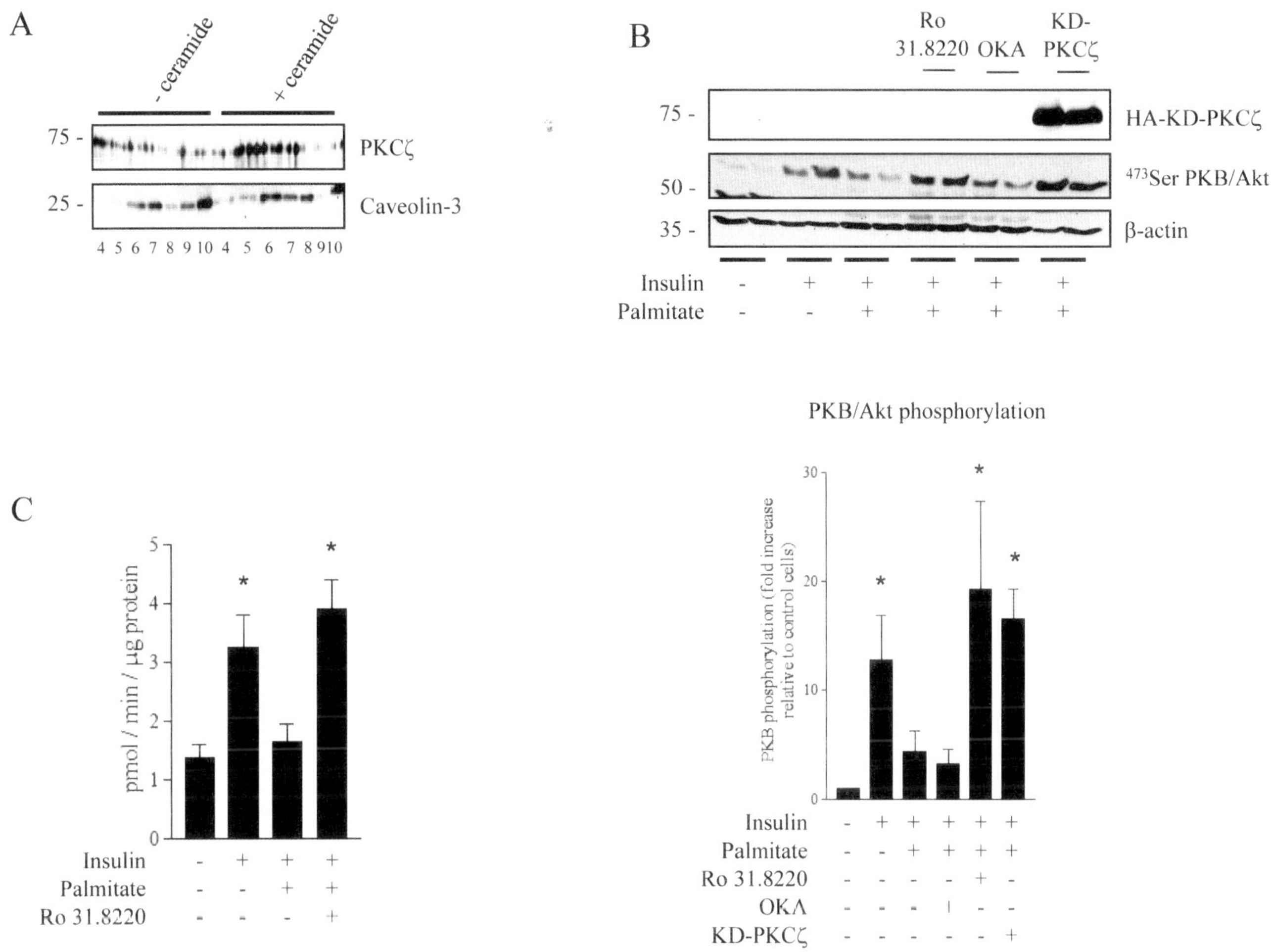

Figure 4. Ceramide action on the insulin signalling pathway in human myotubes. A. Human myotubes were treated with 100 µM C2-ceramide for 2 h before isolation of DRMs. Equal amounts of protein (1 µg) of each fraction were then immunoblotted for the presence of PKCζ and caveolin-3. These are representative immunoblots from three independent experiments. B. Human myotubes from control donors were treated with 0.75 mM palmitate for 48 h in the presence or absence of Ro 31.8220 (5 µM, 48 h) or OKA (500 nM, last 30 min). KD-PKCζ-infected human myotubes were treated with 0.75 mM palmitate for 48 h. Cells were then stimulated with 100 nM insulin for the last 10 min before being lysed. Cell lysates were immunoblotted with antibodies against Ser^{473}PKB/Akt, β-actin and hemagglutinin (HA). Scanning densitometry was performed to quantify changes in Ser^{473}PKB/Akt abundance in cell lysates. Bars represent mean +/− SEM. * denotes significant change $p<0.05$ relative to the untreated control. Blots shown represent at least three separate experiments. C. Human myotubes were incubated with 0.75 mM palmitate for 48 h in the presence or absence of Ro 31.8220. Cells were then treated with 100 nM insulin for the last 30 min prior to the measurement of 2-deoxy-glucose uptake as described in the experimental section. Bars represent mean +/− SEM. * Significant change $p<0.05$ relative to the untreated control ($n=3$).

(C16- and C18-ceramides) have also previously been reported to be increased in myotubes obtained from type 2 diabetic individuals compared to controls [6]. Therefore, these observations suggest that these specific ceramide species may play a key role in mediating the deleterious effects of palmitate upon insulin signal transduction. In accordance with this, we demonstrate that inhibition of endogenous ceramide production with myriocin abolishes palmitate-induced insulin resistance in our human myotubes. Furthermore, in line with our observations in L6 muscle cells [8,9], palmitate-derived ceramide acts to inhibit insulin signalling through activation of the "PKCζ-CEM" pathway in human myotubes. Importantly, we confirmed this by using human myotubes that have been made insulin resistant through palmitate exposure, as well as using primary culture of skeletal muscle cells from diabetic patients. It is important to note that the latter cell model has been extensively studied and displays several metabolic defects that characterize *in vivo* insulin resistance of skeletal muscle such as inhibition of insulin stimulated glucose uptake and glycogen synthesis [24,25,29,30], concomitant with impaired insulin signalling [23,31].

Together, these data implicate the "PKCζ-CEM" pathway as an important therapeutic target to counteract the deleterious effects of saturated fatty acids and their derived lipid intermediates upon insulin signalling in muscle cells. It is important to emphasise that myotubes derived from human subjects used in the present study could present altered membrane structure, gene expression and function due to *in vitro* culture and differentiation. Therefore, it would be interesting to confirm our results in intact muscle.

In summary, our study highlights key mechanistic differences by which ceramide can impair insulin action in rat L6 and mouse C2C12 myotubes. Importantly, our findings suggest that the effectiveness of distinct ceramide-induced pathways to promote insulin resistance in these cell lines, namely through activation of atypical PKC isoforms and PP2A respectively, may be determined by cellular CEM abundance and/or composition. Furthermore, we demonstrate for the first time that ceramide acts to repress

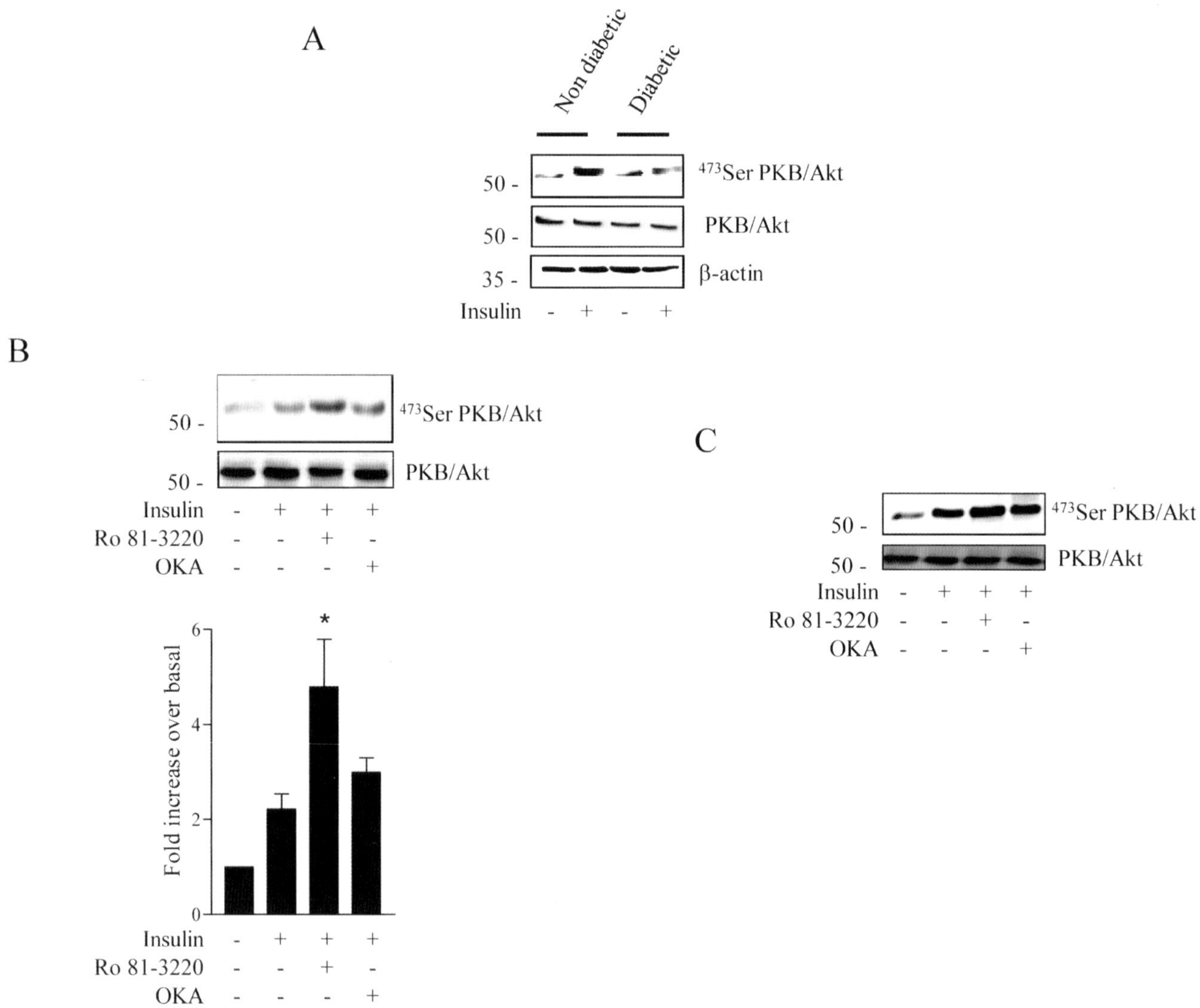

Figure 5. Inhibition of aPKCs sensitizes insulin-resistant human myotubes to insulin. A. Differentiated myotubes from control donors were incubated with Ro 31.8220 (5 μM, 18 h) or OKA (500 nM, last 30 min), then stimulated with 100 nM insulin for the last 10 min before being lysed. Cell lysates were immunoblotted with antibodies against Ser^{473}PKB/Akt, total PKB/Akt and β-actin. B. Differentiated myotubes from diabetic patients were incubated with Ro 31.8220 (5 μM, 18 h) or OKA (500 nM, last 30 min), then stimulated with 100 nM insulin for the last 10 min before being lysed. Cell lysates were immunoblotted with antibodies against Ser^{473}PKB/Akt and total PKB/Akt. Scanning densitometry was performed to quantify changes in Ser^{473}PKB/Akt abundance over total PKB/Akt protein expression in cell lysates. Bars represent mean +/− SEM. * denotes significant change $p<0.05$ relative to the insulin treated cells. Blots represent three separate experiments.

insulin-induced PKB/Akt signalling in primary human myotubes through a pathway dependent on PKCζ. Together, these data raise awareness of the key role that cell membrane structure and/or composition may play in determining the effectiveness and/or predominance of those pathways which can potentially cause insulin resistance in different skeletal muscle cell models. Furthermore, our findings emphasise the need for caution when interpreting and comparing data from different muscle cell lines, particularly when exploring the role of fatty acid derived lipids such as ceramide in the modulation of insulin-regulated signalling and its associated processes.

Acknowledgments

We would like to thank F. Koskas, J. Gaudric, C. Goulfier, C. Jouhannet and T. Khalife (Service de Chirurgie Vasculaire, AP-HP, Hôpital Pitié-Salpêtrière, Paris, France) for the collection of human diabetic samples. We are grateful to J.-T. Vilquin (Groupe Hospitalier Pitié-Salpêtrière, Paris, France) and the tissue bank of the Association Française des Myopathies (AFM) for human control biopsy samples.

Author Contributions

Conceived and designed the experiments: PF FF HSH EH. Performed the experiments: RM RK ST AB-Z NL CL CS. Analyzed the data: PF FF HSH EH. Contributed reagents/materials/analysis tools: OB. Contributed to the writing of the manuscript: CL ST FF EH.

References

1. Sesti G (2006) Pathophysiology of insulin resistance. Best Pract Res Clin Endocrinol Metab 20: 665–679.
2. Lipina C, Hundal HS (2011) Sphingolipids: agents provocateurs in the pathogenesis of insulin resistance. Diabetologia 54: 1596–1607.
3. Turban S, Hajduch E (2011) Protein kinase C isoforms: Mediators of reactive lipid metabolites in the development of insulin resistance. FEBS Lett 585: 269–274.
4. Coen PM, Dube JJ, Amati F, Stefanovic-Racic M, Ferrell RE, et al. (2010) Insulin resistance is associated with higher intramyocellular triglycerides in type I but not type II myocytes concomitant with higher ceramide content. Diabetes 59: 80–88.
5. Amati F, Dube JJ, Carnero EA, Edreira MM, Chomentowski P, et al. (2011) Skeletal-Muscle Triglycerides, Diacylglycerols, and Ceramides in Insulin Resistance: Another Paradox in Endurance-Trained Athletes? Diabetes 60: 2588–97.
6. Bajpeyi S, Myrland CK, Covington JD, Obanda D, Cefalu WT, et al. (2013) Lipid in skeletal muscle myotubes is associated to the donors' insulin sensitivity and physical activity phenotypes. Obesity (Silver Spring) 22(2): 426–34.
7. Hajduch E, Litherland GJ, Hundal HS (2001) Protein kinase B (PKB/Akt)–a key regulator of glucose transport? FEBS Lett 492: 199–203.
8. Hajduch E, Balendran A, Batty IH, Litherland GJ, Blair AS, et al (2001) Ceramide impairs the insulin-dependent membrane recruitment of protein kinase B leading to a loss in downstream signalling in L6 skeletal muscle cells. Diabetologia 44: 173–183.
9. Powell DJ, Hajduch E, Kular G, Hundal HS (2003) Ceramide Disables 3-Phosphoinositide Binding to the Pleckstrin Homology Domain of Protein Kinase B (PKB)/Akt by a PKCzeta-Dependent Mechanism. Mol Cell Biol 23: 7794–7808.
10. Hajduch E, Turban S, Le Liepvre, X, Le Lay S, Lipina C, et al. (2008) Targeting of PKCzeta and PKB to caveolin-enriched microdomains represents a crucial step underpinning the disruption in PKB-directed signalling by ceramide. Biochem J 410: 369–379.
11. Blouin CM, Prado C, Takane KK, Lasnier F, Garcia-Ocana A, et al. (2010) Plasma membrane subdomain compartmentalization contributes to distinct mechanisms of ceramide action on insulin signaling. Diabetes 59: 600–610.
12. Cazzolli R, Carpenter L, Biden TJ, Schmitz-Peiffer C (2001) A role for protein phosphatase 2A-like activity, but not atypical protein kinase Czeta, in the inhibition of protein kinase B/Akt and glycogen synthesis by palmitate. Diabetes 50: 2210–2218.
13. Aas V, Bakke SS, Feng YZ, Kase ET, Jensen J, et al. (2013) Are cultured human myotubes far from home? Cell Tissue Res 354: 671–82.
14. Hajduch E, Alessi DR, Hemmings BA, Hundal HS (1998) Constitutive activation of protein kinase B alpha by membrane targeting promotes glucose and system A amino acid transport, protein synthesis, and inactivation of glycogen synthase kinase 3 in L6 muscle cells. Diabetes 47: 1006–1013.
15. Vilquin JT, Marolleau JP, Sacconi S, Garcin I, Lacassagne MN, et al. (2005) Normal growth and regenerating ability of myoblasts from unaffected muscles of facioscapulohumeral muscular dystrophy patients. Gene Ther 12: 1651–1662.
16. Hage Hassan R, Hainault I, Vilquin JT, Samama C, Lasnier F, et al. (2012) Endoplasmic reticulum stress does not mediate palmitate-induced insulin resistance in mouse and human muscle cells. Diabetologia 55: 204–214.
17. Blachnio-Zabielska AU, Persson XM, Koutsari C, Zabielski P, Jensen MD (2012) A liquid chromatography/tandem mass spectrometry method for measuring the in vivo incorporation of plasma free fatty acids into intramyocellular ceramides in humans. Rapid Commun Mass Spectrom 26: 1134–1140.
18. Blair AS, Hajduch E, Litherland GJ, Hundal HS (1999) Regulation of glucose transport and glycogen synthesis in L6 muscle cells during oxidative stress. Evidence for cross-talk between the insulin and SAPK2/p38 mitogen-activated protein kinase signaling pathways. J Biol Chem 274: 36293–36299.
19. Bradford MM (1976) A rapid and sensitive method for the quantitation of microgram quantities of protein utilizing the principle of protein-dye binding. Anal Biochem 72: 248–254.
20. Parton RG, del Pozo MA (2013) Caveolae as plasma membrane sensors, protectors and organizers. Nat Rev Mol Cell Biol 14: 98–112. nrm3512 [pii]; 10.1038/nrm3512 [doi].
21. Megha, London E (2004) Ceramide selectively displaces cholesterol from ordered lipid domains (rafts): implications for lipid raft structure and function. J Biol Chem 279: 9997–10004.
22. Watson ML, Coghlan M, Hundal HS (2009) Modulating serine palmitoyl transferase (SPT) expression and activity unveils a crucial role in lipid-induced insulin resistance in rat skeletal muscle cells. Biochem J 417: 791–801.
23. Cozzone D, Frojdo S, Disse E, Debard C, Laville M, et al. (2008) Isoform-specific defects of insulin stimulation of Akt/protein kinase B (PKB) in skeletal muscle cells from type 2 diabetic patients. Diabetologia 51: 512–521.
24. Gaster M, Petersen I, Hojlund K, Poulsen P, Beck-Nielsen H (2002) The diabetic phenotype is conserved in myotubes established from diabetic subjects: evidence for primary defects in glucose transport and glycogen synthase activity. Diabetes 51: 921–927.
25. Jackson S, Bagstaff SM, Lynn S, Yeaman SJ, Turnbull DM, et al. (2000) Decreased insulin responsiveness of glucose uptake in cultured human skeletal muscle cells from insulin-resistant nondiabetic relatives of type 2 diabetic families. Diabetes 49: 1169–1177.
26. Lawson MA, Purslow PP (2000) Differentiation of myoblasts in serum-free media: effects of modified media are cell line-specific. Cells Tissues Organs 167: 130–137.
27. Kubo Y (1991) Comparison of initial stages of muscle differentiation in rat and mouse myoblastic and mouse mesodermal stem cell lines. J Physiol 442: 743–759.
28. Blouin CM, Le Lay S, Lasnier F, Dugail I, Hajduch E (2008) Regulated association of caveolins to lipid droplets during differentiation of 3T3-L1 adipocytes. Biochem Biophys Res Commun 376: 331–335.
29. Gaster M, Kristensen SR, Beck-Nielsen H, Schroder HD (2001) A cellular model system of differentiated human myotubes. APMIS 109: 735–744.
30. Ciaraldi TP, Abrams L, Nikoulina S, Mudaliar S, Henry RR (1995) Glucose transport in cultured human skeletal muscle cells. Regulation by insulin and glucose in nondiabetic and non-insulin-dependent diabetes mellitus subjects. J Clin Invest 96: 2820–2827.
31. Bouzakri K, Roques M, Gual P, Espinosa S, Guebre-Egziabher F, et al. (2003) Reduced activation of phosphatidylinositol-3 kinase and increased serine 636 phosphorylation of insulin receptor substrate-1 in primary culture of skeletal muscle cells from patients with type 2 diabetes. Diabetes 52: 1319–1325.

14

Knock-Down of IL-1Ra in Obese Mice Decreases Liver Inflammation and Improves Insulin Sensitivity

Niclas Franck[1], Michael Maris[1,2], Sarah Nalbandian[1], Saswata Talukdar[3], Simon Schenk[4], Hans-Peter Hofmann[3], David Bullough[3], Olivia Osborn[1]*

1 Division of Endocrinology and Metabolism, Department of Medicine, University of California San Diego, La Jolla, California, United States of America, **2** Clinical and Experimental Endocrinology, Catholic University Leuven, Leuven, Belgium, **3** Pfizer Inc. Research Laboratories, Cambridge, Massachusetts, United States of America, **4** Department of Orthopedic Surgery, University of California San Diego, La Jolla, California, United States of America

Abstract

Interleukin 1 Receptor antagonist (IL-1Ra) is highly elevated in obesity and is widely recognized as an anti-inflammatory cytokine. While the anti-inflammatory role of IL-1Ra in the pancreas is well established, the role of IL-1Ra in other insulin target tissues and the contribution of systemic IL-1Ra levels to the development of insulin resistance remains to be defined. Using antisense knock down of IL-1Ra in vivo, we show that normalization of IL-1Ra improved insulin sensitivity due to decreased inflammation in the liver and improved hepatic insulin sensitivity and these effects were independent of changes in body weight. A similar effect was observed in IL1-R1 KO mice, suggesting that at high concentrations of IL-1Ra typically observed in obesity, IL-1Ra can contribute to the development of insulin resistance in a mechanism independent of IL-1Ra binding to IL-1R1. These results demonstrate that normalization of plasma IL-1Ra concentration improves insulin sensitivity in diet- induced obese mice.

Editor: Marc Claret, Institut d'Investigacions Biomèdiques August Pi i Sunyer, Spain

Funding: This work was supported by the National Institutes of Health (NIH) grants: DK-033651, DK-074868, T32-DK-007494, DK-063491 and from a grant from Pfizer. The funders had no role in study design, data collection and analysis, decision to publish, or preparation of the manuscript.

* Email: oosborn@ucsd.edu

Introduction

Insulin resistance is a pathophysiological defect commonly found in obese individuals, and is an important predictor for the progression to type 2 diabetes [1]. The incidence of obesity and associated insulin resistance has risen dramatically in the past 20 years and so understanding the pathways driving the development of insulin resistance is of high importance. Tissue inflammation is now recognized as a major cause of impaired insulin sensitivity in obesity [2,3] and has been observed in all classical insulin target tissues including fat, liver and muscle. Interleukin 1 Beta (IL-1β) is an important proinflammatory cytokine that binds to the type 1 IL-1 Receptor (IL-1R1) and has well described proinflammatory effects [4]. Signal transduction is elicited by interaction of the IL-1R1 with an accessory protein (IL-1RAcP) [5,6]. The endogenous antagonist IL-1R Antagonist (IL-1Ra), also binds to the IL-1R1 but does not initiate signal transduction [7]. IL-1Ra is classically viewed as an anti-inflammatory cytokine that acts as a selective, competitive receptor antagonist at the IL-1R1 by blocking the actions of IL-1β [8] and the balance in expression between IL-1β and IL-1Ra is important in many inflammatory diseases [9].

While the anti-inflammatory role of IL-1Ra in the pancreas is well established in both mice [4,10,11] and humans [12,13], the role of IL-1Ra in other insulin target tissues and the general role of systemic levels of IL-1Ra in the development of obesity and insulin resistance is still unclear. A number of studies over the last decade have raised the question of whether the high levels of IL-1Ra observed in obesity may contribute to the development of insulin resistance. In obese human patients, circulating levels of IL-1Ra are ~6.5 times higher than lean subjects and, interestingly, the levels of IL-1Ra in plasma correlate more closely with insulin resistance than BMI [14], suggesting an important link between IL-1Ra and insulin resistance. Indeed, elevated systemic concentrations of IL-1Ra are associated with an increased risk of developing type 2 diabetes [15,16], and in retrospective studies this increase in IL-1Ra accelerated prior to type 2 diabetes diagnosis [17]. In a recent study IL-1Ra was even identified as a novel biomarker for clinically incident diabetes, over and above the classical risk factors such as BMI and waist: hip ratio [18]. Supporting a possible role in the development of insulin resistance, thiazolidinedione (TZD) treatment significantly reduced levels of IL-1Ra in patients with metabolic syndrome [19], as well as in cell culture studies where TZDs inhibited the production of IL-1Ra from proinflammatory adipocytes [20].

Furthermore, studies in rodents have further confirmed the link between IL-1Ra and insulin resistance. In a short five day study, administration of IL-1Ra led to a decrease in whole body insulin sensitivity in rats [21] while whole body deletion of IL-1Ra significantly improved insulin sensitivity in mice [21–23]. However, the IL-1Ra whole body KO mouse is particularly lean (<20g by 16wks age) which raises the possibility that the complete absence of IL-1Ra from birth may cause growth or sickness issues [23]. Taken together, these results provide a strong link between IL-1Ra and insulin action but to better define the role of IL-1Ra in vivo, in the present study we investigated the hypothesis that normalization of IL-1Ra would improve insulin sensitivity. To address this hypothesis we used antisense oligonucleotides (ASO) to knock down both the secreted and intracellular forms of IL-1Ra in high fat diet (HFD)-fed obese mice. Overall our studies show that reduction of IL-1Ra levels (to approximately half the normal circulating levels in obese mice) improves hepatic insulin sensitivity.

Materials and Methods

Chemicals and Reagents

All chemicals were purchased from Sigma (USA) unless otherwise noted.

In vitro knock-down of IL-1Ra

Antisense oligonucleotides (ASO) against IL-1Ra were a gift from Pfizer Inc. and were synthesized as described by Stanton, 2012 [24]. IL-1Ra ASO-1: 5′ - ßA*ßT*mC*dA*dG*dG*dC*d-A*dG*dT*dT*mG*ßG*ßt - 3′; IL-1Ra ASO-2: 5′-ßT*ßT*dG*d-G*dT*dC*dT*dG*dG*dA*dC*dT*ßG*ßT - 3′; Control ASO: 5′-βZ*ßG*dT*dC*dT*dA*dT*dG*dT*dA*ßT*ßA*ßG - 3′ (*, phosphorothioate backbone link; LNA, locked nucleic acid; Z, 5-methyl cytosine; ß, LNA base; m, 2′-OMethyl nucleoside; A, adenosine monomer; C, cytidine monomer; G, guanosine monomer; T, thymidine monomer).

The efficiency of knock-down of IL-1Ra expression was tested in Hepa 1 6 mouse hepatoma cells by gymnotic delivery. In brief, cells were seeded in 96-well plates at 2,500 cells per well and treated with IL-1Ra ASOs without transfection reagent at varying concentrations. Control cells were incubated with medium only. After 5 days cells were lysed and IL-1Ra mRNA knock-down was analyzed by quantitative PCR.

Mice

All experiments were approved by and conducted in accordance with the Animal Care Program at the University of California, San Diego. All surgery was performed under ketamine anesthesia, and every effort was made to minimize suffering. Male C57BL/6 and IL-1R1 KO were purchased from Jackson Laboratories and at 8 weeks of age. Mice were fed HFD (D12492, Research Diets, 60% of kcal derived from fat) *ad libitum* for 12 weeks to generate diet induced obese (DIO) mice. For acute studies, DIO mice were injected (subcutaneously, 10 mg/kg) once with IL-1Ra ASO (1 or 2) or control ASO and sacrificed one week later. For chronic studies, DIO mice at 20 weeks of age mice were divided into two groups, IL-1Ra ASO-1 or control ASO and both groups were treated twice a week by subcutaneous injection at a dose of 10 mg/kg for 6 weeks while maintained on HFD. At the end of the study (26 wks of age) all the mice were sacrificed.

Metabolic studies

For Glucose tolerance tests (GTT), an intraperitoneal (IP) injection of glucose (1 g/kg) was administered in mice fasted for 6 hours. Blood was collected for measurement of plasma insulin concentration before the injection and 10 and 90 minutes after glucose injection. Blood glucose concentration was assessed at indicated time points. For insulin tolerance tests (ITT), an IP dose of 0.35 U/kg insulin was administered, and blood glucose was measured at the indicated time points. Hyperinsulinemic euglycemic clamp studies were conducted as previously described [25]. Briefly, dual catheters (MRE-025, Braintree Scientific) were implanted in the right jugular vein and mice were allowed to recover for 3 days before the clamp procedure. After 6 hr fasting, the clamp experiments began with a constant infusion (5 μCi/hr) of D-[3-^{3}H] glucose (Du Pont-NEN, Boston, MA). After 90 minutes of tracer equilibration and basal sampling at −10 and 0 minutes, glucose (50% dextrose, variable infusion, Abbott) and tracer (μCi/hr) plus insulin (8 mU/kg/min) was infused via the jugular vein cannulae. Blood was taken from tail clips at 10 minute intervals and analyzed for glucose. Steady-state conditions (120 mg/dl ±5 mg/dl) were confirmed at the end of the clamp by ensuring that glucose infusion and plasma glucose levels were maintained constant for a minimum of 30 min. Blood samples were taken at −10, 0 (basal), 110 and 120 (end of experiment) minutes to determine glucose-specific activity and insulin and FFA levels. Hepatic glucose production (HGP) and glucose disposal rate (GDR) were calculated in the basal state and during the steady-state portion of the clamp. Tracer-determined rates were quantified by using the Steele equation [26]. At steady state, the rate of glucose disappearance, or total GDR, is equal to the sum of the rate of endogenous HGP plus the exogenous (cold) GIR. The IS-GDR is equal to the total GDR minus the basal glucose turnover rate. Glucose was measured using a blood glucose monitor and test strips (Easy Step, Deerfield Beach, FL, USA).

Indirect calorimetry and measurement of core body temperature and activity

After 4 weeks of treatment mice were placed into Comprehensive Lab Animal Monitoring System (CLAMS, Columbus Instruments) metabolic cages. Data were recorded after 48 hours of acclimatization to the chambers under ambient room temperature maintained at 25°C, beginning from the onset of the light cycle 24 hr for three days. Measurement of CBT and locomotor activity was performed as previously described [27]. In brief, radiotelemetry devices (Mini Mitter, Respironics) were surgically implanted into the intraperitoneal cavity and core body temperature and activity was recorded every 15 minutes over a 24 hr period.

RNA Isolation and Quantitative-PCR

Total RNA was isolated using Trizol as described by the manufacturer. (Trizol, Invitrogen, CA). First strand cDNA was synthesized using a High-Capacity cDNA Reverse Transcription Kit (Applied Biosystems, Foster City, CA). For quantitative PCR (qPCR) the samples were run in 20 μl reactions (iTaq SYBRgreen supermix, Biorad) using a stepOnePlus Real Time PCR system, Applied Biosystems). Gene expression levels were calculated after normalization to the standard housekeeping gene *ActB* using the $\Delta\Delta C_T$ method as described previously [28], and results are expressed relative to the control group mean value. Primer sequences are described in table S1).

Measurement of serum parameters

IL-1Ra serum levels were measured using a Mouse IL-1ra/IL-1F3 Quantikine ELISA Kit (R&D Systems, Minneapolis, MN, USA). Plasma concentrations of Interleukin 10 (IL-10), Interleukin 1 beta (IL-1β), Interleukin 6 (IL-6), Monocyte chemotactic protein 1 (MCP-1) and Tumor necrosis factor alpha (TNF-mor necrosis factorleukin 10 (IL-10), Interleukin 1 beta (ILBillerica, MA, USA). Plasma insulin levels were measured by ELISA (ALPCO diagnostics, USA). Plasma free fatty acid (FFA) levels were measured enzymatically using a commercially available kit (NEFA C; Wako Chemicals USA). Triglyceride (TG) levels were measured enzymatically using a commercially available kit (L-Type TG M, Wako Chemicals, USA). Liver enzymes alanine aminotransferase (ALT), aspartate aminotransferase (AST) and glutamate dehydrogenase (GDH) were measured using assay kits (Sigma, MO, USA).

Statistical analyses

Statistical analyses were performed using the Student's *t*-test to compare two groups. One -way ANOVA followed by a Tukey post hoc test was used to assess significance between three groups. Two-way anova with repeated measures followed by the Holm–Sidak test was used to compare two or more groups at different time points. Significance was defined as p value equal or less than less than 0.05 (*). The results are shown as means ± SEM. Graph Pad Prism (Graph Pad, San Diego, CA) was used for all statistical analyses.

Results

IL-1Ra ASO reduces expression of IL-1Ra in vitro and acutely in vivo

In vitro studies in Hepa 1–6 cells using two different ASOs (IL-1Ra ASO-1 and IL-1Ra ASO-2) directed against IL-1Ra revealed a dose dependent knock down of IL-1Ra mRNA(Fig. 1*A*). To determine whether antisense treatment reduced the expression of IL-1Ra in vivo we administered the IL-1Ra ASOs and control ASO by subcutaneous injection, dose 10 mg/kg, to obese mice (fed a 60% HFD for 12 weeks). One week after ASO injection mice were sacrificed IL-1Ra mRNA expression was analyzed by QPCR. Both IL-1Ra ASOs resulted in significant reduction of IL-1Ra in both liver and epididymal adipose tissue (Fig. 1*B*) while closely related family member IL-1β expression was not significantly changed in either tissue (Fig 1B). Furthermore, after 1 week of treatment, both IL-1Ra ASOs resulted in a significant decrease in blood glucose compared with control ASO treatment (Fig 1C), suggesting these ASOs act specifically on IL-1Ra and the glucose lowering effects are less likely to be attributable to off-target secondary effects. IL-1Ra ASO-1 at a dose of 10 mg/kg was selected for use in the chronic studies.

Chronic treatment with IL-1Ra ASO reduces expression of IL-1Ra in vivo

To determine the extent of IL-1Ra knock down in HFD fed mice after chronic treatment (6weeks) with IL-1Ra ASO or control ASO in vivo we measured IL-1Ra mRNA expression levels in tissues as well as circulating protein levels of IL-1Ra. After 6 weeks of treatment the expression of IL-1Ra mRNA was decreased by

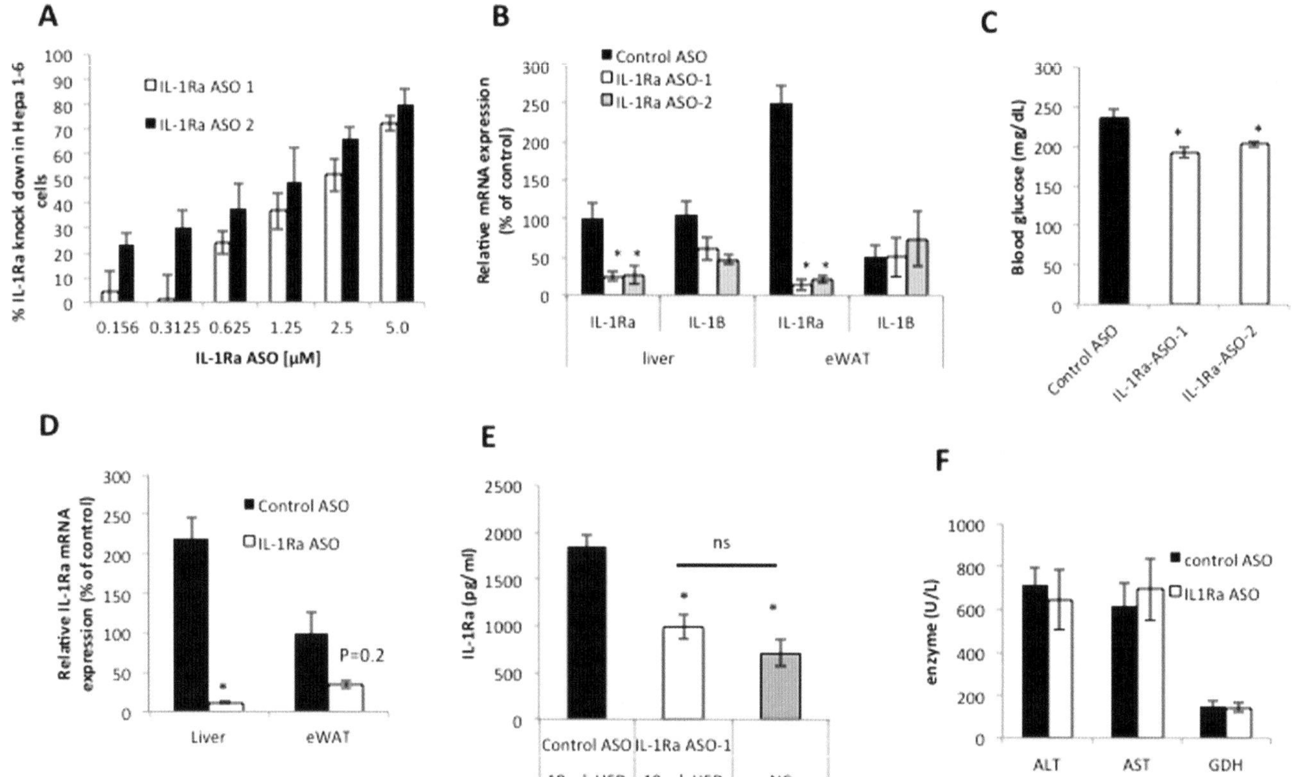

Figure 1. Antisense oligonucleotide (ASO) mediated knock-down of IL-1Ra transcript in vitro and in vivo using locked nucleic acids (LNAs). A) QPCR analysis of IL-1Ra mRNA expression after ASO treatment in Hepa 1–6 cells, each concentration was run in duplicate. B) QPCR analysis of IL-1Ra and IL-1β mRNA levels in liver and epididymal adipose (eWAT) from mice one week after IL-1Ra ASO administration. C) Blood glucose concentration in mice one week after IL-1Ra ASO treatment. D. QPCR analysis of IL-1Ra mRNA expression in liver and eWAT after 6 weeks of treatment of IL-1Ra ASO or control ASO. E. Plasma IL-1Ra concentration in obese mice treated with IL-1Ra ASO or control ASO for 6 weeks compared with aged matched lean control mice fed normal chow (NC). F. Analysis of liver enzyme levels after IL-1Ra ASO treatment in HFD-fed mice (ALT, alanine aminotransferase; AST, aspartate aminotransferase; GDH, glutamate dehydrogenase). *P<0.05 compared with control treated mice, QPCR results are normalized to beta actin mRNA and expressed relative to control treatment. Differences between groups were analyzed by one way ANOVA followed by Tukey post hoc tests, n = 5–8 mice per group, * p<0.05 compared to HFD-fed control treated group; ns, not significant.

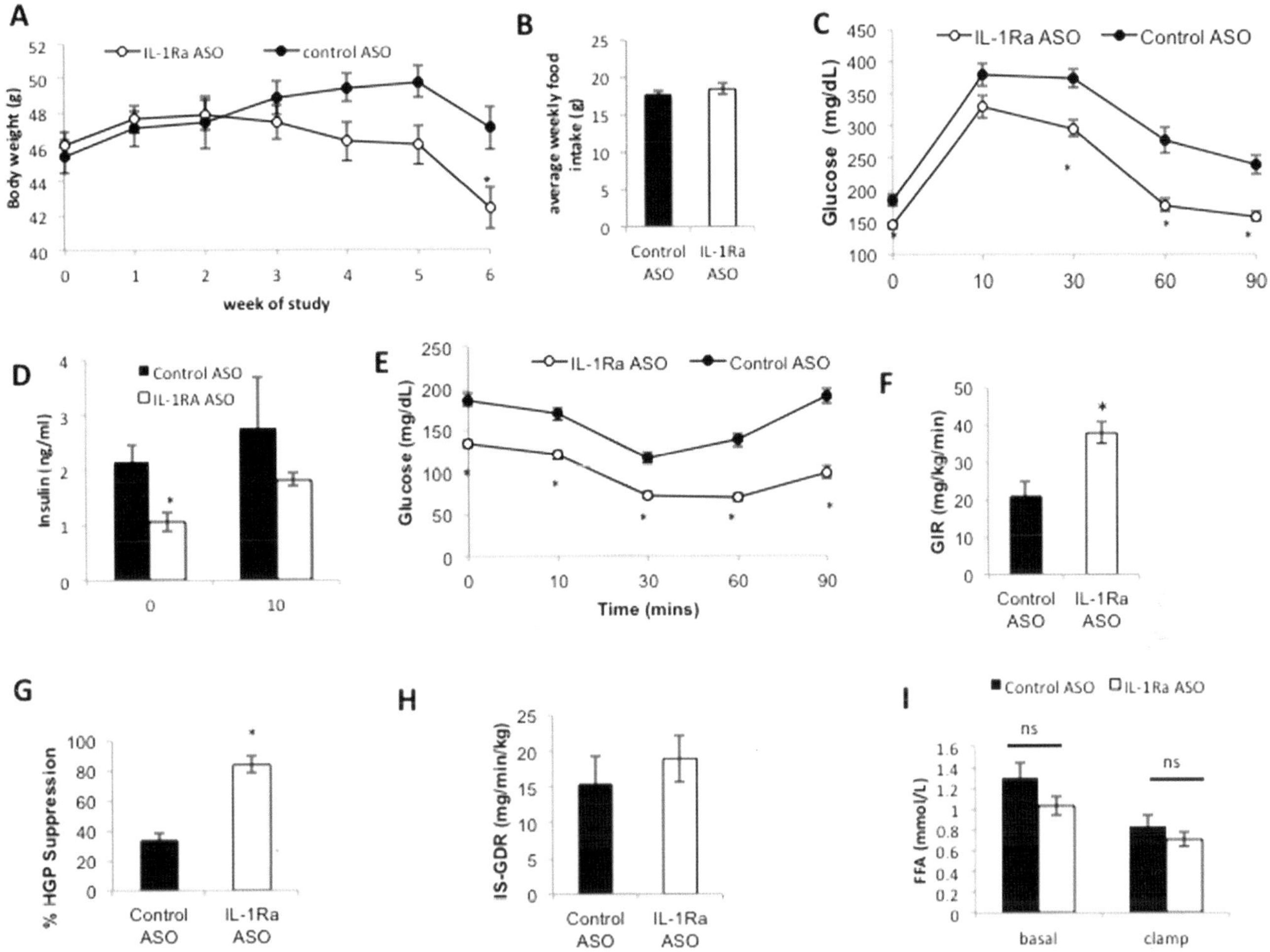

Figure 2. IL-1Ra ASO treatment in HFD-fed obese mice results in decreased body weight (A) despite similar food intake (B) (food intake measured weekly and presented as average food intake over first of 4 weeks of study), improved glucose tolerance (GTT after 3 wks of treatment, treatment $p<0.0001$, time, $p<0.0001$, interaction, $p=0.0285$) (C) with lower fasting insulin levels (D) and improved insulin sensitivity (ITT at 4 wks of treatment, treatment $p<0.001$, time $p<0.0001$, interaction $p<0.0001$) (E). n = 12 mice per group, *$P<0.05$ compared with control treated mice. (F–I) Hyperinsulinemic/euglycemic clamp studies in IL-1Ra ASO treated and control treated HFD mice. F) Glucose infusion rate (GIR), G)% suppression of hepatic glucose production (HGP), H) Insulin stimulated glucose disposal rate (IS-GDR), I) Free fatty acids (FFA). A repeated measures 2-way ANOVA showed a significant effect of treatment, time and interaction in both GTT and ITT experiments. A students t-test was used to asses significance between groups (GIR,% suppression and IS-GDR), a 2-way ANOVA with post hoc Sidak test showed no significant effect on FFA concentration between treatment groups, but a significant effect within groups between basal and clamped samples. n = 5–8 mice per group, * $p<0.05$ compared to HFD-fed control treated group; ns, not significant.

~97% ($p<0.05$) in the liver and 63% ($p=0.2$) in epididymal fat (Fig. 1D) but was not changed in many other tissues (figure S1A). Furthermore, circulating levels of IL-1Ra were reduced by approximately 50% by IL-1Ra ASO treatment compared with control ASO treatment, to similar levels found in normal chow fed, lean mice (Fig. 1E). Circulating levels of other inflammatory mediators including MCP-1, TNF-α and IL-6 were not different between groups (figure S1C), suggesting IL-1Ra ASO treatment did not activate the innate immune system. Importantly, ASO treatment did not cause liver toxicity, as no difference was observed in the circulating levels of liver enzymes alanine aminotransferase (ALT), aspartate aminotransferase (AST) and glutamate dehydrogenase (GDH) after 6 weeks of treatment in HFD-fed obese mice (Fig 1F).

Effect of IL-1Ra knock-down on body weight and insulin resistance in obese-insulin resistant mice

In vivo, IL-1Ra ASO treatment of HFD-fed obese mice resulted in weight loss from approximately 4 weeks of treatment and after 6 weeks of treatment IL-1Ra ASO treated mice were significantly lighter than control ASO treated (Fig. 2*A*), despite no significant difference in food intake (Fig. 2*B*). IL-1Ra ASO treatment resulted in significant improvements in glucose tolerance (Fig. 2*C*, figure *S2B*), largely due to a decrease in basal glucose, as when calculated as percentage change in glucose from initial levels the effect is less pronounced (figure S2A), IL-1Ra ASO treatment reduced fasting insulin (Fig. 2*D*), and improved insulin sensitivity as assessed by an insulin tolerance test (Fig. 2*E* and figure S2C, D).

Despite the differences observed in body weight in the whole cohort we were able to select a subgroup of body weight matched mice (average BW 44 g) from the lighter control ASO treated mice and heavier IL-1Ra ASO-treated mice to study body weight

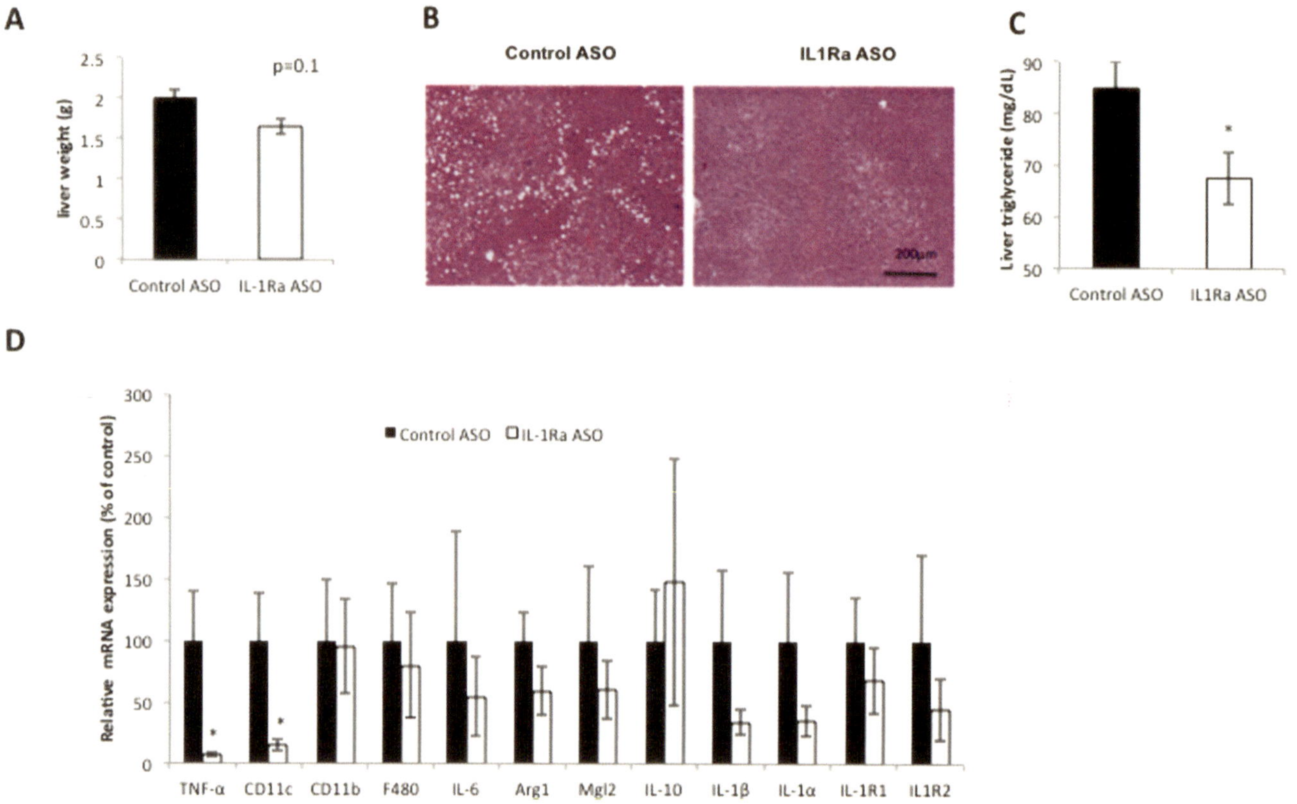

Figure 3. IL1Ra ASO treatment reduces liver triglyceride and improved liver inflammation. A) Liver weight (g), B) H&E stain of liver. C) Liver triglyceride content after 6 weeks of IL-1Ra ASO or control ASO treatment in HFD fed mice. D) QPCR analysis of inflammatory gene expression in the liver of obese mice treated with IL-1Ra ASO or control ASO, results are normalized to beta actin mRNA and expressed relative to control ASO treatment. * $p<0.05$ compared to HFD-fed control treated group, $n=5-8$ mice per group.

independent effects on insulin sensitivity. We performed hyperinsulinemic- euglycemic clamp studies in this body weight matched, HFD-fed, obese cohort of mice ($n=6-7$ per group) (Fig. *2F–I*) to determine which insulin target tissue was responsible for the systemic improvements in insulin sensitivity. These clamp experiments confirmed that the IL-1Ra ASO treated mice have improved systemic insulin sensitivity (Fig. *2F*) that was the result of improved insulin-mediated suppression of hepatic glucose production (Fig. *2G*). No significant difference in insulin sensitivity was observed in muscle (as measured by the insulin-stimulated glucose disposal rate; Fig. *2H*) or adipose tissue (as measured by suppression of plasma FFA concentration; Fig. *2I*). These studies demonstrate that IL-1Ra expression levels play an important role in modulating insulin sensitivity. These clamp results show that, reduced expression of IL-1Ra had beneficial effects to improve hepatic insulin sensitivity as well as systemic insulin sensitivity.

Effect of IL-1Ra ASO treatment in the liver of obese-insulin resistant mice

IL-1Ra ASO treated mice had slightly lighter liver weights ($p=0.1$), significantly reduced triglyceride levels (Fig. *3B,C*). Expression of proinflammatory cytokine tumor necrosis factor alpha (TNF-α) and proinflammatory macrophage marker (CD11c) genes were also significantly reduced (Fig. *3D*), indicating that IL-1Ra ASO treatment results in decreased liver inflammation in HFD- fed mice. These studies were conducted in weight matched obese mice and so IL-1Ra ASO mediated improvement in liver triglyceride levels and reduced inflammation are independent of changes in body weight. Analysis of expression of hepatic gluconeogenic genes after IL-1Ra ASO treatment revealed a slight reduction in PEPCK mRNA but no change in G6Pase (figure S1B).

Effect of IL-1Ra ASO treatment on energy expenditure in obese-insulin resistant mice

The observation that IL-1Ra ASO treatment in obese mice resulted in a decrease in body weight (Fig. 2A) without associated differences in food intake (Fig. *2B*) prompted us to measure the effects of treatment on energy expenditure. IL-1Ra ASO treatment for four weeks in obese mice resulted in an increase in oxygen consumption (Fig. *4A*), and a significant increase in energy expenditure (Fig. *4B*), specifically in the dark cycle. Evaluation of core body temperature (CBT) in the IL-1Ra ASO treated mice revealed an increase in CBT (Fig. *4C*) that was not dependent on changes in locomotor activity (Fig. *4D*). The increase in CBT independent of activity suggests that IL-1Ra ASO treatment may have additional effects driving increased thermogenesis. Indeed, quantitative PCR analysis revealed that transcript levels of *Ucp-1* are increased in the BAT of IL-1Ra ASO treated mice (Fig. 4E).

Effect of IL-1Ra ASO treatment on adipose tissue

Chronic IL-1Ra ASO treatment (for 6 weeks) in obese mice results in decreased body weight (Fig. 5A), and decreased weight of the epididymal fat (eWAT) (Fig. 5B). We observed a significant decrease in adipocyte cell size (Fig. 5C,D,E) consistent with reduction in adipocyte cell size noted in whole body IL-1Ra KO

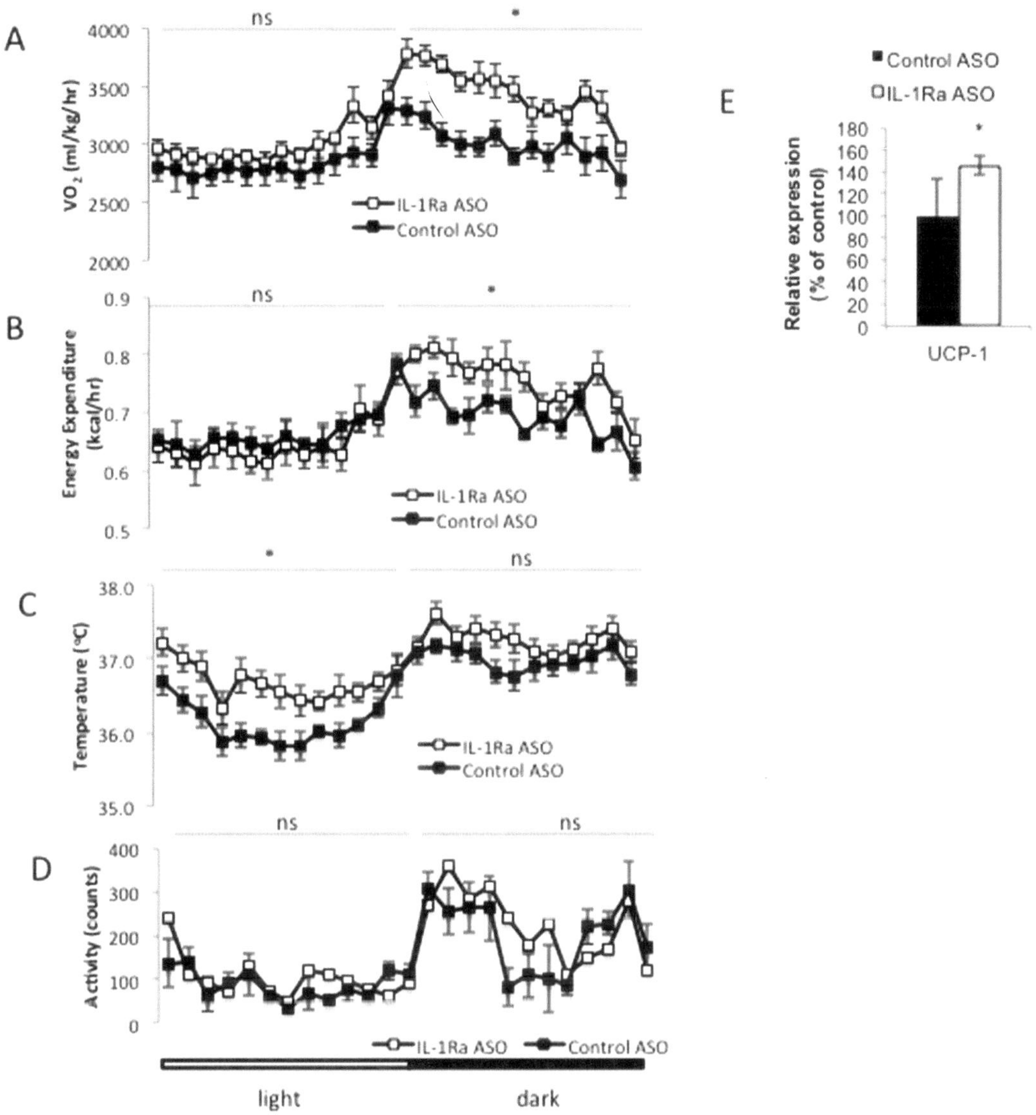

Figure 4. IL-1Ra ASO treatment results in increased energy expenditure. Oxygen consumption (A) and energy expenditure (B) were measured in CLAMS cages over a 48 hr period in week 4 of the study. core body temperature (C) in HFD-fed IL-1Ra ASO treated mice compared with control ASO treated mice. D) Activity is unchanged between groups. E) Quantitative PCR analysis of uncoupling protein 1 (UCP-1) in BAT. * $p<0.05$ compared to HFD-fed control treated group, n = 5 mice per group, ns, not significant.

mice [23]. Expression of proinflammatory markers in adipose tissue was not significantly different in IL-1Ra ASO compared with control ASO treated mice (Fig. 5F).

Effects of IL-1Ra not mediated through Interleukin 1 Receptor 1 (IL-1R1)

To determine if the improvements in insulin sensitivity observed were through the actions of IL-1Ra signaling at IL-1R1 we treated HFD-fed IL-1R1 KO mice with IL-1Ra ASO. Body weight (Fig. 6*A*) and food intake (Fig. 6*B*) were not significantly different between IL-1R1 KO mice treated with IL-1Ra ASO or control ASO. We observed significant improvements in glucose tolerance (GTT, Fig. 6C) and insulin sensitivity (ITT, Fig. 6D) in the IL-1R1 KO treated with IL-1Ra ASO. However, when plotted as percentage change from basal (figure S2 E,G) or as area under the curve (figure S2 F,H) the effects of IL-1Ra ASO treatment in IL-1R1 KO mice were less pronounced. The liver of IL-1R1 KO mice treated with IL-1Ra ASO was significantly lighter than control treated IL-1R1 KO mice (Fig. 6E) and showed less steatosis (Fig. 6F) and significantly reduced inflammation (Fig. 6G). The improved glucose tolerance and reduced liver inflammation observed after IL-1Ra ASO treatment in IL-1R1 KO mice (similar to that observed in WT, diet induced obese mice treated with IL-1Ra ASO) confirm that these insulin sensitizing effects are independent of signaling at the IL-1R1 and occur through an alternate mechanism.

Discussion

IL-1Ra is up-regulated during diet-induced obesity [21] and both adipose tissue and the liver are major sources of IL-1Ra [20,29]. Previous studies have reported that IL-1Ra may play a role in the development of insulin resistance [14–20]. To determine whether decreasing systemic IL-1Ra levels in obesity has therapeutic potential, we treated HFD-fed obese mice with

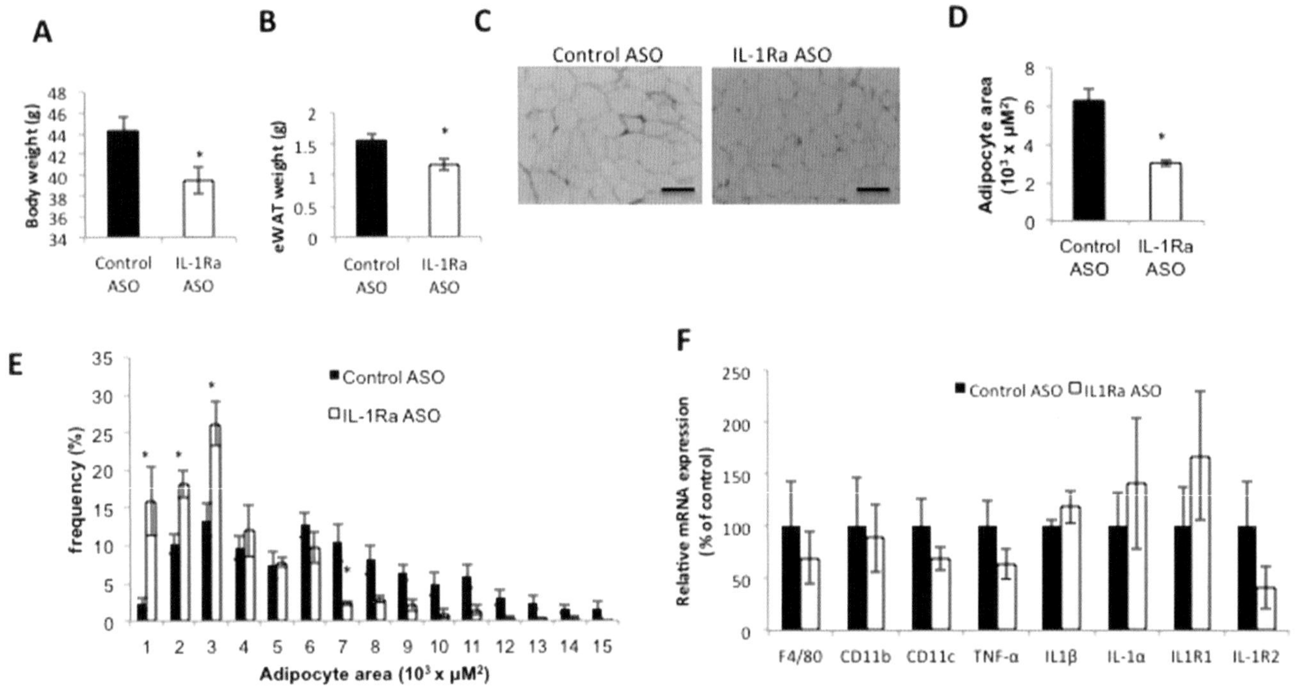

Figure 5. IL-1Ra ASO treatment effect on adipose tissue. After 6 weeks of treatment with IL-1Ra ASO mice have A) significantly reduced body weight, and B) reduced epididymal fat mass. C) H&E staining of visceral adipose tissue shows reduced adipocyte cell size. Scale bars =50 μm. Representative figures are presented from the analyses of five different mice per group. D) Quantification of average adipocyte cell area E) Histogram of adipocyte area in control treated mice (black bars), IL-1Ra ASO treated mice (white bars), using Image Gauge software, version 4 (FujiFilm). (n = 5 mice per group), F) QPCR analysis of inflammatory gene expression in adipose tissue. * $p<0.05$ compared to HFD-fed control treated group, n = 5−8 mice per group.

antisense oligonucleotides (ASOs) resulting in 50% reduction in the systemic concentration of IL-1Ra, to similar levels measured in age matched, lean normal chow fed mice. The extent of reduction in expression levels is comparable with may other published reports on the use of locked nucleic acid ASOs to inhibit gene expression [30–33]. We report for the first time that normalization of IL-1Ra by antisense-mediated knock-down of IL-1Ra expression improves hepatic insulin sensitivity and decreases body weight in diet induced obese mice. Importantly, studies in IL-1R1 KO mice revealed that the IL-1Ra ASO mediated improvement in insulin sensitivity was independent of IL-1R1.

Differences in body weight and the degree of obesity strongly impact insulin action. An important finding was that in HFD-fed mice, IL-1Ra ASO treatment not only improved insulin action, but also reduced body weight by ~10% after 6 weeks of treatment. Thus, it is possible that improvement in insulin sensitivity in IL-1Ra ASO-treated mice was simply due to the lower body weight. To address this confounding variable we performed detailed measurements of whole-body and tissue specific insulin action using hyperinsulinemic-euglycemic clamps in body weight matched mice using the lighter control ASO treated mice and heavier IL 1Ra ASO treated mice in the cohort. Significantly, our results revealed that the improvements in whole-body insulin sensitivity were independent of changes in body weight. In addition, these improvements were due to significantly enhanced hepatic insulin sensitivity, with no improvements in muscle or adipose insulin sensitivity. Furthermore, inflammatory gene expression (TNF-α and CD11c) and triglyceride levels were also significantly and specifically reduced in the liver of IL-1Ra ASO treated mice compared with control treated HFD mice.

The balance of IL-1β and IL-1Ra is particularly important [9] and as IL-1β expression increases with obesity it induces the expression of IL-1Ra [20]. IL-1Ra and IL-1β share conserved sequences that allow them to both bind to the IL-1R1 but also have areas of low sequence and structural similarity which mediate their distinct biologic activities [34]. We measured IL-1Ra and IL-1β mRNA expression and noted no significant difference in IL-1β expression in liver or adipose tissue of mice treated with IL-1Ra ASO compared with control ASO suggesting IL-1Ra knockdown was specific and did not have off-target effects on IL-1β.

Importantly, we show that these insulin sensitizing effects are not mediated through the IL-1R1 as antisense knock-down of IL-1Ra in mice lacking the IL-1R1 still show improved insulin sensitivity. Although the receptor through which IL-1Ra exerts these effects in the liver remains to be identified, other studies have also reported that IL-1Ra has agonist effects at another receptor other than IL-1R1 [35,36]. For example, Loscher et al (2003) show that incubation of IL-1Ra with synaptosomes from IL-1R1 KO resulted in decreased glutamate release while IL-1β had no effect, thus demonstrating that IL-1Ra can also signal through an alternate receptor other than the IL-1R1 [36]. At high concentrations, as found in obesity, IL-1Ra could have deleterious effects independent of IL-1R1 since IL-1R1 KO mice display improved insulin sensitivity after IL-1Ra knock-down.

Targeted IL-1 therapy is a major focus point of current anti-inflammatory approaches in the treatment of type 2 diabetes [37]. Therapeutics targeting IL-1 signaling are based on the selective blockade of IL-1R1 activation with either IL-1Ra or specific neutralizing antibodies to IL-1β, which result in lower blood glucose levels and improves β-cell secretory function [10,38]. However, clinical studies have revealed that although anti-

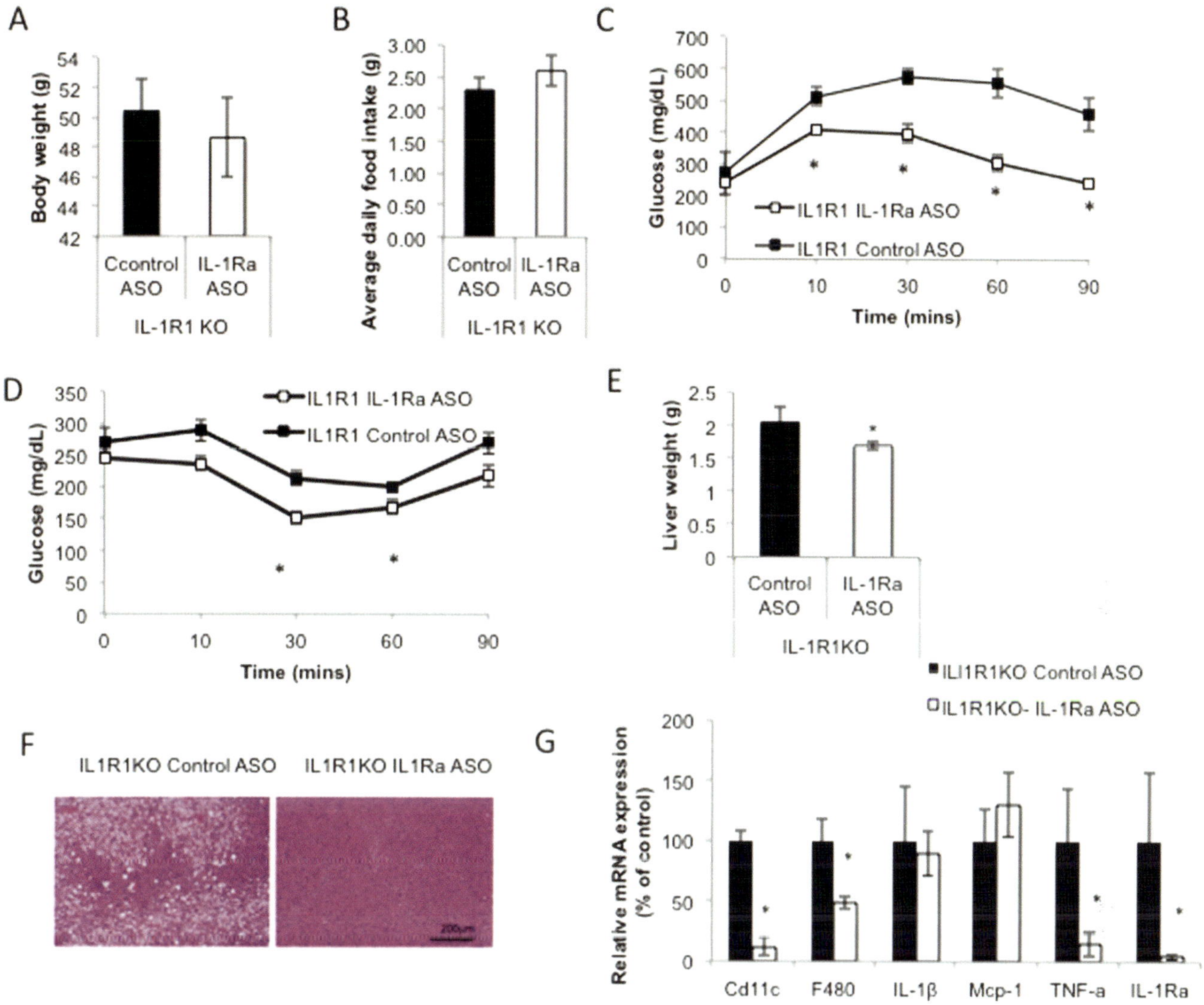

Figure 6. IL-1Ra ASO treatment improves glucose tolerance and insulin sensitivity independent of IL-1R1 signaling. A) Body weight, B) Average food intake, (measured weekly for 6 weeks). C. GTT after 5 weeks of treatment, (treatment $p<0.035$ time $p<0.0001$, interaction, 0.5554), D. ITT after 5.5 wks of treatment, (treatment $p<0.0188$, time $p<0.0001$, interaction $p=0.0058$). E) Liver weight, F) H&E stain of liver, G) QPCR analysis of inflammatory gene expression, in IL-1R1KO mice fed with HFD for 12 weeks and then treated with IL-1Ra ASO or control ASO for 6 weeks, ($n=4$ mice per group, * $p<0.05$ compared to HFD-fed control treated group). A repeated measures 2-way ANOVA was used to compare the effect of IL-1Ra ASO and Control ASO on GTT and ITT experiments.

inflammatory treatment of type 2 diabetic patients with recombinant IL-1Ra (Anakinra) produced modest reductions in glycated hemoglobin, no difference in insulin sensitivity was observed compared with placebo [12,13]. We propose that this can be explained by the tissue specific effects of IL-1Ra on the development of insulin resistance.

Previous studies have demonstrated an important interplay between IL-1 signaling, energy homeostasis and body weight regulation. For example, IL-1R1 deficient mice develop mature onset obesity [39,40] while IL-1Ra KO mice are leaner than their littermates [22,23]. High levels of IL-1Ra may be linked to the development of obesity-induced leptin resistance, as direct injection of IL-1Ra to the cerebral ventricle can inhibit the suppressive effects of leptin on food intake and blunt leptin mediated increase in core body temperature [14,41]. Interestingly, we found that IL-1Ra ASO treatment decreased body weight of HFD-fed, obese mice, despite similar food intake and thus is unlikely to have affected appetite. Our energy expenditure data suggest that the leaner body weight is at least in part due to higher oxygen consumption, as well as a higher CBT. IL-1Ra knock-down in HFD-fed mice resembles the phenotype previously observed in IL-1Ra KO mice, whom display increased energy expenditure, increased oxygen consumption and higher CBT [22,23,42]. The reasons for these effects on energy expenditure could be due, in part, to the noted up-regulation of UCP1 in BAT in IL-1Ra-ASO treated HFD mice and the pyrogenic effects of IL-1β [43].

In summary, we show that normalization of IL-1Ra improves insulin sensitivity in obese, insulin resistant mice. This mechanism is independent of the classical IL-1R1 signaling and we hypothesize that at high concentrations, as observed in chronic obesity, IL-1Ra also binds to another, yet to be identified, receptor and drives the development of hepatic insulin resistance. These findings have important consequences in current and future anti-inflammatory approaches in the treatment of Type 2 diabetes.

Supporting Information

Figure S1 A. QPCR analysis of IL-1Ra expression after 6 wks of treatment in various tissues, B. QPCR analysis of Glucose 6-phosphatase(G6Pase) and PCK1 liver expression in IL-1a ASO and control ASO treated mice after 6 wks of treatment. C. Plasma concentration of Interleukin 10 (IL-10), Interleukin 1 beta (IL-1β), Interleukin 6 (IL-6), Monocyte chemotactic protein 1 (MCP-1) and Tumor necrosis factor alpha (TNF-α) after 6 weeks of IL-1Ra ASO or control ASO treatment.

Figure S2 A–D: GTT and ITT in WT IL1Ra ASO or control ASO treated mice. A) GTT, presented as % change from initial blood glucose (Treatment $p = 0.5084$, Time $p < 0.0001$, Interaction $p = 0.0103$), B) Area under the curve for GTT, C) ITT presented as % change from initial blood glucose, (Treatment $p = 0.0034$, Time $p < 0.0001$, Interaction, $p < 0.0001$) D) Area under the curve for ITT. E–H, GTT and ITT in IL-1R1 KO mice treated with IL-1Ra or control ASO E) GTT, presented as % change from initial blood glucose, (Treatment $p = 0.274$, Time $p < 0.0001$, Interaction, $p = 0.0219$. F) Area under the curve for GTT, G) ITT, presented as % change from initial blood glucose ASO (Treatment $p = 0.2169$, Time $p < 0.0001$, Interaction, $p = 0.1212$. H) Area under the curve for ITT.

Table S1 Primer information.

Acknowledgments

This work was supported by the National Institutes of Health (NIH) grants: DK-033651, DK-074868, T32-DK-007494, DK-063491 and from a grant from Pfizer Inc. MM is a postdoctoral fellow supported by the Flemish Research Foundation (FWO). The authors thank Dr. Tamas Bartfai (The Scripps Research Institute) and Dr. Jerrold M. Olefsky (University of California, San Diego) for guidance.

Author Contributions

Conceived and designed the experiments: HH DB OO. Performed the experiments: NF SN MM. Analyzed the data: OO. Contributed reagents/materials/analysis tools: HH DB ST. Wrote the paper: OO SS.

References

1. Moller DE, Kaufman KD (2005) Metabolic syndrome: a clinical and molecular perspective. Annu Rev Med 56: 45–62.
2. Gregor MF, Hotamisligil GS (2011) Inflammatory mechanisms in obesity. Annu Rev Immunol 29: 415–445.
3. Lumeng CN, Saltiel AR (2011) Inflammatory links between obesity and metabolic disease. J Clin Invest 121: 2111–2117.
4. Dinarello CA (1996) Biologic basis for interleukin-1 in disease. Blood 87: 2095–2147.
5. Greenfeder SA, Nunes P, Kwee L, Labow M, Chizzonite RA, et al. (1995) Molecular cloning and characterization of a second subunit of the interleukin 1 receptor complex. J Biol Chem 270: 13757–13765.
6. Martin MU, Wesche H (2002) Summary and comparison of the signaling mechanisms of the Toll/interleukin-1 receptor family. Biochim Biophys Acta 1592: 265–280.
7. Arend WP (1990) Interleukin-1 receptor antagonist: discovery, structure and properties. Prog Growth Factor Res 2: 193–205.
8. Arend WP, Malyak M, Guthridge CJ, Gabay C (1998) Interleukin-1 receptor antagonist: role in biology. Annu Rev Immunol 16: 27–55.
9. Arend WP (2002) The balance between IL-1 and IL-1Ra in disease. Cytokine Growth Factor Rev 13: 323–340.
10. Osborn O, Brownell SE, Sanchez-Alavez M, Salomon D, Gram H, et al. (2008) Treatment with an Interleukin 1 beta antibody improves glycemic control in diet-induced obesity. Cytokine 44: 141–148.
11. Sauter NS, Schulthess FT, Galasso R, Castellani LW, Maedler K (2008) The antiinflammatory cytokine interleukin-1 receptor antagonist protects from high-fat diet-induced hyperglycemia. Endocrinology 149: 2208–2218.
12. Larsen CM, Faulenbach M, Vaag A, Volund A, Ehses JA, et al. (2007) Interleukin-1-receptor antagonist in type 2 diabetes mellitus. N Engl J Med 356: 1517–1526.
13. van Asseldonk EJ, Stienstra R, Koenen TB, Joosten LA, Netea MG, et al. (2011) Treatment with Anakinra improves disposition index but not insulin sensitivity in nondiabetic subjects with the metabolic syndrome: a randomized, double-blind, placebo-controlled study. J Clin Endocrinol Metab 96: 2119–2126.
14. Meier CA, Bobbioni E, Gabay C, Assimacopoulos-Jeannet F, Golay A, et al. (2002) IL-1 receptor antagonist serum levels are increased in human obesity: a possible link to the resistance to leptin? J Clin Endocrinol Metab 87: 1184–1188.
15. Herder C, Brunner EJ, Rathmann W, Strassburger K, Tabak AG, et al. (2009) Elevated levels of the anti-inflammatory interleukin-1 receptor antagonist precede the onset of type 2 diabetes: the Whitehall II study. Diabetes Care 32: 421–423.
16. Saltevo J, Laakso M, Jokelainen J, Keinanen-Kiukaanniemi S, Kumpusalo E, et al. (2008) Levels of adiponectin, C-reactive protein and interleukin-1 receptor antagonist are associated with insulin sensitivity: a population-based study. Diabetes Metab Res Rev 24: 378–383.
17. Carstensen M, Herder C, Kivimaki M, Jokela M, Roden M, et al. (2010) Accelerated increase in serum interleukin-1 receptor antagonist starts 6 years before diagnosis of type 2 diabetes: Whitehall II prospective cohort study. Diabetes 59: 1222–1227.
18. Salomaa V, Havulinna A, Saarela O, Zeller T, Jousilahti P, et al. (2010) Thirty-one novel biomarkers as predictors for clinically incident diabetes. PLoS One 5: e10100.
19. Halvorsen B, Heggen E, Ueland T, Smith C, Sandberg WJ, et al. (2010) Treatment with the PPARgamma agonist rosiglitazone downregulates interleukin-1 receptor antagonist in individuals with metabolic syndrome. Eur J Endocrinol 162: 267–273.
20. Juge-Aubry CE, Somm E, Giusti V, Pernin A, Chicheportiche R, et al. (2003) Adipose tissue is a major source of interleukin-1 receptor antagonist: upregulation in obesity and inflammation. Diabetes 52: 1104–1110.
21. Somm E, Cettour-Rose P, Asensio C, Charollais A, Klein M, et al. (2006) Interleukin-1 receptor antagonist is upregulated during diet-induced obesity and regulates insulin sensitivity in rodents. Diabetologia 49: 387–393.
22. Matsuki T, Horai R, Sudo K, Iwakura Y (2003) IL-1 plays an important role in lipid metabolism by regulating insulin levels under physiological conditions. J Exp Med 198: 877–888.
23. Somm E, Henrichot E, Pernin A, Juge-Aubry CE, Muzzin P, et al. (2005) Decreased fat mass in interleukin-1 receptor antagonist-deficient mice: impact on adipogenesis, food intake, and energy expenditure. Diabetes 54: 3503–3509.
24. Stanton R, Sciabola S, Salatto C, Weng Y, Moshinsky D, et al. (2012) Chemical modification study of antisense gapmers. Nucleic Acid Ther 22: 344–359.
25. Oh DY, Talukdar S, Bae EJ, Imamura T, Morinaga H, et al. (2010) GPR120 is an omega-3 fatty acid receptor mediating potent anti-inflammatory and insulin-sensitizing effects. Cell 142: 687–698.
26. Steele R, Wall JS, De Bodo RC, Altszuler N (1956) Measurement of size and turnover rate of body glucose pool by the isotope dilution method. Am J Physiol 187: 15–24.
27. Sanchez-Alavez M, Osborn O, Tabarean IV, Holmberg KH, Eberwine J, et al. (2011) Insulin-like growth factor 1-mediated hyperthermia involves anterior hypothalamic insulin receptors. J Biol Chem 286: 14983–14990.
28. Yoshizaki T, Milne JC, Imamura T, Schenk S, Sonoda N, et al. (2009) SIRT1 exerts anti-inflammatory effects and improves insulin sensitivity in adipocytes. Mol Cell Biol 29: 1363–1374.
29. Gabay C, Smith MF, Eidlen D, Arend WP (1997) Interleukin 1 receptor antagonist (IL-1Ra) is an acute-phase protein. J Clin Invest 99: 2930–2940.
30. Di Martino MT, Gulla A, Gallo Cantafio ME, Altomare E, Amodio N, et al. (2014) In vitro and in vivo activity of a novel locked nucleic acid (LNA)-inhibitor-miR-221 against multiple myeloma cells. PLoS One 9: e89659.
31. Gupta N, Fisker N, Asselin MC, Lindholm M, Rosenbohm C, et al. (2010) A locked nucleic acid antisense oligonucleotide (LNA) silences PCSK9 and enhances LDLR expression in vitro and in vivo. PLoS One 5: e10682.
32. Koch T, Rosenbohm C, Hansen HF, Hansen B, Straarup EM, et al. (2008) Locked Nucleic Acid: Properties and Therapeutic Aspects. Therapeutic Oligonucleotides: 103–141.
33. Moschos SA, Frick M, Taylor B, Turnpenny P, Graves H, et al. (2011) Uptake, efficacy, and systemic distribution of naked, inhaled short interfering RNA (siRNA) and locked nucleic acid (LNA) antisense. Mol Ther 19: 2163–2168.
34. Boraschi D, Bossu P, Ruggiero P, Tagliabue A, Bertini R, et al. (1995) Mapping of receptor binding sites on IL-1 beta by reconstruction of IL-1ra-like domains. J Immunol 155: 4719–4725.
35. Boutin H, Kimber I, Rothwell NJ, Pinteaux E (2003) The expanding interleukin-1 family and its receptors: do alternative IL-1 receptor/signaling pathways exist in the brain? Molecular Neurobiology 27: 239–248.

36. Loscher CE, Mills KH, Lynch MA (2003) Interleukin-1 receptor antagonist exerts agonist activity in the hippocampus independent of the interleukin-1 type I receptor. J Neuroimmunol 137: 117–124.
37. Donath MY, Shoelson SE (2011) Type 2 diabetes as an inflammatory disease. Nat Rev Immunol 11: 98–107.
38. Owyang AM, Maedler K, Gross L, Yin J, Esposito L, et al. (2010) XOMA 052, an anti-IL-1{beta} monoclonal antibody, improves glucose control and {beta}-cell function in the diet-induced obesity mouse model. Endocrinology 151: 2515–2527.
39. Garcia MC, Wernstedt I, Berndtsson A, Enge M, Bell M, et al. (2006) Mature-onset obesity in interleukin-1 receptor I knockout mice. Diabetes 55: 1205–1213.
40. McGillicuddy FC, Harford KA, Reynolds CM, Oliver E, Claessens M, et al. (2011) Lack of interleukin-1 receptor I (IL-1RI) protects mice from high-fat diet-induced adipose tissue inflammation coincident with improved glucose homeostasis. Diabetes 60: 1688–1698.
41. Luheshi GN, Gardner JD, Rushforth DA, Loudon AS, Rothwell NJ (1999) Leptin actions on food intake and body temperature are mediated by IL-1. Proc Natl Acad Sci U S A 96: 7047–7052.
42. Chida D, Hashimoto O, Kuwahara M, Sagara H, Osaka T, et al. (2008) Increased fat: carbohydrate oxidation ratio in Il1ra (-/-) mice on a high-fat diet is associated with increased sympathetic tone. Diabetologia 51: 1698–1706.
43. Luheshi GN (1998) Cytokines and fever. Mechanisms and sites of action. Ann N Y Acad Sci 856: 83–89.

15

Combined Vildagliptin and Metformin Exert Better Cardioprotection than Monotherapy against Ischemia-Reperfusion Injury in Obese-Insulin Resistant Rats

Nattayaporn Apaijai[1,2], Kroekkiat Chinda[1,2], Siripong Palee[1,5], Siriporn Chattipakorn[1,3], Nipon Chattipakorn[1,2,4]*

1 Cardiac Electrophysiology Research and Training Center, Faculty of Medicine, Chiang Mai University, Chiang Mai, Thailand, **2** Cardiac Electrophysiology Unit, Department of Physiology, Faculty of Medicine, Chiang Mai University, Chiang Mai, Thailand, **3** Department of Oral Biology and Diagnostic Sciences, Faculty of Dentistry, Chiang Mai University, Chiang Mai, Thailand, **4** Biomedical Engineering Center, Chiang Mai University, Chiang Mai, Thailand, **5** School of Medicine, Mae FahLuang University, Chiang Rai, Thailand

Abstract

Background: Obese-insulin resistance caused by long-term high-fat diet (HFD) consumption is associated with left ventricular (LV) dysfunction and increased risk of myocardial infarction. Metformin and vildagliptin have been shown to exert cardioprotective effects. However, the effect of these drugs on the hearts under obese-insulin resistance with ischemia-reperfusion (I/R) injury is unclear. We hypothesized that combined vildagliptin and metformin provide better protective effects against I/R injury than monotherapy in obese-insulin resistant rats.

Methodology: Male Wistar rats were fed either HFD or normal diet. Rats in each diet group were divided into 4 subgroups to receive vildagliptin, metformin, combined vildagliptin and metformin, or saline for 21 days. Ischemia due to left anterior descending artery ligation was allowed for 30-min, followed by 120-min reperfusion. Metabolic parameters, heart rate variability (HRV), LV function, infarct size, mitochondrial function, calcium transient, Bax and Bcl-2, and Connexin 43 (Cx43) were determined. Rats developed insulin resistance after 12 weeks of HFD consumption. Vildagliptin, metformin, and combined drugs improved metabolic parameters, HRV, and LV function. During I/R, all treatments improved LV function, reduced infarct size and Bax, increased Bcl-2, and improved mitochondrial function in HFD rats. However, only combined drugs delayed the time to the first VT/VF onset, reduced arrhythmia score and mortality rate, and increased p-Cx43 in HFD rats.

Conclusion: Although both vildagliptin and metformin improved insulin resistance and attenuate myocardial injury caused by I/R, combined drugs provided better outcomes than single therapy by reducing arrhythmia score and mortality rate.

Editor: Shang-Zhong Xu, University of Hull, United Kingdom

Funding: This work was supported by the Thailand Research Fund RTA5580006 (NC), BRG (SC), the Thailand Research Fund Royal Golden Jubilee Program (NC and NA), and the Chiang Mai University Excellent Center Award (NC). Vildagliptin was kindly provided by Novartis (Thailand). The funders had no role in study design, data collection and analysis, decision to publish, or preparation of the manuscript.

Competing Interests: This work was supported by the Thailand Research Fund RTA5580006 (NC), BRG (SC), the Thailand Research Fund Royal Golden Jubilee Program (NC and NA), and the Chiang Mai University Excellent Center Award (NC). Vildagliptin was kindly provided by Novartis (Thailand). These funders had no role in study design, data collection and analysis, decision to publish, or preparation of the manuscript.

* Email: nchattip@gmail.com

Introduction

Long-term high-fat diet consumption is known to cause obesity, insulin resistance, and cardiac dysfunction [1], and have been shown to increase the risk of having ischemic heart disease [2]. While revascularization is the goal of myocardial ischemia treatment, reperfusion therapy is known to induce reperfusion injury and lead to greater myocardial damage. This adverse effect has been shown to be even more severe in obese insulin resistance, resulting in increased infarct size and increased myocardial susceptibility to ischemia-reperfusion (I/R) injury [3,4]. I/R injury has been shown to associate with fatal cardiac arrhythmias [5]. Cardiac mitochondrial damage has been implicated as one of the major factors responsible for myocardial cell death from I/R injury [6]. Several lines of evidence showed that increased intracellular and mitochondrial calcium accumulation can trigger cell apoptosis [6,7]. Previous studies also demonstrated that decreased Connexin 43 (Cx43), the principal gap junction protein, is found in acute myocardial infarction [8]. Many studies demonstrated that loss of Cx43expression in the heart could result in a markedly increase in incidence of arrhythmia [9,10].

Several anti-diabetic drugs including dipeptidyl peptidase 4 (DPP-4) inhibitors and metformin have been shown to exert cardioprotective effects in addition to their glycemic control [11,12]. A recent study reported the beneficial effects of combined DPP-4 inhibitor and metformin on metabolic parameters in type 2

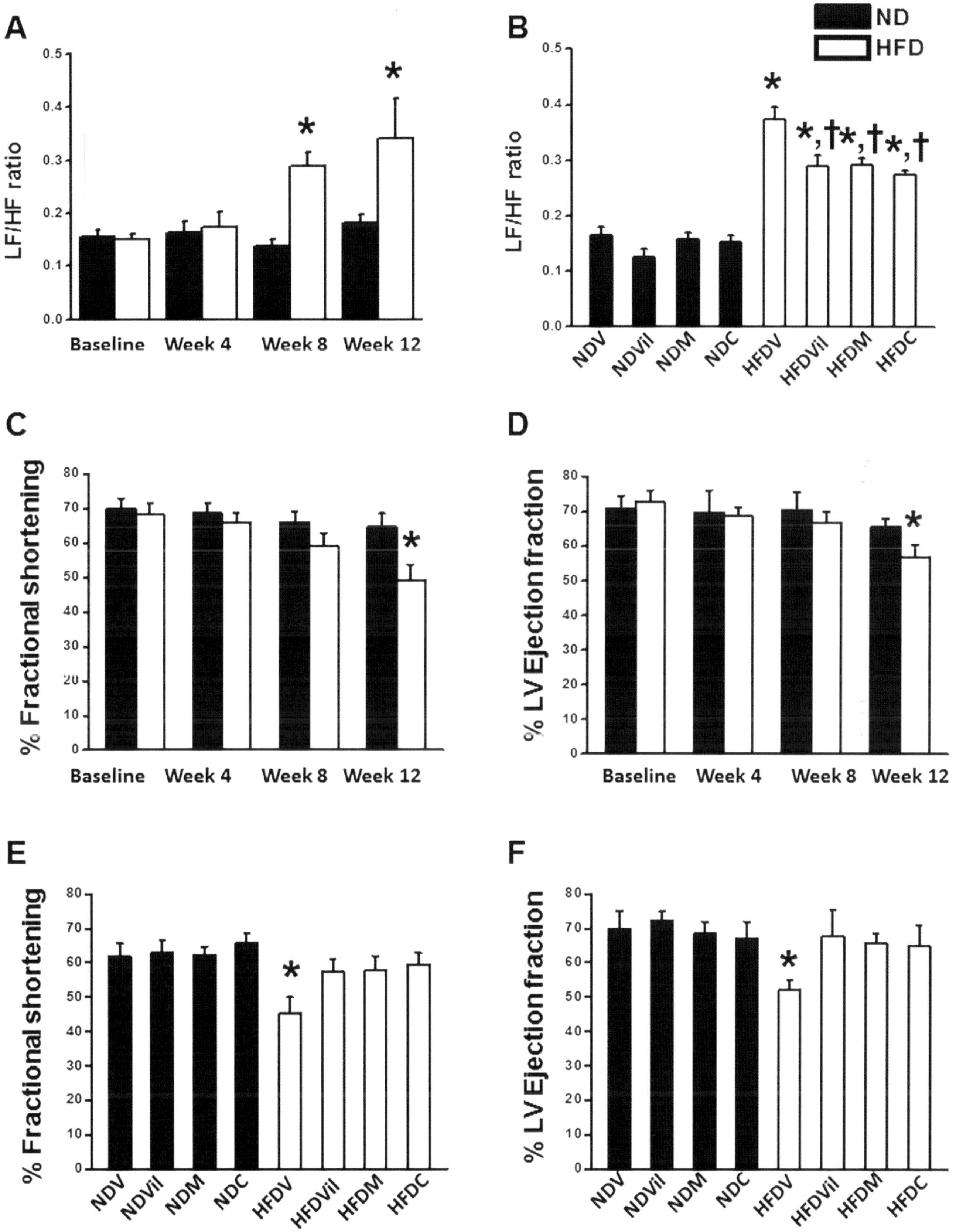

Figure 1. Effects of HFD consumption, vildagliptin, metformin, and combined drugs on HRV and echocardiographic parameters. (A) The LF/HF ratio was increased at week 8th and week 12th of HFD consumption.*$p<0.05$ vs. baseline, n = 11/group. (B) Vildagliptin, metformin, and combined drugs reduced the LF/HF ratio in HFD rats. *$p<0.05$ vs. NDV, †$p<0.05$ vs. HFDV, n = 11/group, (C) %FS was decreased after 12 weeks of HFD

consumption.*$p<0.05$ vs. ND, n = 11/group. (D) LVEF was decreased after 12 weeks of HFD consumption.*$p<0.05$ vs. ND, n = 11/group. (E) Vildagliptin, metformin, and combined drugs increased %FS in HFD rats. *$p<0.05$ vs. HFDV, n = 11/group. (F) Vildagliptin, metformin, and combined drugs increased LVEF in HFD rats. *$p<0.05$ vs. HFDV, n = 11/group.

diabetic patients [13]. However, the role of these drugs including combined drugs therapy on cardiac function, heart rate variability (HRV), cardiac mitochondrial function, and intracellular calcium regulation during I/R in long-term HFD-induced obese insulin resistant rats have not been investigated.

We have previously reported the protective effects of vildagliptin and metformin on metabolic parameters and LV function in obese-insulin resistant rats [14]. In the present study, we determine the effects of a DPP-4 inhibitor vildagliptin, metformin, and combined drugs on the hearts of obese-insulin resistant rats underwent I/R injury. We hypothesized that vildagliptin and metformin provide cardioprotective effects against I/R injury in obese-insulin resistant rats, and we demonstrate that combined drugs exert better cardioprotection than either single drug regimen.

Materials and Methods

Animals and diet

All experiments in this study were approved by the Faculty of Medicine, Chiang Mai University Institutional Animal Care and Use Committee (Permit No. 29/2555), in compliance with NIH guidelines, and in accordance with the ARRIVE guidelines for reporting experiments involving animals [15]. Male Wistar rats weighing 180–200 g were obtained from the National Animal Center, Salaya Campus, Mahidol University, Bangkok, Thailand. Rats were allowed to acclimate for seven days and housed in 12/12 hour dark/light cycle with controlled temperature (25°C). They were divided into 2 groups to receive either normal diet (ND; a standard laboratory pelleted diet containing 19.8% energy from fat) or high-fat diet (HFD; a diet containing 59.3% energy from fat) [1,16]. Rats were fed with their diet for 15 weeks. At week 12, rats in each dietary group were divided into 4 subgroups to receive vildagliptin 3-mg/kg/day (Galvus, Novartis, Bangkok, Thailand) [14], metformin 30-mg/kg/day (Glucophage, Merkserono, Bangkok, Thailand) [14], combination of vildagliptin and metformin, or vehicle (0.9% normal saline solution in an equal volume) for another 21 days via gavage feeding. Body weight and food intake were recorded weekly, and blood samples were collected from the tail vein at baseline, 12th week, and at the end of treatment (15th week). HRV was determined at baseline, 4th week, 8thweek, 12thweek, and 15thweek (the end of pharmacological interventions).

Metabolic parameters

Plasma glucose, total cholesterol, and triglyceride levels were determined using a commercial colorimetric assay kit (Erba Diagnostics Mannheim GmbH, Mannheim, Germany) [16]. Plasma HDL level was determined using a commercial colorimetric assay kit (Biovision, California, USA) [1], and plasma LDL level was calculated using Friedewald equation [17]. Plasma insulin level was determined using a commercial sandwich ELISA kit (LINCO research, Missouri, USA) [1]. The Homeostasis Model Assesment (HOMA) index was used to assess insulin resistance. Increased HOMA index indicates a higher degree of insulin resistance [18].

Plasma and cardiac malondialdehyde (MDA) level

Plasma and cardiac MDA level was determined using high performance liquid chromatography (HPLC) based assay (Thermo scientific, Bangkok, Thailand) [1]. Plasma was mixed with H_3PO_4 and thiobarbituric acid (TBA) to produce thiobarbituric acid reactive substances (TBARS). Plasma TBARS was determined from a standard curve and reported as equivalent to the MDA concentration [1].

Heart rate variability (HRV)

Lead II electrocardiogram (ECG) was recorded for 20 minutes in conscious rats using PowerLab (AD instruments, Sydney, Australia) with Chart 5.0 program. Power spectra of R-R interval variability were obtained using Fast Fourier Transform (FFT) algorithm [1,19]. High-frequency band (HF; 0.6–3 Hz), Low-frequency band (LF; 0.2–0.6 Hz), and Very low-frequency band (VLF; below 0.2 Hz) were detected and calculated as integrals under the respective part of the power spectral density function. To minimize the effect of changes in total power on the LF and HF bands, LF and HF bands were expressed as normalized units by dividing them with the total power minus VLF [19]. LF/HF ratio was analyzed using analytical program [1]. The LF/HF ratio was considered a measure of cardiac sympathovagal balance. Increased LF/HF ratio indicated depressed HRV [19].

Echocardiography

At baseline, 4thweek, 8thweek, 12thweek, and 15th week (post-treatment), echocardiographic parameters were measured in each rat using a HP/Agilent Philips Sonos 4500 (Agilent technologies, Massachusetts, USA). An echocardiography probe was placed in gentle contact with the chest, and images were collected along the parasternal short axis of the heart [20]. M-mode echocardiography was performed at the level of the papillary muscles. %Fractional shortening (%FS) and left ventricular ejection fraction (LVEF) were determined.

Ischemia-reperfusion injury protocol

At the end of treatment, rats were subject to I/R injury protocol (Figure 1). Rats were anesthetized using Zoletil (50 mg/kg, Virbac Laboratories, Carros, France) and Xylazine (0.15 mg/kg, LaboratoriosCalier, Barcelona, Spain), intramuscularly. Zoletil is a combination of a dissociative anesthetic agent, tiletamine hypochloride, and a tranquilizer, zolazepam hydrochloride. The onset of action is 3–5 minutes by intramuscular route. We checked the depth of anesthesia by testing the absence of eyelid reflex and the tail pinch reflex. To maintain anesthesia, we used xylazine (0.15 mg/kg) which is an $\alpha 2$ adrenergic receptor agonist results in sedation, analgesia, and muscle relaxation and provides a sedative effect within 1–3 hours. Tracheostomy was performed and rats were ventilated with room air from a positive pressure rodent ventilator (CWE, Inc, Ardmore, Pennsylvania, USA). Lead II ECG was recorded throughout the experiment to determine the time to the 1st ventricular tachycardia/ventricular fibrillation (VT/VF) onset, VT/VF incidence, and arrhythmia scores. Arrhythmia score was characterized in accordance with the Lambeth conventions and using a score as described by Curtis and Walker [21]. A left-side thoracotomy was performed at the fourth intercostal space, and the pericardium was incised to expose the

Table 1. Effects of HFD consumption on metabolic parameters at baseline and 12-week after HFD consumption.

Metabolic parameters	Baseline		Week 12	
	ND	HFD	ND	HFD
Body weight (g)	191±2	190±9	480±10*	595±28*,†
Food intake (g/day)	26±1	29±1	29±2	26±2
Plasma insulin (ng/ml)	1.8±0.2	1.7±0.3	1.6±0.5	4.4±0.7*,†
Plasma glucose (mg/dl)	130±9	135±6	131±6	137±8
HOMA index	15±2	14±3	14±4	35±9*,†
Plasma total cholesterol (mg/dl)	41±5	42±4	41±2	53±3*,†
Plasma triglyceride (mg/dl)	70±6	72±8	80±8	87±5
Plasma HDL (mg/dl)	9.6±1	8.3±0.8	10.7±1	7.4±1.7*,†
Plasma LDL (mg/dl)	17.4±1	19.4±0.8	14.3±1.3	28.2±1.7*,†
Plasma MDA (μmol/ml)	2.9±0.2	3.1±0.1	3.3±0.2	6.4±0.1*,†

ND = normal diet, HFD = high-fat diet. *$P<0.05$ vs. Baseline, †$P<0.05$ vs. ND week 12.

heart. Left anterior descending (LAD) coronary artery was identified and ligated at approximately 2 mm distal to its origin [5,22]. The end of a ligature was passed through a small vinyl tube, which is used to occlude the LAD by pulling the thread. ST elevation was used to confirm ischemia. The heart was subject to ischemia for 30 minutes, then the ligature was loosened for the ischemic myocardium to be reperfused for 120 minutes.

Left-ventricular (LV) function

The right carotid artery was identified and the pressure-volume (P-V) catheter (Scisense, Ontario, Canada) was inserted and advanced into the left ventricle to determine the cardiac function during I/R injury. Heart rate (HR), end-systolic pressure (ESP), end-diastolic pressure (EDP), maximum pressure (Pmax), minimum pressure (Pmin), dP/dtmax, dP/dtmin, stroke work (SW), and stroke volume/body weight (SV/BW) were determined prior to I/R injury protocol, at the end of occlusion, and at the end of reperfusion using analytical software program (Labscribe, Dover, New Hampshire, USA).

Infarct size determination

After 150 minutes of I/R period, the heart was excised and mount on the modified Langendorff apparatus via the aorta. Cold saline solution was used to flush out the blood, after which the LAD was re-occluded and 1-ml of 0.5% (w/v) Evans blue dye was injected to define the area at risk. Evans blue dye stained the perfused myocardium, whereas the LAD occlusion area did not stained with Evans blue dye, after which the heart was sliced into pieces with approximately 1-mm thickness for each slice and incubated with 1% buffered 2,3,5-triphenyltetrazolium chloride (TTC) (Sigma-Aldrich, St. Louis, Missouri, USA), followed by placing them in 10% formalin overnight [5,22]. The infarct and remote areas were determined using the image tool software version 3.0. The infarct size was calculated depending on the weight of each slice according to Reiss et al.'s formula [5,11,23].

Determination of cardiac mitochondrial function

For mitochondrial study, mitochondria were obtained from the ischemic myocardium and remote myocardium from fresh hearts. Ischemic area was obtained from left ventricular apex and remote area was obtained from right ventricle. The heart was minced and homogenized in the mitochondrial isolation buffer, pH 7.2, containing 300 mM sucrose, 0.2 mM EGTA, 5 mM TES. Homogenates was centrifuged at 800 g, 4°C for 5 min. The supernatant was collected and centrifuged at 8800 g, 4°C for 5 min. Then, the mitochondrial pellet was resuspended in the mitochondrial isolation buffer and centrifuged at 8800 g, 4°C for 5 min. The mitochondria were collected and the protein concentration was determined by the bicinchoninic acid method [22]. Cardiac mitochondrial function was assessed by determining cardiac mitochondrial reactive oxygen species (ROS) production, cardiac mitochondrial membrane potential change, and cardiac mitochondrial swelling [11,14,24].

Cardiac mitochondrial ROS production. Cardiac mitochondria were incubated with2 μM DCFH-DA dye at 25°C for 20 minutes. The dye was excited at λ_{ex} 485 nm and detected at λ_{em} 530 nm using fluorescent microplate reader (BioTek Instruments, Winooski, Vermont, USA). An increase in the fluorescent intensity indicated an increased mitochondrial ROS production [1,11,24].

Cardiac mitochondrial membrane potential changes. Cardiac mitochondrial membrane potential changes were determined using 5- μM JC-1 dye as described previously [1,24]. In brief, cardiac mitochondria were incubated with JC-1 at 37°C for 30 minutes. JC-1 monomer form (green fluorescent) was excited at λ_{ex} 485 nm and detected at λ_{em} 590 nm, and JC-1 aggregate form (red fluorescent) was excited at λ_{ex} 485 nm and detected at λ_{em} 530 nm using a fluorescent microplate reader. An increase in the red/green fluorescent intensity ratio indicates cardiac mitochondrial membrane depolarization [1,11,24].

Cardiac mitochondrial swelling. Cardiac mitochondria were incubated with 1.5-mM respiration buffer containing 100 mMKCl, 10 mM HEPES, 5 mM KH2PO4, and the absorbance was determined using a spectrophotometer as described previously [1,24]. Cardiac mitochondrial swelling is indicated by a decrease in the detected absorbance [1,11,24].

Cardiac mitochondria morphology. Cardiac mitochondria were fixed with 2.5% glutaraldehyde in a 0.1-M phosphate buffer overnight and post fixed in a 1% cacodylate-buffer osmium tetroxide for 2 hours, then dehydrated with graded series of ethanol [24]. Cardiac mitochondria were embedded in Epon-Araldite, cut with a diamond knife, and stained with uranyl acetate and lead acetate[24]. Cardiac mitochondria morphology were detected using a transmission electron microscope [24].

Table 2. Effects of vildagliptin, metformin, and combination of vildagliptin and metformin on metabolic parameters (n = 11/group).

Parameters	NDV	NDVil	NDM	NDC	HFDV	HFDVil	HFDM	HFDC
Body weight (g)	478±11	454±14	439±12	472±14	608±18*	567±28*	566±7*	586±36*
Visceral fat (g)	22±1	23±2	22±3	22±1	50±4*	42±4*	46±3*	56±5*
Food intake (g/day)	22±1	25±1	22±3	23±2	22±2	25±1	19±2	19±1
Plasma glucose (mg/dl)	135±12	143±12	130±14	139±13	138±9	132±5	134±16	135±11
Plasma insulin (ng/ml)	2.3±0.3	1.7±0.4	2.1±0.4	2.3±0.3	5.4±0.6*	3.1±0.5†	3.8±0.2†	3.3±0.2†
HOMA index	19±3	18±5	16±4	20±3	32±5*	23±4†	26±2†	22±1†
Plasma total cholesterol (mg/dl)	49±6	44±4	49±2	54±3	63±4*	43±3†	51±2†	42±3†
Plasma triglyceride (mg/dl)	86±5	79±1	85±4	86±2	88±4	80±2	87±4	84±2
Plasma HDL (mg/dl)	12.1±1	10.9±2	11.8±2	10±1	7.6±1*	10.6±2†	10.9±1†	12±2†
Plasma LDL (mg/dl)	19.7±1	17.2±2	20.2±2	20±3	37±1*	20.4±2†	22.7±1†	23.2±1†
Plasma MDA (µmol/ml)	3.6±0.1	3.5±0.1	3.7±0.1	3.1±0.1	6.8±0.1*	6.1±0.2*,†	6.3±0.2*,†	6.3±0.1*,†
Cardiac MDA (µmol/mgprotein)	23.5±3.4	12.8±3.9*	14.5±2.8*	11.8±2.9*	32.7±4.6*	12.8±1.6†	14.2±1.7†	12.5±2.7†

*$P<0.05$ vs. NDV, †$P<0.05$ vs. HFDV.

Western blot analysis

The myocardial tissues for western blot study was obtained from the fresh heart at the end of the I/R protocol. The ischemic myocardium was obtained from the left ventricular apex and intact myocardium was obtained from the right ventricle. Myocardial protein extracts were prepared by a homogenization of nitrogen-frozen myocardial tissues (ischemia and remote area) in a 300- µl extraction buffer containing 20-mMTris-HCl (pH 6.8), 1-mM Sodium orthovanadate, 5-mMSodium fluoride, and protease inhibitor. Total protein concentration was determined using a Bio-Rad protein assay kit (Bio-Rad Laboratories, Hercules, California, USA). Fifty to 80 µg of total protein were mixed with loading buffer (5% betamercaptoethanol, 0.05% bromophenol blue, 75 mMTris-HCl (pH 6.8), 2% SDS and 10% glycerol), and loaded onto the 10% SDS-Acrylamide gels. Proteins were transferred to polyvinylidenedifluoride (PVDF) membrane in a glycine/methanol transferred buffer [5,22] in a Wet/Tank blotting system (Bio-Rad Laboratories, Hercules, California, USA). Membranes were blocked in 5% skim milk in Tris-Buffered Saline and Tween (TBST) buffer. Western blot analysis for Bax, Bcl-2, total Connexin-43, and Connexin43 phosphorylated at Ser368 was done in myocardial tissues. Membranes were exposed to mouse polyclonal anti-rat Bax and Bcl-2 (1:1000 dilution, Santa Cruz Biotechnology, Dallas, Texas, USA), Phospho-Cx43(Ser368), Cx43 (1:1000 dilution, Cell Signaling Technology, Danvers, Massachusetts, USA). Bound antibody was detected by horseradish peroxidase conjugated with anti-rabbit IgG (1:2000 dilution, Cell Signaling Technology, Danvers, Massachusetts, USA). The membranes were developed using the Amersham enhanced chemiluminescence Prime Western Blotting Detection Reagent (GE healthcare, Buckinghamshire, UK) and densitometric analysis was carried out [5].

Ventricular cardiomyocyte isolation

A separated group of thirty-two male Wistar rats was used in the intracellular calcium transient study. Rats were anesthetized by intraperitoneal injection of thiopental (1 ml/kg, Research institute of antibiotics and biotransformation, Prague, Czechoslovakia), and 0.2-ml heparin (LEO pharma, Ballerup, Denmark) was injected into the femoral vein. The heart was excised quickly with decent length of aorta and mounted on the cannula and tied with suture. The blood was washed out with solution 1 (Tyrode's solution and 750 µM $CaCl_2$) then switched to solution 2 (Tyrode's solution and 100 µM ethylene glycol tetraacetic acid (EGTA) for 4 minutes, and switched to solution 3 (Tyrode's solution, 100 µM $CaCl_2$, and 1 mg/ml collagenase (Worthington, Lakewood, New Jersey, USA)) for 10 minutes. The ventricles were cut and triturated in solution 3 at 37°C for 30 minutes, and were then filtered with a nylon mesh. The cells were left to settle down for 10 minutes and solution 3 was removed. Cells were resuspened in solution 4 (Tyrode's solution, 0.5 mM $CaCl_2$, and 1% BSA) for 10 minutes. Cells were resuspened in 10 ml of solution 5 (Tyrode's solution, 1 mM $CaCl_2$) and were ready for calcium transient study [22].

Intracellular calcium transient

The measurement of cardiomyocyte calcium transient was performed using a modified method from Wongchareon*et al.* [25] as described previously [22]. Isolated cardiomyocytes were incubated with 25- µM Fura-2/AM (Sigma Chemical, St. Louis, Massachusetts, USA) in 37°C, 5% CO_2, for 30 minutes. Fura-2 was excited at ultraviolet light wavelength of 340 nm and 387 nm by monochromator from xenon arc lamp controlled by a microfluorometry system (OSP 100-CA, Olympus, Tokyo, Japan). The excitation light was directed into an inverted microscope (IX-

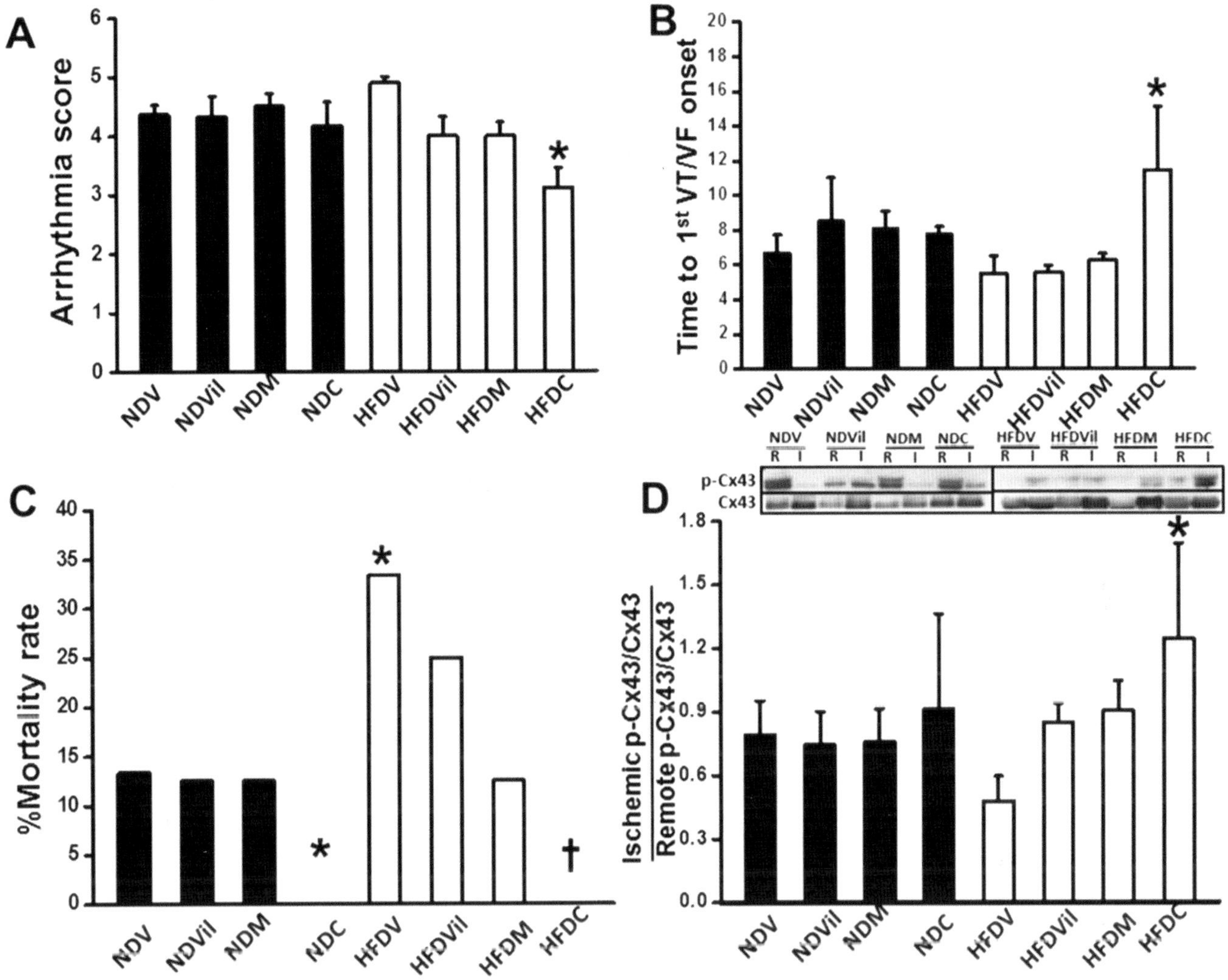

Figure 2. Effects of vildagliptin, metformin, combined drugs on arrhythmia, mortality rate, and phosphorylation of Cx43 level. (A) Combined drugs reduced arrhythmia score in HFD rats.*$p<0.05$ vs. HFDV, n = 11/group. (B) Combined drugs delayed time to the 1st VT/VF onset in HFD rats. *$p<0.05$ vs. HFDV, n = 11/group. (C) Mortality rate was higher in HFDV, and combined drugs reduced mortality rate in both ND and HFD rats. *$p<0.05$ vs. NDV, †$p<0.05$ vs. HFDV, n = 11/group. (D) Combined drugs increased p-Cx43 in HFD rats. *$p<0.05$ vs. HFDV, n = 5/group.

70, Olympus, Tokyo, Japan). The emitted fluorescent intensity from Fura-2 was detected at wavelength 500 nm and digitized at 200 Hz. The ratio of fluorescent emission of two wavelengths was recorded as the index of intracellular calcium. The intracellular calcium transient peak amplitude and decay rate were measured during 1-Hz field-stimulation with a 10-ms twice-threshold strength square-pulse wave [22]. After baseline recording, 2-mM hydrogen peroxide (H_2O_2) was applied onto cardiomyocytes to induce oxidative stress (mimicking the ischemic process), after which the ratio of fluorescent emission of two wavelengths was recorded to determine the differences on intracellular calcium transient under oxidative stress condition among cardiomyocytes taken from the hearts of rats treated with vildagliptin, metformin, combined drugs, and vehicle.

Statistical Analysis

Data were expressed as mean ± SEM. One-way ANOVA followed by Fisher's least significant difference post hoc was used to test the different among the group. Mortality rate and VT/VF incidence were analyzed using Chi-square test. Mitochondrial function was analyzed using Kruskal-Wallis H followed by Mann-Whitney U test. $P<0.05$ was considered statistical significant.

Results

Effects of metformin and vildagliptin on metabolic parameters

At baseline, metabolic parameters were not different between ND and HFD group (Table 1). After 12 weeks of HFD consumption, the body weight, plasma insulin, plasma cholesterol, plasma MDA levels and HOMA index were increased in HFD rats, compared with ND rats (Table 1). Vildagliptin, metformin, and combined drugs reduced plasma insulin, plasma total cholesterol, plasma LDL, plasma and cardiac MDA levels and increased plasma HDL level in HFD rats, compared with HFD rats treated with vehicle (HFDV) (Table 2). No difference on these parameters was found between monotherapy and combined drugs.

Table 3. Effects of metformin, vildagliptin, and combination of vildagliptin and metformin on cardiac function before I/R injury (n = 11/group).

Cardiac function	NDV	NDVil	NDM	NDC	HFDV	HFDVil	HFDM	HFDC
Heart rate (bpm)	237±15	199±17	221±12	213±28	241±18	244±11	209±7	230±15
ESP (mmHg)	85±6	83±9	81±3	94±7	68±5*	93±10†	90±10†	91±9†
EDP (mmHg)	10±2	9±3	6±1	9±5	21±6*	8±2†	8±2†	10±1†
Pmax (mmHg)	108±7	87±9	82±11	101±5	93±8	117±15	94±11	114±14
Pmin (mmHg)	11±5	5±3	3±1	8±3	14±4	9±3	8±2	10±2
dP/dtmax (mmHg/s)	10090±1501	9487±442	10189±369	10561±781	8439±393	10081±1945	9077±737	11626±1974
dP/dtmin (mmHg/s)	−6378±1281	−4557±1162	−4119±891	−6205±454	−5388±428	−5226±800	−4714±632	−5761±1292
SW (mmHg/ml)	14653±784	12541±1440	14528±1106	14813±935	13698±1433	14929±1893	13495±1568	15446±1268
SV/BW (µl)	1.06±0.12	1.06±0.13	1.12±0.10	1.16±0.15	0.65±0.05*	1.08±0.14†	1.10±0.09†	1.04±0.2†

*$P<0.05$ vs. NDV, †$P<0.05$ vs. HFDV.

Effects of metformin and vildagliptin on HRV

At baseline, the LF/HF ratio was not different between ND and HFD rats (Figure 1A). The LF/HF ratio was increased after 8 weeks of HFD consumption (Figure 1A). After treatment, the LF/HF ratio was not different in ND groups (Figure 1B). Treatments with vildagliptin, metformin, and combined drugs significantly reduced the LF/HF ratio in HFD rats (Figure 1B), indicating an improved cardiac sympathovagal balance in HFD rats.

Effects of metformin and vildagliptin on left ventricular function prior to I/R

At baseline, %FS and LVEF were not different between ND and HFD. We found that %FS and LVEF were decreased after 12 weeks of HFD consumption, compared with ND (Figure 1C–D). After treatment, vildagliptin, metformin, and combined drugs restored %FS and LVEF in HFD rats, compared with HFDV (Figure 1E–F).

Effects of metformin and vildagliptin on arrhythmia score during I/R

Arrhythmia score tended to be higher during I/R in HFDV than NDV rats, but the value did not reach statistical significance (Figure 2A). Only HFD rats treated with combined drugs had reduced arrhythmia score (Figure 2A). The time to 1st VT/VF onset was not different between NDV and HFDV. In ND rats, time to 1st VT/VF onset was not different among different treatment groups. In HFD rats, only combined drugs delayed time to the first VT/VF onset in HFD rats (Figure 2B). We also found that HFDV rats had a higher mortality rate, compared with the NDV group (Figure 2C). The mortality rate was reduced only in ND and HFD rats treated with combined drugs (Figure 2C). We determined the levels of Cx43 phosphorylation in heart tissues since it has been shown to closely associate with arrhythmia during I/R, and found that Cx43 phosphorylation was not different among the different treatments in ND groups (Figure 2D). However, in HFD rats, the phosphorylation of Cx43 was increased only in HFD rats treated with combined drugs (Figure 2D).

Effects of metformin and vildagliptin on left ventricular function during I/R

Baseline LV function data by P-V loop assessment prior to I/R are shown in Table 3. LV function was not different among ND groups prior to I/R injury. ESP, SV/BW were decreased and EDP was increased in HFDV rats, compared with NDV group ($p<0.05$ vs. NDV, Table 3). All treatments increased ESP and SV/BW and reduced EDP in HFD rats ($p<0.05$ vs. HFDV, Table 3).

LV function data at the end of LAD occlusion are shown in Table 4. At the end of LAD occlusion, all treatments increased the dP/dt_{max}, and combined drugs also increased the ESP in ND rats, compared with the NDV group ($p<0.05$ vs. NDV). In HFDV rats, the HR and EDP were increased and the ESP and SV/BW was decreased ($p<0.05$ vs. NDV). All treatments reduced the EDP, and increased the ESP, dP/dt_{max}, and SV/BW in HFD rats ($p<0.05$ vs. HFDV, Table 4).

LV function data at the end of reperfusion are shown in Table 5. At the end of reperfusion, LV function was not different among ND groups. In HFD groups, the ESP and SV/BW was decreased and the EDP was increased in the HFDV group ($p<0.05$ vs. NDV). All treatments reduced the EDP and increased the ESP and SV/BW in HFD rats ($p<0.05$ vs. HFDV, Table 5).

Table 4. Effects of vildagliptin, metformin, and combination of vildagliptin and metformin on cardiac function at the end of Occlusion (n = 11/group).

Cardiac function	NDV	NDVil	NDM	NDC	HFDV	HFDVil	HFDM	HFDC
Heart rate (bpm)	214±11	200±12	227±17	213±12	266±23*	249±14	243±23	242±26
ESP (mmHg)	74±4	82±7	83±20	103±3*	66±7*	90±8†	93±6†	90±7†
EDP (mmHg)	15±4	10±1	11±2	9±2	26±4*	13±2†	12±1†	14±2†
Pmax (mmHg)	95±5	96±9	99±20	105±3	106±11	94±8	102±6	109±10
Pmin (mmHg)	10±4	5±1	6±1	12±2	11±3	9±3	13±2	14±2
dP/dtmax (mmHg/s)	7709±1049	12088±2244*	12245±1716*	13906±2385*	4849±394	11060±2295†	12040±2132†	12565±1091†
dP/dtmin (mmHg/s)	−4002±475	−4077±572	−5724±912	−5252±395	−4411±561	−3982±813	−4005±460	−4038±844
SW (mmHg/ml)	10941±1492	12886±1162	12004±2505	13998±637	10020±1456	10620±1937	9776±1553	10237±2322
SV/BW (µl)	1.28±0.38	1.58±0.19	1.13±0.27	0.89±0.20	0.60±0.04*	0.89±0.16†	0.98±0.10†	0.93±0.08†

*$P<0.05$ vs. NDV, $^{\dagger}P<0.05$ vs. HFDV.

Effects of metformin and vildagliptin on the infarct size

In this study, the area at risk (AAR) was not different among all groups. We found that the infarct size/AAR was increased in the HFDV group, compared with the NDV group (Figure 3A–B). All treatments reduced the infarct size in both ND and HFD rats (Figure 3A–B). The western blot analysis revealed that the Bax expression was not different among groups of ND rats (Figure 3C). However, the Bax expression was increased in the HFDV rats, compared with the NDV group. In HFD rats, vildagliptin and metformin reduced the Bax expression, compared with the HFDV group. Moreover, Bax expression was markedly decreased in HFD rats treated with combined drugs, compared with the HFDV group (Figure 3C). The Bcl-2 expression was not different among ND groups (Figure 3D). The Bcl-2 expression was decreased in the HFDV rats, compared with the NDV group, and all treatments increased Bcl-2 expression in HFD rats (Figure 3D).

Effects of metformin and vildagliptin on cardiac mitochondrial function and morphology

Our data demonstrated that mitochondrial ROS production was increased in the ischemic area of both NDV and HFDV groups, compared to the remote (non-ischemic) area (Figure 4A). Moreover, the ROS level in the ischemic area was also significantly higher in the HFDV rats, compared to the NDV rats. All treatments reduced mitochondrial ROS production in the ischemic area of HFD rats (Figure 4A).For mitochondrial membrane potential change, the red/green fluorescent intensity ratio was decreased in the ischemic area of both NDV and HFDV groups, compared with their remote areas, indicating mitochondrial membrane depolarization (Figure 4B). All treatments could attenuate mitochondrial depolarization (Figure 4B). For mitochondrial swelling assessment, we found that the absorbance was decreased in the ischemic area of both NDV and HFDV groups, compared with their remote areas, indicating mitochondrial swelling (Figure 4C). Moreover, mitochondrial swelling was significantly greater in the HFDV rats, compared to the NDV rats. All treatments increased the absorbance in both ND and HFD rats (Figure 4C).

Representative images of cardiac mitochondria from the transmission electron microscopy showed the unfolded cristae which is an indicator of mitochondrial swelling. Compared to the intact cardiac mitochondria in the remote area of the NDV rat (Figure 4D), we found that unfolded cristae were mostly found in the ischemic area of the NDV (Figure 4E) and HFDV rats (Figure 4J). Moreover, cardiac mitochondria in the remote area of the HFDV rat (Figure 4I) also had unfolded cristae compared to that in the NDV group, indicating mitochondrial swelling. The marked unfolded cristae were found in the ischemic area of

Table 5. Effects of vildagliptin, metformin, and combination of vildagliptin and metformin on cardiac function at the end of Reperfusion (n = 11/group).

Cardiac function	NDV	NDVil	NDM	NDC	HFDV	HFDVil	HFDM	HFDC
Heart rate (bpm)	281±23	248±18	286±63	237±25	343±48	252±30	281±31	264±25
ESP (mmHg)	82±3	82±14	86±30	96±8	65±4*	91±18†	94±6†	97±8†
EDP (mmHg)	9±3	8±2	11±3	9±3	23±1*	9±3†	9±2†	11±1†
Pmax (mmHg)	117±8	126±10	109±19	97±9	102±10	116±17	110±5	123±9
Pmin (mmHg)	7±2	8±2	8±3	9±4	10±2	6±2	10±2	9±2
dP/dtmax (mmHg/s)	9216±553	12625±2759	10536±1899	10593±2807	8285±1089	9732±1806	10855±816	10776±1761
dP/dtmin (mmHg/s)	−6621±657	−6715±1673	−6431±651	−6551±1434	−7858±1440	−8777±850	−7945±1243	−7550±684
SW (mmHg/ml)	11823±2519	13943±846	10847±743	11095±1073	12374±1219	11775±1270	11434±313	10228±414
SV/BW (µl)	1.02±0.28	1.74±0.26	0.92±0.12	1.00±0.13	0.67±0.02*	1.04±0.18†	0.97±0.07†	0.94±0.18†

*$P<0.05$ vs. NDV, $^{\dagger}P<0.05$ vs. HFDV.

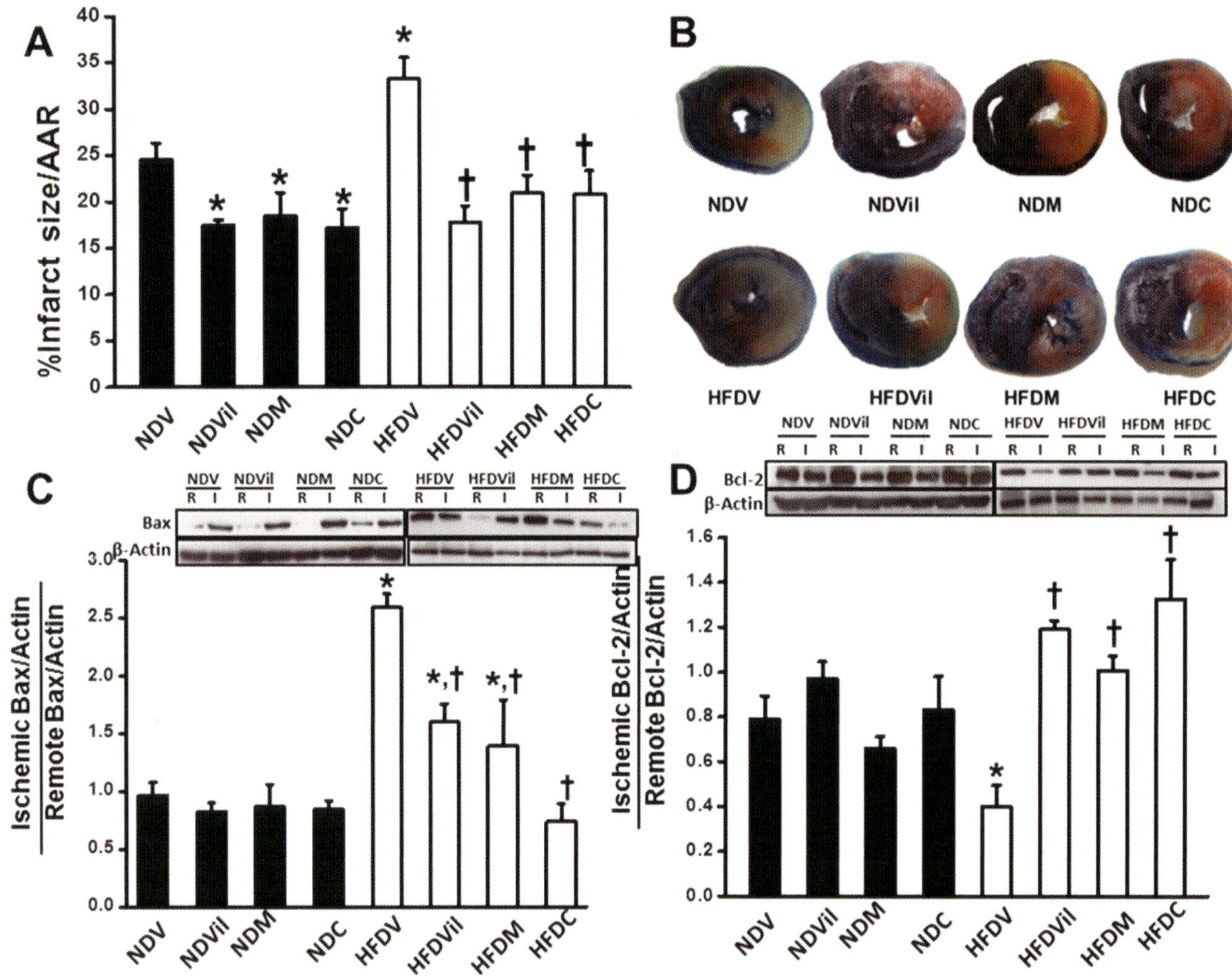

Figure 3. Effects of vildagliptin, metformin, and combined drugs on infarct size, Bax, and Bcl-2 expression. (A) Infarct size was increased in HFDV, and all treatments reduced infarct size in both ND and HFD rats. *$p<0.05$ vs. NDV, $^{\dagger}p<0.01$ vs. HFDV, n = 6/group. (B) Representative images showing TTC staining for infarct size determination. (C) Bax expression was increased in HFDV, and all treatments reduced Bax expression in HFD rats. *$p<0.05$ vs. NDV, $^{\dagger}p<0.05$ vs. HFDV, n = 5/group. (D) Bcl-2 expression was decreased in HFDV, and all treatments increased Bcl-2 expression in HFD rats. *$p<0.05$ vs. NDV, $^{\dagger}p<0.05$ vs. HFDV, n = 5/group.

HFDV. All treatments prevented unfolded cristae in both ND (Figure 4F–H) and HFD rats (Figure 4K–M).

Effects of metformin and vildagliptin on intracellular calcium transient

Our results demonstrated that the intracellular diastolic calcium level was increased in HFDV hearts, compared with the NDV group (Figure 5A). After treated with H_2O_2, intracellular diastolic calcium level was increased in both NDV and HFDV groups, compared with their control. We found that all treatments prevented a change in the intracellular diastolic calcium under oxidative stress condition (Figure 5A).

Calcium transient amplitude was significantly decreased in the HFDV group, compared with the NDV group (Figure 5B). After treated with H_2O_2, calcium transient amplitude was not different from baseline of its own group for both NDV and HFDV rats. However, cardiomyocytes from HFD rats treated with vildagliptin, metformin, and combined drugs had a significant increase in calcium transient amplitude both at baseline and with the presence of H_2O_2 (Figure 5B).

Calcium transient decay rate was significantly decreased in the HFDV cardiomyocytes, compared with the NDV group (Figure 5C). Calcium transient decay rate in the HFDV group was not different from baseline after treated with H_2O_2. All treatments significantly increased calcium decay rate in HFD cardiomyocytes both at baseline and with the presence of H_2O_2 (Figure 5C). Representatives of signals of intracellular calcium transients from cardiomyocytes from each group are shown in Figure 5D.

Discussion

Findings from the present study demonstrated that HFD caused obese-insulin resistance, increased oxidative stress level, depressed HRV, and LV dysfunction. Treatment with vildagliptin, metformin, and combined drugs improved insulin resistance, reduced oxidative stress level, improved HRV, and attenuated LV dysfunction in obese-insulin resistant rats prior to I/R. Under I/R condition, all treatments improved LV dysfunction, reduced the infarct size, prevented cardiac mitochondrial dysfunction, decreased Bax and increased Bcl-2 expression, and reduced cardiac

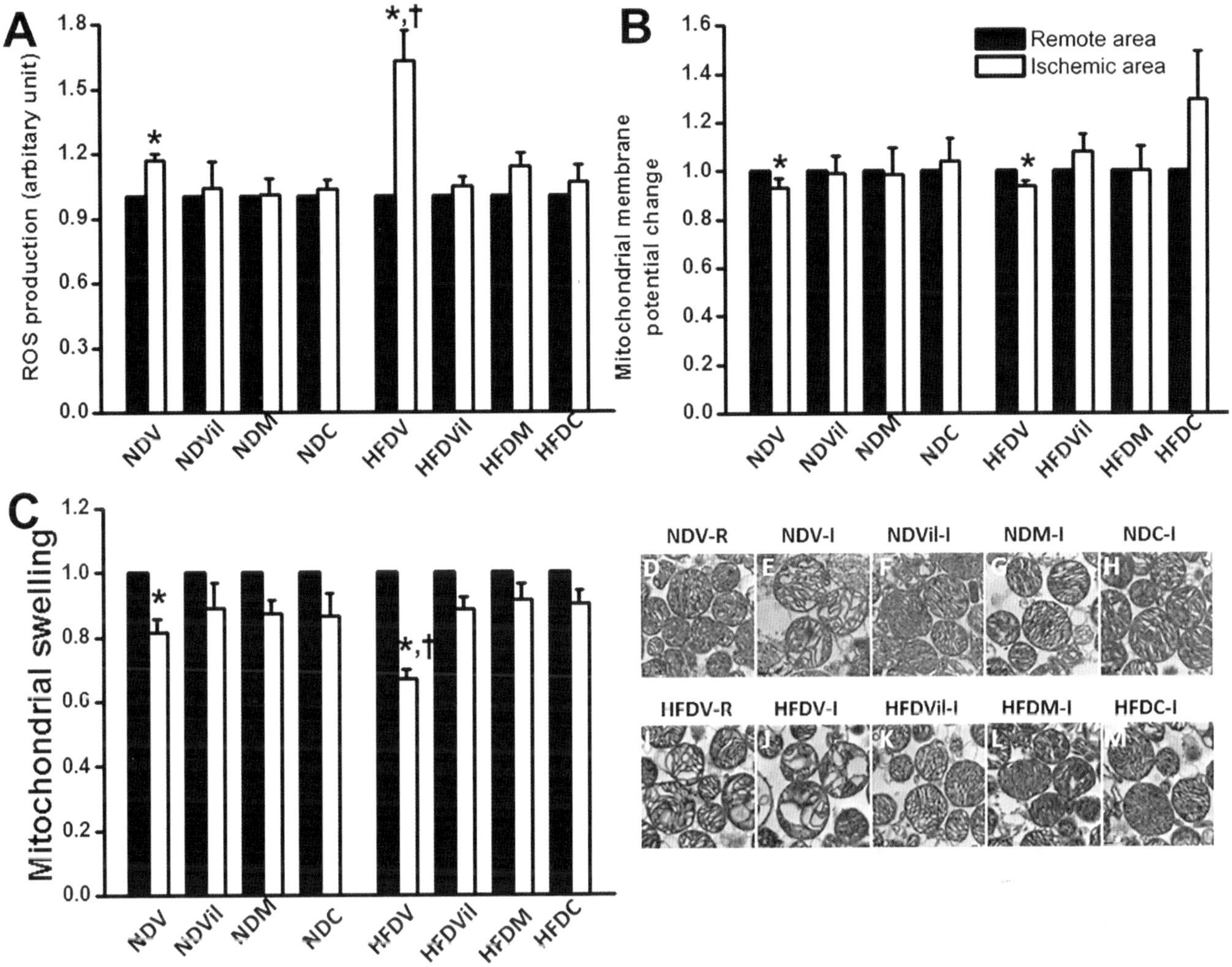

Figure 4. Effects of vildagliptin, metformin, and combined drugs on cardiac mitochondrial function and morphology. (A) Mitochondrial ROS production was increased in ischemic area of NDV and HFDV, Mitochondrial ROS production was higher in HFDV than NDV, and all treatments reduced mitochondrial ROS production. *$p<0.05$ vs. remote area, †$p<0.05$ vs. ischemic area of NDV, n = 5/group. (B) Mitochondrial membrane depolarization was found in ischemia area of NDV and HFDV, all treatment prevented mitochondrial membrane depolarization. *$p<0.05$ vs. remote area of NDV, n = 5/group. (C) An absorbance was decreased in ischemic area of NDV and HFDV. The reduction of absorbance was greater in HFDV than NDV, and all treatments prevented mitochondrial swelling, *$p<0.05$ vs. remote area of NDV, n = 5/group. (D–M) Cardiac mitochondrial morphology

oxidative stress level. Furthermore, all treatments improved intracellular calcium transient regulation in the absence and presence of H_2O_2 in the obese-insulin resistant rats. However, only combined drugs could reduce the arrhythmia score, mortality rate, delayed the time to the 1st VT/VF onset, and increased Cx-43 phosphorylation.

In this study, rats developed insulin resistance after 12 weeks of HFD consumption. This finding is consistent with previous studies in which long-term HFD consumption could induce hyperinsulinemia and increased HOMA index, indicating insulin resistance, as well as oxidative stress after 12 weeks of HFD consumption [1,14,16,26]. Previous studies have shown the beneficial effects of vildagliptin and metformin on metabolic parameters [14,27,28]. Our data showed that vildagliptin and metformin improved insulin resistance and metabolic parameters as well as oxidative stress in obese-insulin resistant rats. Clinical study reported that vildagliptin in addition to metformin reduced fasting plasma insulin level and HOMA-IR in type 2 diabetic patients [13]. Our study showed that all treatment reduced plasma cholesterol levels. However, the levels of cholesterol in this study were lower than that reported in our previous study [14]. Although these differences could be due to different kits and methods used, all drugs could still decrease the cholesterol levels, compared to the control. Moreover, clinical studies as well as studies in diabetic and insulin resistant animal models reported that vildagliptin and metformin could ameliorate oxidative stress levels [14,29,30]. In the present study, rats in all treatment groups had reduced plasma MDA level (prior to I/R) and reduced cardiac MDA level (after I/R), suggesting that vildagliptin and metformin improved insulin resistance and exerted an anti-oxidative stress benefit in obese-insulin resistant rats.

HRV is an indicator of cardiac sympathovagal balance [19]. Previous studies demonstrated that cardiac sympathovagal imbalance was observed in long-term HFD fed rats [14,31]. Consistent with previous studies, we found that the LF/HF ratio was increased after 8 weeks of HFD consumption, indicating cardiac

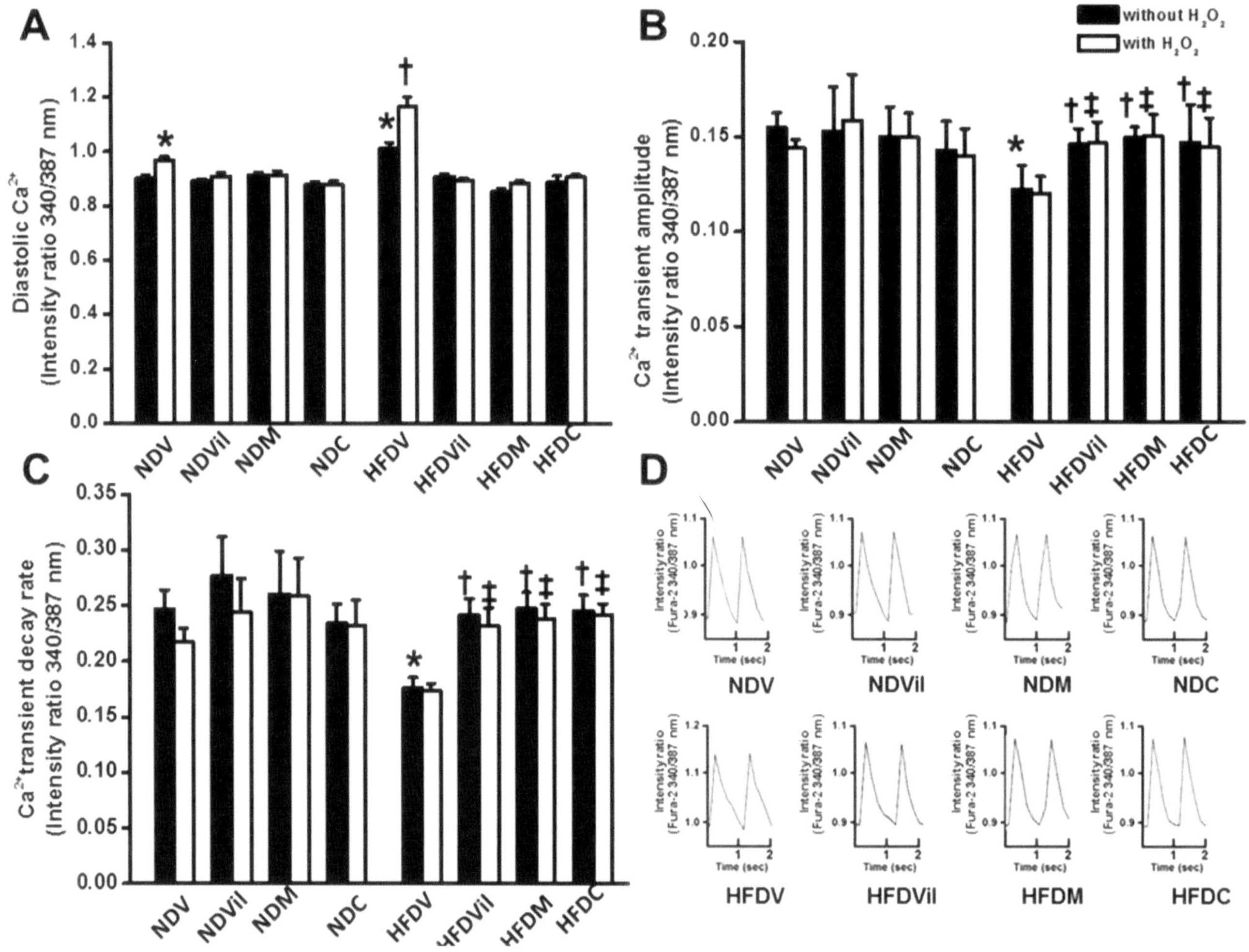

Figure 5. Effects of vildagliptin, metformin, and combined drugs on intracellular calcium regulation. (A) Intracellular diastolic calcium was increased in HFDV. All treatments reduced intracellular diastolic calcium in HFD rats. (B) Calcium transient amplitude was decreased in HFDV. All treatments improved calcium transient amplitude in HFD rats. (C) Calcium transient decay rate was reduced in HFDV. All treatments increased the calcium transient decay rate in HFD rats. (D) Representative calcium transient tracing for calcium transient parameters determination. $^{*}p<0.05$ vs. baseline NDV, $^{\dagger}p<0.01$ vs. baseline HFDV, $^{\ddagger}p<0.05$ vs. HFDV with H_2O_2 n=8 cells/group

sympathovagal imbalance. Vildagliptin, metformin, and combined drugs improved the HRV by decreasing LF/HF ratio in obese-insulin resistant rats. Since depressed HRV has been reported to be associated with increased oxidative stress such as an increased MDA level [32], the improved HRV in obese-insulin resistant rats by the drugs found in our study could be due to the reduced oxidative stress caused by these drugs.

Previous studies have shown that long-term HFD consumption caused LV dysfunction [14,31], and that vildagliptin and metformin could improve LV function in obese-insulin resistant rats [14]. Consistent with previous studies, we found that LV ejection fraction and fractional shortening were reduced after 12 weeks of HFD consumption. Vildagliptin and metformin improved the LV ejection fraction and fractional shortening in the present study. Moreover, we also found that these drugs reduced intracellular diastolic calcium, improved intracellular calcium transient amplitude and decay rate in obese-insulin resistant rats. These findings suggested that one of the mechanisms responsible for improved LV function by vildagliptin and metformin could be attributed to their role in the improved intracellular calcium regulation.

In the present study, vildagliptin and metformin reduced the infarct size caused by I/R injury in obese-insulin resistant rats. Chinda and colleagues reported previously that vildagliptin reduced the infarct size in swine hearts with I/R injury [11], and several studies have demonstrated that metformin also reduced the infarct size in both non-diabetic and diabetic animals [33,34,35]. Our results further demonstrated that both vildagliptin and metformin also exerted infarct size reduction benefit in the obese-insulin resistant rat model. The mechanism responsible for this benefit of both drugs could partly due to their anti-apoptotic effects as indicated by reduced Bax and increased Bcl-2 expression. Bax is a pro-apoptotic protein, whereas Bcl-2 is an anti-apoptotic protein, both of which are known to regulate apoptosis during I/R. Furthermore, we demonstrated in the present study that both metformin and vildagliptin could attenuate cardiac mitochondrial dysfunction caused by I/R injury. It has been shown previously that both Bax and Bcl-2 are associated with mitochondrial ROS level [36]. Several studies have shown that metformin improved cardiac mitochondrial function and ultrastructure in insulin resistant rats, diabetic rats, and normal rats with I/R injury [14,37,38]. In the present study, we demonstrated that vildagliptin and metformin improved cardiac mitochondrial function and ultrastructure in obese-insulin resistant rats. All of these findings suggested that vildagliptin and metformin reduced the infarct sized by attenuating myocardial apoptosis and cardiac mitochondrial dysfunction. The improved cardiac mitochondrial function as well as infarct size reduction could also be responsible for improved LV function during I/R.

Despite the beneficial effects of metformin and vildagliptin as a single therapy in the present study, we found that only vildagliptin and metformin giving as combined therapy reduced fatal arrhythmias as well as delayed time to the first VT/VF onset during I/R in this obses-insulin resistant rats. This antiarrhythmic effect could be due to the fact that only rats treated with combined metformin and vildagliptin had increased Cx43 phosphorylation. Cx 43 is a cardiac gap junction protein, and it has been shown previously that the engraftment of Cx43 expressing cells could protect the heart against the induction of ventricular tachycardia in mice with myocardial infarction model [39]. Cx 43 phosphorylation at serine 368 has been shown to protect against cardiac arrhythmias during I/R [5,40]. Our data suggested that the increased Cx43 phosphorylation by combined metformin and vildagliptin could be a mechanism responsible for arrhythmia reduction and leading to decrease arrhythmic death from I/R in obese-insulin resistant rats.

Conclusions

In conclusion, long-term HFD consumption induced obese-insulin resistance, oxidative stress, cardiac autonomic imbalance, and LV dysfunction. Vildagliptin, metformin, and combined drugs attenuated these adverse effects. Under I/R, these drugs prevented LV dysfunction and reduced infarct size, that was associated with decreased mitochondrial function, improved intracellular calcium regulation, increased anti-apoptotic protein, and reduced pro-apoptotic protein. Only combined metformin and vildagliptin exert better benefits by reduced cardiac arrhythmia score and arrhythmic death during I/R injury in obese-insulin resistant rats by increasing Cx-43 phosphorylation.

Acknowledgments

The authors would like to thank Dr. Wanpitak Pongkan, Ms. Sivaporn Sivasinprasasn and Ms. Piangkwan Sa-nguanmoo for their technical assistance on ventricular cardiomyocyte isolation.

Author Contributions

Conceived and designed the experiments: SC NC. Performed the experiments: NA KC SP. Analyzed the data: NA KC SP SC NC. Contributed reagents/materials/analysis tools: SC NC. Wrote the paper: NA SC NC.

References

1. Apaijai N, Pintana H, Chattipakorn SC, Chattipakorn N (2013) Effects of vildagliptin versus sitagliptin, on cardiac function, heart rate variability and mitochondrial function in obese insulin-resistant rats. Br J Pharmacol 169: 1048–1057.
2. Shibata R, Sato K, Pimentel DR, Takemura Y, Kihara S, et al. (2005) Adiponectin protects against myocardial ischemia-reperfusion injury through AMPK- and COX-2-dependent mechanisms. Nat Med 11: 1096–1103.
3. du Toit EF, Smith W, Muller C, Strijdom H, Stouthammer B, et al. (2008) Myocardial susceptibility to ischemic-reperfusion injury in a prediabetic model of dietary-induced obesity. Am J Physiol Heart Circ Physiol 294: H2336–2343.
4. Wensley I, Salaveria K, Bulmer AC, Donner DG, Du Toit EF (2013) Myocardial Structure, Function, and Ischaemic Tolerance in a Rodent Model of Obesity with Insulin Resistance. Exp Physiol. (in press)
5. Surinkaew S, Kumphune S, Chattipakorn S, Chattipakorn N (2013) Inhibition of p38 MAPK during ischemia, but not reperfusion, effectively attenuates fatal arrhythmia in ischemia/reperfusion heart. J Cardiovasc Pharmacol 61: 133–141.
6. Honda HM, Korge P, Weiss JN (2005) Mitochondria and ischemia/reperfusion injury. Ann N Y Acad Sci 1047: 248–258.
7. Di Lisa F, Bernardi P (2006) Mitochondria and ischemia-reperfusion injury of the heart: fixing a hole. Cardiovasc Res 70: 191–199.
8. Jackson PE, Feng QP, Jones DL (2008) Nitric oxide depresses connexin 43 after myocardial infarction in mice. Acta Physiol (Oxf) 194: 23–33.
9. Danik SB, Rosner G, Lader J, Gutstein DE, Fishman GI, et al. (2008) Electrical remodeling contributes to complex tachyarrhythmias in connexin43-deficient mouse hearts. FASEB J 22: 1204–1212.
10. Poelzing S, Rosenbaum DS (2004) Altered connexin43 expression produces arrhythmia substrate in heart failure. Am J Physiol Heart Circ Physiol 287: H1762–1770.
11. Chinda K, Palee S, Surinkaew S, Phornphutkul M, Chattipakorn S, et al. (2013) Cardioprotective effect of dipeptidyl peptidase-4 inhibitor during ischemia-reperfusion injury. Int J Cardiol 167: 451–457.
12. Whittington HJ, Hall AR, McLaughlin CP, Hausenloy DJ, Yellon DM, et al. (2013) Chronic metformin associated cardioprotection against infarction: not just a glucose lowering phenomenon. Cardiovasc Drugs Ther 27: 5–16.
13. Derosa G, Ragonesi PD, Carbone A, Fogari E, D'Angelo A, et al. (2013) Evaluation of the positive effects on insulin-resistance and beta-cell measurements of vildagliptin in addition to metformin in type 2 diabetic patients. Pharmacol Res 73: 20–26.
14. Apaijai N, Pintana H, Chattipakorn SC, Chattipakorn N (2012) Cardioprotective effects of metformin and vildagliptin in adult rats with insulin resistance induced by a high-fat diet. Endocrinology 153: 3878–3885.
15. Kilkenny C, Browne W, Cuthill IC, Emerson M, Altman DG (2010) Animal research: reporting in vivo experiments: the ARRIVE guidelines. Br J Pharmacol 160: 1577–1579.
16. Pratchayasakul W, Kerdphoo S, Petsophonsakul P, Pongchaidecha A, Chattipakorn N, et al. (2011) Effects of high-fat diet on insulin receptor function in rat hippocampus and the level of neuronal corticosterone. Life Sci 88: 619–627.
17. Friedewald WT, Levy RI, Fredrickson DS (1972) Estimation of the concentration of low-density lipoprotein cholesterol in plasma, without use of the preparative ultracentrifuge. Clin Chem 18: 499–502.
18. Pipatpiboon N, Pratchayasakul W, Chattipakorn N, Chattipakorn SC (2012) PPARgamma agonist improves neuronal insulin receptor function in hippocampus and brain mitochondria function in rats with insulin resistance induced by long term high-fat diets. Endocrinology 153: 329–338.
19. Chattipakorn N, Incharoen T, Kanlop N, Chattipakorn S (2007) Heart rate variability in myocardial infarction and heart failure. Int J Cardiol 120: 289–296.
20. Lekawanvijit S, Kompa AR, Zhang Y, Wang BH, Kelly DJ, et al. (2012) Myocardial infarction impairs renal function, induces renal interstitial fibrosis, and increases renal KIM-1 expression: implications for cardiorenal syndrome. Am J Physiol Heart Circ Physiol 302: H1884–1893.
21. Curtis MJ, Hancox JC, Farkas A, Wainwright CL, Stables CL, et al. (2013) The Lambeth Conventions (II): Guidelines for the study of animal and human ventricular and supraventricular arrhythmias. Pharmacol Ther 139: 213–248.
22. Palee S, Weerateerangkul P, Chinda K, Chattipakorn SC, Chattipakorn N (2013) Mechanisms responsible for beneficial and adverse effects of rosiglitazone in a rat model of acute cardiac ischaemia-reperfusion. Exp Physiol 98: 1028–1037.
23. Riess ML, Rhodes SS, Stowe DF, Aldakkak M, Camara AK (2009) Comparison of cumulative planimetry versus manual dissection to assess experimental infarct size in isolated hearts. J Pharmacol Toxicol Methods 60: 275–280.
24. Thummasorn S, Kumfu S, Chattipakorn S, Chattipakorn N (2011) Granulocyte-colony stimulating factor attenuates mitochondrial dysfunction induced by oxidative stress in cardiac mitochondria. Mitochondrion 11: 457–466.
25. Wongcharoen W, Chen YC, Chen YJ, Chang CM, Yeh HI, et al. (2006) Effects of a Na+/Ca2+ exchanger inhibitor on pulmonary vein electrical activity and ouabain-induced arrhythmogenicity. Cardiovasc Res 70: 497–508.
26. Pintana H, Apaijai N, Pratchayasakul W, Chattipakorn N, Chattipakorn SC (2012) Effects of metformin on learning and memory behaviors and brain mitochondrial functions in high fat diet induced insulin resistant rats. Life Sci 91: 409–414.
27. Mari A, Sallas WM, He YL, Watson C, Ligueros-Saylan M, et al. (2005) Vildagliptin, a dipeptidyl peptidase-IV inhibitor, improves model-assessed beta-cell function in patients with type 2 diabetes. J Clin Endocrinol Metab 90: 4888–4894.
28. Bikman BT, Zheng D, Kane DA, Anderson EJ, Woodlief TL, et al. (2010) Metformin Improves Insulin Signaling in Obese Rats via Reduced IKKbeta Action in a Fiber-Type Specific Manner. J Obes 2010.
29. Esteghamati A, Eskandari D, Mirmiranpour H, Noshad S, Mousavizadeh M, et al. (2013) Effects of metformin on markers of oxidative stress and antioxidant reserve in patients with newly diagnosed type 2 diabetes: a randomized clinical trial. Clin Nutr 32: 179–185.
30. Avila Dde L, Araujo GR, Silva M, Miranda PH, Diniz MF, et al. (2013) Vildagliptin ameliorates oxidative stress and pancreatic beta cell destruction in type 1 diabetic rats. Arch Med Res 44: 194–202.
31. Supakul L, Pintana H, Apaijai N, Chattipakorn S, Shinlapawittayatorn K, et al. (2013) Protective effects of garlic extract on cardiac function, heart rate

variability, and cardiac mitochondria in obese insulin-resistant rats. Eur J Nutr. (in press)
32. Pavithran P, Nandeesha H, Sathiyapriya V, Bobby Z, Madanmohan T (2008) Short-term heart variability and oxidative stress in newly diagnosed essential hypertension. Clin Exp Hypertens 30: 486-496.
33. Bhamra GS, Hausenloy DJ, Davidson SM, Carr RD, Paiva M, et al. (2008) Metformin protects the ischemic heart by the Akt-mediated inhibition of mitochondrial permeability transition pore opening. Basic Res Cardiol 103: 274-284.
34. Gundewar S, Calvert JW, Jha S, Toedt-Pingel I, Ji SY, et al. (2009) Activation of AMP-activated protein kinase by metformin improves left ventricular function and survival in heart failure. Circ Res 104: 403-411.
35. Calvert JW, Gundewar S, Jha S, Greer JJ, Bestermann WH, et al. (2008) Acute metformin therapy confers cardioprotection against myocardial infarction via AMPK-eNOS-mediated signaling. Diabetes 57: 696-705.
36. Zhang Y, Dong Y, Wu X, Lu Y, Xu Z, et al. (2010) The mitochondrial pathway of anesthetic isoflurane-induced apoptosis. J Biol Chem 285: 4025-4037.
37. Barreto-Torres G, Parodi-Rullan R, Javadov S (2012) The Role of PPARalpha in Metformin-Induced Attenuation of Mitochondrial Dysfunction in Acute Cardiac Ischemia/Reperfusion in Rats. Int J Mol Sci 13: 7694-7709.
38. Whittington HJ, Hall AR, McLaughlin CP, Hausenloy DJ, Yellon DM, et al. (2013) Chronic metformin associated cardioprotection against infarction: not just a glucose lowering phenomenon. Cardiovasc Drugs Ther 27: 5-16.
39. Roell W, Lewalter T, Sasse P, Tallini YN, Choi BR, et al. (2007) Engraftment of connexin 43-expressing cells prevents post-infarct arrhythmia. Nature 450: 819-824.
40. Srisakuldee W, Nickel BE, Fandrich RR, Jiang ZS, Kardami E (2006) Administration of FGF-2 to the heart stimulates connexin-43 phosphorylation at protein kinase C target sites. Cell Commun Adhes 13: 13-19.

16

The Apolipoprotein-AI Mimetic Peptide L4F at a Modest Dose Does Not Attenuate Weight Gain, Inflammation, or Atherosclerosis in LDLR-Null Mice

Michelle M. Averill[1], Eung Ju Kim[2], Leela Goodspeed[2], Shari Wang[2], Savitha Subramanian[2], Laura J. Den Hartigh[2], Chongren Tang[2], Yilei Ding[2], Catherine A. Reardon[3], Godfrey S. Getz[3], Alan Chait[2]*

1 Department of Environmental and Occupational Health, University of Washington, Seattle, Washington, United States of America, **2** Department of Medicine, University of Washington, Seattle, Washington, United States of America, **3** Department of Pathology, University of Chicago, Chicago, Illinois, United States of America

Abstract

Objective: High density lipoprotein (HDL) cholesterol levels are inversely related to cardiovascular disease risk and associated with a reduced risk of type 2 diabetes. Apolipoprotein A-I (apoA-I; major HDL protein) mimetics have been reported to reduce atherosclerosis and decrease adiposity. This study investigated the effect of L4F mimetic peptide and apoA-I overexpression on weight gain, insulin resistance, and atherosclerosis in an LDL receptor deficient ($Ldlr^{-/-}$) model fed a high fat high sucrose with cholesterol (HFHSC) diet.

Methods: Studies in differentiated 3T3-L1 adipocytes tested whether L4F could inhibit palmitate-induced adipocyte inflammation. *In vivo* studies used male $Ldlr^{-/-}$ mice fed a HFHSC diet for 12 weeks and were injected daily with L4F (100 μg/mouse) subcutaneously during the last 8 weeks. Wild-type and apoA-I overexpressing $Ldlr^{-/-}$ mice were fed HFHSC diet for 16 weeks.

Results: Neither L4F administration nor apoA-I overexpression affected weight gain, total plasma cholesterol or triglycerides in our studies. While pre-treatment of 3T3-L1 adipocytes with either L4F or HDL abolished palmitate-induced cytokine expression *in vitro*, L4F treatment did not affect circulating or adipose tissue inflammatory markers *in vivo*. Neither L4F administration nor apoA-I overexpression affected glucose tolerance. ApoA-I overexpression significantly reduced atherosclerotic lesion size, yet L4F treatment did not affect atherosclerosis.

Conclusion: Our results suggest that neither L4F (100 μg/day/mouse) nor apoA-I overexpression affects adiposity or insulin resistance in this model. We also were unable to confirm a reduction in atherosclerosis with L4F in our particular model. Further studies on the effect of apoA-I mimetics on atherosclerosis and insulin resistance in a variety of dietary contexts are warranted.

Editor: Esther Lutgens, University of Amsterdam Academic Medical Center, Netherlands

Funding: This work was supported by National Institutes of Health (www.nih.gov) grants RO1 HL094352 (AC), P01 HL092969 (AC),P30 DK-035816 (AC), and R01 HL 106145 (CR, GG). The funder had no role in study design, data collection and analysis, decision to publish, or preparation of the manuscript.

Competing Interests: The authors have declared that no competing interests exist.

* Email: achait@u.washington.edu

Introduction

The strong inverse relationship between high density lipoprotein (HDL) cholesterol levels and coronary heart disease [1] has been known for over three decades. HDL's role in reverse cholesterol transport has been hypothesized to inhibit atherogenesis [2], and has been thought to contribute to HDL's role as a negative cardiovascular risk factor. Recent research also has highlighted other functional properties of HDL, including its anti-inflammatory and anti-oxidant activities, as additional mechanisms to reduce atherosclerosis [3]. Low HDL cholesterol levels are also associated with development of type 2 diabetes mellitus (T2DM) [4]. Inflammation has been suggested to be responsible for the reduction in HDL levels seen in the setting of insulin resistance and obesity [5]. However, recent data have also highlighted anti-inflammatory properties of HDL [6], suggesting HDL may improve insulin sensitivity [7].

Apolipoprotein A-I (apoA-I) is the main protein in HDL and contributes to the cholesterol efflux, anti-oxidant, and anti-inflammatory potential of HDL [2]. ApoA-I mimetic peptides are 18 amino acid peptides modeled after the amphipathic α-helical structure of apoA-I [8]. The 4F peptide, the most widely studied mimetic, has been shown to promote cholesterol efflux, have anti-inflammatory properties, and to reduce atherosclerosis and adiposity in some murine models [8–10]. Early phase trials of 4F use in humans have been reported [11]. The majority of murine studies with the 4F mimetic peptide have been conducted in apolipoprotein E deficient ($apoE^{-/-}$) mice, a common model of hyperlipidemia associated with development of premature atherosclerosis [9]. The *apoE*$^{-/-}$ model does not lend itself to the study of obesity or insulin resistance, whereas the *Ldlr*$^{-/-}$ mouse, another common model of atherosclerosis, allows for the combined study of diet induced obesity, insulin resistance, and atherosclerosis [12]. Thus further investigation of the effect of the 4F mimetic peptide in the *Ldlr*$^{-/-}$ model is warranted.

The purpose of the current study was to determine the effect of 4F mimetic peptide on atherosclerosis and obesity in *Ldlr*$^{-/-}$ mice fed an obesogenic diet. We also determined the effect of either apoA-I overexpression or the 4F mimetic peptide on insulin resistance and inflammation. We used a previously validated model of diet-induced obesity (DIO) to induce atherosclerosis and insulin resistance, i.e., male *Ldlr*$^{-/-}$ mice fed a high fat high sucrose diet with added cholesterol (HFHSC) [13]. The L4F version of the peptide, synthesized using L amino acids, was used based on our previous studies [10].

Methods

L4F Mimetic Peptides

N-terminally acetylated and C-terminally amidated L4F peptide was purchased from BioSynthesis. The "4F" denotes the following peptide: Ac-DWFKAFYDKVAEKFKEAF-NH2. Lyophilized peptide was stored at −20°C and solubilized in sterile PBS immediately prior to use. The L4F peptide does not form precipitates upon extended storage at 4°C in PBS [14].

In Vitro Adipocyte Studies

The effect of HDL and L4F peptide on adipocyte inflammation was determined using 3T3-L1 adipocytes exposed to palmitate. HDL (d = 1.063 to 1.210 g/mL) was isolated from plasma of healthy human volunteers by ultracentrifugation. 3T3-L1 murine pre-adipocytes (American Type Tissue Culture Collection) were differentiated into adipocytes according to standard procedures [15]. Fully differentiated 3T3-L1 adipocytes, cultured in DMEM media containing 5 mmol/L glucose and 10% fetal bovine serum, were pre-treated with 50 µg/ml HDL or 25 µg/ml L4F for 6 h. After the pre-treatment, cells were washed three times with PBS. Adipocytes were incubated with 250 µmol/L palmitate (16:0; Sigma) for 24 h (DMEM media containing 5 mmol/L glucose and 10% fetal bovine serum), as described previously [6]. At the end of the study RNA was isolated from the 3T3 cells using a lipid specific RNA isolation kit (Qiagen) and gene expression was determined using RT-PCR.

Real-time quantitative reverse-transcription polymerase chain reaction (RT-PCR)

Specific gene expression was determined using specific primers and TaqMan probes obtained from Applied Biosystems Assay-on-Demand and the TaqMan Master kit (Applied Biosystems). GAPDH was used as the control housekeeping gene. Samples were run using the ABI prism 7900HT system. Each sample was analyzed in triplicate and relative amounts of target genes calculated using the ΔΔCT formula.

Animals and Diet

Male *Ldlr*$^{-/-}$ mice originally purchased from Jackson Labs (Sacramento, CA, USA) on the C57BL/6 background, were 10-weeks-old when started on a HFHSC diet (35.5% calories as fat and 36.6% as carbohydrate, 0.15% added cholesterol, BioServ No. F4997). Mice used for the mimetic study were on diet for 12 weeks, an early time point chosen to model our previous data showing the L4F peptide works on early rather than on advanced lesions [10]. After 4 weeks of diet, either saline or L4F peptide (100 µg/mouse) was injected subcutaneously daily for the remaining 8 weeks of the study, the injection duration used in our previous study [10].

ApoA-I^{tg} (mice overexpressing human apoA-I) mice were purchased from the Jackson laboratory. *Ldlr*$^{-/-}$*apoA-I*^{tg} and control *Ldlr*$^{-/-}$*apoA-I*^{wt} mice were generated from these homozygous mice. Confirmation of apoA-I overexpression was done using quantitative RT-PCR to confirm homozygous overexpression and an ELISA for human apoA-I confirmed appropriate genotype for all mice used in breeding and in the study. From this breeding colony adult (10-week-old) male *Ldlr*$^{-/-}$ mice overexpressing human apoA-I (*apoA-I*^{tg}) and control *Ldlr*$^{-/-}$ mice (*apoA-I*^{wt}) were fed the HFHSC diet for 16 weeks. A longer time on diet was chosen to analyze more advanced stages of atherosclerosis and more dramatic differences in insulin sensitivity, corresponding with several of our recent studies [16]. The *apoA-I*^{tg} mice are the same as reported previously [6]. Data in this current manuscript is additional to that previously reported. However a limited amount of data from that report is reproduced here for direct comparison of the response with that seen after peptide treatment.

At sacrifice, epididymal adipose tissues were snap-frozen at −70°C for isolation of total RNA using lipid specific isolation kit (Qiagen). Aortic tissue were excised at the time of sacrifice and prepared for atherosclerosis analysis (described below).

Ethics Statement

All experimental procedures were undertaken with approval from the Institutional Animal Care and Use Committee of the University of Washington (Protocol Number: 3104-01). The study was carried out in accordance with the National Institutes of Health recommendations based on the published *Guide for the Care and Use of Laboratory Animals* [17]. All efforts were made to minimize animal suffering.

Analytic Procedures for Mimetic and apoA-I overexpression study

At both 4 weeks into the diet and the end of each study blood was collected after a 4–6 hour fast. Analysis of plasma insulin was done using a commercially available kit (Linco Research Inc). Plasma triglycerides and cholesterol were assayed using colorimetric assay kits, and levels of lipoproteins were analyzed by fast-phase liquid chromatography (FPLC) as described previously [13]. Plasma SAA levels (isoforms 1 and 2) were measured by enzyme-linked immunosorbent assay (ELISA) [13]. Glucose tolerance testing (GTT) was performed as previously described [13] at week 11 in mimetic study and week 14 in apoA-I overexpression study. Plasma was collected at the 30 minute time point of the GTT to analyze glucose stimulated insulin levels. Body composition was determined in the mimetic study using quantitative magnetic resonance (qMRI) (EchoMRI 3-in-1 machine whole body composition analyzer; Echo MRI, LLC, Houston, TX) after 10 weeks on diet [18,19].

Atherosclerosis Quantification

The en face technique was used to quantify the extent of atherosclerosis as described previously [20]. Additional atherosclerosis quantification was done in the mimetic study by analyzing atherosclerosis in the brachiocephalic artery [21]. The brachiocephalic artery was dissected, fixed, embedded, and serial sectioned. Every fourth section was stained with a Movat pentachrome stain. Atherosclerotic lesion area in the brachiocephalic artery was determined in a masked fashion by calculating maximal and average lesion area.

Statistical analysis

Data shown are expressed as means± standard deviation unless noted otherwise. With the exception of atherosclerotic lesions data, mean values were compared using ANOVA and post-hoc testing with Bonferroni correction for multiple comparisons for parametric data using GraphPad Prism program (Version 3.03, GraphPad Software Inc). As the atherosclerotic lesion data was not normally distributed (D'Agostino and Pearson omnibus normality test) this analysis employed the Mann-Whitney non-parametric test. Significance was denoted at p-value less than 0.05.

Results

L4F inhibits palmitate induced chemokine expression in 3T3-L1 adipocytes

We previously have shown that palmitate induces chemotactic factor expression in 3T3-L1 adipocytes [15] and this can be inhibited by pre-treatment with HDL [6]. Thus, we investigated if L4F peptide can similarly inhibit chemokine expression in 3T3-L1 cells. After palmitate exposure 3T3-L1 cells pre-treated with L4F peptide expressed significantly less MCP-1 and SAA3 (figure 1), two chemokines present in inflamed obese adipose tissue [13]. This effect was comparable to that seen with HDL pre-treatment.

Neither L4F (100 μg/day/mouse) nor apoA-I overexpression attenuate weight gain in *Ldlr*$^{-/-}$ mice fed HFHSC diet

The diet employed in this study is one intended to induce a large gain in weight. Treatment of *Ldlr*$^{-/-}$ mice with L4F peptide given at 100 μg/day/mouse had no impact on the extent of weight gain (figure 2A), compared with the saline injected animals. Further, there was no impact of L4F treatment on fat mass measured by qMRI (36.4%±3.3% saline versus 35.6%±5.1% L4F). Similarly, gain in body weight was no different for human apoA-I overexpressing mice on the *Ldlr*$^{-/-}$ background than in mice expressing murine apoA-I at wild type levels (figure 2B). Also the weight gain was very similar for the *Ldlr*$^{-/-}$ animals in the mimetic study and the apoA-I study over the first 12 weeks of diet.

Neither L4F (100 μg/day/mouse) nor apoA-I overexpression affected plasma total cholesterol or triglycerides

The *Ldlr*$^{-/-}$ HFHSC fed mouse develops hyperlipidemia with increased VLDL and LDL cholesterol, which promotes atherosclerosis [22]. However, in *Ldlr*$^{-/-}$ mice fed the HFHSC diet, neither L4F nor apoA-I overexpression affected plasma total cholesterol or triglyceride levels (figure 3 A through D). There were also no differences noted in plasma cholesterol or triglycerides after 4 weeks on diet (figure 3 A through D), a time point chosen as the baseline before the initiation of peptide injections. In both the peptide study and the apoA-I overexpression study plasma cholesterol and triglyceride did significantly increase over the remaining time on diet (figure 3 A through D). There was no indication that L4F alters the lipoprotein profile (figure 3E). FPLC profiles do suggest apoA-I overexpression increases HDL cholesterol content (figure 3F), yet we were unable to assess the statistical significance of this difference since the FPLC profiles represent pooled samples.

L4F (100 μg/day/mouse) did not attenuate systemic or adipose tissue inflammation

One mechanism potentially linking obesity to insulin resistance is through adipose tissue inflammation. We have shown in previous studies that the HFHSC diet in *Ldlr*$^{-/-}$ mice results in increased macrophage content in adipose tissue and increased expression of inflammatory cytokines [13]. We have also shown that overexpression of apoA-I in C57BL/6 mice or *Ldlr*$^{-/-}$ mice inhibit adipose tissue macrophage content and inflammatory gene expression [6]. Given that L4F elicits an anti-inflammatory response in 3T3-L1 cells we examined the effect of L4F on SAA, a marker of systemic inflammation and on adipose tissue inflammatory gene expression. In contrast to our previous results in the apoA-I overexpression model [6], we did not see any effect of L4F (100 μg/day/mouse) on circulating SAA, or adipose tissue gene expression (figure 4A and B).

Neither L4F (100 μg/day/mouse) nor apoA-I overexpression improve glucose tolerance in *Ldlr*$^{-/-}$ mice fed HFHSC diet

Our original hypothesis was that the L4F mimetic would decrease adipose tissue inflammation and thus improve glucose

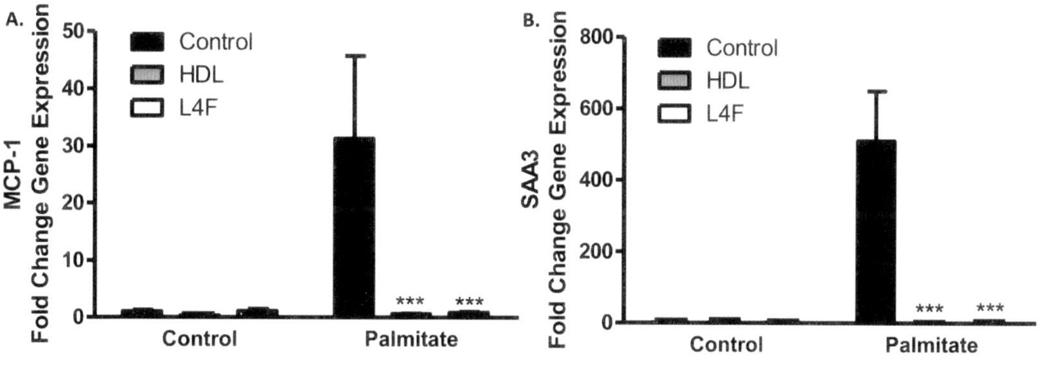

Figure 1. L4F mimetic peptide blocks palmitate-induced chemokine factor expression in 3T3-L1 adipocytes. MCP-1 (A) and SAA3 (B) gene expression in 3T3-L1 cells exposed to control (fatty acid free albumin) or palmitate (250 μmol/l). Prior to fatty acid exposure cells were pre-incubated with control, HDL (50 μg/ml), and L4F (25 μg/ml) containing media. Fold gene expression was determined using the ΔΔCT fold change method normalized to GAPDH. Each graph is representative of three independent experiments. ***P<0.001 vs control in palmitate treated cells using 2-way ANOVA and Bonferroni adjustment for multiple comparisons.

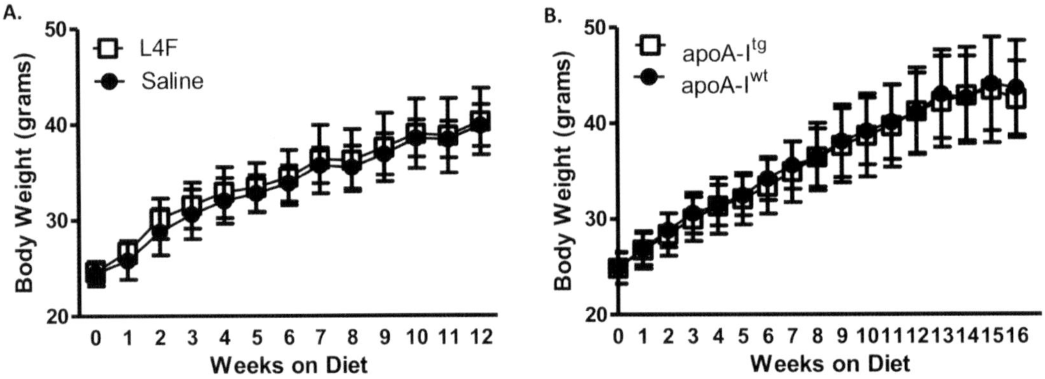

Figure 2. 100 μg/day/mouse L4F mimetic peptide and apoA-I overexpression do not affect weight gain. Body weights for the peptide study (A; n = 5) and the apoA-I overexpression study (B; n = 15–17). No significant differences were identified.

homeostasis. In order to test this, glucose tolerance tests and glucose-stimulated insulin levels were examined. There was no significant effect of L4F peptide given at 100 μg/day/mouse on glucose tolerance or glucose-stimulated insulin secretion (figure 4C and E). As with the response to L4F, apoA-I overexpression did not improve glucose tolerance (figure 4D). In addition, there was no effect of apoA-I overexpression on glucose-stimulated plasma insulin levels (figure 4F).

L4F (100 μg/day/mouse) did not attenuate atherosclerosis

Our final objective was to determine if L4F peptide could inhibit atherosclerosis similarly in the *Ldlr*$^{-/-}$ model as has been described for the *ApoE*$^{-/-}$ model. We examined the extent of atherosclerosis using the *en face* method as previously described [20]. Given the small size of the lesions our final analysis was based only on the arch and not the entire aorta for the mimetic study. Our results suggest there was no effect on lesion size with the L4F mimetic provided at 100 μg/day/mouse in *Ldlr*$^{-/-}$ mice (figure 5A, representative images in figure 5D). We also assessed lesion area in the brachiocephalic artery and found no difference in maximum lesion area (figure 5B) or average lesion area (data not shown). Morphological assessment of these lesions revealed the lesions were characterized by foam cell accumulation with no evidence of fibrosis or necrotic core formation, characteristic of early fatty streaks. No differences in lesion morphology were identified and representative images are shown in figure 5E. To validate our model and methods, the effect of apoA-I overexpression on lesion area was examined by the *en face* method. As expected and supporting previous research [23], a significant reduction in atherosclerosis was observed (figure 5C; representative images in figure 5F). It is important to note that the absolute extent of lesions differed between the mimetic and apoA-I overexpression studies due to the fact that the mimetic study focused on the arch while the apoA-I study included the entire aorta.

Discussion

In this manuscript we report several new findings. Our results suggest that while L4F can markedly reduce adipocyte inflammation *in vitro* similar to HDL, this does not carry through to improvements in inflammation, glucose tolerance, or atherosclerosis in *Ldlr*$^{-/-}$ male mice fed the HFHSC diet using an LF4 dose of 100 μg/day/mouse. Further, despite our previous studies showing that apoA-I overexpression can reduce adipose tissue inflammation, our current data suggests this does not confer improvements in glucose tolerance.

Our *in vitro* studies demonstrated a novel ability of L4F to mimic apoA-I function in adipocytes. ApoA-I [6], HDL and L4F (figure 1) exposure markedly reduced the expression of inflammatory markers in 3T3L1 cultured adipocytes. The dramatic efficacy of L4F in these *in vitro* experiments suggests that the peptide is functioning in culture in a similar fashion to apoA-I in HDL. As the L4F peptide was developed to mimic apoA-I function, and this appears to be borne out by our *in vitro* studies, we have compared apoA-I overexpression with L4F treatment in several pathophysiological endpoints in *Ldlr*$^{-/-}$ male mice fed the HFHSC diet. The effect of apoA-I overexpression on insulin resistance in the *Ldlr*$^{-/-}$ DIO model has not been reported on previously, and thus an important dataset for comparison to L4F treatment. Provided chronic inflammation which is associated with obesity related insulin resistance [24], our *in vitro* findings suggest that L4F and apoA-I overexpression could potentially improve glucose tolerance in an *in* vivo model of DIO. In our previous study apoA-I overexpression relieved some of the adipose tissue inflammation [6]. However, in the present study L4F treatment of 100 μg/day/mouse had no impact on adipose tissue or systemic inflammatory markers (figure 4). Further, neither the overexpression of apoA-I nor treatment with L4F had an impact on glucose tolerance nor glucose stimulated insulin levels (figure 4). Note that neither apoA-I overexpression nor L4F treatment had an impact on weight gain or adiposity in this model (figure 2), confirmed in the peptide study by body composition analysis. ApoA-I and L4F mimetics are often cited for their anti-atherosclerotic properties. This effect of apoA-I overexpression in *Ldlr*$^{-/-}$ mice fed a high fat diet has been documented [23] and confirmed in the present study (figure 5). Yet, L4F treatment had no such effect at a dosage of 100 μg/day/mouse.

It is striking that despite the dramatic effect of L4F on 3T3L1 cells, the peptide is without influence on the measured parameters studied *in vivo* at 100 μg/day/mouse. One limitation of this study is that the absence of any *in vivo* effect of peptide treatment raises questions about the efficacy of the dose and route of administration of the peptide. We have followed protocols and dosages that have been shown in *apoE*$^{-/-}$ and *ob/ob* mice to be effective [10,25]. The dose we employed (4–5 mg/kg/day), is equal to the effective dose of 4.5 mg/kg/day shown by Navab and colleagues to reduce plasma SAA levels [26]. Importantly, they have found the dose was determining rather than the concentration in the plasma [26]. This group has further suggested that the primary function of the

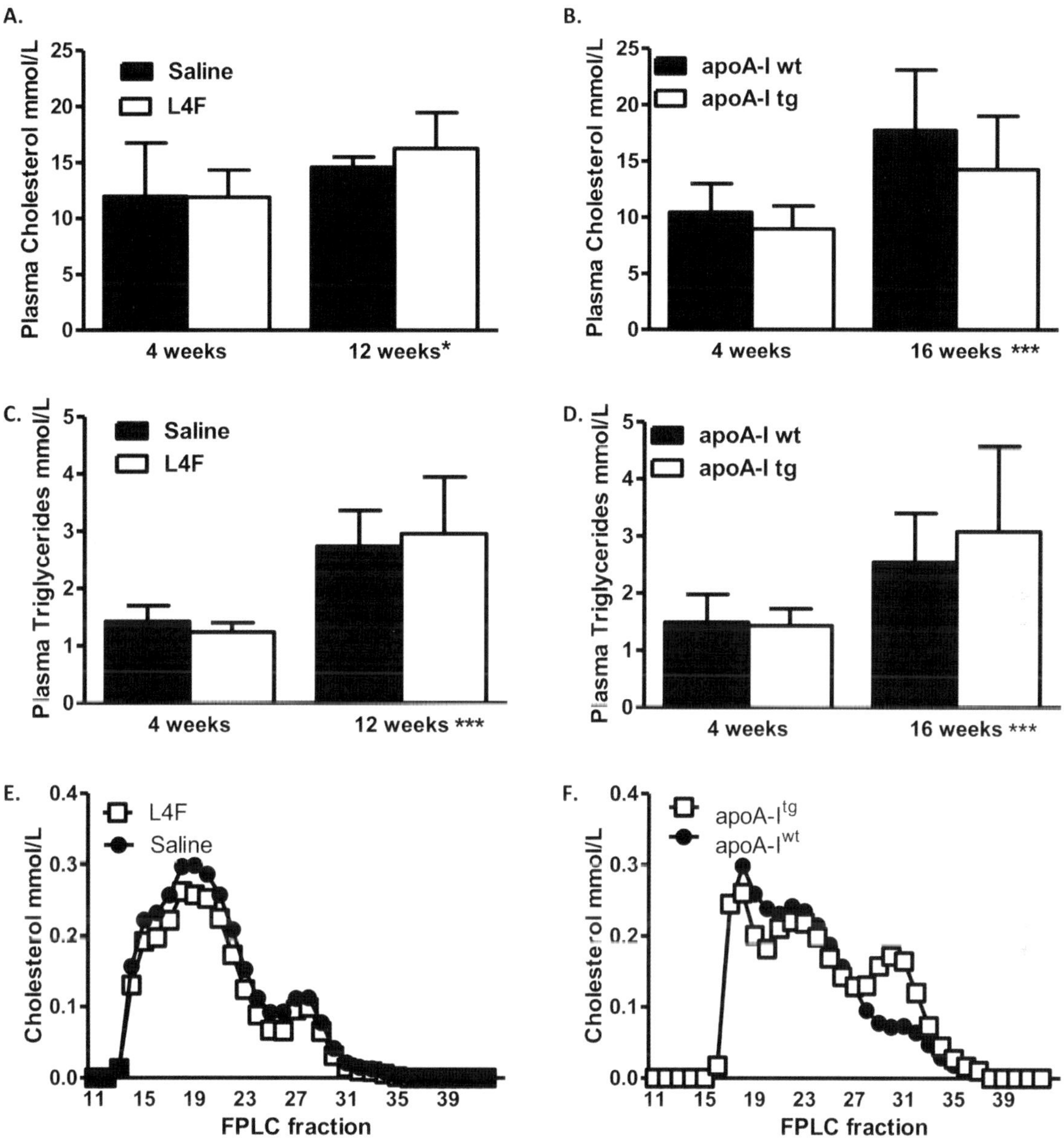

Figure 3. 100 μg/day/mouse L4F mimetic peptide and apoA-I overexpression do not affect plasma total cholesterol or triglycerides. Total plasma cholesterol and triglycerides are shown for the peptide (A,C; n = 5) and the apoA-I overexpression study (B,D, n = 9–13) after 4 weeks on the diet and at the end of the study protocol. FPLC cholesterol analysis on pooled plasma samples from the peptide study (E) and the apoA-I overexpression study (F). Differences in cholesterol eluting times, as noted by the different starting peaks for cholesterol, are due to a newer FPLC column used with the apoA-I overexpression study. No significant differences were identified. *$P<0.05$ 4 week versus 12 weeks on diet peptide study, ***$P<0.0001$ 4 week vs 16 weeks on diet apoA-I study by paired two-way ANOVA.

peptides is to attenuate the oxidized lipid and unsaturated lysophosphatidic acid concentrations in the intestine [27]. The current study utilized the L version of the peptide injected subcutaneously as it is not stable for oral delivery while other studies have used the D version of the peptide which is stable for oral delivery. However, data suggests that neither the route of administration nor the enantiomer version of the peptide determines effectiveness. One study directly compared L4F versus D4F delivered subcutaneously in rabbits and found similar reductions in atherosclerosis [28]. While studies suggest the site of action is primarily in the intestine, Navab and colleagues have shown D4F is similarly effective when delivered subcutaneously or orally and equivalent amounts appear in the feces [29]. L4F delivered orally with niclosamide (which protects the peptide from degradation) was equally effective in reducing SAA in *apoE*$^{-/-}$ mice as L4F delivered subcutaneously [26]. This suggests that the effect of 4F peptide on inflammation and atherosclerosis is independent of route of administration and the enantiomer version of the peptide, and thus does not explain the lack of effect in the current study. Given the above discussion, it is possible that either L4F does not influence obesity, inflammation, or atherosclerosis in this model or that a higher dose of peptide is required to affect these outcomes in this model. In addition, we have no information on the role of oxidized lipids in the intestine in our model. Further work is needed to address the effectiveness of 4F peptide, optimal

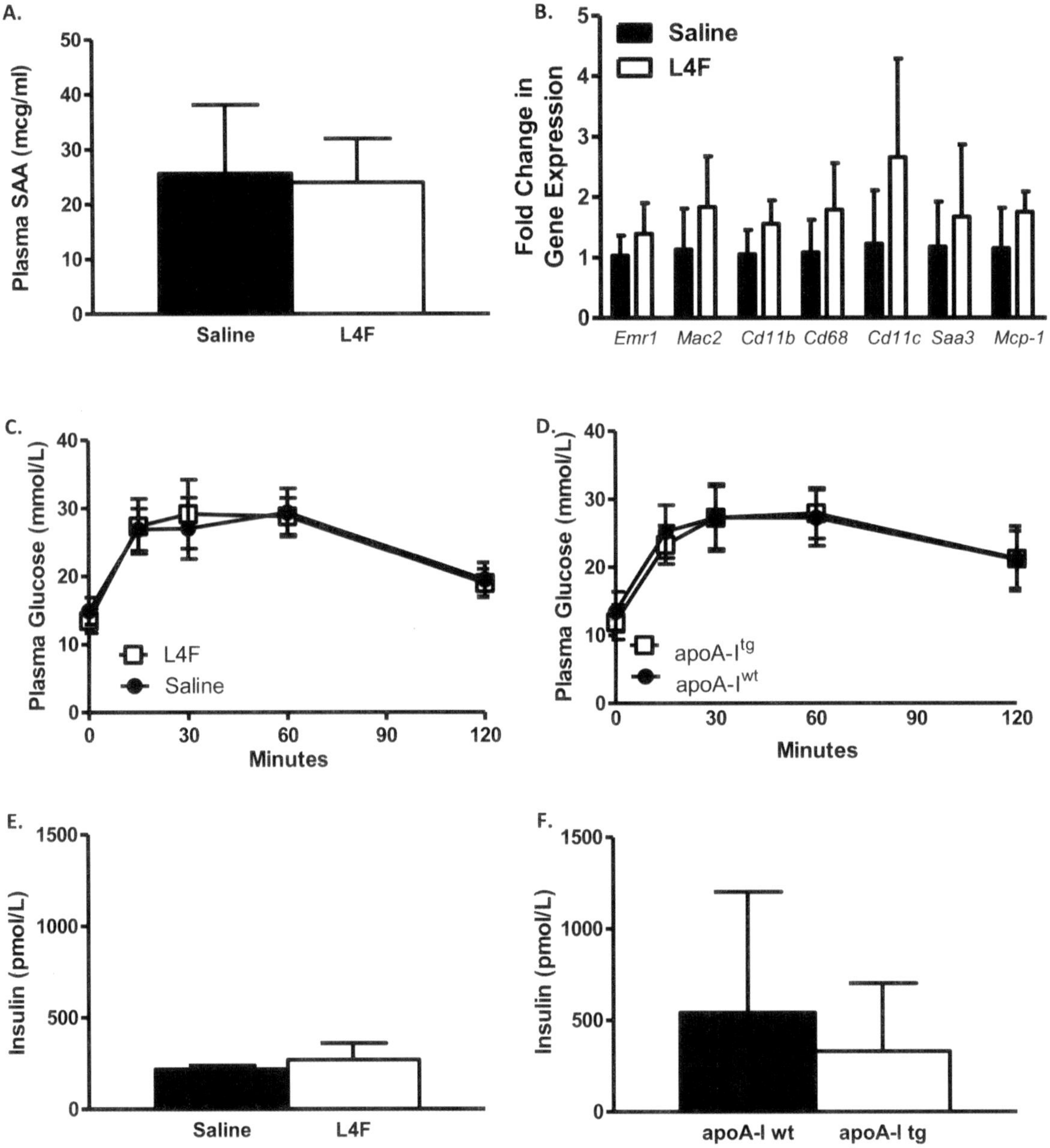

Figure 4. 100 μg/day/mouse L4F did not attenuate inflammation, and neither L4F nor apoA-I overexpression improved glucose tolerance. SAA was measured in the plasma (A, n = 5) and inflammatory gene expression was analyzed in epididymal adipose tissue extracts (B, n = 4–5). GTTs are shown for the peptide study (C: n = 5) and the apoA-I overexpression study (D: n = 10–12). Plasma was collected at the 30 minute time point of the GTT and insulin was measured in both studies (E, F). No significant differences were noted.

dosage, route of administration, and potential mode of action in *Ldlr*$^{-/-}$ male mice fed the HFHSC diet.

Another recognized limitation of our study is the small sample size in the peptide group (n = 5). To determine the extent to which this limitation impacts the ability to draw conclusions from the data power analysis and sample size calculations were performed (Graphpad StatMate 2.00). The sample size calculation was based on the observed standard deviation of 5.54% for the percent of total arch that contains lesion and an observed difference in the means of 2%. Considering these statistics and a desired power > 80%, a sample size of greater than 100 per group would be needed to identity significant differences. Based on these sample size calculations it is not expected that doubling or tripling the sample size of the current study would result in significant differences.

Most studies with mimetic peptides have been performed with *apoE*$^{-/-}$ mice, which has been responsive in several respects to L4F treatment, especially on early atherosclerotic lesions [10]. Relatively few experiments have addressed the role of the peptide on inflammation and atherosclerosis in *Ldlr*$^{-/-}$ mice. Of the studies investigating the effect of 4F peptide in *Ldlr*$^{-/-}$ mice, the dosages used which resulted in a reduction of inflammation or atherosclerosis were 9–25 times greater than the dosages employed in the current study [30], [27], [31]. Thus it is possible that *Ldlr*$^{-/-}$ mice are less sensitive to peptide treatment than are *apoE*$^{-/-}$ mice and a higher dose may be required to observe reductions in inflamma-

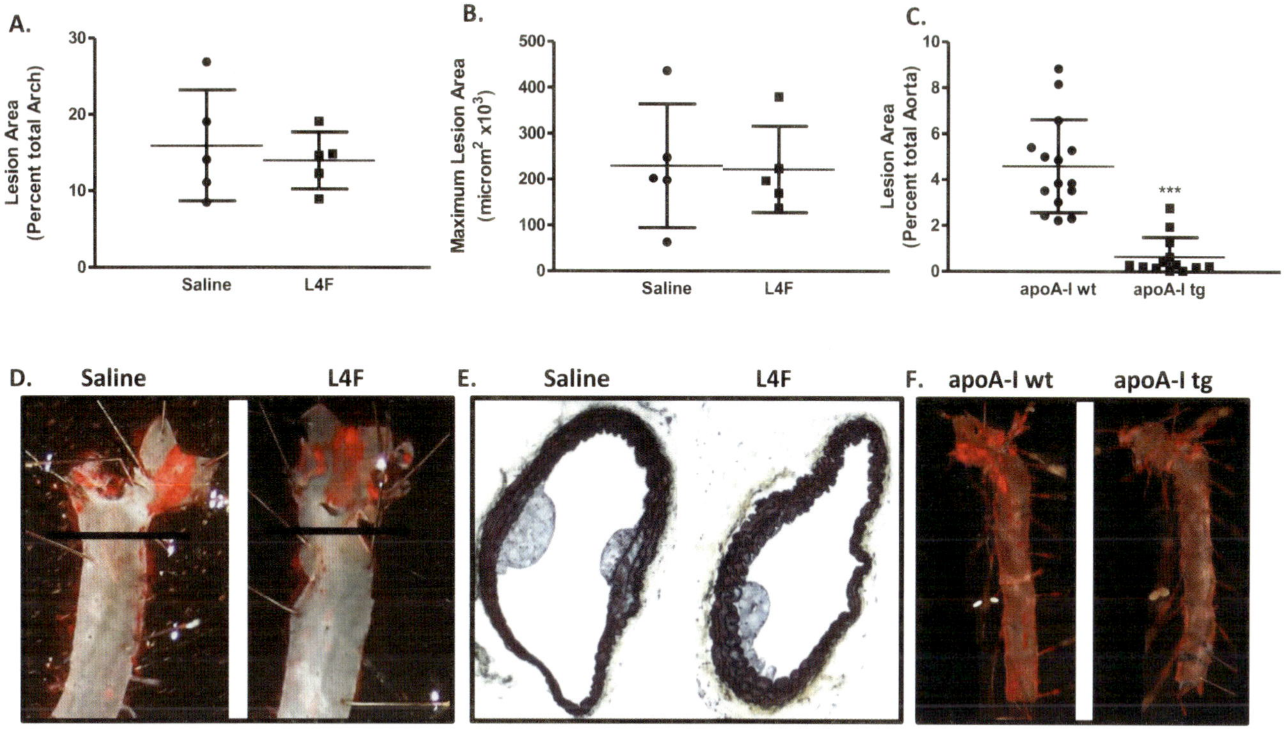

Figure 5. 100 μg/day/mouse L4F did not while apoA-I overexpression did reduce atherosclerosis, in *Ldlr*$^{-/-}$ mice fed HFHSC diet. Atherosclerotic lesion area was determined using the *en face* method. Given the small lesion size the percent lesion area was calculated for the arch section in the peptide study (A, n = 5) and calculated as a percent of the total aorta in the apoA-I overexpression study (C, n = 13-15). Analysis of the maximum lesion area in the brachiocephalic artery lesions is shown for the peptide study (B, n = 5). Representative lesions are shown for the peptide study for both the en face (D) and the brachiocephalic artery (E). Note the black line in the en face image (D) indicated the bottom of the arch indicating the boundary of the analysis. Representative en face images for the apoA-I study are also shown (F). ***P<0.0001 vs apoA-I wt by Mann-Whltney.

tion and atherosclerosis. Possible contributors to reduced sensitivity to peptide in this model may be not only the absence of the LDLR but also the interaction with the highly obesogenic diet.

With respect to adiposity and glucose tolerance, one study used chow-fed ob/ob mice injected with L4F at the dose of 2 mg/kg/day and demonstrated attenuated obesity and adipose inflammation [25,32]. In that study, L4F treatment also improved both glucose and insulin tolerance tests. While the ob/ob model consistently develops obesity related insulin resistance, the hyperlipidemia is characterized by elevations in HDL and this does not associate with atherosclerosis development [12]. We are the first to have reported effects on weight gain, inflammation, insulin resistance, and atherosclerosis in a model of DIO with lipid profiles similar to humans [12]. Our ability to compare the effects of L4F treatment directly to that of apoA-I overexpression is another strength of this research. We have shown using the HFHSC diet in C57BL/6 mice that were either wild type or transgenic with respect to apoA-I expression, apoA-I overexpression reduced adipose tissue inflammation [6]. Similar reductions of adipose tissue inflammation by apoA-I overexpression were also seen in the *Ldlr*$^{-/-}$ background [6], with no change in total plasma cholesterol or triglyceride levels. It is generally thought that adipose tissue inflammation is related to several systemic perturbations, such as glucose intolerance [24]. In the present study, despite the reduction of adipose tissue inflammation, apoA-I overexpression did not influence weight gain or glucose sensitivity in the DIO *Ldlr*$^{-/-}$ male model. This suggests that the gain of adipose tissue mass is not strictly correlated with the degree of inflammation in this tissue. These data argue that the relationship between adiposity, weight gain, adipose tissue inflammation, and glucose intolerance is more complex than has been thought and are not directly correlated. Peptide treatment of *Ldlr*$^{-/-}$ mice on the HFHSC diet also did not influence glucose tolerance [24] at a moderate dose of 100 μg/day/mouse.

Peptide treatment could have two major actions: influence on cholesterol homeostasis and reduced oxidized lipid concentrations [9]. In our model, there is no evidence of these actions of peptide being operative *in vivo*. Perhaps the drive of our dietary model toward atherogenesis and glucose intolerance is so strong as to be beyond the reach of the peptide at the level we employed, which was dosed based on studies in *apoE*$^{-/-}$ and *ob/ob* mice [10,25]. It is not clear whether obesity in this model would indeed be responsive to higher doses of peptide. While a majority of the studies have been conducted in *apoE*$^{-/-}$ mice, this model is driven by hyperlipidemia and does not lend itself to investigation of several other aspects of the metabolic syndrome, namely DIO and insulin resistance. Further study in models that incorporate obesity and insulin resistance, including the *Ldlr*$^{-/-}$ mice fed a HFHSC diet, will improve our understanding of the potential to utilize mimetic peptides in all aspects of the metabolic syndrome.

There continues to be a strong relationship between increased apoA-I and HDL in animal models and reduced atherosclerosis. However, the true potential of mimetic peptides as a means to harness the positive properties of apoA-I remain uncertain. Further, there is some question as to the most appropriate model of insulin resistance and atherosclerosis and it is likely studies in multiple models are needed to identify the true potential of mimetics. Results presented in the current paper do not support a protective role for apoA-I mimetic L4F at a dose of 100 μg/day/mouse in weight gain, inflammation, insulin resistance, or atherosclerosis in a model of DIO ($Ldlr^{-/-}$ male mice fed HFHSC). Future research needs to verify the mechanism of protection and identify an appropriate dosage, route of delivery and timing to effect change on atherosclerosis progression in appropriate models of human disease. The ability for HDL to prevent insulin resistance remains an intriguing idea, and despite results in the current model it warrants further research.

Author Contributions

Conceived and designed the experiments: MMA SS CAR GSG AC. Performed the experiments: MMA EJK LG SW SS LJDH CT YD. Analyzed the data: MMA. Contributed reagents/materials/analysis tools: CT CAR GSG AC. Wrote the paper: MMA SS CAR GSG AC.

References

1. Gordon T, Castelli WP, Hjortland MC, Kannel WB, Dawber TR (1977) High density lipoprotein as a protective factor against coronary heart disease. The Framingham Study. Am J Med 62: 707–714.
2. Gordon SM, Hofmann S, Askew DS, Davidson WS (2011) High density lipoprotein: it's not just about lipid transport anymore. Trends Endocrinol Metab 22: 9–15.
3. Rosenson RS, Brewer HB, Ansell B, Barter P, Chapman MJ, et al. (2013) Translation of High-Density Lipoprotein Function Into Clinical Practice: Current Prospects and Future Challenges. Circulation 128: 1256–1267.
4. Wilson PW, Anderson KM, Kannel WB (1986) Epidemiology of diabetes mellitus in the elderly. The Framingham Study. Am J Med 80: 3–9.
5. Navab M, Anantharamaiah GM, Reddy ST, Van Lenten BJ, Fogelman AM (2009) HDL as a biomarker, potential therapeutic target, and therapy. Diabetes 58: 2711–2717.
6. Umemoto T, Han CY, Mitra P, Averill MM, Tang C, et al. (2013) Apolipoprotein AI and High-Density Lipoprotein Have Anti-Inflammatory Effects on Adipocytes via Cholesterol Transporters: ATP-Binding Cassette A-1, ATP-Binding Cassette G-1, and Scavenger Receptor B-1. Circ Res 112: 1345–1354.
7. Olefsky JM, Glass CK (2010) Macrophages, inflammation, and insulin resistance. Annu Rev Physiol 72: 219–246.
8. Getz GS, Reardon CA (2011) Apolipoprotein A-I and A-I mimetic peptides: a role in atherosclerosis. J Inflamm Res 4: 83–92.
9. Getz G, Wool G, Reardon C (2010) Biological Properties of Apolipoprotein A-I Mimetic Peptides. Current Atherosclerosis Reports 12: 96–104.
10. Wool GD, Cabana VG, Lukens J, Shaw PX, Binder CJ, et al. (2011) 4F Peptide reduces nascent atherosclerosis and induces natural antibody production in apolipoprotein E-null mice. FASEB J 25: 290–300.
11. Bloedon LT, Dunbar R, Duffy D, Pinell-Salles P, Norris R, et al. (2008) Safety, pharmacokinetics, and pharmacodynamics of oral apoA-I mimetic peptide D-4F in high-risk cardiovascular patients. Journal of Lipid Research 49: 1344–1352.
12. Kennedy AJ, Ellacott KL, King VL, Hasty AH (2010) Mouse models of the metabolic syndrome. Dis Model Mech 3: 156–166.
13. Subramanian S, Han CY, Chiba T, McMillen TS, Wang SA, et al. (2008) Dietary cholesterol worsens adipose tissue macrophage accumulation and atherosclerosis in obese LDL receptor-deficient mice. Arterioscler Thromb Vasc Biol 28: 685–691.
14. Wool GD, Reardon CA, Getz GS (2008) Apolipoprotein A-I mimetic peptide helix number and helix linker influence potentially anti-atherogenic properties. Journal of Lipid Research 49: 1268–1283.
15. Yeop Han C, Kargi AY, Omer M, Chan CK, Wabitsch M, et al. (2010) Differential effect of saturated and unsaturated free fatty acids on the generation of monocyte adhesion and chemotactic factors by adipocytes: dissociation of adipocyte hypertrophy from inflammation. Diabetes 59: 386–396.
16. Montes VN, Turner MS, Subramanian S, Ding Y, Hayden-Ledbetter M, et al. (2013) T cell activation inhibitors reduce CD8+ T cell and pro-inflammatory macrophage accumulation in adipose tissue of obese mice. PLoS One 8: e67709.
17. Committee for the Update of the Guide for the Care and Use of Laboratory Animals (2011) Guide for the Care and Use of Laboratory Animals: Eighth Edition: The National Academies Press.
18. Taicher GZ, Tinsley FC, Reiderman A, Heiman ML (2003) Quantitative magnetic resonance (QMR) method for bone and whole-body-composition analysis. Anal Bioanal Chem 377: 990–1002.
19. Tinsley FC, Taicher GZ, Heiman ML (2004) Evaluation of a quantitative magnetic resonance method for mouse whole body composition analysis. Obes Res 12: 150–160.
20. Schreyer SA, Lystig TC, Vick CM, LeBoeuf RC (2003) Mice deficient in apolipoprotein E but not LDL receptors are resistant to accelerated atherosclerosis associated with obesity. Atherosclerosis 171: 49–55.
21. Averill MM, Barnhart S, Becker L, Li X, Heinecke JW, et al. (2011) S100A9 Differentially Modifies Phenotypic States of Neutrophils, Macrophages, and Dendritic Cells: Implications for Atherosclerosis and Adipose Tissue Inflammation. Circulation 123: 1216–1226.
22. Ishibashi S, Goldstein JL, Brown MS, Herz J, Burns DK (1994) Massive xanthomatosis and atherosclerosis in cholesterol-fed low density lipoprotein receptor-negative mice. J Clin Invest 93: 1885–1893.
23. Valenta DT, Bulgrien JJ, Banka CL, Curtiss LK (2006) Overexpression of human ApoAI transgene provides long-term atheroprotection in LDL receptor-deficient mice. Atherosclerosis 189: 255–263.
24. Lumeng CN, Saltiel AR (2011) Inflammatory links between obesity and metabolic disease. J Clin Invest 121: 2111–2117.
25. Peterson SJ, Drummond G, Kim DH, Li M, Kruger AL, et al. (2008) L-4F treatment reduces adiposity, increases adiponectin levels, and improves insulin sensitivity in obese mice. J Lipid Res 49: 1658–1669.
26. Navab M, Reddy ST, Anantharamaiah GM, Imaizumi S, Hough G, et al. (2011) Intestine may be a major site of action for the apoA-I mimetic peptide 4F whether administered subcutaneously or orally. J Lipid Res 52: 1200–1210.
27. Navab M, Reddy ST, Anantharamaiah GM, Hough G, Buga GM, et al. (2012) D-4F-mediated reduction in metabolites of arachidonic and linoleic acids in the small intestine is associated with decreased inflammation in low-density lipoprotein receptor-null mice. J Lipid Res 53: 437–445.
28. Van Lenten BJ, Wagner AC, Navab M, Anantharamaiah GM, Hama S, et al. (2007) Lipoprotein inflammatory properties and serum amyloid A levels but not cholesterol levels predict lesion area in cholesterol-fed rabbits. Journal of Lipid Research 48: 2344–2353.
29. Navab M, Ruchala P, Waring AJ, Lehrer RI, Hama S, et al. (2009) A novel method for oral delivery of apolipoprotein mimetic peptides synthesized from all L-amino acids. J Lipid Res 50: 1538–1547.
30. Navab M, Anantharamaiah GM, Hama S, Garber DW, Chaddha M, et al. (2002) Oral Administration of an Apo A-I Mimetic Peptide Synthesized From D-Amino Acids Dramatically Reduces Atherosclerosis in Mice Independent of Plasma Cholesterol. Circulation 105: 290–292.
31. Navab M, Hough G, Buga GM, Su F, Wagner AC, et al. (2013) Transgenic 6F tomatoes act on the small intestine to prevent systemic inflammation and dyslipidemia caused by Western diet and intestinally derived lysophosphatidic acid. J Lipid Res 54: 3403–3418.
32. Marino JS, Peterson SJ, Li M, Vanella L, Sodhi K, et al. (2012) ApoA-1 mimetic restores adiponectin expression and insulin sensitivity independent of changes in body weight in female obese mice. Nutr Diabetes 2: e33.

Intestine-Targeted DGAT1 Inhibition Improves Obesity and Insulin Resistance without Skin Aberrations in Mice

Naoto Tsuda[1,2]*, Shin Kumadaki[1], Chika Higashi[1], Makoto Ozawa[1], Mikihiko Shinozaki[1], Yutaka Kato[1], Koutarou Hoshida[1], Satomi Kikuchi[1], Yoshihisa Nakano[1], Yoshihiro Ogawa[2], Shoji Furusako[1]

1 Discovery Research, Mochida Pharmaceutical Company Limited, Shizuoka, Japan, **2** Department of Molecular Endocrinology and Metabolism, Graduate School of Medical and Dental Sciences, Tokyo Medical and Dental University, Tokyo, Japan

Abstract

Objective: Diacylglycerol O acyltransferase 1 (DGAT1) catalyzes the final committed step in triglyceride biosynthesis. DGAT1 null mice are known to be resistant to diet-induced obesity, and more insulin sensitive relative to the wild-type; however, the mice exhibit abnormalities in the skin. This work determined whether the intestine-targeted DGAT1 inhibitor could improve obesity and insulin resistance without skin aberrations in mice.

Design and Methods: We synthesized 2 DGAT1 inhibitors: Compound A, described in the patent application from the Japan Tobacco, and Compound B (A-922500), reported by Abbott Laboratories. Both compounds were evaluated for inhibitory activities against DGAT1 enzymes and effects on the skin in mice *in vivo*. Compound B was further investigated for effects on obesity and insulin resistance in diet-induced-obese (DIO) mice.

Results: The 2 compounds comparably inhibited the DGAT1 enzyme activity and the cellular triglyceride synthesis *in vitro*, while they showed different distribution patterns in mice *in vivo*. Compound A, which distributed systemically, caused skin aberrations, while Compound B, which preferentially distributed to the intestine, improved obesity and insulin resistance without skin aberrations in DIO mice.

Conclusions: Our results suggest that the intestine is the key tissue in which DGAT1 plays a role in promoting obesity and insulin resistance.

Editor: Yanqiao Zhang, Northeast Ohio Medical University, United States of America

Funding: Mochida Pharmaceutical provided all funds for this work. NT, SK, CH, MO, MS, YK, KH, SK, YN, and SF are current employees of Mochida Pharmaceutical and may own stock or hold stock options in Mochida Pharmaceutical. The funders had no role in study design, data collection and analysis, decision to publish, or preparation of the manuscript.

Competing Interests: Mochida Pharmaceutical provided all funds for this work. NT, SK, CH, MO, MS, YK, KH, SK, YN, and SF are current employees of Mochida Pharmaceutical and may own stock or hold stock options in Mochida Pharmaceutical.

* Email: naoto.tsuda@mochida.co.jp

Introduction

Diacylglycerol O-acyltransferase (DGAT) 1 and DGAT2 catalyze the final committed step in triglyceride biosynthesis [1]. DGAT1 null mice are resistant to diet-induced obesity, and exhibit higher insulin sensitivity compared to the wild-type [2–4]. These results have revealed that DGAT1 plays important roles in the triglyceride synthesis and regulation of energy metabolism. Similarly, DGAT2 also plays a role in mammalian triglyceride synthesis. Although plasma glucose, triglyceride, free fatty acid levels and liver glycogen are decreased in DGAT2 null mice, these mice are lipopenic and die soon after birth due to reduction in substrates for energy metabolism and profound skin aberrations [5]. Thus, the DGAT1 inhibitor is expected to become a novel treatment option for obesity and type-2 diabetes mellitus (T2DM) without the severe adverse events associated with the DGAT2 inhibition. However, DGAT1 null mice exhibit skin aberrations, presumably due to depletion of essential lipids within the skin [3], and thus the DGAT1 inhibitor could induce skin aberrations when systemically administered for the treatment of obesity and diabetes.

Orally taken triglycerides go through hydrolysis and then are rearranged within the enterocyte into triglyceride-rich chylomicrons destined for systemic circulation. Since DGAT1 catalyzes this triglyceride rearrangement, the improvement of metabolic disorders observed in DGAT1 null mice seems to be derived from lack of DGAT1 activity in the intestine. Moreover, the metabolic phenotypes of DGAT1 null mice such as resistance to hepatic steatosis and diet-induced obesity are reported to be lost when DGAT1 is reintroduced into the intestine [6]. Thus the inhibition of the intestinal DGAT1 may be sufficient to improve metabolic disorders, suggesting that the intestine-targeted DGAT1 inhibitor shows beneficial metabolic effects without skin aberrations. Indeed, a previous report [7] aimed for discovery and optimization of intestine-targeted DGAT1 inhibitors. However, detailed comparisons between systemic delivery and intestine-targeted delivery of DGAT1 inhibitors have not been made so far.

In this study, we evaluated the effects of 2 DGAT1 inhibitors with different distribution patterns on skin aberrations in mice. As a result, we have found that the predominantly intestine-targeted DGAT1 inhibitor attenuates metabolic disorders without inducing skin aberrations.

Materials and Methods

Compounds

Compound A (4-[4-(4-amino-2,7,7-trimethyl-7H-pyrimido[4,5-b][1,4]oxazin-6-yl)phenyl]-trans-Cyclohexaneacetic acid, Figure 1A), described in the patent application from the Japan Tobacco [8], has been reported as a potent DGAT1 inhibitor by AstraZeneca [9]. Compound B (A-922500, (1R, 2R)-2-[[4′-[[(Phenylamino)carbonyl]amino][1,1′-biphenyl]-4-yl]carbonyl]cyclopentanecarboxylic acid, Figure 1B) has also been reported as a potent DGAT1 inhibitor by Pfizer and Abbott Laboratories [10,11]. Compound A and B act on the acyl-CoA binding site of DGAT1 and that they compete each other for the binding to DGAT1 [10]. These compounds were synthesized in our laboratory and used for the present study.

Animals

Male C57BL/6J mice were purchased from Charles River Japan. Mice were fed ad libitum with either a standard rodent chow (CE-2; CLEA Japan, Tokyo, Japan) or a high-fat diet (D12492; Research Diets, New Brunswick, NJ). All animals were housed under a 12-h light-dark cycle (lights on from 7:30 am to 7:30 pm) with free access to food and tap water.

All experimental procedures were approved by the Institutional Animal Care and Use Committee of Mochida Pharmaceutical Research Center. Blood sample was withdrawn from venous blood vessels using heparinized syringe. All surgery was performed under isoflurane anesthesia, and all efforts were made to minimize suffering.

Enzyme assays

The effects of the DGAT1 inhibitors were assessed using human (BC015762 from HeLa cell) and mouse DGAT1 (NM_010046 from mouse testis) in Sf9 insect microsomes. To collect the cell S9 fraction, sf9 cells were infected with the recombinant baculovirus containing human DGAT1 coding sequences and harvested after 72 h. The Sf9 cells were homogenized and centrifuged at 600 g for 20 min. Thereafter, the supernatant was centrifuged at 10000 g for 1 h and the precipitate was collected as the S9 fraction.

The reaction was started by adding ^{14}C decanoyl CoA (0.85 kBq; American Radiolabeled Chemicals Inc., Saint Louis, MO) to 5 μg/ml protein of the S9 fraction with Compound A or B, 150 mM $MgCl_2$, 0.01% BSA and 0.15 mM dioleoyl-glycerol in a total volume of 100 μl in 96-well plates. The mixture was incubated at room temperature for 45 min. The reaction was stopped by adding 0.5 M HCl and the incubated mixture was filtered using Multiscreen$_{HTS}$-FB (Millipore, Billerica, MA). The human DGAT1 activity was quantified by counting the radioactivity of synthesized ^{14}C triglycerides by the Microbeta scintillation counter (PerkinElmer, Waltham, MA) in duplicate. The 50% inhibitory concentration (IC_{50}) was calculated using the sigmoidal curve-fitting program (Symyx Assay Explorer 3.1 SP2; Symyx Technologies Inc., Santa Clara, CA). Mouse DGAT1 enzyme assays were carried out in the same way.

Triglyceride synthesis in HT-29 cells and HepG2 cells

The HT-29 cell line (American Type Culture Collection, Manassas, VA) was maintained in the McCoy's 5A medium (Life Technologies, Carlsbad, CA) containing 10% fetal bovine serum. The HepG2 cell line (American Type Culture Collection) was maintained in the Dulbecco's Modified Eagle Medium (Sigma-Aldrich, St. Louis, MO) containing 10% fetal bovine serum. For the experiments, the HT-29 cells were plated in 12-well plates at 3×10^5 cells, the HepG2 cells were plated in 12-well plates at 5×10^5 cells. The cells were cultured in serum-free media for 24 h, and incubated with a compound and oleic acid-albumin (Sigma-Aldrich) solubilized in dimethyl sulfoxide (final 0.1%) for 30 min. The triglyceride synthesis was initiated by the addition of ^{14}C oleic acid (0.2 μCi). The cells were washed in PBS and harvested into the organic phase using hexane:2-propanol (3:2) 30 min after initiation of the triglyceride synthesis. The solvent was evaporated, the extracts were solubilized in chloroform, and lipids were separated via TLC. Incorporation of the radiolabel into the triglyceride fraction was analyzed using BAS2000 in triplicate. The IC_{50} of each compound was calculated using GraphPad Prism.

Compound distribution in mice

Exposure was analyzed using blood, skin, and intestine samples from the C57BL/6J mice orally treated with 30 mg/kg of a compound. At 1, 4, 8, and 24 h after the administration, mice were anesthetized with isoflurane, and blood, skin, and intestine samples were collected. Three mice were used in each group. The blood samples were collected with sodium heparin, subjected to centrifugation, and plasma samples were collected. The skin and the intestine were homogenized and centrifuged to collect samples. The compound concentrations in each tissue sample with values equal to or greater than the lower limit of quantification (LLOQ; 0.005 μg/ml) were used for analyses (HPLC-MS/MS: Shiseido, Tokyo, Japan, Thermofisher Scientific, Waltham, MA).

Effects of Compound A and B on the skin in diet-induced-obese (DIO) mice

After 10 weeks on high-fat diet, mice became obese (36±0.24 g). Mice showed resistance to diet-induced obesity were excluded from the experiment. Fourteen-week-old male DIO mice were orally administered the vehicle (10% Pluronic F-68 for Compound A, 1% Tween 80 for Compound B), 30 mg/kg

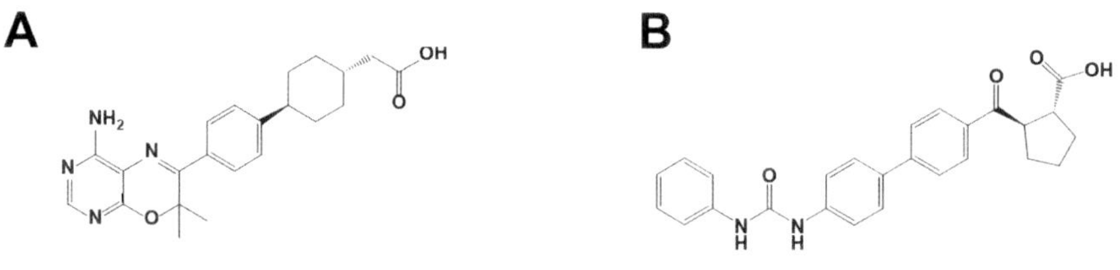

Figure 1. Chemical structures of Compound A (A) and Compound B (B).

Compound A once daily or 30 mg/kg Compound B twice daily. These dosing regimens were decided based on the ratios of concentration at 24 h after the compound administration (C_{24}) in the intestine/the IC50 for mDGAT1 (3.7 for Compound A and 1.2 for Compound B; Table 1) so that both compounds inhibit the intestinal DGAT1 to the same extent at 24 h after their administration. After 4 weeks of the treatment, all the animals were sacrificed. The skin (dorsolateral lesion) was removed and then fixed in 10% neutral buffered formalin, processed, embedded in paraffin, cut into thin sections and stained with Hematoxylin and Eosin. Histopathological examinations were performed. The size of the sebaceous glands were measured using WinROOF (Mitani Corporation, Tokyo, Japan).

Effects of Compound B on postprandial hyperlipidemia in mice

Eight-week-old male C57BL/6J mice were divided into treatment groups, each consisting of 7–8 mice, based on the body weight for the purpose of simplification of dose calculation. Mice were orally administered 1% Tween 80 (vehicle), 0.3, 1, 3, 10, or 30 mg/kg Compound B. Twelve h after administration, mice were orally given 3 ml/kg corn oil. Blood samples were collected 1, 2, and 3 h later, and the plasma triglyceride level was determined by using WAKO TG H (Wako, Osaka, Japan). The area under the curve (AUC) of plasma triglyceride (AUCtriglyceride) was calculated.

Effects of Compound B on glucagon-like peptide-1 (GLP-1) secretion in mice

Mice were divided into treatment groups, each consisting of 6–8 mice, based on the body weight for the purpose of simplification of dose calculation. Mice were orally administered 1% Tween 80 (vehicle), 10, or 30 mg/kg Compound B. Thirty minute after administration, mice were orally given 3 ml/kg corn oil. Blood samples were collected 2 h later, and the plasma GLP-1 level was determined by using Glucagon Like Peptide-1 (Active) ELISA Kit (Linco Research, Inc., St. Charles, MO).

Long-time treatment with Compound B in DIO mice

For evaluation of efficacy of long-time treatment with Compound B, after 10 weeks on high-fat diet, 14-week-old male mice were divided into treatment groups, each consisting of 9–10 animals, based on the body weight and glucose levels. Mice were orally administered 1% Tween 80 (vehicle), 1, 3, 10 or 30 mg/kg Compound B twice daily for 4 weeks. The DIO mice were fed with high-fat diet during the 4-week treatment period. Mice were fasted for 4 hours prior to blood collection. Plasma glucose, insulin, triglyceride, and free fatty acid concentrations were determined by using Glucose CII Test Wako (Wako), ultra sensitive mouse ELISA (Morinaga, Yokohama, Japan), L type WAKO TG H, and HA test WAKO NEFA (Wako), respectively.

Statistical analyses

Data were expressed as means ± SEM or means ± SD. Statistical analyses between the vehicle-treated group and each compound-treated group were performed with the Dunnett's multiple comparison test, and those between the vehicle-treated group and the control group were performed by the t-test, using SAS version 9.1 (SAS Institute Inc, Cary, NC).

Results

Characteristics of the tested compounds *in vitro*

Compound A and B were potent DGAT1 inhibitors for mouse and human DGAT1 (Table 2). These results were consistent with those in the previous reports [9–11].

Inhibition of triglyceride synthesis *in vitro*

In the cellular assay, Compound A was evaluated at concentrations of 0.3 to 3 μM. Compound A inhibited the cellular triglyceride synthesis with the increase in concentrations, and significant inhibition was observed at 1 and 3 μM in HT-29 human colon (Figure 2A) and at all the concentrations tested in HepG2 human liver cells (Figure 2B). Compound B was evaluated at concentrations of 0.1 to 3 μM. Compound B also inhibited the cellular triglyceride synthesis with the increase in concentrations, and significant inhibition was observed at 1 and 3 μM in HT-29 human colon and at all the concentrations tested in HepG2 human liver cells.

Distribution of DGAT1 inhibitors in mice

Figure 3A and 3B show the concentrations of Compound A and B in the plasma, skin, and the intestine of the mice after its oral

Table 1. Pharmacokinetic properties of Compound A and Compound B in mice.

	Compound A	Compound B
T_{max} (h)	1	1
C_{max} in plasma (μM)	240±59	9.1±2.3
plasma/IC_{50}	38±9.2	0.59±0.15
C_{max} in skin (μmol/kg)	14±0.62	1.3±0.51
skin/IC_{50}	2.2±0.097	0.084±0.033
C_{max} in intestine (μmol/kg)	77±37	92±36
intestine/IC_{50}	12±5.8	5.9±2.3
C_{24} in intestine (μmol/kg)	24±1.6	19±3.7
C_{24} in intestine/mDGAT1 IC_{50}	3.7±0.24	1.2±0.24
Intestine/Plasma ratio at T_{max}	0.32±0.090	10±2.8
Intestine/Skin ratio at T_{max}	5.6±2.5	74±8.4

plasma/IC_{50} = C_{max} in plasma/mDGAT1 IC_{50}, skin/IC_{50} = C_{max} in skin/mDGAT1 IC_{50}, intestine/IC_{50} = C_{max} in intestine/mDGAT1 IC_{50}, Three mice were used in each group. Data were expressed as means ± SD.

Table 2. Summary of the effects of Compound A and Compound B.

	Compound A	Compound B
mDGAT1 IC_{50}[a]	6.4 nM	15.5 nM
hDGAT1 IC_{50}[a]	2.6 nM	8.4 nM
Log D	<0.9	<0.9
m plasma protein binding	3.2% free	0.1% free

[a]The 50% inhibitory concentration (IC_{50}) for each compound in the enzymes expressed in insect microsomes.

administration at 30 mg/kg. The time to reach the maximum concentration (Tmax) for Compound A was 1 h, and Compound A exhibited higher concentrations in the plasma and the skin as compared to Compound B (Table 1). The Tmax of Compound B was also 1 h. Compound B exhibited a higher concentration in the intestine in spite of its relatively low concentrations in the plasma and skin. The intestine/plasma and intestine/skin ratios for Compound B (10 and 74) were much higher than those for Compound A (0.32 and 5.6).

Effects of DGAT1 inhibitors on the skin in diet-induced-obese (DIO) mice

The DIO mice treated with Compound A showed skin aberrations derived from atrophy of the sebaceous gland which were characterized by decrease amount and size of sebaceous gland acini (Figure 4A and 4C). All the mice treated with Compound A exhibited skin aberrations, while such aberrations were not observed in the mice treated with the vehicle. Compound A induced no injurious or inflammatory changes, and the skin aberrations recovered 2 weeks after the compound withdrawal. On the other hand, the changes in the skin were not observed in all the DIO mice treated with Compound B, which displayed higher distribution to the intestine over plasma or the skin (Figure 4B and 4C).

Effects of short-time treatment with the intestine-targeted DGAT1 inhibitor on postprandial hyperlipidemia in mice

Compound B was evaluated in a model of postprandial hyperlipidemia by measuring chylomicron-derived triglycerides. Compound B at 0.3, 1, 3, or 10 mg/kg, when orally administered 12 h before the corn oil administration, reduced plasma triglyceride levels with a dose-dependent tendency (Figure 5). The maximum efficacy was achieved at 10 mg/kg. In addition, compound B at 10 and 30 mg/kg also increased plasma glucagon-like peptide-1 (GLP-1) levels after corn oil administration (Figure 5C).

Effects of long-time treatment with the intestine-targeted DGAT1 inhibitor on diet induced obesity in mice

As short-time treatment with Compound B improved postprandial hyperlipidemia, potential anti-obesity effects of Compound B were examined in DIO mice. Following the feeding on high-fat diet for 10 weeks, mice became obese, and exhibited significant increases in the body weight, plasma glucose level, plasma insulin concentration, insulin resistance (HOMA-IR: control vs. DIO = 0.70 vs. 2.0), mesenteric adipose tissue weight, epididymal adipose tissue weight, content of hepatic triglyceride and the content of hepatic total-cholesterol, indicating the development of diet-induced obesity in mice (i.e., DIO mice), as compared to the control mice fed on normal diet. In DIO mice, long-time treatment with Compound B attenuated the body weight gain with the increase in doses (Figure 6A). After the 4-week treatment period, significant attenuation and significant reduction were observed at 10 mg/kg and 30 mg/kg, respectively (Figure 6B). Compound B reduced plasma glucose levels (Figure 6C), and significant reduction was observed at 30 mg/kg. Insulin concentrations tended to decrease in the DIO mice treated with Compound B (Figure 6D). There were also differences in the weight of white adipose tissue (WAT) among the groups.

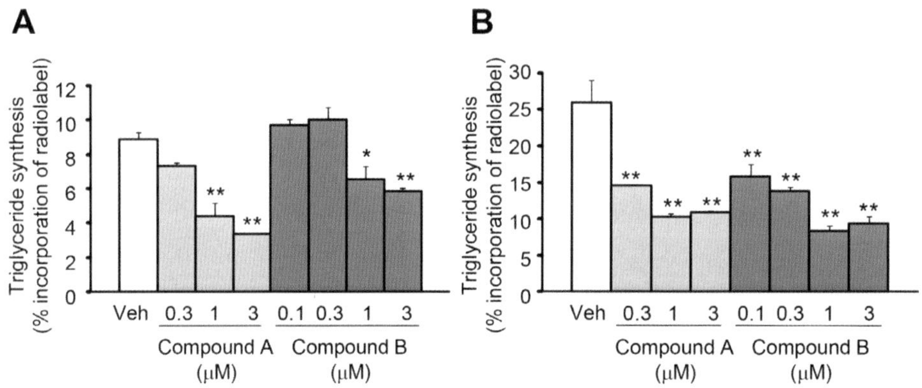

Figure 2. Effects of Compound A and Compound B on the triglyceride synthesis. The effects of Compound A and Compound B on the triglyceride synthesis in HT-29 human colon cells (A) and in HepG2 human liver cells (B). Data are expressed as means + SEM of 3 assays. *$P<0.05$ and **$P<0.01$. Statistical analyses between the vehicle (Veh) group and compound-treated groups were performed by the Dunnett's multiple comparison test.

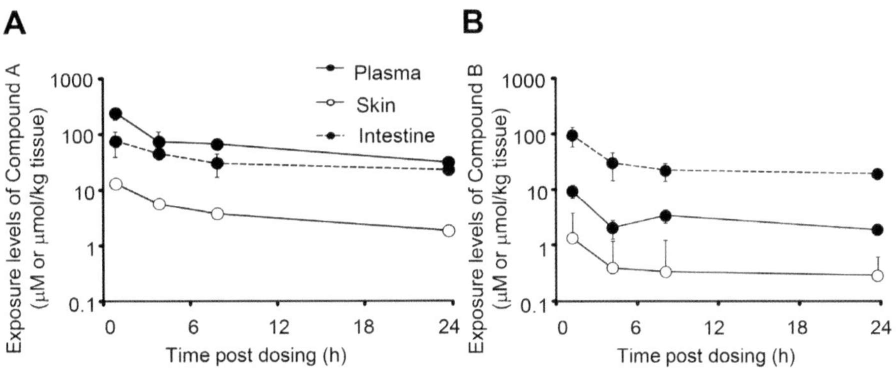

Figure 3. Plasma and tissue concentrations after single oral dosing of Compound A and Compound B. Plasma, skin, and intestine samples were collected from the mice orally administered 30 mg/kg Compound A (A) or B (B). Data are expressed as means ± SD of 3 animals.

Treatment with Compound B reduced the weight of mesenteric (Figure 6E) and epididymal (Figure 6F) fat with the increase in doses and significant reduction was observed at 30 mg/kg. Furthermore, despite lack of differences in the liver weight among the groups (Figure 6G), Compound B reduced concentrations of triglyceride and total-cholesterol in the liver with the increase of doses, and significant reduction was observed at 30 mg/kg (Figure 6H, 6I). Histological analysis also indicated that Compound B attenuated fatty liver (Figure S1).

Discussion

DGAT1 is an endoplasmic membrane bound enzyme which catalyzes the final committed step in triglyceride biosynthesis, distributed in various tissues such as the skeletal muscle, liver, adipose tissue, intestine and the skin. In addition to the metabolic phenotypes of DGAT1 null mice such as resistance to hepatic steatosis and diet-induced obesity, they exhibit skin aberrations owing to lack of DGAT1 in the skin [3]. As the metabolic phenotypes of DGAT1 null mice are lost when DGAT1 is reintroduced into the intestine [6], we raised a hypothesis that the intestine-targeted DGAT1 inhibitor would improve metabolic disorders with minimizing the adverse effect that may be driven by systemic DGAT1 inhibition. In this study, we focused on effects of the 2 DGAT1 inhibitors with different distribution patterns on skin aberrations in mice. Consequently, we found that the predominantly intestine-targeted DGAT1 inhibitor Compound B did not exhibit skin aberrations, while the systemically distributed Compound A caused skin aberrations in DIO mice. We also indicated that the intestine-targeted DGAT1 inhibitor improved metabolic disorders in DIO mice.

The present result showed that Compound A and B similarly inhibited the activities of the mouse and the human DGAT1 enzyme *in vitro* as previously reported [9–11]. Moreover, both compounds inhibited the cellular triglyceride synthesis in HT-29, HepG2, and mouse skin homogenates. In spite of similar profiles *in vitro*, we identified that orally administered Compound A and B exhibited different distribution patterns in mice *in vivo*. The recent publication [12] indicates that distribution of DGAT1 inhibitors to the skin did correlate with its lipophilicity. However lipophilicity (Log D) of Compound A and B were similarly low. Although the precise reason for the difference of distribution has not yet been identified, the intestine-targeted distribution of Compound B may potentially be due to its transporter-mediated efflux from the intestine in the same way as previously discussed with another intestine-targeted DGAT1 inhibitor [7]. It is noteworthy that the intestine/plasma and intestine/skin ratios for Compound B (10 and 74) were much higher than those for Compound A (0.32 and 5.6). Since there is a report that Compound A shows beneficial metabolic effects [10], we focused on whether the predominantly intestine-targeted DGAT1 inhibitor could improve obesity and insulin resistance without skin aberrations in mice in the present study.

In a model of postprandial hyperlipidemia measuring chylomicron-derived triglycerides in mice, single oral administration of Compound B reduced plasma triglyceride levels. This is consistent with the previous observations on the suppression by other DGAT1 inhibitors of postprandial hyperlipidemia [9–11] and the delayed fat absorption in DGAT1 null mice [13–14]. Furthermore, Compound B also increased plasma GLP-1 levels after corn oil administration. The present results support the hypothesis that intestinal DGAT1 might directly regulate the releases of GLP-1 [15]. It might be possible that diacylglycerol accumulated in the intestinal cells following oil administration stimulates the release of GLP-1, since it has been known that the activation of phorbol ester-sensitive protein kinase C leads to GLP-1 release. These results highlighted that pharmacological as well as genetic inhibition of DGAT1 in the intestine would reduce dietary fat absorption and increase plasma GLP-1 levels.

Long-time treatment with Compound B, which selectively inhibits intestinal DGAT1, reduced the body weight gain, weight of white adipose tissues, hepatic triglyceride and the hepatic cholesterol content in DIO mice. In addition, long-time treatment with Compound B reduced plasma glucose levels and tended to reduce insulin concentrations, suggesting that Compound B would improve insulin resistance. In the recent publication [12], the pharmacokinetic/pharmacodynamic relationship of DGAT1 inhibitors between tissue concentration/IC_{50} and its effects was reported. High value (>1) of intestine/IC_{50} of Compound B in spite of its relatively low values of skin/IC_{50} and plasma/IC_{50} supports the consideration that the effects of DGAT1 inhibitors are achieved by the compound in intestine. The beneficial metabolic effects of Compound B may, at least partly, be ascribed to suppressed fat absorption from the intestine via inhibited intestinal DGAT1, as postprandial hyperlipidemia is assumed to promote hepatic steatosis [16] and insulin resistance. In addition to reduction of fat absorption, since it is known that GLP-1 has beneficial metabolic effects such as reduction of body weight gain and improvement of insulin resistance, increased GLP-1 secretion via the inhibition of intestinal DGAT1 would also contribute to the favorable metabolic effects of Compound B.

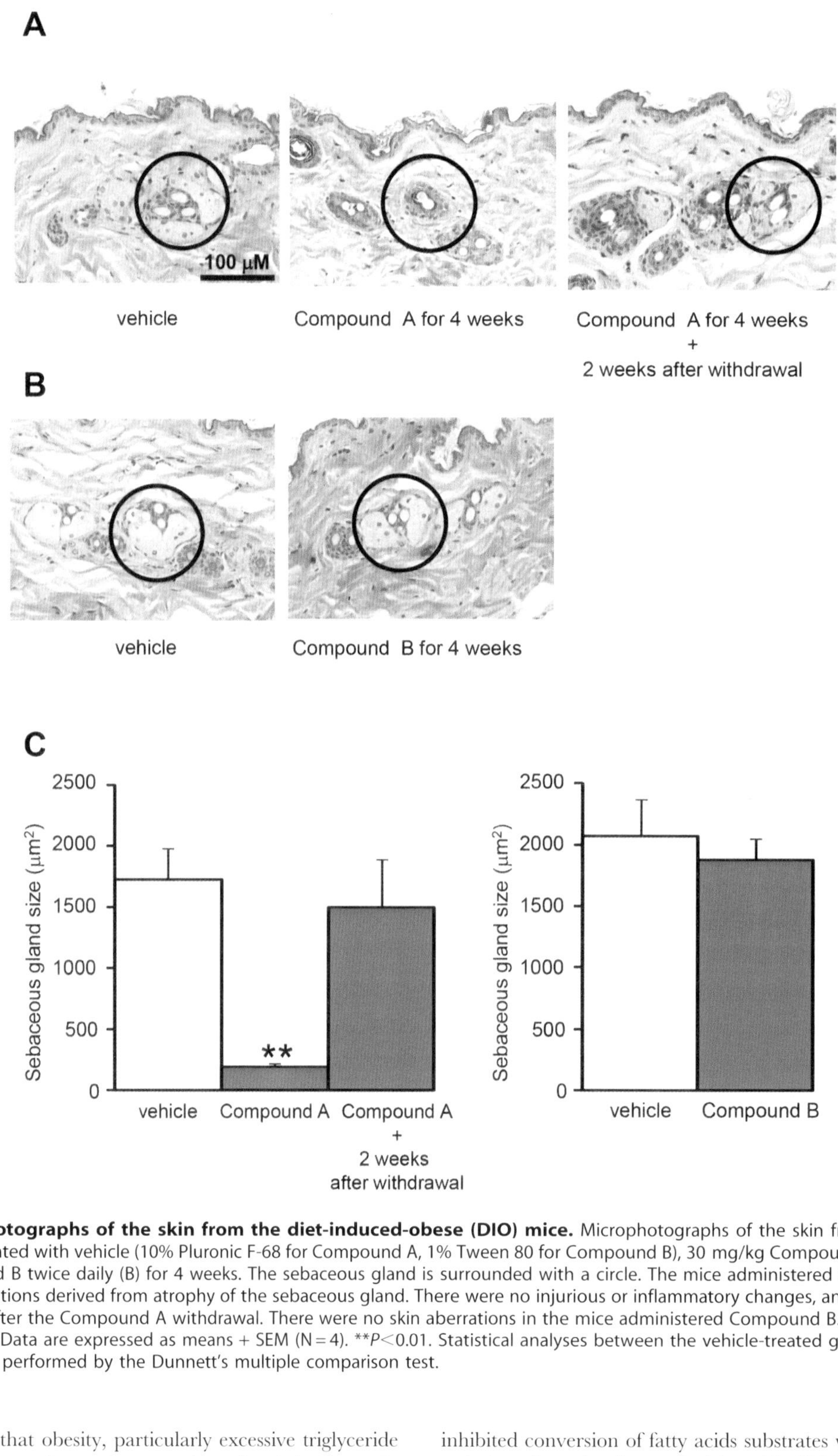

Figure 4. Microphotographs of the skin from the diet-induced-obese (DIO) mice. Microphotographs of the skin from the diet-induced-obese (DIO) mice treated with vehicle (10% Pluronic F-68 for Compound A, 1% Tween 80 for Compound B), 30 mg/kg Compound A once daily (A), or 30 mg/kg Compound B twice daily (B) for 4 weeks. The sebaceous gland is surrounded with a circle. The mice administered Compound A showed moderate skin aberrations derived from atrophy of the sebaceous gland. There were no injurious or inflammatory changes, and the skin aberrations recovered 2 weeks after the Compound A withdrawal. There were no skin aberrations in the mice administered Compound B. The sebaceous gland sizes are plotted (C). Data are expressed as means + SEM (N = 4). $^{**}P<0.01$. Statistical analyses between the vehicle-treated group and Compound-treated groups were performed by the Dunnett's multiple comparison test.

It is well known that obesity, particularly excessive triglyceride deposition in the non-adipose tissues such as the skeletal muscle and the liver, is related to diabetes and insulin resistance [17–21]. DGAT1 inhibition in the whole body may reduce excessive triglyceride deposition in the non-adipose tissues including the skeletal muscle [22], resulting in amelioration of metabolic disorders. In contrast, however, the inhibition of DGAT1 activities in the skeletal muscle or macrophage may cause insulin resistance, leading to aggravation of metabolic disorders, as a result of inhibited conversion of fatty acids substrates which induce insulin resistance into the form of triglyceride [23,24]. Those opposing actions of DGAT1 may explain the reasons why the reintroduction of DGAT1 into the intestine of DGAT1 null mice is sufficient to lose metabolic phenotypes such as resistance to hepatic steatosis and diet-induced obesity, and why long-time treatment with Compound B showed beneficial metabolic effects such as insulin-sensitization and reduction of the body weight gain and hepatic lipids.

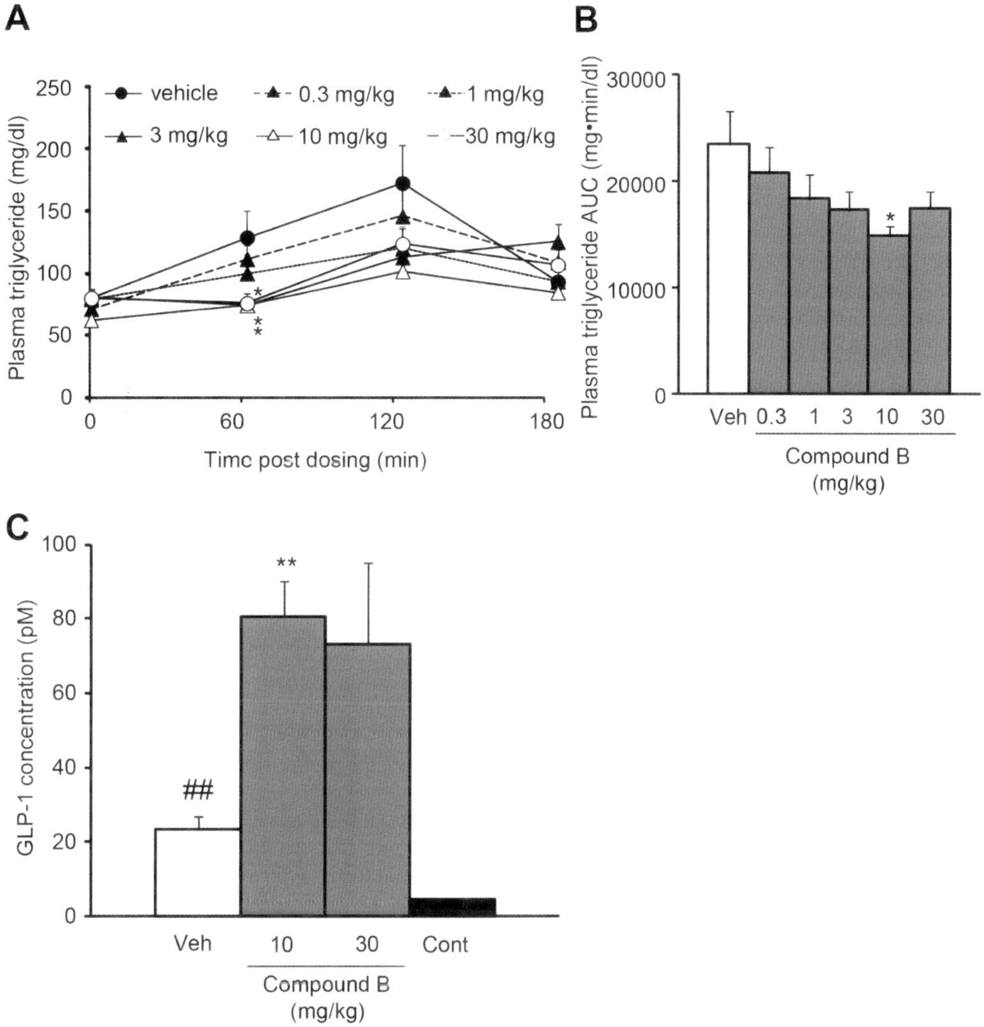

Figure 5. Effects of Compound B on the plasma triglyceride (A, B) and glucagon-like peptide-1 (C) levels. The changes in plasma triglyceride (A) and AUCtriglyceride (−5−180 min) of plasma triglyceride (B), and the plasma GLP-1 levels 2 h following corn oil administration (C) are indicated. The plasma GLP-1 levels of the mice given corn oil are higher than the control mice (Cont). Data are expressed as means + SEM of 6–8 animals. *$P<0.05$ and **$P<0.01$. Statistical analyses between the vehicle (Veh)-treated group and Compound B-treated groups were performed by the Dunnett's multiple comparison test. ##$P<0.01$. Statistical analyses between the vehicle-treated group and the control group were performed by the t-test.

Long-time treatment with Compound B for 4 weeks did not cause any skin aberrations in DIO mice. Long-time treatment with Compound A, in contrast to that with Compound B, caused moderate skin aberrations derived from atrophy of the sebaceous gland which were characterized by decrease amount and size of sebaceous gland acini. The skin aberrations associated with Compound A were not injurious or inflammatory changes, and the aberrations recovered 2 weeks after the compound withdrawal. As these skin aberrations resemble the observations in DGAT1 null mice, depletion of essential lipids due to DGAT1 inhibition is likely to be responsible for the aberrations. The results from the present study and DGAT1 null mice demonstrate that congenital DGAT1 is involved in maintenance and/or development of the sebaceous gland, producing fur essential lipids. As both Compound A and B inhibited the triglyceride synthesis, the lack of skin aberrations in the DIO mice treated with Compound B seems to be due to its minimal distribution to the skin.

Clinical data [25,26] indicate that profound gastrointestinal (GI) adverse events such as nausea, diarrhea, and vomiting appear likely related to DGAT1 inhibition/loss of function in the GI tract. Ideally, a DGAT1 inhibitor as an oral therapeutic agent should overcome those adverse events. In the present study, we cannot deny the possibility that the DGAT1 inhibitor with intestine-restricted distribution may have the same problems in human. Although adverse events would, at least partly, be caused by the inhibition of intestinal DGAT1, their precise mechanisms are unclear. Further clinical studies of intestine-targeted compounds would clarify the therapeutic window of this type of DGAT1 inhibitors.

In conclusion, this study has shown for the first time that the intestine-targeted delivery of the DGAT1 inhibitor improves postprandial hyperlipidemia, body adiposity, hepatic lipid accumulation and insulin resistance without skin aberrations. The presently-observed improvement of metabolic abnormalities is in agreement with other reported results of the studies using DGAT1 inhibitors with different chemical structures [9–11,27–28] or DGAT1 null mice. Collectively, our results provide pharmacological support for the hypothesis that the intestine is the key tissue

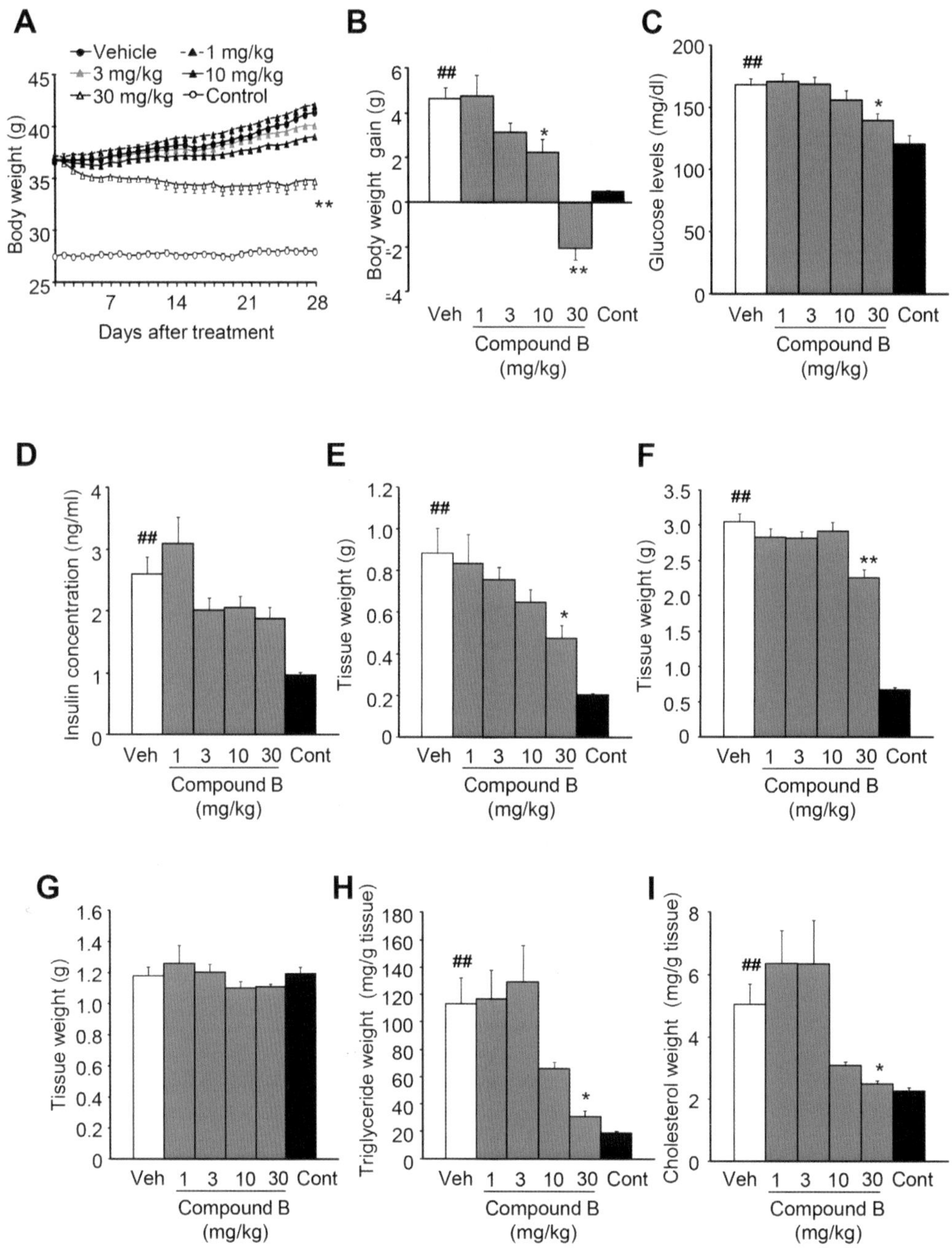

Figure 6. Effects of Compound B in diet-induced-obese (DIO) mice. Mice were orally treated with 1% Tween 80 (vehicle; Veh) or 30 mg/kg Compound B twice daily for 4 weeks. The time-course of body weight changes (A) and the body weight gain at 4 weeks of Compound B treatment (B) are indicated respectively. The body weight of the mice fed a high-fat diet is significantly higher than the control mice (Cont) fed a standard rodent chow during the 4-week treatment period. The plasma glucose level (C), plasma insulin concentration (D), mesenteric adipose tissue weight (E), epididymal adipose tissue weight (F), liver weight (G), content of hepatic triglyceride (H), and the content of hepatic total-cholesterol (I) at 4 weeks of Compound B treatment are indicated respectively. Data are expressed as means ± SEM of 9–10 animals. *$P<0.05$ and **$P<0.01$. Statistical analyses between the vehicle-treated group and Compound B-treated groups were performed by the Dunnett's multiple comparison test. ##$P<0.01$. Statistical analyses between the vehicle-treated group and the control group were performed by the t-test.

in which DGAT1 plays a role in promoting obesity and insulin resistance when exposed to high fat food.

Acknowledgments

We thank the members of the discovery research division of Mochida Pharmaceutical Company Limited, including Akira Karasawa and Junji Takada for their writing assistant and general support. All authors were involved in writing the paper and have approved the final manuscript.

Author Contributions

Conceived and designed the experiments: NT SK CH MO MS YK KH SK YN YO SF. Performed the experiments: NT SK CH MO MS YK KH SK YN. Analyzed the data: NT SK CH MO KH SK YN. Contributed reagents/materials/analysis tools: NT SK CH MS YK SK YN. Contributed to the writing of the manuscript: NT YK.

References

1. Cases S, Smith SJ, Zheng YW, Myers HM, Lear SR, et al. (1998) Identification of a gene encoding an acyl CoA:diacylglycerol acyltransferase, a key enzyme in triacylglycerol synthesis. Proc. Natl. Acad. Sci. U. S. A. 95: 13018–23.
2. Smith SJ, Cases S, Jensen DR, Chen HC, Sande E, et al. (2000) Obesity resistance and multiple mechanisms of triglyceride synthesis in mice lacking Dgat. Nat Genet. 25: 87–90.
3. Chen HC, Smith SJ, Ladha Z, Jensen DR, Ferreira LD, et al. (2002) Increased insulin and leptin sensitivity in mice lacking acyl CoA:diacylglycerol acyltransferase 1. J. Clin. Invest. 109: 1049–55.
4. Chen HC, Farese RV Jr (2005) Inhibition of triglyceride synthesis as a treatment strategy for obesity: lessons from DGAT1-deficient mice. Arterioscler. Thromb. Vasc. Biol. 25: 482–6.
5. Stone SJ, Myers HM, Watkins SM, Brown BE, Feingold KR, et al. (2004) Lipopenia and skin barrier abnormalities in DGAT2-deficient mice. J. Biol. Chem. 279: 11767–76.
6. Lee B, Fast AM, Zhu J, Cheng JX, Buhman KK (2010) Intestine-specific expression of acyl CoA:diacylglycerol acyltransferase 1 reverses resistance to diet-induced hepatic steatosis and obesity in Dgat1 −/− mice. J. Lipid Res. 51: 1770–80.
7. Michael HSW, Gary MC, Yongjin G, Alan DN, Ricardo C, et al. (2012) Intestinally Targeted Diacylglycerol Acyltransferase 1 (DGAT1) Inhibitors Robustly Suppress Postprandial Triglycerides. ACS Med. Chem. Lett. 3: 411–5.
8. Brian MF, Furukawa N, Hao X, Iio K, Inaba T, et al (2004) Fused bicyclic nitrogen-containing heterocycles. International Patent Application. WO 2004047755 A2.
9. Birch AM, Birtles S, Buckett LK, Kemmitt PD, Smith GJ, et al. (2009) Discovery of a potent, selective, and orally efficacious pyrimidinooxazinyl bicyclooctaneacetic acid diacylglycerol acyltransferase-1 inhibitor. J. Med. Chem. 52: 1558–68.
10. Cao J, Zhou Y, Peng H, Huang X, Stahler S, et al. (2011) Targeting Acyl-CoA:diacylglycerol acyltransferase 1 (DGAT1) with small molecule inhibitors for the treatment of metabolic diseases. J. Biol. Chem. 286: 41838–51.
11. King AJ, Segreti JA, Larson KJ, Souers AJ, Kym PR, et al. (2009) Diacylglycerol acyltransferase 1 inhibition lowers serum triglycerides in the Zucker fatty rat and the hyperlipidemic hamster. J. Pharmacol. Exp. Ther. 330: 526–31.
12. Muise ES, Zhu Y, Verras A, Karanam BV, Gorski J, et al. (2014) Identification and characterization of sebaceous gland atrophy-sparing DGAT1 inhibitors. PLoS One. 18: e88908.
13. Buhman KK, Smith SJ, Stone SJ, Repa JJ, Wong JS, et al. (2002) DGAT1 is not essential for intestinal triacylglycerol absorption or chylomicron synthesis. J. Biol. Chem. 277: 25474–9.
14. Ables GP, Yang KJ, Vogel S, Hernandez-Ono A, Yu S, et al. (2012) Intestinal DGAT1 deficiency reduces postprandial triglyceride and retinyl ester excursions by inhibiting chylomicron secretion and delaying gastric emptying. J. Lipid Res. 53: 2364–79.
15. Okawa M, Fujii K, Ohbuchi K, Okumoto M, Aragane K, et al. (2009) Role of MGAT2 and DGAT1 in the release of gut peptides after triglyceride ingestion. Biochem. Biophys. Res. Commun. 390: 377–81.
16. Musso G, Gambino R, Durazzo M, Biroli G, Carello M, et al. (2005) Adipokines in NASH: postprandial lipid metabolism as a link between adiponectin and liver disease. Hepatology 42: 1175–83.
17. Phillips DI, Caddy S, Ilic V, Fielding BA, Frayn KN, et al. (1996) Intramuscular triglyceride and muscle insulin sensitivity: evidence for a relationship in nondiabetic subjects. Metabolism 45: 947–50.
18. Pan DA, Lillioja S, Kriketos AD, Milner MR, Baur LA, et al. (1997) Skeletal muscle triglyceride levels are inversely related to insulin action. Diabetes 46: 983–8.
19. Ebeling P, Essen-Gustavsson B, Tuominen JA, Koivisto VA. (1998) Intramuscular triglyceride content is increased in IDDM. Diabetologia 41: 111–5.
20. Manco M, Mingrone G, Greco AV, Capristo E, Gniuli D, et al. (2000) Insulin resistance directly correlates with increased saturated fatty acids in skeletal muscle triglycerides. Metabolism 49: 220–4.
21. Virkamaki A, Korsheninnikova E, Seppala-Lindroos A, Vehkavaara S, Goto T, et al. (2001) Intramyocellular lipid is associated with resistance to in vivo insulin actions on glucose uptake, antilipolysis, and early insulin signaling pathways in human skeletal muscle. Diabetes 50: 2337–43.
22. Yamamoto T, Yamaguchi H, Miki H, Kitamura S, Nakada Y, et al. (2011) A novel coenzyme A:diacylglycerol acyltransferase 1 inhibitor stimulates lipid metabolism in muscle and lowers weight in animal models of obesity. Eur. J. Pharmacol. 650: 663–72.
23. Liu L, Zhang Y, Chen N, Shi X, Tsang B, et al. (2007) Upregulation of myocellular DGAT1 augments triglyceride synthesis in skeletal muscle and protects against fat-induced insulin resistance. J. Clin. Invest. 117: 1679–89.
24. Koliwad SK, Streeper RS, Monetti M, Cornelissen I, Chan L, et al. (2010) DGAT1-dependent triacylglycerol storage by macrophages protects mice from diet-induced insulin resistance and inflammation. J. Clin. Invest. 120: 756–67.
25. Haas JT, Winter HS, Lim E, Kirby A, Blumenstiel B, et al. (2012) DGAT1 mutation is linked to a congenital diarrheal disorder. J. Clin. Invest. 122: 4680–8.
26. Denison H, Nilsson C, Löfgren L, Himmelmann A, Mårtensson G, et al. (2014) Diacylglycerol acyltransferase 1 inhibition with AZD7687 alters lipid handling and hormone secretion in the gut with intolerable side effects: a randomized clinical trial. Diabetes Obes. Metab. 16: 334–43.
27. Zhao G, Souers AJ, Voorbach M, Falls HD, Droz B, et al. (2008) Validation of diacyl glycerolacyltransferase I as a novel target for the treatment of obesity and dyslipidemia using a potent and selective small molecule inhibitor. J. Med. Chem. 51: 380–3.
28. Yamamoto T, Yamaguchi H, Miki H, Shimada M, Nakada Y, et al. (2010) Coenzyme A: diacylglycerol acyltransferase 1 inhibitor ameliorates obesity, liver steatosis, and lipid metabolism abnormality in KKAy mice fed high-fat or high-carbohydrate diets. Eur. J. Pharmacol. 640: 243–9.

Metformin Reduces Thyroid Cancer Risk in Taiwanese Patients with Type 2 Diabetes

Chin-Hsiao Tseng[1,2,3]*

1 Department of Internal Medicine, National Taiwan University College of Medicine, Taipei, Taiwan, 2 Division of Endocrinology and Metabolism, Department of Internal Medicine, National Taiwan University Hospital, Taipei, Taiwan, 3 Division of Environmental Health and Occupational Medicine of the National Health Research Institutes, Taipei, Taiwan

Abstract

Background: Whether metformin may affect thyroid cancer risk has not been studied. This study investigated the association between metformin use and thyroid cancer risk in Taiwanese patients with type 2 diabetes mellitus.

Methods: The reimbursement databases of all diabetic patients from 1996 to 2009 were retrieved from the National Health Insurance. An entry date was set at 1 January 2006 and 1,414,723 patients with type 2 diabetes were followed for thyroid cancer incidence until the end of 2009. Incidences for ever-users, never-users and subgroups of metformin exposure using tertile cutoffs for cumulative duration of therapy and cumulative dose were calculated and adjusted hazard ratios were estimated by Cox regression. Additional sensitivity analyses were conducted.

Results: There were 795,321 ever-users and 619,402 never-users, with respective numbers of incident thyroid cancer of 683 (0.09%) and 1,614 (0.26%), and respective incidence of 24.09 and 87.33 per 100,000 person-years. The overall fully adjusted hazard ratio (95% confidence interval) was 0.683 (0.598–0.780), and all categories of the dose-response parameters showed significantly lower risk with *P*-trends <0.0001. The protective effect of metformin on thyroid cancer incidence was also supported by sensitivity analyses, disregarding age (<50 or ≥ 50 years) and sex; and was not affected by excluding users of insulin, sulfonylurea, and insulin and/or sulfonylurea respectively, by previous diagnosis of other cancers or by potential detection examinations that might lead to differential diagnosis of thyroid cancer.

Conclusions: This study provides evidence for the first time that metformin use in patients with type 2 diabetes may reduce the risk of thyroid cancer.

Editor: Suminori Akiba, Kagoshima University Graduate School of Medical and Dental Sciences, Japan

Funding: The study was supported by the National Science Council (NSC102-2314-B-002-067) of Taiwan. The funders had no role in study design, data collection and analysis, decision to publish, or preparation of the manuscript.

Competing Interests: The author has declared that no competing interests exist.

* Email: ccktsh@ms6.hinet.net

Introduction

Patients with type 2 diabetes have a higher risk of cancer involving the breast, endometrium, stomach, colorectum, liver, pancreas, urinary bladder, and non-Hodgkin's lymphoma [1–8]. The mechanisms may be related to insulin resistance, hyperinsulinemia, proinflammatory status and increased oxidative stress [1,2,9]. With regards to thyroid cancer, there has been an increasing trend of its incidence over the past decades worldwide; and this has been ascribed to the increasing prevalence of insulin resistance [10].

Although insulin resistance may lead to an increased risk of thyroid cancer in patients with type 2 diabetes, our recent population-based study did not support a higher risk of thyroid cancer in these patients [11]. Recent studies suggested that antidiabetic drugs may play some role in the development of cancers. For example, metformin may reduce [12–16], while insulin and sulfonylureas may increase [1,17–19] the risk of various types of cancer. On the other hand, the use of pioglitazone [20–22], but not rosiglitazone [21–23], may increase the risk of bladder cancer. Therefore, a lack of association between diabetes and thyroid cancer as observed in our previous study [11] can be a composite outcome of the interaction between the mechanisms that lead to a higher risk (e.g., insulin resistance) and the effects of the use of metformin that lead to a lower risk.

Whether metformin use can reduce the risk of thyroid cancer in patients with type 2 diabetes remains to be confirmed. Some recent *in vitro* studies suggested that metformin may inhibit the growth of thyroid cancer cells through inhibition of the mammalian target of rapamycin (mTOR) pathway by activating the AMP-activated protein kinase (AMPK) [24] or by diminishing the growth stimulation by insulin [25]. In humans, an earlier observational report of 4 cases showed that metformin might suppress thyroid stimulating hormone (TSH) without causing clinical hyperthyroidism [26], but this can not be confirmed in a later large sample-sized retrospective study comparing 250 patients on metformin therapy to 578 diabetic patients without metformin treatment [27]. A recent small clinical study conducted in 66 women with insulin resistance and thyroid nodular hyperplasia for 6 months suggested that metformin alone or better in combination with levothyroxine may reduce the size of the nodule [28].

All of the above *in vitro* and preliminary human studies suggested a potential usefulness of metformin on the prevention of thyroid cancer. However, large human observational studies are still lacking [16,29]. Therefore, the purpose of the present study was to evaluate whether metformin use in Taiwanese patients with type 2 diabetes could affect the risk of thyroid cancer by using the National Health Insurance (NHI) database obtained from the whole nation.

Materials and Methods

A retrospective cohort analysis using the NHI databases including all patients with a diagnosis of diabetes during the period from 1996 (the earliest database available) to 2009 in Taiwan was conducted. The study using the NHI database was approved by an ethic review board of the National Health Research Institutes with registered approval number 99274. Written informed consent from the participants was not required according to local regulations because the identification information of the individuals was scrambled and de-identified prior to analysis for the protection of privacy.

Since March 1995 a compulsory and universal system of health insurance (the so-called NHI) was implemented in Taiwan. All contracted medical institutes must submit computerized and standard claim documents for reimbursement. More than 99% of citizens are enrolled in the NHI, and >98% of the hospitals nationwide are under contract with the NHI. The average number of annual physician visits in Taiwan is one of the highest around the world, at approximately 15 visits per year per capita in 2009.

The databases contain detailed records on every visit for each patient, including outpatient visits, emergency department visits and hospital admission; and include principal and secondary diagnostic codes, prescription orders, and claimed expenses. Diabetes was coded 250.00–250.93 and thyroid cancer 193, based on the *International Classification of Diseases, Ninth Revision, Clinical Modification* (ICD-9-CM).

We first retrieved the databases of all patients who had been diagnosed as having diabetes and/or under treatment with either oral anti-diabetic agents or insulin during the period of 1996–2009 from the whole nation ($n = 3,756,511$). The selected entry date was 1 January 2006. After excluding patients who had a diagnosis of diabetes after the year 2006 ($n = 773,801$), patients who held a Severe Morbidity Card as having type 1 diabetes ($n = 7182$, in Taiwan, patients with type 1 diabetes were issued a so-called "Severe Morbidity Card" after certified diagnosis and they were waived for much of the co-payments), patients having a diagnosis of thyroid cancer before 2006 ($n = 8,252$), those who died ($n = 169,509$) or withdrew from the NHI ($n = 23,784$) before entry date, duplicated identification number ($n = 216$), unclear information on date of birth or sex ($n = 14,284$), and diabetic patients without any reimbursement record after the entry date ($n = 1,556,791$), a total of 1,414,723 patients with a diagnosis of type 2 diabetes and/or under therapy with oral anti-diabetic agents or insulin were recruited.

Those who had ever been prescribed metformin before entry date were defined as ever-users; and never-users were defined as those who had never been prescribed metformin before entry date. To evaluate whether a dose-response relationship could be seen between metformin and thyroid cancer, the tertile cutoffs for the following parameters were applied: 1) cumulative duration of therapy in months; and 2) cumulative dose in mg.

Baseline characteristics of ever- and never-users of metformin at entry were compared by Chi square test. Age and all comorbidities and covariates were determined as a status/diagnosis before the entry date. The ICD-9-CM codes for the comorbidities were [11–14,30]: nephropathy 580–589, hypertension 401–405, chronic obstructive pulmonary disease (a surrogate for smoking) 490–496, stroke 430–438, ischemic heart disease 410–414, peripheral arterial disease 250.7, 785.4, 443.81 and 440–448, eye disease 250.5, 362.0, 369, 366.41 and 365.44, obesity 278, dyslipidemia 272.0–272.4, benign thyroid disease 240–246, and cancer other than thyroid cancer 140–208 (excluding 193). Medications included sulfonylurea, insulin, acarbose, pioglitazone, rosiglitazone, statin, fibrate, angiotensin-converting enzyme inhibitor and/or angiotensin receptor blocker, calcium channel blocker, aspirin, ticlopidine, clopidogrel, dipyridamole and non-steroidal anti-inflammatory drugs (excluding aspirin).

The incidence density of thyroid cancer was calculated for ever-users and never-users and for different subgroups of exposure. The numerator for the incidence was the number of patients with incident thyroid cancer during the 4-year follow-up from January 1, 2006 to December 31, 2009, and the denominator was the person-years of follow-up. For ever-users, the follow-up duration was either censored at the date of thyroid cancer diagnosis or at the date of the last record of the available reimbursement databases in individuals without incident thyroid cancer. In the lack of information on the vital status or migration of the patients, the last reimbursement record may serve as a surrogate because patients who die or migrate out of the country should be withdrawn from the NHI in Taiwan. For never-users, the follow-up was censored at the date of metformin initiation or thyroid cancer diagnosis or the last reimbursement record, depending on whichever occurring first. This ensured no exposure to metformin throughout the whole follow-up period until censor in the referent group of never-users.

Cox proportional hazards regression was performed to estimate the hazard ratios for thyroid cancer for ever-users versus never-users, and for the various subgroups of dose-response parameters. The following fully adjusted models were created with consideration of all covariates mentioned above: 1) Models I conducted in the whole original cohort; 2) Models II conducted after excluding users of both metformin and sulfonylurea, in order to avoid the potential bias resulted from multi-collinearity because a very high proportion of metformin users were also users of sulfonylurea; and 3) Models III conducted after excluding users of antidiabetic drugs other than metformin, in order to create a "cleaner" comparison for metformin only versus diabetic patients without use of antidiabetic drugs (i.e., on diet control only).

Additional sensitivity analyses were conducted by creating the following Cox regression models to estimate the fully adjusted hazard ratios for metformin users versus non-users: 1) In subgroups of men, women, age <50 years and age ≥50 years, respectively; 2) Excluding patients with a diagnosis of cancer other than thyroid cancer; 3) Excluding users of insulin, sulfonylurea, and insulin and/or sulfonylurea, respectively; 4) Additional adjustment for potential detection examinations including thyroid sonography, thyroid aspiration and thyroid function test (described previously [30]) that might have led to differential detection of thyroid cancer between ever-users and never-users of metformin.

Analyses were conducted using SAS statistical software, version 9.3 (SAS Institute, Cary, NC). $P<0.05$ was considered statistically significant.

Table 1. Baseline characteristics between never-users and ever-users of metformin.

Variables	Metformin				*P* value
	Never users		Ever users		
	n	%	*n*	%	
n = 1414723	619402		795321		
Age (years)					
<0	43229	6.98	30708	3.86	<0.0001
40–49	90027	14.53	100815	12.68	
50–59	155055	25.03	210883	26.52	
60–69	143566	23.18	214320	26.95	
≥70	187525	30.28	238595	30.00	
Sex (men)	291424	47.05	397316	49.96	<0.0001
Diabetes duration (years)					
<1	76021	12.27	39395	4.95	<0.0001
1–3	122049	19.70	97004	12.20	
3–5	109316	17.65	108390	13.63	
>5	312016	50.37	550532	69.22	
Hypertension	193690	31.27	536498	67.46	<0.0001
Chronic obstructive pulmonary disease	43116	6.96	149644	18.82	<0.0001
Stroke	37674	6.08	151546	19.05	<0.0001
Nephropathy	45351	7.32	124597	15.67	<0.0001
Ischemic heart disease	57508	9.28	238766	30.02	<0.0001
Peripheral arterial disease	21408	3.46	135384	17.02	<0.0001
Eye disease	10859	1.75	106035	13.33	<0.0001
Obesity	4015	0.65	15647	1.97	<0.0001
Dyslipidemia	196607	31.74	466909	58.71	<0.0001
Benign thyroid disease	21855	3.53	43401	5.46	<0.0001
Other cancer	106265	17.16	93978	11.82	<0.0001
Statin	63535	10.26	309483	38.91	<0.0001
Fibrate	40065	6.47	221696	27.88	<0.0001
Angiotensin converting enzyme inhibitor/angiotensin receptor blocker	101931	16.46	451197	56.73	<0.0001
Calcium channel blocker	83733	13.52	329741	41.46	<0.0001
Sulfonylurea	149415	24.12	722015	90.78	<0.0001
Insulin	17198	2.78	172418	21.68	<0.0001
Acarbose	14592	2.36	170206	21.40	<0.0001
Pioglitazone	2716	0.44	55662	7.00	<0.0001
Rosiglitazone	8381	1.35	165822	20.85	<0.0001
Aspirin	67805	10.95	320342	40.28	<0.0001
Ticlopidine	4643	0.75	29727	3.74	<0.0001
Clopidogrel	5491	0.89	32008	4.02	<0.0001
Dipyridamole	40354	6.51	210556	26.47	<0.0001
Non-steroidal anti-inflammatory drugs (excluding aspirin)	229967	37.13	596320	74.98	<0.0001

Results

Among the patients 317,508 (22.4%) were on diet control without any pharmacological intervention, 907,599 (64.2%) were using oral antidiabetic drugs only, 179,847 (12.7%) were using oral antidiabetic drugs plus insulin, and 9,769 (0.7%) were using insulin only.

Table 1 compares the baseline characteristics between ever- and never-users of metformin. All variables differed significantly between the two groups. Ever-users are characterized by older age distribution, higher proportion with a diabetes duration >5 years, higher proportions of all comorbidities except with a lower proportion of a diagnosis with other cancer, and higher proportions of using other medications.

Table 2 shows the incidences of thyroid cancer between ever-users and never-users of metformin, and among the different categories of the dose-response parameters for metformin exposure. During follow-up, a total of 2,297 (0.16%) patients developed

Table 2. Incidence of thyroid cancer by metformin exposure at entry.

Metformin use	Case number	Incident thyroid cancer	%	Person-years	Incidence rate (per 100,000 person-years)
Never users	619402	1614	0.26	1848266.92	87.33
Ever users	795321	683	0.09	2835264.08	24.09
P value			0.0222		
Cumulative duration of therapy (months)					
Never users	619402	1614	0.26	1848266.92	87.33
<9.13	262339	257	0.10	905836.25	28.37
9.13–37.00	262486	211	0.08	945139.58	22.32
>37.00	270496	215	0.08	984288.25	21.84
P value			0.0067		
Cumulative dose (mg)					
Never users	619402	1614	0.26	1848266.92	87.33
<264,000	262425	258	0.10	908265.75	28.41
264,000–1,263,000	262430	217	0.08	943853.92	22.99
>1,263,000	270466	208	0.08	983144.42	21.16
P value			0.0043		

thyroid cancer. Among them, 1,614 were never-users and 683 were ever-users of metformin at entry. The incidence rate in never- and ever-users of metformin was 87.33 and 24.09 per 100,000 person-years, respectively.

Table 3 shows the fully adjusted hazard ratios with regards to different categories of metformin exposure in Models I, II and III. In the models evaluating the overall hazard ratios for ever-users versus never-users, all of the hazard ratios showed a significantly lower risk associated with metformin use. In the models evaluating the dose-response exposure to metfomrin, a lower risk could be seen in all tertiles of the dose-response parameters, with significant *P*-values for the trend. The dose-response effect in Models I was not as remarkable as in Models II, suggesting potentially biased estimates resulting from the high correlation between use of metformin and sulfonylurea in Models I.

Table 4 shows the fully adjusted hazard ratios for thyroid cancer in the additional sensitivity analyses. The results suggested that the protective effect of metformin on thyroid cancer was not restricted to a certain group of age or sex; and was not affected by excluding users of insulin, sulfonylurea, and insulin/and or sulfonylurea, respectively, by previous diagnosis of other cancers or by potential detection examinations.

Discussion

Observational studies suggested that metformin may be associated with a reduced risk of some cancer involving the bladder, breast, liver, and colorectum [14–16]. However, whether metformin use can be associated with a reduced risk of thyroid cancer has not been investigated previously [16,29]. This is the first observational study that clearly demonstrated a protective effect of metformin on thyroid cancer risk in patients with type 2 diabetes (Tables 2, 3 and 4).

Several randomized clinical trials are being conducted to evaluate the potential usefulness of metformin as an adjuvant to other chemotherapeutic agents on some solid cancers like the breast, endometrial, prostate, and lung cancer [31]. However, clinical trials focusing specifically on the effect of metformin on thyroid cancer are still lacking. This study provided an important rationale for future in-depth investigation on metformin for the prevention and treatment of thyroid cancer.

A large number ($n = 1,556,791$) of the patients with a diagnosis of diabetes did not have reimbursement data after study entry and had been excluded from the analyses. This could be a main source of bias in the study. It is assumable that this population of excluded diabetic patients might have mainly composed of patients being on diet control without any pharmacological intervention. The consistent finding in the comparison of metformin-treated patients to patients on diet control alone conducted in Models III of Table 3 would obviate the concern of this potential bias.

The present study suggested that a significantly lower risk of thyroid cancer could be observed with a cumulative duration of 9 months or a cumulative dose of 263,000 mg (Table 3). This time window for a protective effect of metformin may be supported by a small clinical trial showing that metformin use for 6 months may significantly reduce the size of thyroid nodules [28], and by another study showing that the adjusted hazard ratio for prostate cancer-specific mortality was 0.76 (95% confidence interval: 0.64–0.89) for each additional 6 months of metformin use [32].

If insulin resistance is the underlying cause of thyroid cancer as advocated by Gursoy [10] and metformin treatment in patients with type 2 diabetes would reduce the incidence of thyroid cancer (Tables 2, 3 and 4), it is expected that the incidence of thyroid cancer should be increased gradually from obesity, impaired glucose tolerance through the early stage of type 2 diabetes when they were put on diet control without pharmacological intervention, but the risk would decrease when metformin was initiated. However, such a temporal change in thyroid cancer incidence becomes more complicated when the disease progresses to the development of diabetes complications, when other clinical comorbidities set in, or when multiple drugs are used. Because most patients with type 2 diabetes require multiple antidiabetic drugs for controlling their blood glucose [33], the joint effects and interactions among the various antidiabetic drugs are interesting

Table 3. Metformin exposure at entry and hazard ratios for thyroid cancer.

Metformin use	Models I			Models II			Models III		
	HR	95% CI	*P*	HR	95% CI	*P*	HR	95% CI	*P*
Ever-users	0.683	(0.598–0.780)	<0.0001	0.421	(0.334–0.530)	<0.0001	0.432	(0.336–0.555)	<0.0001
Cumulative duration of therapy (months)									
<9.1	0.699	(0.601–0.813)	<0.0001	0.439	(0.336–0.574)	<0.0001	0.461	(0.347–0.611)	<0.0001
9.1–36.9	0.655	(0.547–0.785)	<0.0001	0.396	(0.249–0.630)	<0.0001	0.426	(0.253–0.717)	0.0013
>36.9	0.677	(0.554–0.826)	0.0001	0.339	(0.150–0.765)	0.0092	0.159	(0.039–0.642)	0.0098
P-trend			<0.0001			<0.0001			<0.0001
Cumulative dose (mg)									
<263,000	0.691	(0.594–0.803)	<0.0001	0.433	(0.333–0.564)	<0.0001	0.439	(0.331–0.583)	<0.0001
263,000–1,260,000	0.675	(0.564–0.808)	<0.0001	0.408	(0.257–0.650)	0.0002	0.475	(0.287–0.788)	0.0039
>1,260,000	0.667	(0.543–0.819)	0.0001	0.314	(0.117–0.848)	0.0222	0.123	(0.017–0.880)	0.0369
P-trend			<0.0001			<0.0001			<0.0001

Referent group: never-users of metformin; HR: hazard ratio, CI: confidence interval.
Models I: Fully adjusted models conducted in the whole cohort.
Models II: Fully adjusted models conducted after excluding users of both metformin and sulfonylurea.
Models III: Fully adjusted models conducted after excluding users of antidiabetic drugs other than metformin.

Table 4. Additional sensitivity analyses for metformin and thyroid cancer.

Model	Fully adjusted HR	95% CI	*P*-value
Men	0.770	(0.602–0.985)	0.0379
Women	0.651	(0.555–0.762)	<0.0001
Age <50 years	0.576	(0.437–0.759)	<0.0001
Age ≥50 years	0.732	(0.628–0.853)	<0.0001
Excluding patients with a diagnosis of cancers other than thyroid cancer	0.613	(0.538–0.699)	<0.0001
Excluding users of insulin	0.682	(0.594–0.782)	<0.0001
Excluding users of sulfonylurea	0.434	(0.344–0.548)	<0.0001
Excluding users of insulin and/or sulfonylurea	0.436	(0.344–0.552)	<0.0001
Additional adjustment for potential detection examination	0.667	(0.584–0.761)	<0.0001

Referent group: never-users of metformin.
HR: hazard ratio, CI: confidence interval.

and important. However, these are out of the scope of the present study and await future investigations.

The anti-cancer effects of metformin may probably involve the activation of the AMPK, inhibition of the mTOR pathway, and inhibition of insulin-like growth factors [34]. All of these have been demonstrated in *in vitro* studies conducted in thyroid cancer cell lines [24,25], in women with insulin resistance and benign thyroid nodules [28] and in patients with type 2 diabetes [35]. The suppression on TSH by metformin observed in humans [26,36] may also contribute to the lower risk of thyroid cancer in metformin users, although this beneficial effect can not be confirmed by another recent study [27].

Leptin, a hormone produced by adipocytes and regulates energy balance in the brain, signals the expression of thryotropin-releasing hormone, leading to increased secretion of TSH [37]. Therefore, one of the possible mechanisms explaining the inhibitory effect of metformin on TSH secretion may be through its leptin inhibition [37]. Recent basic researches also suggested that metformin may sensitize thyroid cancer cells to oxidative stress [38], inhibit thyroid cancer stem cells [25,39], cause cell cycle arrest at G0/G1 phase [25], induce apoptosis [25], inhibit colony formation [25], inhibit stimulation of mitogen-activated protein kinase by insulin [25], and inhibit growth of doxorubicin-resistant thyroid carcinoma cells [25]. The growth inhibitory effect of metformin is not only demonstrated in thyroid carcinoma cells, a recent study also demonstrates such a growth inhibitory effect on medullary thyroid cancer cells [24]. Metformin may have an advantage of inducing growth arrest specifically in cancer stem cells through the inhibition of Akt, which is not affected in differentiated cells [40,41].

There are several strengths in the present study. First, we made a special request to include all patients diagnosed as having diabetes from the NHI database covering the whole period since its availability in 1996. Such an approach avoided the possibility of selection bias and insufficient cases of thyroid cancer for subgroup analyses. In the absence of a special request, the usually provided NHI database is a 1 million random sample of the general population, and the number of diabetic patients derived from such a 1 million sample is surely too small for the analyses of the association between the use of anti-diabetic drugs and some cancers. Second, the consistency of a lower risk of thyroid cancer in metformin users in the sensitivity analyses strengthened the preventive role of metformin on thyroid cancer. Third, the database included outpatients and inpatients, and we included diagnoses from both sources. The use of medical records also reduced the bias related to self-reporting.

The limitations of the study may include a lack of the histological types of thyroid cancer for analysis. However, because thyroid papillary cancer represents 80.5% and 87.1% of thyroid cancer in men and women, respectively, in Taiwan [42], the findings should better be applied to thyroid papillary cancer. Second, although some cases of thyroid cancer may have been misclassified, such an occurrence was probably low because labeled diagnoses should be printed on all prescriptions handed out to patients in Taiwan. Mislabeling of a cancer diagnosis would not be acceptable to the patients when they saw the diagnosis. Third, ionizing radiation has been implicated as a risk factor for thyroid cancer [43]. A confounding effect due to the lack of such data collection could not be excluded. Fourth, we did not have biochemical data for evaluating their impacts.

In summary, this study supports a protective effect of metformin on the development of thyroid cancer in Taiwanese patients with type 2 diabetes. The uses of metformin for reversing the increasing trend of thyroid cancer incidence in the general population and for the treatment of thyroid cancer are worthy of further investigation.

Author Contributions

Conceived and designed the experiments: CHT. Performed the experiments: CHT. Analyzed the data: CHT. Contributed reagents/materials/analysis tools: CHT. Wrote the paper: CHT.

References

1. Arcidiacono B, Iiritano S, Nocera A, Possidente K, Nevolo MT, et al. (2012) Insulin resistance and cancer risk: an overview of the pathogenetic mechanisms. Exp Diabetes Res 2012: 789174.
2. Nicolucci A (2010) Epidemiological aspects of neoplasms in diabetes. Acta Diabetol 47: 87–95.
3. Tseng CH (2011) Diabetes conveys a higher risk of gastric cancer mortality despite an age-standardised decreasing trend in the general population in Taiwan. Gut 60: 774–779.
4. Tseng CH, Chong CK, Tseng CP, Chan TT (2009) Age-related risk of mortality from bladder cancer in diabetic patients: A 12-year follow-up of a national cohort in Taiwan. Ann Med 41: 371–379.

5. Tseng CH (2011) Diabetes and risk of bladder cancer: A study using the National Health Insurance database in Taiwan. Diabetologia 54: 2009–2015.
6. Tseng CH (2012) Diabetes and non-Hodgkin's lymphoma: Analyses of prevalence and annual incidence in 2005 using the National Health Insurance database in Taiwan. Ann Oncol 23: 153–158.
7. Tseng CH (2012) Diabetes, insulin use, and non-Hodgkin lymphoma mortality in Taiwan. Metabolism 61: 1003–1009.
8. Tseng CH (2013) New-onset diabetes with a history of dyslipidemia predicts pancreatic cancer. Pancreas 42: 42–48.
9. Dong X, Li Y, Tang H, Chang P, Hess KR, et al. (2012) Insulin-like growth factor axis gene polymorphisms modify risk of pancreatic cancer. Cancer Epidemiol 36: 206–211.
10. Gursoy A (2010) Rising thyroid cancer incidence in the world might be related to insulin resistance. Med Hypotheses 74: 35–36.
11. Tseng CH (2012) Thyroid cancer risk is not increased in diabetic patients. PLoS One 7: e53096.
12. Tseng CH (2012) Diabetes, metformin use, and colon cancer: A population-based cohort study in Taiwan. Eur J Endocrinol 167: 409–416.
13. Tseng CH (2013) Benign prostatic hyperplasia is a significant risk factor for bladder cancer in diabetic patients: a population-based cohort study using the National Health Insurance in Taiwan. BMC Cancer 13: 7.
14. Tseng CH (2014) Metformin may reduce bladder cancer risk in Taiwanese patients with type 2 diabetes. Acta Diabetol 51: 295–303.
15. Tseng CH (2014) Metformin may reduce breast cancer risk in Taiwanese women with type 2 diabetes. Breast Cancer Res Treat 145: 785–790.
16. Franciosi M, Lucisano G, Lapice E, Strippoli GF, Pellegrini F, et al. (2013) Metformin therapy and risk of cancer in patients with type 2 diabetes: systematic review. PLoS One 8: e71583.
17. Tseng CH (2013) Diabetes, insulin use, smoking, and pancreatic cancer mortality in Taiwan. Acta Diabetol 50: 879–886.
18. Tseng CH (2013) Type 2 diabetes, smoking, insulin use and mortality from hepatocellular carcinoma: a 12-year follow-up of a national cohort in Taiwan. Hepatol Int 7: 693–702.
19. Tseng CH (2013) Insulin use and smoking jointly increase the risk of bladder cancer mortality in patients with type 2 diabetes. Clin Genitourin Cancer 11: 508–514.
20. Tseng CH (2012) Pioglitazone and bladder cancer: a population-based study of Taiwanese. Diabetes Care 35: 278–280.
21. Tseng CH, Tseng FH (2012) Peroxisome proliferator-activated receptor agonists and bladder cancer: lessons from animal studies. J Environ Sci Health C Environ Carcinog Ecotoxicol Rev 30: 368–402.
22. Tseng CH (2014) A review on thiazolidinediones and bladder cancer in human studies. J Environ Sci Health C Environ Carcinog Ecotoxicol Rev 32: 1–45.
23. Tseng CH (2013) Rosiglitazone is not associated with an increased risk of bladder cancer. Cancer Epidemiol 37: 385–389.
24. Klubo-Gwiezdzinska J, Jensen K, Costello J, Patel A, Hoperia V, et al. (2012) Metformin inhibits growth and decreases resistance to anoikis in medullary thyroid cancer cells. Endocr Relat Cancer 19: 447–456.
25. Chen G, Xu S, Renko K, Derwahl M (2012) Metformin inhibits growth of thyroid carcinoma cells, suppresses self-renewal of derived cancer stem cells, and potentiates the effect of chemotherapeutic agents. J Clin Endocrinol Metab 97: E510–520.
26. Vigersky RA, Filmore-Nassar A, Glass AR (2006) Thyrotropin suppression by metformin. J Clin Endocrinol Metab 91: 225–227.
27. Díez JJ, Iglesias P (2013) Relationship between serum thyrotropin concentrations and metformin therapy in euthyroid patients with type 2 diabetes. Clin Endocrinol (Oxf) 78: 505–511.
28. Rezzónico J, Rezzónico M, Pusiol E, Pitoia F, Niepomniszcze H (2011) Metformin treatment for small benign thyroid nodules in patients with insulin resistance. Metab Syndr Relat Disord 9: 69–75.
29. Rizos CV, Elisaf MS (2013) Metformin and cancer. Eur J Pharmacol 705: 96–108.
30. Tseng CH (2014) Treatment with human insulin does not increase thyroid cancer risk in patients with type 2 diabetes. Eur J Clin Invest 44: 736–742.
31. Kourelis TV, Siegel RD (2012) Metformin and cancer: new applications for an old drug. Med Oncol 29: 1314–1327.
32. Margel D, Urbach DR, Lipscombe LL, Bell CM, Kulkarni G, et al. (2013) Metformin use and all-cause and prostate cancer-specific mortality among men with diabetes. J Clin Oncol 31: 3069–3075.
33. Willey CJ, Andrade SE, Cohen J, Fuller JC, Gurwitz JH (2006) Polypharmacy with oral antidiabetic agents: an indicator of poor glycemic control. Am J Manag Care 12: 435–440.
34. Aljada A, Mousa SA (2012) Metformin and neoplasia: Implications and indications. Pharmacol Ther 133: 108–115.
35. Ittermann T, Markus MR, Schipf S, Derwahl M, Meisinger C, et al. (2013) Metformin inhibits goitrogenous effects of type 2 diabetes. Eur J Endocrinol 169: 9–15.
36. Cappelli C, Rotondi M, Pirola I, Agosti B, Formenti A, et al. Thyreotropin levels in diabetic patients on metformin treatment. Eur J Endocrinol 167: 261–265.
37. Nar A, Gedik O (2009) The effect of metformin on leptin in obese patients with type 2 diabetes mellitus and nonalcoholic fatty liver disease. Acta Diabetol 46: 113–118.
38. Klubo-Gwiezdzinska J, Costello J Jr, Patel A, Bauer A, Jensen K, et al. (2013) Treatment with metformin is associated with higher remission rate in diabetic patients with thyroid cancer. J Clin Endocrinol Metab 98: 3269–3279.
39. Malaguarnera R, Frasca F, Garozzo A, Gianì F, Pandini G, et al. (2011) Insulin receptor isoforms and insulin-like growth factor receptor in human follicular cell precursors from papillary thyroid cancer and normal thyroid. J Clin Endocrinol Metab 96: 766–774.
40. Würth R, Pattarozzi A, Gatti M, Bajetto A, Corsaro A, et al. (2013) Metformin selectively affects human glioblastoma tumor-initiating cell viability: A role for metformin-induced inhibition of Akt. Cell Cycle 12: 145–156.
41. Würth R, Barbieri F, Florio T (2014) New molecules and old drugs as emerging approaches to selectively target human glioblastoma cancer stem cells. Biomed Res Int 2014: 126586.
42. Tseng CH (2013) Diabetes and thyroid cancer mortality: a 12-year prospective follow-up of Taiwanese. Eur J Clin Invest 43: 595–601.
43. Shih SR, Chiu WY, Chang TC, Tseng CH (2012) Diabetes and thyroid cancer risk: literature review. Exp Diabetes Res 2012: 578285.

19

Can Evidence from Genome-Wide Association Studies and Positive Natural Selection Surveys Be Used to Evaluate the Thrifty Gene Hypothesis in East Asians?

Xuan-Han Koh[1], Xuanyao Liu[2,3], Yik-Ying Teo[2,3,4,5,6]*

1 Department of Biological Sciences, National University of Singapore, Singapore, Singapore, **2** NUS Graduate School for Integrative Science and Engineering, National University of Singapore, Singapore, Singapore, **3** Saw Swee Hock School of Public Health, National University of Singapore, Singapore, Singapore, **4** Life Sciences Institute, National University of Singapore, Singapore, Singapore, **5** Department of Statistics and Applied Probability, National University of Singapore, Singapore, Singapore, **6** Genome Institute of Singapore, Agency for Science, Technology and Research, Singapore, Singapore

Abstract

Body fat deposition and distribution differ between East Asians and Europeans, and for the same level of obesity, East Asians are at higher risks of Type 2 diabetes (T2D) and other metabolic disorders. This observation has prompted the reclassifications of body mass index thresholds for the definitions of "overweight" and "obese" in East Asians. However, the question remains over what evolutionary mechanisms have driven the differences in adiposity morphology between two population groups that shared a common ancestor less than 80,000 years ago. The Thrifty Gene hypothesis has been suggested as a possible explanation, where genetic factors that allowed for efficient food-energy conversion and storage are evolutionarily favoured by conferring increased chances of survival and fertility. Here, we leveraged on the existing findings from genome-wide association studies and large-scale surveys of positive natural selection to evaluate whether there is currently any evidence to support the Thrifty Gene hypothesis. We first assess whether the existing genetic associations with obesity and T2D are located in genomic regions that are reported to be under positive selection, and if so, whether the risk alleles sit on the extended haplotype forms. In addition, we interrogate whether these risk alleles are the derived forms that differ from the ancestral alleles, and whether there is significant evidence of population differentiation at these SNPs between East Asian and European populations. Our systematic survey did not yield conclusive evidence to support the Thrifty Gene hypothesis as a possible explanation for the differences observed between East Asians and Europeans.

Editor: Fengfeng Zhou, Shenzhen Institutes of Advanced Technology, China

Funding: XHK, XYL and YYT acknowledge support from the Saw Swee Hock School of Public Health from the National University of Singapore and the National Research Foundation Singapore (NRF-RF-2010-05). YYT also acknowledges the support from the Life Sciences Institute, National University of Singapore. The funders had no role in study design, data collection and analysis, decision to publish, or preparation of the manuscript.

Competing Interests: The authors have declared that no competing interests exist.

* Email: statyy@nus.edu.sg

Introduction

The past decade has seen a precipitous surge in obesity and diabetes globally, where the bulk of the increase has been in Asian populations such as China and India [1]. For example, a systematic review of 22 studies reported an increase in prevalence of Type 2 diabetes (T2D) in adults in China from 2.6% in 2000 to 9.7% in 2010 [2]. Epidemiologically, for the same body mass index (BMI), an East Asian individual is more susceptible to insulin resistance, and is more predisposed to body fat and visceral adiposity than a European individual [3]. The observations that East Asians tend to develop T2D at a less severe stage of obesity compared to Europeans have contributed in part to the reclassification of the definitions of "overweight" and "obese" for East Asians. Overweight and obese are defined as possessing a BMI $\geq$23 kg/m^2 and BMI $\geq$28 kg/m^2 respectively for East Asians, compared to corresponding thresholds of 25 kg/m^2 and 30 kg/m^2 for non-East Asians [3].

While the global surge in obesity and T2D has undoubtedly been attributed to the shift towards a high-fat high-sugar diet coupled with increasingly sedentary lifestyles, a fundamental question exists around the physiological differences in T2D etiology between East Asians and other populations. What are the molecular mechanisms that have resulted in the different types and location of adiposity, and what evolutionary processes could have driven these changes?

The Thrifty Gene hypothesis has been posited as a possible explanation for the steep increase in the prevalence of obesity and T2D in modern populations, particularly amongst East Asians. This hypothesizes that periods of famine in the history of modern humans presented a significant evolutionary force in favour of genes involved in fat storage, by increasing fertility and survival [4]. Even during fluctuating periods of abundance and scarcity, these individuals with metabolically thrifty genes were able to utilize food, store fat and gain weight more efficiently such that they were likely to survive better than those without the thrifty genes during periods of famine. The comparative perpetual abundance of food in modern societies means that the advantageous genes are preparing the hosts for famines that do not occur, which subsequently manifests as obesity and increases the risk to T2D [5]. A famine-like incident is believed to have occurred during the human migration to East Asia (and subsequently onwards to the Americas) in the last 20,000 years that is believed to have led to further enhancements of metabolically thrifty genes amongst East Asians than in the Europeans [6–9].

Presently, there have not been many concrete reports validating or refuting the Thrifty Gene hypothesis despite an ongoing debate and growing literature that focused on the role of natural selection in this hypothesis [5,10]. One of the metrics to appraise the evidence of positive selection is by measuring the length of haplotypes in the genome. Recombination breaks down long haplotypes, and an uncharacteristically long haplotype at a locus often indicates that the particular genetic background has been preferred over other shorter haplotypes. This is thus indicative that a "hard sweep", defined as a selection event with very high evolutionary fitness, has occurred.

The availability of high-density genetic data across multiple populations, coupled with recent discoveries from genome-wide association studies (GWAS) on obesity and T2D, confers an unprecedented opportunity to explore the Thrifty Gene hypothesis. Here, we combine findings from positive selection analyses and GWAS to evaluate whether there is any evidence to support the Thrifty Gene hypothesis in East Asians. This utilizes a recently developed method (haploPS) to locate genomic signatures of positive selection in humans [11], which additionally identifies the haplotype form that the advantageous allele sits on. This allows us to evaluate whether the selected haplotype form actually carries known variants that have been reported to increase the risk to obesity or T2D, which is vital given the reliance on tagging SNPs in GWAS to discover phenotypic associations.

Specifically, we adopted a four-step qualitative approach in evaluating the evidence to support the Thrifty Gene hypothesis in East Asians that is otherwise absent outside East Asia and the Americas. (i) We first examined the GWAS catalogue to identify SNPs that have been indisputably associated with obesity and T2D onset, and to compare these against the set of positive selection signals that were present only in the East Asian populations of the International HapMap Project [12] and the Singapore Genome Variation Project [13] (CHB, CHD, CHS, JPT). (ii) The selected haplotype forms were then checked to see whether they carried the reported risk alleles. (iii) In addition, we interrogated whether the reported risk alleles were the derived alleles by comparing against the chimpanzee genome sequence from dbSNP Build 138, as would have been supported under the Thrifty Gene hypothesis. (iv) Finally, we evaluated the degree of population differentiation using F_{ST} at the reported SNPs between East Asian and European populations, with the expectation of significant differentiation between the two ancestry groups if the East Asian-specific evolutionary events under the Thrifty Gene hypothesis did occur.

Methods

Datasets

We used the genome-wide genotype data for 11 populations from Phase 3 of the International HapMap Project (abbreviated subsequently as HapMap) [12], and for the three populations in the Singapore Genome Variation Project (SGVP) [13]. All 14 populations were genotyped on the Affymetrix SNP 6.0 and Illumina 1M genotyping microarrays. We only considered unrelated individuals from the HapMap and these consisted of: (i) 53 individuals of African ancestry in Southwest USA (ASW); (ii) 113 Utah residents with Northern and Western European ancestry from the CEPH collection (CEU); (iii) 84 Han Chinese from Beijing, China (CHB); (iv) 85 Chinese in Metropolitan Denver, Colorado (CHD); (v) 88 Gujarati Indians in Houston, Texas (GIH); (vi) 86 Japanese from Tokyo, Japan (JPT); (vii) 90 Luhyas from Webuye, Kenya (LWK); (viii) 50 individuals with Mexican ancestry in Los Angeles, California (MXL); (ix) 143 Maasai in Kinyawa, Kenya (MKK); (x) 88 Toscani in Italia (TSI); and (xi) 113 Yoruban from Ibadan, Nigeria (YRI). We considered a consensus set of 1,525,445 SNPs that was present across all eleven populations, and the phased haplotypes downloaded from the HapMap resource were thinned to consist of only this set of SNPs. The SGVP resource comprised 268 individuals from the three major ethnic groups in Singapore consisting of 96 Southern Han Chinese (CHS), 89 Southeast Asian Malays (MAS) and 83 South Asian Indians (INS). We considered the phased haplotypes of the post-QC set of autosomal SNPs that were available from the SGVP resource, which consisted of 1,584,040 SNPs for CHS, 1,580,905 SNPs for MAS and 1,583,454 SNPs for INS.

Analysis of positive selection

Genomic evidence of positive selection was quantified with the use of the haploPS algorithm [11]. Briefly, haploPS explicitly locates uncharacteristically long haplotypes in the genome at a given frequency, which is defined against the distribution of haplotypes for that particular frequency across the genome by performing an exhaustive search across the SNPs. The length of each haplotype is measured by the genetic distance (in cM) spanned and by the number of SNPs on the haplotype. These two metrics are ranked against all other haplotypes across the genome of the same frequency in other to derive two empirical p-values: (i) the proportion of haplotypes that span a genetic distance at least as large as the target haplotype; and (ii) the proportion of haplotypes that span as many SNPs as the target haplotype. The haploPS score is defined as the product of these two empirical p-values and the total number of haplotypes across the genome at that particular frequency, and haplotypes with scores <0.05 are interpreted as exhibiting evidence of positive selection. This analysis is performed for each of the 14 populations, with the haplotype frequencies ranging from 0.05 to 0.95 in increments of 0.05. Since a site that is found to possess an uncharacteristically long haplotype at a particular frequency is similarly likely to possess long haplotypes at lower frequencies as well, we report only the evidence found at the highest haplotype frequency, and identify the specific haplotype form at this frequency as the one that is expected to carry the advantageous functional allele. Population-average recombination rates from the HapMap were used in the calculation of genetic distance [14].

Quantifying similarity of positively selected haplotypes

A positive selection signal in a particular genomic region can be present across multiple populations, either by stemming from the same mutation event in the common ancestor of these multiple populations, or through convergent evolution where different mutation events in response to the same environmental trigger have happened independently in these populations. HaploPS quantifies the presence of positive selection by locating the longest haplotype form in a particular genomic region, and we can differentiate between the two scenarios above by comparing the selected haplotype forms from the multiple populations: in the former scenario where the selection seen in multiple populations is attributed to the same mutation event, we expect a significant degree of similarity between the haplotype forms; whereas in the latter scenario, we expect the advantageous alleles (either at the same site or at different sites) to have arisen on different haplotype backgrounds such that the longest haplotypes from different populations will exhibit a significant degree of discordance. As such, the haplotype similarity index (HSI), as described in the formulation of haploPS [11], is used to distinguish between the two scenarios, where a HSI >0.98 is indicative of a single mutation event in the common ancestor of the multiple populations, and a HSI <0.9 is indicative that convergent evolution is likely to have happened.

Mapping GWAS signals to positively selected haplotypes

We considered the GWAS findings for obesity and T2D from the GWAS catalogue maintained by the National Human Genome Research Institute (NHGRI) at http://www.genome.gov/gwastudies/, which was accessed on 30th June 2013. Specifically, we considered 56 loci for T2D from 31 GWAS studies and nine loci for obesity from four GWAS studies, where for each locus there was at least one SNP reported to be associated with the phenotype where the statistical significance of the association was more significant than 5×10^{-8} (**Tables S1, S2 in File S1**). Note that we did not require these associations to be specific to or have been reported in East Asian populations. In searching for uncharacteristically long haplotypes, haploPS explicitly identifies the specific haplotype form that is expected to be carrying the functional allele that confers an evolutionary advantage. We thus interrogated whether there was any evidence of positive selection in East Asian populations that overlapped with any of the 35 loci reported to be associated with T2D and obesity, and if so, whether the reported risk alleles were found on the selected haplotype forms in the East Asian populations. The loci are considered to be overlapping with the selection signals if they are located within the selection regions.

Measurement of population differentiation

We used the locus-specific fixation index F_{ST} to quantify the extent of genetic differences between populations at a particular SNP [15]. This measures the divergence in the population-specific allele frequencies from the population-averaged allele frequency, and is defined as the ratio of the observed variance for the allele frequencies across the populations to the maximum possible variance under the global allele frequency.

Results

Starting with the list of 405 positively selected genomic regions in the 14 populations from HapMap and SGVP, we identified six T2D-associated index SNPs in or around nine genes from the GWAS catalogue (**Table 1**) that overlapped with evidence of positive selection in the East Asian populations in HapMap and SGVP (**Table 2**) [16–24]. Three of these SNPs were located in six genes (*ARF5, PAX4, SND1, GCC1, C2CD4A, C2CD4B*) that were identified to be associated with T2D in only East Asian populations, while *HHEX* was common to both East Asian and Europeans, and two genes (*THADA, IDE*) were specific to the Europeans. In particular, we noted that the specific allele for rs7578597 in *THADA* that was identified to increase the risk of T2D was almost fixed in the two East Asian populations (CHD, CHS). Strikingly, even though we started with the intention to consider both obesity and T2D-associated loci, only the T2D-associated loci met our criteria for being East Asian specific in both trait association and positive selection signals.

Table 1. Positively selected Type 2 diabetes associated SNPs from genome-wide association studies (GWAS).

SNP	Chr	Pos. NCBI 36.3 (bp)	No-risk allele	Risk allele	Risk allele frequency	Nearest gene(s)	*p*-value	Odds ratio	Reported in East Asians	Reported in Europeans
rs7578597	2	43,586,327	C	T[a]	0.9	THADA	1×10^{-9}	1.15	N	Y
rs10229583	7	127,034,139	A	G[a]	0.825	ARF5, PAX4, SND1	2×10^{-10}	1.14	Y	N
rs6467136	7	126,952,194	A	G[a]	0.79	GCC1, PAX4	5×10^{-11}	1.11	Y	N
rs5015480	10	94,455,539	T	C[a]	NR	HHEX, IDE	1×10^{-15}	1.18	N	Y
rs1111875	10	94,452,862	T[a]	C	0.52	HHEX	7×10^{-12}	1.21	Y	Y
rs7172432	15	60,183,681	G[a]	A	0.58	C2CD4A, C2CD4B	9×10^{-14}	1.11	Y	N

Summary of six SNPs reported to be associated with Type 2 diabetes from the GWAS catalogue maintained by the National Human Genome Research Institute (NHGRI), accessed on 30th June 2013, that are located in genomic regions that are putatively under positive selection in at least one of 14 populations from the International HapMap Project and the Singapore Genome Variation Project.
[a]Ancestral allele.

For *THADA*, the T2D risk allele was located on the positively selected haplotype identified by haploPS (**Figure 1**, **Table 2**). The evidence of positive selection was present in two of the four East Asian populations (CHD, CHS), and the selected haplotype forms from both populations were identical with a haplotype similarity index (HSI) of 1.00. We observed that haploPS inferred the frequency of the selected haplotype to be 45% for both populations, although the frequencies of the risk alleles were at 99.4% and 100% in CHD and CHS respectively. However, it was noted that the associated risk allele was in fact an ancestral allele identical to that found in the chimpanzee genome.

We observed the same evidence for the two index SNPs (rs10229583, rs6467136) located in the cluster of genes (*ARF5*, *PAX4*, *SND1*, *GCC1*) on chromosome 7, where the specific risk alleles were located on the positively selected haplotypes identified by haploPS (**Figure 2**, **Table 2**). The selection evidence was present in all four East Asian populations (CHB, CHD, CHS, JPT), and the selected haplotype forms from all four populations were identical with a HSI of 1.00. HaploPS inferred the frequency of the selection to be between 40% and 50% in the four populations, although the frequencies of the risk alleles ranged between 77% and 86%. Both risk alleles were ancestral and common with the chimpanzee genome.

The risk alleles for the remaining three index SNPs (rs5015480, rs1111875, rs7172432) did not sit on the positively selected haplotype. For rs7172432 on chromosome 15, it was also clear from the frequencies of the risk allele and the selected haplotypes that the selected haplotypes did not uniquely carry the risk or the protective allele (**Table 2, Figure S1 in File S1**).

With the evidence of positive selection and trait association converging for only *THADA* and the gene cluster on chromosome 7, the analysis of genetic differentiation thus focused on only the three relevant index SNPs. We observed that while both rs7578597 and rs10229583 were not significantly differentiated between East Asian and European populations, rs6467136 exhibited F_{ST} scores that were in excess of 8.2% (**Table 3**), indicating significant degree of genetic differentiation.

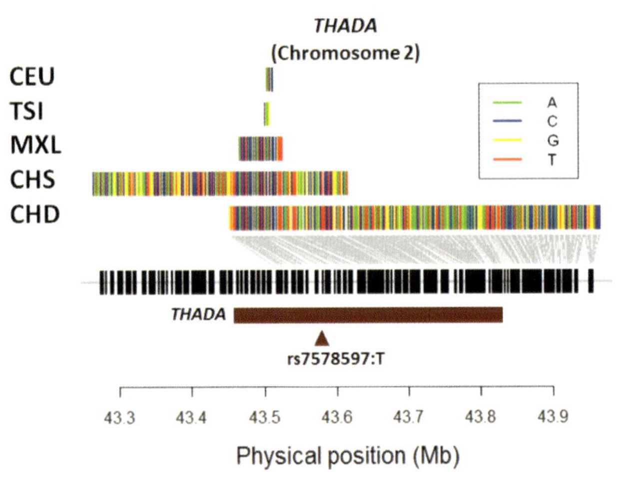

Figure 1. Long haplotypes around *THADA* in East Asian and European populations. Illustration of haplotype forms identified by haploPS that span the longest genetic distances around *THADA* (brown horizontal bar) on chromosome 2. Uncharacteristically long haplotypes were found at the same frequency of 45% in two East Asian populations (CHD, CHS) to span *THADA*, whereas at the same frequency, the longest haplotypes present in European populations (CEU, TSI, MXL) were comparatively much shorter. The haplotypes for the two East Asian populations also carried the thymine allele at rs7578597 that has been reported in association studies to increase the risk to Type 2 diabetes.

Discussion

We started with the intention to evaluate whether genetics can explain the disparity in risk to T2D and other cardiovascular diseases between East Asians and Europeans, where for the same level of obesity as measured by BMI, East Asians are more likely than their European counterparts to experience a cardiac event or to be diabetic. One possible explanation centers around the Thrifty Gene hypothesis, and we attempted to evaluate whether current findings from GWAS and genetic surveys of positive selection can provide the genetic evidence to support this hypothesis. We observed that only six T2D-associated loci were found in regions undergoing positive selection in East Asian populations, and while the risk alleles of three of these loci sat on the positively selected haplotypes, they were all ancestral alleles that, despite acknowledging the reliance of GWAS on identifying tagging SNPs, did not conform to the notion that these alleles are derived from specific mutation events that have occurred recently to confer greater survivability. Similar to a previous report [25], we did not find consistent evidence to unambiguously support the Thrifty Gene hypothesis as it pertains to East Asians.

There has been considerable confusion as to what constitutes a 'thrifty gene'. While it is most commonly associated with a metabolic trait related to the frugal utilization of fuel [7], various researchers have broadened the concept to encompass multiple notions of thrift, such as behavioral and physiological traits that might be adaptive during periods of food shortages [7,26]. In this paper, we adopted the definition of 'thrift' as five broad categories that favor sustained positive energy balance as suggested by Bouchard [27], encompassing (a) metabolism or thermogenesis, (b) regulation of appetite, (c) physical inactivity, (d) lipid oxidization, and (e) lipid storage capacity of adipocytes, for practical purposes of testability. As such, the central assumption is that individuals possessing thrifty genes may exhibit high adiposity in modern society, and thus be identified among populations of people with obesity and/or type 2 diabetes. While obesity and type 2 diabetes are not perfect surrogate measures of the modern day effects of metabolic thrift, they represent objective measures of the biological system that can be tested and compared across populations.

It is interesting to note that, despite explicitly searching for obesity and T2D-associated loci, none of the obesity-associated SNPs displayed evidence of position selection that was specific to East Asians even though obesity is commonly regarded as upstream of T2D pathogenesis and would have been a better surrogate measure for the presence of thrifty genes. Although obesity is a major predictor of T2D, most obese individuals do not develop T2D, and conversely T2D patients are not necessarily obese. The complexity of the interaction between both diseases illustrates the difficulty in using T2D as a surrogate for the modern day effect of thrifty genes.

A gene that shows evidence of positive selection and an association with T2D is not necessarily a thrifty gene, as it may have been selected for reasons other than thrift. For example, the thymine allele of rs7903146 in *TCF7L2* increases T2D risk with an odds ratio of 1.37 [28], representing the T2D susceptibility gene with the largest effect size discovered to date that has been successfully replicated across multiple populations. However, the $HapB_{T2D}$ haplotype containing the risk allele is found to be negatively associated with BMI in T2D patients and is not the variant that displays evidence of recent positive selection, contrary to predictions of the thrifty gene hypothesis [29]. If thrifty genes

Table 2. Long haplotype regions (specific to East Asians) containing trait associated SNPs.

Chr	Start position	End position	HaploPS score	Pop.	Pos. NCBI 36.3 (bp)	rsID	Risk allele	Hap. freq.	All. freq.	Found on hap.	Nearest gene(s)
2	43,282,562	43,910,360	0.017	CHD	43,586,327	rs7578597 (3′ UTR)	T[a]	0.45	0.994	Y	THADA
2	43,301,270	43,958,429	0.008	CHS	43,586,327	rs7578597 (3′ UTR)	T[a]	0.45	1	Y	THADA
7	126,647,066	127,610,096	0.021	CHB	127,034,139	rs10229583 (downstream)	G[a]	0.40	0.798	Y	ARF5, PAX4, SND1
7	126,647,066	127,610,096	0.021	CHB	126,952,194	rs6467136 (intergenic)	G[a]	0.40	0.775	Y	GCC1, PAX4
7	126,716,840	127,589,178	0.022	CHS	127,034,139	rs10229583 (downstream)	G[a]	0.45	0.775	Y	ARF5, PAX4, SND1
7	126,716,840	127,589,178	0.022	CHS	126,952,194	rs6467136 (intergenic)	G[a]	0.45	0.801	Y	GCC1, PAX4
7	126,720,180	127,631,331	0.024	CHD	127,034,139	rs10229583 (downstream)	G[a]	0.45	0.829	Y	ARF5, PAX4, SND1
7	126,720,180	127,631,331	0.024	CHD	126,952,194	rs6467136 (intergenic)	G[a]	0.45	0.780	Y	GCC1, PAX4
7	126,735,606	127,628,256	0.015	JPT	127,034,139	rs10229583 (downstream)	G[a]	0.50	0.866	Y	ARF5, PAX4, SND1
7	126,735,606	127,628,256	0.015	JPT	126,952,194	rs6467136 (intergenic)	G[a]	0.50	0.818	Y	GCC1, PAX4
10	92,947,202	95,385,717	0.032	JPT	94,455,539	rs5015480 (downstream)	C[a]	0.05	0.186	N	HHEX, IDE
10	92,947,202	95,385,717	0.032	JPT	94,452,862	rs1111875 (intergenic)	C	0.05	0.349	N	HHEX
15	61,999,328	62,941,185	0.033	CHS	60,183,681	rs7172432 (intergenic)	A	0.60	0.330	N	C2CD4A, C2CD4B
15	62,122,278	62,938,688	0.003	JPT	60,183,681	rs7172432 (intergenic)	A	0.70	0.552	N	C2CD4A, C2CD4B
15	62,303,982	62,934,451	0.012	CHD	60,183,681	rs7172432 (intergenic)	A	0.80	0.631	N	C2CD4A, C2CD4B

Three SNPs from three genomic regions associated with T2D in or near *ARF5, PAX4, SND1, GCC1, C2CD4A,* and *C2CD4B* genes, which meet the criteria that both the evidence of T2D association and positive selection (haploPS score <0.05) were specific to only East Asians. The allele that increases the risk of T2D is identified and interrogated whether it (i) matches the ancestral allelic form on the chimpanzee genome, and/or (ii) sits on the positively selected haplotype form.

[a]Ancestral allele.

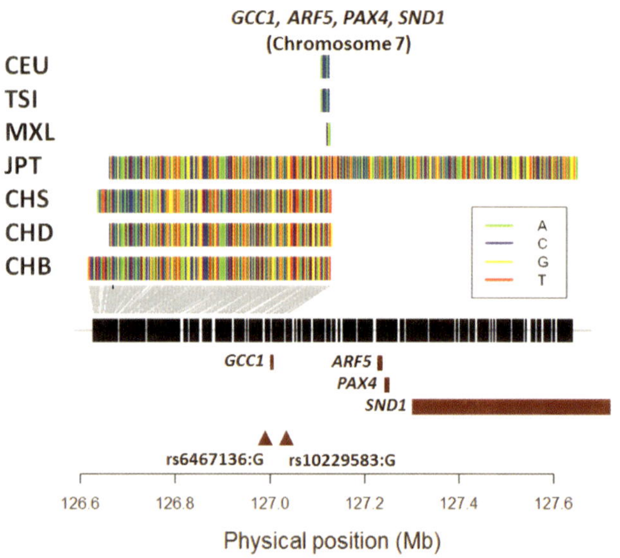

Figure 2. Long haplotypes around two T2D-associated SNPs in East Asian and European populations. Illustration of haplotype forms identified by haploPS that span the longest genetic distance around two SNPs rs6467136 and rs10229583 that are located around a cluster of four genes on chromosome 7 (brown horizontal bars: *GCC1, ARF5, PAX4, SND1*). The figure shows the uncharacteristically long haplotypes that were present at a haplotype frequency of 40% in the four East Asian populations (CHB, CHD, CHS, JPT), together with the longest haplotypes present in the European populations (CEU, TSI, MXL) that were comparatively much shorter and did not yield significant evidence of positive selection. The haplotypes for the four East Asian populations carried both risk alleles at the two SNPs that have been reported in association studies to increase the risk to Type 2 diabetes.

indeed exist, functional evidence that the T2D risk alleles are involved in a mechanism consistent with thrift is essential.

One challenge to testing the Thrifty Gene theory is the lack of clarity behind the mechanisms linking obesity, T2D, and insulin resistance. It has been proposed that the phenotypic expression of the thrifty gene may be hyperinsulinemia or insulin resistance [30], although this appears to be paradoxical as a decrease in insulin sensitivity suggests a negative impact on fat storage ability. For normal individuals without pancreatic islet β-cell dysfunction, the β-cells increase insulin secretion sufficiently to compensate for the reduced sensitivity to insulin action, thereby maintaining normal glucose tolerance [31]. It is hypothesized that this increase in blood insulin is responsible for a greater net tendency towards fat storage. However, some have proposed that the evidence behind insulin resistance as the phenotypic expression of the thrifty gene is inconsistent [32], citing evidence that Pima Indians have the greatest prevalence of diabetes in the world and ought to be an obvious candidate for carriers of thrifty genes given the population genetic history, except that in non-diabetic Pima Indians, insulin resistance is instead associated with a reduced risk of weight gain [33] which is contrary to what one would expect under the Thrifty Gene hypothesis.

One proposed mechanism linking obesity, insulin resistance, and T2D suggests that a defect in the ability of β-cells to secrete insulin is sufficient to lead to decreased insulin signaling in the hypothalamus, resulting in increased food intake and thus weight gain [34]. In this way, a thrifty allele that causes β-cell dysfunction and results in decreased insulin secretion can potentially be selected for thrift through its effects on increased food intake, consistent with the Thrifty Gene hypothesis. However, a decrease

Table 3. F_{ST} scores between pairs of East Asian and European populations at three index SNPs around *THADA* and on chromosome 7 in the cluster of genes containing *GCC1, ARF5, PAX4* and *SND1*.

F_{ST} score	CHB-CEU	CHB-TSI	CHB-MXL	CHD-CEU	CHD-TSI	CHD-MXL	JPT-CEU	JPT-TSI	JPT-MXL
rs7578597	–	–	–	0.057	0.024	0.004	–	–	–
rs10229583	0.012	0.007	<0.001	0.011	0.006	<0.001	0.024	0.016	0.006
rs6467136	0.082	0.131	0.113	0.085	0.135	0.116	0.113	0.168	0.147

Population abbreviations represent: CEU – Utah residents with Northern and Western European ancestry from the CEPH collection; CHB – Han Chinese in Beijing, China; CHD – Chinese in Metropolitan Denver, Colorado; JPT – Japanese in Toyko, Japan; MXL – Mexican ancestry in Los Angeles, California; TSI – Toscani in Italia.

in insulin secretion also impairs the storage of glucose as triglycerides in adipocytes, leading to increased lipolysis and elevated plasma non-esterified fatty acids (NEFA) levels [31]. The increase in NEFA and glucose levels in the plasma, together with increased food intake due to brain signaling processes can result in insulin resistance, further aggravating β-cell function [31]. Interestingly, the convergence of events towards increased insulin resistance may hint at thrifty genes with different phenotypic expressions that function along a similar pathway. It thus remains an open question as to whether thrifty genes directly affect β-cell function, insulin resistance, fat storage upstream of any T2D-related event, or if a more plausible thrifty genotype exists where numerous genes involved in different functions at various points along the carbohydrate and fat regulation pathway account for an aggregate effect towards fat storage. Even then, a possibility maintains that thrift is also accounted for by mechanisms other than increased fat storage.

Though it remains to be demonstrated that the genes at which the index SNPs are located in are functionally responsible for the GWAS signals for obesity and T2D, there is a great amount of evidence supporting the roles of the identified genes, particularly for *THADA* and *PAX4*. The *THADA* risk allele is linked to decreased glucagon-like peptide-1-induced and arginine-induced insulin release [35], while studies have shown that the early expression of *PAX4* is involved in the differentiation of β-cells in the pancreas, thus affecting insulin secretion [36,37]. It has to be noted that both genes affect pancreatic insulin secretion and/or plasma insulin levels that is upstream of fat storage. Ideally, we would expect a thrifty allele to be directly involved in efficient fat storage. However, it remains to be seen if genes that affect fat storage indirectly have less of an impact on fertility and/or survival, and thus selection.

Perhaps one of the most plausible explanations on the lack of evidence thus far for the Thrifty Gene hypothesis is the fact that the search for genomic signatures of positive selection with recent genome-wide data has primarily focused on locating hard sweeps, given the reliance on methods that capitalise on variance in allele frequencies or the presence of long haplotypes. These methods are capable of identifying selection signals that leave distinctive imprints in the genome, but are unfortunately poorly powered to locate evidence arising from polygenic soft sweeps. This is compounded by the fact that obesity and T2D are complex phenotypes, where even the genetic determinants are multi-factorial and exert at best a modest impact, unlike the classical situation where genetic mutations confer a strong fitness against an infectious disease that produces a rapid proliferation of the advantageous mutations in a population. If indeed thrifty genes do exist, these are highly likely to be working in tandem in a polygenic manner to alter phenotype expression, where any evolutionary advantage they confer will similarly be visible only by explicitly searching for polygenic soft selection sweeps.

Author Contributions

Conceived and designed the experiments: YYT. Performed the experiments: XHK XYL. Analyzed the data: XHK XYL. Contributed reagents/materials/analysis tools: XHK XYL. Contributed to the writing of the manuscript: XHK YYT.

References

1. Hu FB (2011) Globalization of diabetes: the role of diet, lifestyle, and genes. Diabetes Care 34: 1249 1257.
2. Li H, Oldenburg B, Chamberlain C, O'Neil A, Xue B, et al. (2012) Diabetes prevalence and determinants in adults in China mainland from 2000 to 2010: a systematic review. Diabetes Res Clin Pract 98: 226 235.
3. Ma RC, Chan JC (2013) Type 2 diabetes in East Asians: similarities and differences with populations in Europe and the United States. Ann N Y Acad Sci 1281: 64 91.
4. Prentice AM, Hennig BJ, Fulford AJ (2008) Evolutionary origins of the obesity epidemic: natural selection of thrifty genes or genetic drift following predation release? Int J Obes (Lond) 32: 1607 1610.
5. Speakman JR (2008) Thrifty genes for obesity, an attractive but flawed idea, and an alternative perspective: the drifty gene' hypothesis. Int J Obes (Lond) 32: 1611 1617.
6. Diamond J (2003) The double puzzle of diabetes. Nature 423: 599 602.
7. Prentice AM, Rayco-Solon P, Moore SE (2005) Insights from the developing world: thrifty genotypes and thrifty phenotypes. Proc Nutr Soc 64: 153 161.
8. Prentice AM (2005) Early influences on human energy regulation: thrifty genotypes and thrifty phenotypes. Physiol Behav 86: 640 645.
9. Benyshek DC, Watson JT (2006) Exploring the thrifty genotype's food-shortage assumptions: a cross-cultural comparison of ethnographic accounts of food security among foraging and agricultural societies. Am J Phys Anthropol 131: 120 126.
10. Prentice AM (2005) Starvation in humans: evolutionary background and contemporary implications. Mech Ageing Dev 126: 976 981.
11. Liu X, Ong RT, Pillai EN, Elzein AM, Small KS, et al. (2013) Detecting and Characterizing Genomic Signatures of Positive Selection in Global Populations. Am J Hum Genet.
12. Altshuler DM, Gibbs RA, Peltonen L, Dermitzakis E, Schaffner SF, et al. (2010) Integrating common and rare genetic variation in diverse human populations. Nature 467: 52 58.
13. Teo YY, Sim X, Ong RT, Tan AK, Chen J, et al. (2009) Singapore Genome Variation Project: a haplotype map of three Southeast Asian populations. Genome Res 19: 2154 2162.
14. Frazer KA, Ballinger DG, Cox DR, Hinds DA, Stuve LL, et al. (2007) A second generation human haplotype map of over 3.1 million SNPs. Nature 449: 851 861.
15. Qian W, Deng L, Lu D, Xu S (2013) Genome-wide landscapes of human local adaptation in Asia. PLoS One 8: e54224.
16. Zeggini E, Scott LJ, Saxena R, Voight BF, Marchini JL, et al. (2008) Meta-analysis of genome-wide association data and large-scale replication identifies additional susceptibility loci for type 2 diabetes. Nat Genet 40: 638 645.
17. Ma RC, Hu C, Tam CH, Zhang R, Kwan P, et al. (2013) Genome-wide association study in a Chinese population identifies a susceptibility locus for type 2 diabetes at 7q32 near PAX4. Diabetologia 56: 1291 1305.
18. Cho YS, Chen CH, Hu C, Long J, Ong RT, et al. (2012) Meta-analysis of genome-wide association studies identifies eight new loci for type 2 diabetes in east Asians. Nat Genet 44: 67 72.
19. Voight BF, Scott LJ, Steinthorsdottir V, Morris AP, Dina C, et al. (2010) Twelve type 2 diabetes susceptibility loci identified through large-scale association analysis. Nat Genet 42: 579 589.
20. Perry JR, Voight BF, Yengo L, Amin N, Dupuis J, et al. (2012) Stratifying type 2 diabetes cases by BMI identifies genetic risk variants in LAMA1 and enrichment for risk variants in lean compared to obese cases. PLoS Genet 8: e1002741.
21. Scott LJ, Mohlke KL, Bonnycastle LL, Willer CJ, Li Y, et al. (2007) A genome-wide association study of type 2 diabetes in Finns detects multiple susceptibility variants. Science 316: 1341 1345.
22. Saxena R, Voight BF, Lyssenko V, Burtt NP, de Bakker PI, et al. (2007) Genome-wide association analysis identifies loci for type 2 diabetes and triglyceride levels. Science 316: 1331 1336.
23. Takeuchi F, Serizawa M, Yamamoto K, Fujisawa T, Nakashima E, et al. (2009) Confirmation of multiple risk Loci and genetic impacts by a genome-wide association study of type 2 diabetes in the Japanese population. Diabetes 58: 1690 1699.
24. Yamauchi T, Hara K, Maeda S, Yasuda K, Takahashi A, et al. (2010) A genome-wide association study in the Japanese population identifies susceptibility loci for type 2 diabetes at UBE2E2 and C2CD4A-C2CD4B. Nat Genet 42: 864 868.
25. Southam L, Soranzo N, Montgomery SB, Frayling TM, McCarthy MI, et al. (2009) Is the thrifty genotype hypothesis supported by evidence based on

confirmed type 2 diabetes- and obesity-susceptibility variants? Diabetologia 52: 1846–1851.
26. Wells JC (2009) Thrift: a guide to thrifty genes, thrifty phenotypes and thrifty norms. Int J Obes (Lond) 33: 1331–1338.
27. Bouchard C (2007) The biological predisposition to obesity: beyond the thrifty genotype scenario. Int J Obes (Lond) 31: 1337–1339.
28. Frayling TM (2007) Genome-wide association studies provide new insights into type 2 diabetes aetiology. Nat Rev Genet 8: 657–662.
29. Helgason A, Palsson S, Thorleifsson G, Grant SF, Emilsson V, et al. (2007) Refining the impact of TCF7L2 gene variants on type 2 diabetes and adaptive evolution. Nat Genet 39: 218–225.
30. Wendorf M, Goldfine ID (1991) Archaeology of NIDDM. Excavation of the "thrifty" genotype. Diabetes 40: 161–165.
31. Kahn SE, Hull RL, Utzschneider KM (2006) Mechanisms linking obesity to insulin resistance and type 2 diabetes. Nature 444: 840–846.
32. Watve MG, Yajnik CS (2007) Evolutionary origins of insulin resistance: a behavioral switch hypothesis. BMC Evol Biol 7: 61.
33. Swinburn BA, Nyomba BL, Saad MF, Zurlo F, Raz I, et al. (1991) Insulin resistance associated with lower rates of weight gain in Pima Indians. J Clin Invest 88: 168–173.
34. Schwartz MW, Woods SC, Porte D Jr, Seeley RJ, Baskin DG (2000) Central nervous system control of food intake. Nature 404: 661–671.
35. Simonis-Bik AM, Nijpels G, van Haeften TW, Houwing-Duistermaat JJ, Boomsma DI, et al. (2010) Gene variants in the novel type 2 diabetes loci CDC123/CAMK1D, THADA, ADAMTS9, BCL11A, and MTNR1B affect different aspects of pancreatic beta-cell function. Diabetes 59: 293–301.
36. Blyszczuk P, Czyz J, Kania G, Wagner M, Roll U, et al. (2003) Expression of Pax4 in embryonic stem cells promotes differentiation of nestin-positive progenitor and insulin-producing cells. Proc Natl Acad Sci U S A 100: 998–1003.
37. Sosa-Pineda B, Chowdhury K, Torres M, Oliver G, Gruss P (1997) The Pax4 gene is essential for differentiation of insulin-producing beta cells in the mammalian pancreas. Nature 386: 399–402.

20

The Dual-Specificity Phosphatase 2 (DUSP2) Does Not Regulate Obesity-Associated Inflammation or Insulin Resistance in Mice

Graeme I. Lancaster[1]*, Michael J. Kraakman[1], Helene L. Kammoun[1], Katherine G. Langley[1], Emma Estevez[1], Ashish Banerjee[3], Raelene J. Grumont[2], Mark A. Febbraio[1¶], Steve Gerondakis[2¶]

1 Cellular and Molecular Metabolism Laboratory, Baker IDI Heart and Diabetes Institute, Melbourne, Victoria, Australia, **2** The Australian Centre for Blood Diseases and Department of Clinical Hematology, Monash University Central Clinical School, Melbourne, Victoria, Australia, **3** Centre for Cancer Research, MIMR-PHI Institute of Medical Research, Monash University, Victoria, Australia

Abstract

Alterations in the immune cell profile and the induction of inflammation within adipose tissue are a hallmark of obesity in mice and humans. Dual-specificity phosphatase 2 (DUSP2) is widely expressed within the immune system and plays a key role promoting immune and inflammatory responses dependent on mitogen-activated protein kinase (MAPK) activity. We hypothesised that the absence of DUSP2 would protect mice against obesity-associated inflammation and insulin resistance. Accordingly, male and female littermate mice that are either wild-type (*wt*) or homozygous for a germ-line null mutation of the *dusp2* gene (*dusp2*$^{-/-}$) were fed either a standard chow diet (SCD) or high fat diet (HFD) for 12 weeks prior to metabolic phenotyping. Compared with mice fed the SCD, all mice consuming the HFD became obese, developed glucose intolerance and insulin resistance, and displayed increased macrophage recruitment and markers of inflammation in epididymal white adipose tissue. The absence of DUSP2, however, had no effect on the development of obesity or adipose tissue inflammation. Whole body insulin sensitivity in male mice was unaffected by an absence of DUSP2 in response to either the SCD or HFD; however, HFD-induced insulin resistance was slightly, but significantly, reduced in female *dusp2*$^{-/-}$ mice. In conclusion, DUSP2 plays no role in regulating obesity-associated inflammation and only a minor role in controlling insulin sensitivity following HFD in female, but not male, mice. These data indicate that rather than DUSP2 being a pan regulator of MAPK dependent immune cell mediated inflammation, it appears to differentially regulate inflammatory responses that have a MAPK component.

Editor: Shree Ram Singh, National Cancer Institute, United States of America

Funding: This study was supported by the Victorian Government Operational Infrastructure Support Program. M.A.F. and S.G. are Research Fellows of the National Health & Medical Research Council of Australia. K.G.L. is supported by a Baker IDI Bright Sparks Stipend and a Monash University Faculty of Medicine, Nursing and Health Sciences Postgraduate Research Scholarship. M.J.K. is supported by an Australian Postgraduate Award. The funders had no role in study design, data collection and analysis, decision to publish, or preparation of the manuscript.

Competing Interests: The authors have declared that no competing interests exist.

* Email: Graeme.lancaster@bakeridi.edu.au

¶ MAF and SG are joint senior authors on this work.

Introduction

Research over the last two decades has identified that chronic, low-grade inflammation plays a critical role in initiating insulin resistance, a key step in the development of type 2 diabetes [1]. Underpinning obesity-associated WAT inflammation is a marked shift in the immune cell profile of the WAT during the transition from a lean to obese state [2]. A loss of anti-inflammatory immune cells, concomitant with the accumulation of pro-inflammatory immune cells, initiates a state of local inflammation within the WAT that contributes to insulin resistance [2]. Studies in which particular immune cells or pro-inflammatory molecules have been genetically or pharmacologically targeted underscore the important role specific immune cells, and inflammation more generally, play in systemic insulin resistance [3–8].

Amongst the different classes of molecules shown to influence metabolism are protein tyrosine phosphatases [9]. The protein tyrosine phosphatase (PTP) superfamily is divided into classical PTPs and dual specificity phosphatases (DUSPs), the products of which catalyze the hydrolysis of phospho-tyrosine and phospho-threonine substrates [10]. Classical PTPs such as PTP1B and T-cell PTP have been identified as critical regulators of insulin and leptin signalling, serving important roles in the development of obesity and insulin resistance [11–14]. Of the many DUSPs described to date are the class I sub-family of DUSP proteins. The class I DUSPs specifically recognize and de-phosphorylate the conserved TxY motif present in the activation loop of the 4 major classes of mitogen-activated protein kinases (MAPK); ERK (1 and 2), ERK5, p38 (α, β, γ and δ) plus JNK (1, 2 and 3), and, accordingly, are also referred to as MAPK phosphatases (MKPs) [15]. Based on sequence homology, substrate specificity and subcellular localization, these MKPs can be further sub-divided into three groups. The first includes DUSP1/MKP-1, DUSP2

(PAC1), DUSP4/MKP-2 and DUSP5, all of which serve as mitogen- and stress-inducible nuclear MKPs. The second group includes DUSP6/MKP-3, DUSP7/MKP-X and DUSP9/MKP-4, which are ERK-specific MKPs localized exclusively in the cytoplasm. The final group comprising DUSP8 (M3/6), DUSP10/MKP-5 and DUSP16/MKP-7 are JNK/p38-specific phosphatases found in both the cytoplasm and nucleus [10].

Consistent with the numerous roles MAPKs serve regulating diverse processes in immune cells that encounter growth factors, pathogens and inflammatory cytokines or undergo stress [10], DUSPs provide a critical level of spatiotemporal control over these responses. For example, in the absence of either DUSP1 [16] or DUSP10 [17], lipopolysaccharide (LPS) treated macrophages display increased JNK activation and elevated pro-inflammatory cytokine production, whereas LPS activated macrophages isolated from DUSP2-deficient (*dusp2*$^{-/-}$) mice exhibit reduced pro-inflammatory cytokine production [18]. The roles DUSPs play controlling MAPK-dependent innate immune and inflammatory responses has prompted an examination of their individual functions in the context of obesity and insulin resistance. Specifically, over-expression of DUSP9 decreases ERK and JNK phosphorylation and improves glucose tolerance in genetically obese ob/ob mice [19]. DUSP1-deficient mice by contrast do not have improved glucose tolerance, despite being protected from HFD-induced obesity [20].

However, the regulatory roles other DUSPs play in inflammation-induced obesity and insulin resistance remains unclear. One candidate of interest is DUSP2. First cloned as an immediate early gene in human T lymphocytes [21], DUSP2 belongs to the subfamily of nuclear specific DUSPs that includes DUSP1, 4 and 5 [10]. DUSP2 is primarily expressed within the immune system [21,22] and is further up-regulated in diverse immune cells following activation [18,22]. Importantly, a lack of DUSP2 in immune cells suppresses the production of a variety of pro-inflammatory mediators *in vitro* [18] and reduces inflammation and disease pathology in a murine model of inflammatory arthritis [18].

Based on the key role of immune cells and inflammation in obesity-associated insulin resistance, the roles ascribed to certain DUSPs in the regulation of obesity and insulin resistance, high level DUSP2 expression in various activated immune cells, plus reduced inflammation *in vitro* and *in vivo* in DUSP2-deficient cells, we have examined the role of DUSP2 in the context of obesity-associated inflammation and insulin resistance. We hypothesized that a loss of DUSP2 function would reduce obesity-associated inflammation and, consequently, would improve insulin sensitivity in mice fed a HFD.

Materials and Methods

Generation of the *dusp2*$^{-/-}$ mice were described previously [18] and this strain has been backcrossed to the C57Bl6J background for>10 generations. Wild-type (*wt*) and the DUSP2 deficient (*dusp2*$^{-/-}$) male and female littermates used in this study were generated by mating mice heterozygous for a *dusp2* null allele. Mice were housed at 22±1°C and maintained on a 12/12 h light/dark cycle, with free access to drinking water and food. Mice were fed either a SCD containing 5% of energy from fat or a HFD containing 43% of energy from fat (both diets were supplied by Specialty Feeds, Glen Forrest, WA, Australia). All procedures were approved by the AMREP Animal Ethics Committee and were in accordance with the National Health and Medical Research Council of Australia guidelines.

Bone marrow-derived macrophages (BMDM) were generated from the hind limb bones of *dusp2*$^{-/-}$ and *wt* C57Bl6J mice. After 7 days of culture in RPMI media containing 15% fetal bovine serum (FBS) and 20% L-cell conditioned media, BMDM were changed overnight to RPMI media containing 5% FBS and 2% bovine serum albumin (BSA) prior to experimental treatment. Palmitate (P0500; Sigma Aldrich) was dissolved in 100% ethanol at a stock concentration of 100 mM and was then conjugated to bovine serum albumin (BSA) (2% weight per volume; A6003; Sigma Aldrich) in RPMI media containing 5% FBS to create a final concentrations of 1 mM. The vehicle contained BSA and ethanol, but no palmitate. Media was collected after 8 h of treatment with either palmitate or vehicle and the concentrations of the pro-inflammatory cytokines IL-1β and TNF were then determined by enzyme-linked immunosorbent assay (R&D Systems, Minneapolis, USA). For the analysis of intracellular signaling molecules, cells were lysed after 4 h of treatment with palmitate or vehicle, protein concentrations determined and samples examined by Western blotting as described below.

Mice were administered 2 g of glucose per kg of lean mass by oral gavage following a 5 h fast to assess glucose tolerance. Blood was obtained prior to and at the indicated intervals for the proceeding 2 h from the tip of the tail. Blood glucose concentrations were determined using a glucometer (Accu-Check, Roche, NSW, Australia). Fat and lean mass were determined using an EchoMRI 4-in-1 (Echo Medical Systems, Houston, TX, USA). Plasma insulin concentrations were determined using a mouse ultrasensitive plasma insulin ELISA (ALPCO, Salem, NH, USA).

For quantitative RT-PCR, RNA was extracted from epididymal WAT using Trizol (Invitrogen, Carlsbad, CA, USA) and total RNA measured using the ND-1000 NanoDrop Spectrophotometer (Thermo Scientific, Waltham, MA, USA). RNA samples were treated with DNase I (Invitrogen) and cDNA generated using the Tetro cDNA synthesis kit (Bioline). Gene expression studies were performed by RT-PCR using TaqMan primers and probes for genes of interest and 18S rRNA (Applied Biosystems, Foster City, CA, USA). For cytokine and DUSP2 gene expression, 40 ng of cDNA was used, whereas *f4/80* and *cd11c* expression was determined using 20 ng of cDNA. The comparative C_T method was used to quantify results from RT-PCR.

Genotyping of tail or ear clip DNA samples was performed using the following primers. WT: Forward 5′-ATTTGCTCTCCCTTCTTCGA-3′ and Reverse 5′-TGACACACACACGTCACTTCCT-3′. DUSP2 KO: Forward 5′-ATTTGCTCTCCCTTCTTCGA-3′ and Reverse 5′-GCCTGCTCTTTACTGAAGGC-3′. The following cycling conditions were used: 1 cycle of 3 min at 95°C, 60 s at 57°C, 45 s at 72°C, followed by 39 cycles of 60 s at 95°C, 60 s at 57°C, 45 s at 72°C. Products were resolved on a 2% agarose gel containing ethidium bromide.

For Western blotting, epididymal WAT was removed from mice under anesthesia, snap frozen in liquid N_2 and stored at −80°C. WAT was lysed and protein concentrations determined using the BCA method (Thermo Scientific). Samples (20 ug total protein per sample) were solubilized in Laemmli's buffer and heated at 95°C for 5 min, then western blotting performed as described previously [23]. Antibodies against phosphorylated (4671) and total (9258) forms of JNK, phosphorylated (9211) and total (9212) forms of p38, and total ERK1/2 (9102) were from Cell Signalling Technology Inc (Danvers, MA, USA). The antibody against phosphorylated ERK1/2 (sc-7383) was from Santa-Cruz Biotechnology, Inc.

Statistical analysis was performed using SigmaStat version 3.5. Statistical significance was determined using a Student's t-test or 2 way ANOVA analysis, where appropriate. Data are presented as the mean ± the standard deviation. A p-value of less than 0.05 was considered statistically significant; although we have indicated where the p-values were lower than 0.05. Quantification of western blots was done using Quantity One (Bio-Rad Laboratories).

Results

DUSP2 expression is markedly increased in many immune cell types following activation [18,22]. Given activated immune cells accumulate in the adipose tissue of obese mice, we first determined whether *dusp2* gene expression was increased in the epididymal WAT of obese mice. Consistent with the links between immune cell dependent inflammation and obesity, *dusp2* mRNA expression was significantly higher in WAT from *wt* mice fed a HFD compared with *wt* mice fed a SCD (Figure 1).

To investigate the role of DUSP2 in the context of obesity-associated inflammation and insulin resistance, we exploited a mutant strain of mice that lack DUSP2 [18]. Male and female *wt* and *dusp2*$^{-/-}$ litter mates were fed either a SCD or HFD for 12 weeks commencing at 8 weeks of age. DUSP2-deficient mice have no known lymphoid or myeloid developmental abnormalities and have normal longevity free from any spontaneous immunopathology [18]. Both male (Figure 2a–c) and female (Figure 2 d–f) *wt* and *dusp2*$^{-/-}$ mice responded as expected to the HFD. The HFD resulted in an increase in total body mass (Figure 2a and d), an effect entirely attributable to an increase in fat mass (Figure 2b and e). While male mice appeared to gain fat mass more rapidly than female mice fed a HFD, at the end of the dietary period both male and female mice, irrespective of genotype, had gained similar amounts of fat mass (Figure 2b and e).

To assess glucose tolerance and insulin sensitivity, we performed oral glucose tolerance tests (OGTT) and assessed plasma insulin levels during the OGTT in both male and female mice after 4 and 12 weeks of either SCD or HFD. Compared with those fed the SCD, male mice fed the HFD were glucose intolerant (Figure 3a and d) and had higher plasma insulin levels, indicative of insulin resistance, during the OGTT (Figure 3 b, c, e and f) after both 4 and 12 weeks of HFD. No differences were observed in oral glucose tolerance or plasma insulin levels during the OGTT between *wt* and *dusp2*$^{-/-}$ male mice on either the SCD or HFD (Figure 3a–f). In female mice, 12 weeks of a HFD induced glucose intolerance and elevated plasma insulin levels compared to female mice fed the SCD (Figure 4a–f). As with the male mice, no differences were observed with oral glucose tolerance between *wt* and *dusp2*$^{-/-}$ female mice on either the SCD or HFD (Figure 4a and d). However, after 12 weeks of HFD, female *dusp2*$^{-/-}$ mice had lower plasma insulin levels during the OGTT than *wt* mice (Figure 4e and f), a finding indicative of an improvement in insulin sensitivity.

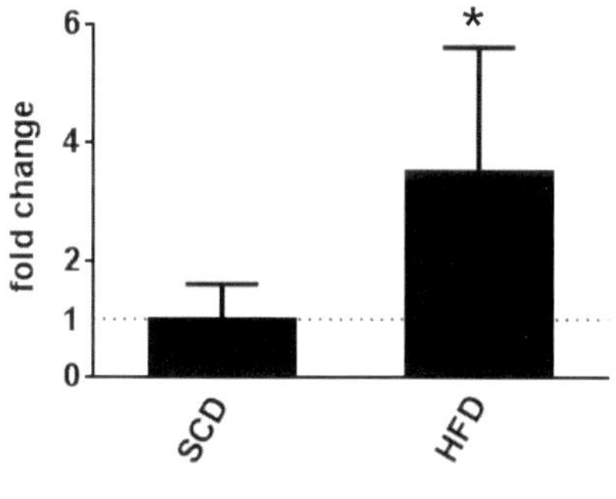

Figure 1. HFD increases *dusp2* mRNA expression. *Dusp2* mRNA expression in the WAT of *wt* C57Bl6J mice fed either SCD or HFD for 12 weeks. * $p<0.05$. Data are mean ± SD. N = 5 for SCD and 8 for HFD.

The data described thus far provided no evidence that an absence of DUSP2 activity in male mice affected obesity or measures of glucose tolerance and insulin sensitivity, whereas female *dusp2*$^{-/-}$ fed a HFD displayed a small, but significant improvement in insulin sensitivity when compared to *wt* controls. Given the published data ascribing an important role to DUSP2 in promoting inflammation and immune cell activation, we next investigated whether the absence of DUSP2 influenced epididymal adipose tissue inflammation. Total macrophage numbers, which included the recruitment of pro-inflammatory macrophages, inferred from the levels of *f480* and *cd11c* gene expression, were markedly elevated following 12 weeks of HFD (Figure 5a and b). Consistent with this finding, levels of gene expression for monocyte chemo-attractant protein 1 (*mcp1*), the pro-inflammatory cytokines tumour necrosis factor (*tnf*) and interleukin 1β (*il1b*), plus the anti-inflammatory cytokine *il10*, were all significantly higher following 12 weeks of HFD (Figure 5c–f), emphasizing the potent pro-inflammatory environment in adipose tissue induced by obesity. Although the HFD led to significant increases in the expression of *f480*, *cd11c*, *tnf*, *il1b* and *mcp*1 in female mice (Figures 5a–e), these differences were markedly lower than those observed in male mice. Notably, an absence of DUSP2 did not affect macrophage markers, pro-inflammatory cytokine or *il10* expression in male mice (Figures 5a–f). A near identical expression pattern for these genes was observed in female mice, the exception being *il10*, for which a small, but significant genotype-dependent difference was observed (Figure 5f). Furthermore, with the exception of *il1b*, the recruitment of macrophages and the increases in pro-inflammatory gene expression were markedly lower in female compared with male mice. This trend is consistent with the known anti-inflammatory effects of estrogen [24] and the finding that a loss of estrogen receptor α expression in the myeloid cells of female mice exacerbates obesity-associated WAT inflammation [25]. Finally, while DUSP1 expression was increased in both male and female mice following the HFD we observed no compensatory increases in DUSP1 expression in epididymal WAT of either male or female *dusp2*$^{-/-}$ mice (Figure 5g).

The activation of JNK and subsequent serine phosphorylation of insulin receptor substrate 1 (IRS1) in adipose tissue is postulated to be a key nexus by which a number of obesity-associated stimuli can directly impair insulin-dependent signaling [1]. A report that JNK phosphorylation is abnormally elevated in *dusp2*$^{-/-}$ cells following stimulation [18] prompted us to examine the impact of DUSP2 on JNK activation in epididymal adipose tissue. We observed a significant increase in the level of JNK phosphorylation in the WAT of male mice following 12 weeks of HFD (Figure 6a). However, the absence of DUSP2 had no additional impact on the levels of JNK phosphorylation in WAT (Figure 6a). We also determined ERK1/2 (Figure 6b) and p38 (Figure 6c) phosphorylation levels in WAT by western blotting. Neither the HFD nor DUSP2 deletion affected ERK1/2 or p38 phosphorylation in WAT.

A loss of DUSP2 activity in immune cells was previously reported to reduce LPS-induced pro-inflammatory cytokine production, but potentiate LPS-induced JNK phosphorylation [18]. Accordingly, we investigated whether pro-inflammatory cytokine production and JNK activation in BMDM activated by the long chain saturated fatty acid palmitate was also affected by an absence of DUSP2. While palmitate treatment resulted in increased TNF and IL-1β secretion as well as elevated JNK

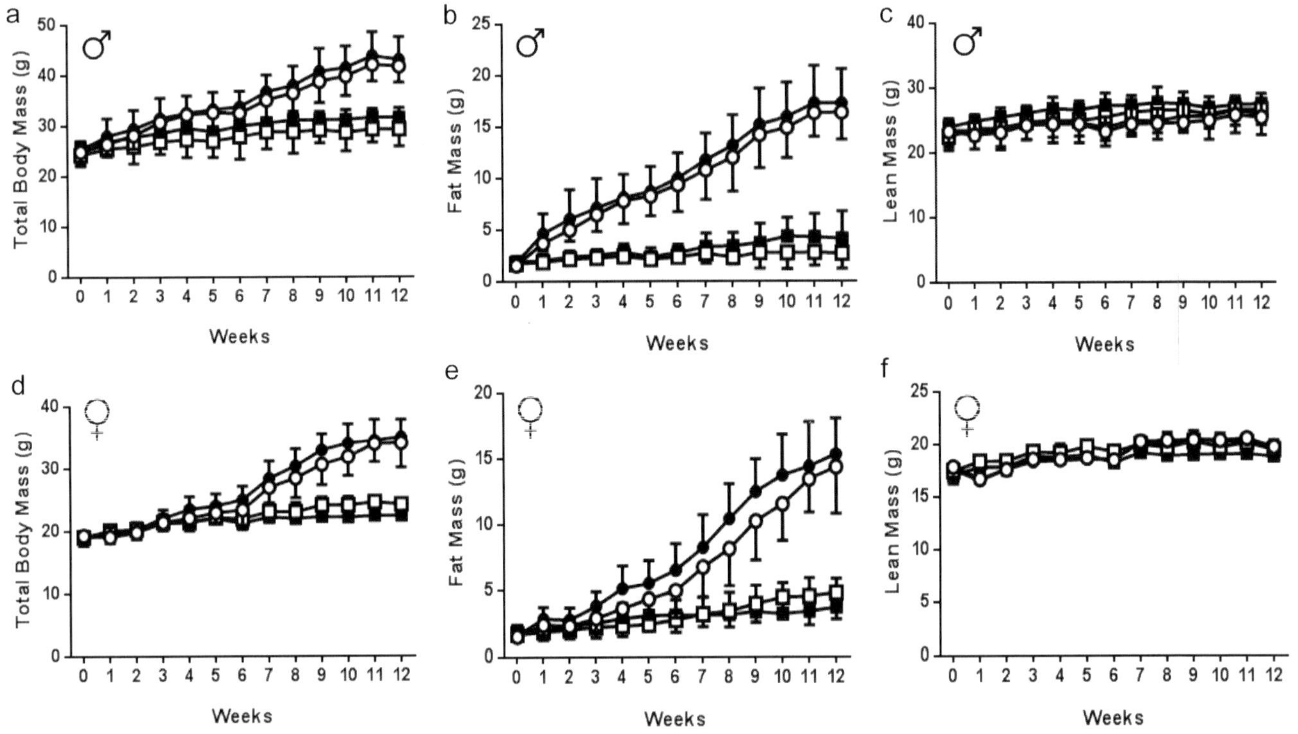

Figure 2. The development of obesity in *wt* and *dusp2*$^{-/-}$ male and female mice. (**a** and **d**) Total body mass; (**b** and **e**) fat mass; and (**c** and **f**) lean mass in *wt* and *dusp2*$^{-/-}$ male and female mice fed either a SCD or HFD for 12 weeks. Data are mean ± SD. White squares are *wt* mice fed SCD; Black squares are *dusp2*$^{-/-}$ mice fed SCD; White circles are *wt* mice fed HFD; Black circles are *dusp2*$^{-/-}$ mice fed HFD. For male mice, Ns are 5, 8, 8 and 8, for *wt* SCD, *dusp2*$^{-/-}$ SCD, *wt* HFD and *dusp2*$^{-/-}$ HFD, respectively. For female mice Ns are 9, 8, 7 and 7 for *wt* SCD, *dusp2*$^{-/-}$ SCD, *wt* HFD and *dusp2*$^{-/-}$ HFD, respectively.

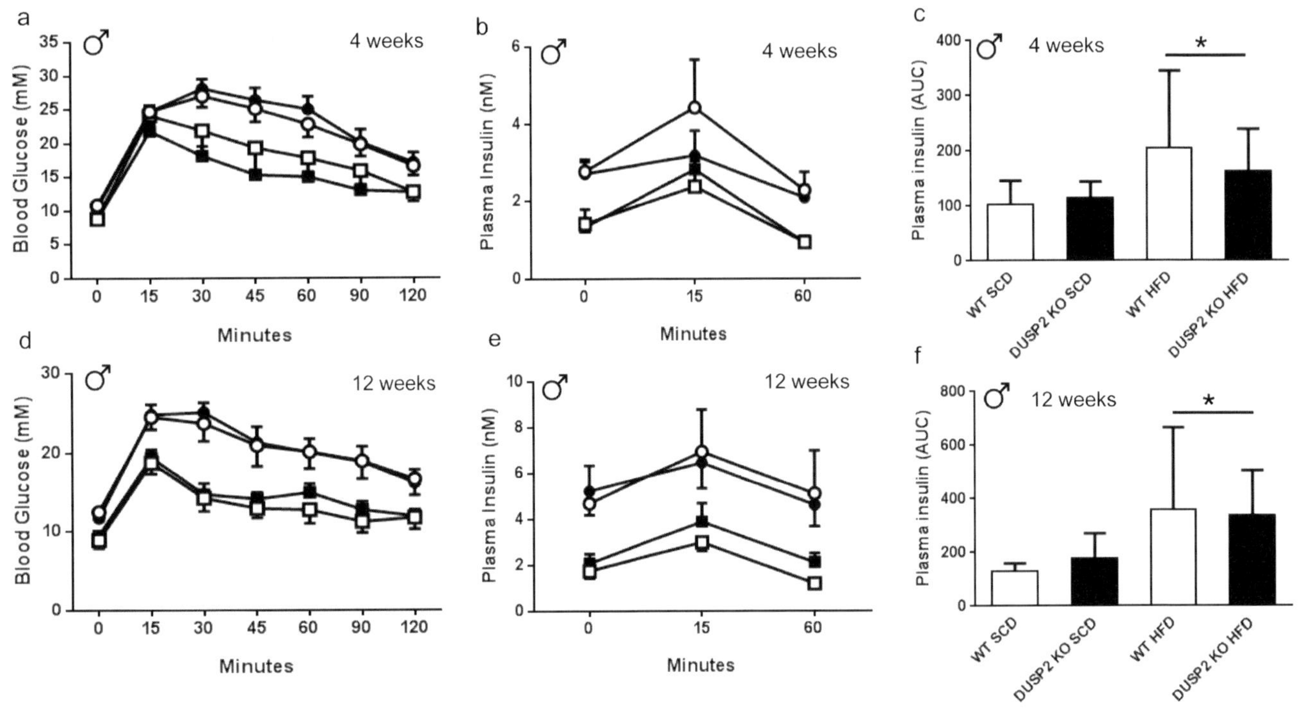

Figure 3. Glucose tolerance and insulin sensitivity in *wt* and *dusp2*$^{-/-}$ male mice after 4 and 12 weeks of diet. (**a** and **d**) oral glucose tolerance; (**b** and **e**) plasma insulin during the OGTT; and (**c** and **f**) plasma insulin area under the curve (AUC). * $p<0.05$; Main Effect for HFD vs SCD. Data are mean ± SD. White squares are *wt* mice fed SCD; Black squares are *dusp2*$^{-/-}$ mice fed SCD; White circles are *wt* mice fed HFD; Black circles are *dusp2*$^{-/-}$ mice fed HFD. Ns are 5, 8, 8 and 8, for *wt* SCD, *dusp2*$^{-/-}$ SCD, *wt* HFD and *dusp2*$^{-/-}$ HFD, respectively.

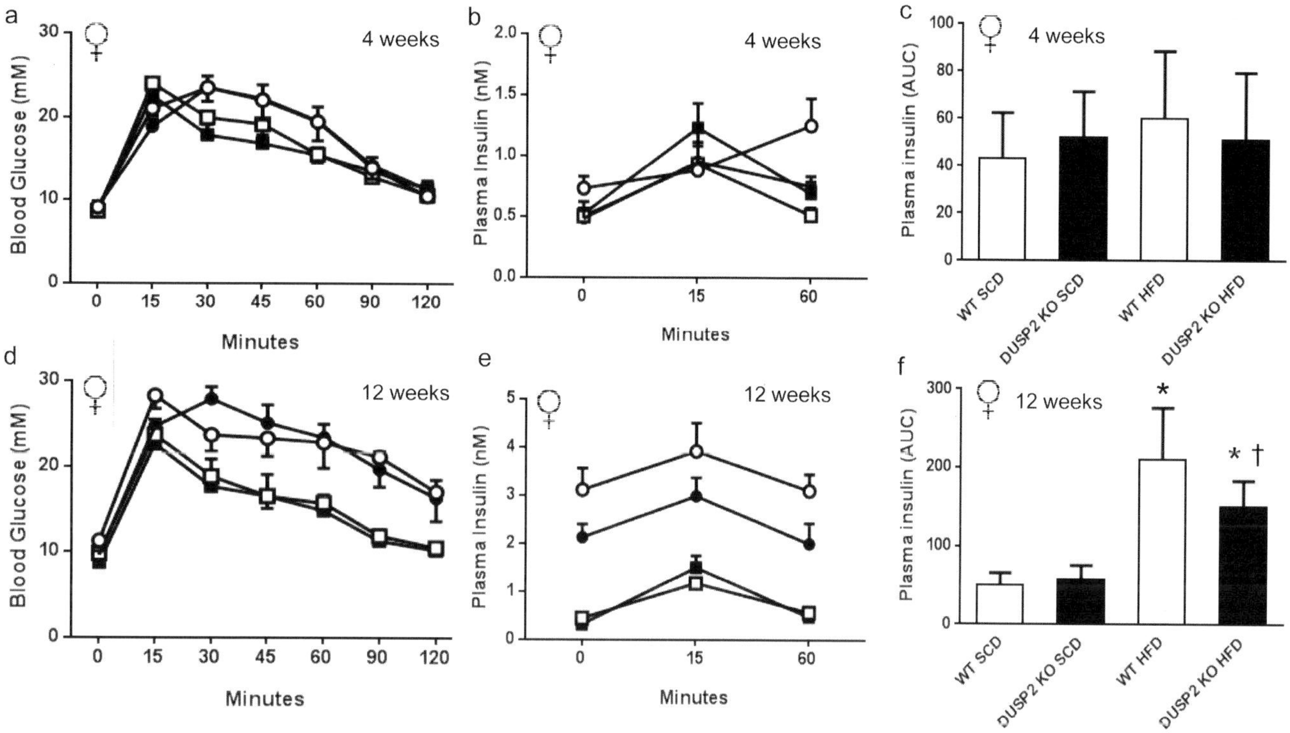

Figure 4. Glucose tolerance and insulin sensitivity in *wt* and *dusp2*$^{-/-}$ female mice. (**a** and **d**) oral glucose tolerance; (**b** and **e**) plasma insulin during the OGTT; and (**c** and **f**) plasma insulin area under the curve (AUC). *$p<0.05$; Interaction Effect *wt* SCD vs. *wt* HFD and *dusp2*$^{-/-}$ SCD vs. *dusp2*$^{-/-}$ HFD. † $p<0.05$ Interaction Effect *wt* HFD vs. *dusp2*$^{-/-}$ HFD. Data are mean ± SD. White squares are *wt* mice fed SCD; Black squares are *dusp2*$^{-/-}$ mice fed SCD; White circles are *wt* mice fed HFD; Black circles are *dusp2*$^{-/-}$ mice fed HFD. Ns are 9, 8, 7 and 7 at 4 weeks and 9, 7, 6 and 7 at 12 weeks for *wt* SCD, *dusp2*$^{-/-}$ SCD, *wt* HFD and *dusp2*$^{-/-}$ HFD, respectively.

phosphorylation, we observed no differences in these responses between *wt* and *dusp2*$^{-/-}$ BMDM (Figure 7a–d).

Discussion

Studies reporting roles for the MAPK dual specificity phosphatases DUSP1 and DUSP9 during inflammation, obesity and insulin sensitivity, prompted us to investigate what function DUSP2 might play in these processes. DUSP2, a nuclear specific DUSP that is mainly expressed in immune cells, had been shown in macrophages and mast cells to promote the production of various inflammatory mediators [18] that included key mediators of obesity-induced metabolic disease. Based on these properties of DUSP2, we examined whether obesity driven inflammation in WAT and its associated impact on glucose intolerance and insulin resistance would be reduced in mice lacking DUSP2. In contrast to the previously ascribed role for DUSP2 regulating inflammatory responses in culture and *in vivo*, our findings reported here demonstrate that DUSP2 plays no role in the development of obesity or obesity-associated inflammation. Furthermore, a lack of DUSP2 activity does not prevent the development of obesity-associated glucose intolerance or insulin resistance in male mice, although it does appear to have a small protective effect in female mice.

Previous studies have demonstrated roles for DUSP family members in the development of obesity, and obesity-associated inflammation and insulin sensitivity. DUSP1-deficient (*dusp1*$^{-/-}$) mice, which exhibit elevated MAPK activity in several metabolically important tissues including skeletal muscle, liver and adipose tissue [20] have significantly less fat mass than control animals when fed a HFD for 12 weeks [20]. Nevertheless, they are still not protected from the deleterious effects a HFD has on glucose metabolism [20]. DUSP9 over-expression in genetically obese *ob/ob* mice on the other hand, improved glucose tolerance [19], while DUSP9 over-expression in 3T3-L1 adipocytes suppressed ERK1/2 and JNK activation, with a concomitant reduction in IRS1 serine phosphorylation that prevented the induction of insulin resistance [19]. A comparative evaluation of the biochemical properties of DUSP1 and DUSP9 with those of DUSP2, in conjunction with the impact their loss of function or over-expression has on obesity, inflammation and insulin sensitivity, provides valuable insight into the different mechanisms by which certain DUSPs, but not others, appear to regulate metabolism. For example, both DUSP1 and DUSP2, which are localized to the nucleus, are induced by stress or mitogenic signals and share overlapping substrate specificities for ERK and p38 [26], have different impacts on whole body metabolism, with DUSP1, but not DUSP2, controlling fat mass. This difference in the regulation of fat mass may reflect the broader pattern of DUSP1 expression and the ability of DUSP1 to also dephosphorylate JNK [27]. Although DUSP2 and DUSP9 can both dephosphorylate ERK, these DUSPs are restricted to the nucleus and cytoplasm respectively [27]. In the context of inflammation-induced insulin resistance seen in obesity, the subcellular localization of these DUSPs may be a critical point of difference, with serine phosphorylation of IRS1 by various serine kinases including ERK1/2 and JNK thought to be a key effector mechanism by which pro-inflammatory stimuli induce cellular insulin resistance [1]. As the phosphorylation of IRS1 occurs at the plasma

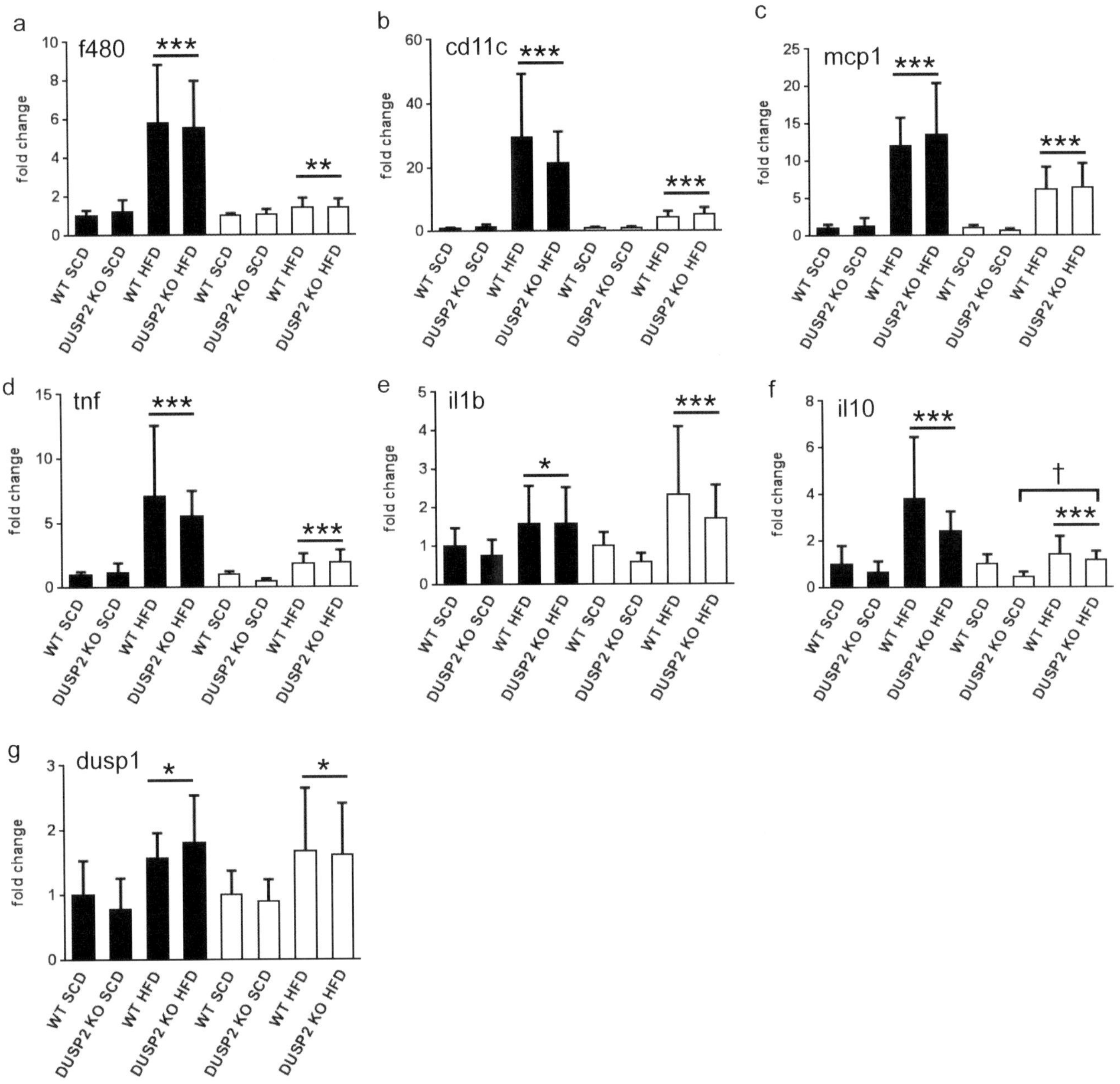

Figure 5. Inflammation in the WAT of *wt* and *dusp2*$^{-/-}$ male and female mice. The mRNA expression of (**a**) *f480*; (**b**) *cd11c*; (**c**) *mcp1*; (**d**) *tnf*; (**e**) *il1b*; (**f**) *il10* and (**g**) *dusp1* in epididymal adipose tissue. *$p<0.05$ Main Effect SCD vs. HFD; **$p<0.01$ Main Effect SCD vs. HFD; ***$p<0.005$ Main Effect SCD vs. HFD; †$p<0.05$ Main Effect *wt* vs. *dusp2*$^{-/-}$. Data are mean ± SD. Black bars are male mice, white bars are female mice. Ns are 5, 8, 8 and 8 for male mice and Ns are 8, 8, 6 and 7 for female mice for *wt* SCD, *dusp2*$^{-/-}$ SCD, *wt* HFD and *dusp2*$^{-/-}$ HFD, respectively.

membrane, it is DUSP9 rather than DUSP2 that has access to cytoplasmic ERK.

Given the importance of inflammation and the accumulation of numerous immune cell types in the WAT of obese mice, we hypothesized that a loss of DUSP2 function might reduce obesity-associated macrophage recruitment or inflammation in WAT. However, unlike the previous role ascribed to DUSP2 in positively regulating inflammatory responses, our data reveal that DUSP2 has no effect on obesity-associated inflammation. Several explanations could account for these differences in the roles of DUSP2 *in vivo*. For example, the qualitative and/or quantitative features of an inflammatory response may be important in dictating the involvement of DUSP2. Whereas DUSP2 was found to promote pathology in an arthritis model that rapidly induces leukocyte recruitment and pronounced inflammation within several days [18], obesity-associated inflammation in mice, by contrast, often takes weeks to months to manifest and is typically a low grade inflammatory response. Therefore, it is possible that the low-grade inflammation associated with obesity is not a sufficiently strong stimulus to employ DUSP2 as a means of modulating MAPK dependent inflammatory responses. Indeed, this may be reflected in the relatively modest increase in DUSP2 expression in the WAT of mice fed a HFD. Functional redundancy amongst the nuclear specific DUSPs, which in addition to DUSP2 include DUSP1, DUSP4 and DUSP5, may also be a contributing factor in DUSP2 not playing a unique role in obesity-associated WAT inflamma-

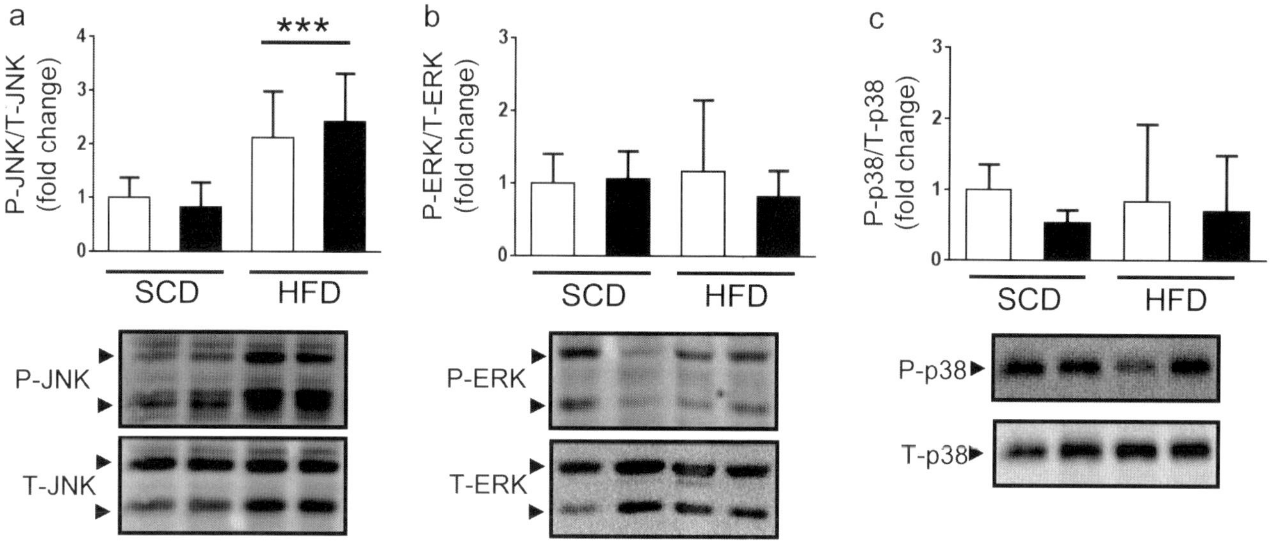

Figure 6. MAPK analysis in epididymal adipose tissue. JNK (**a**), ERK (**b**) and p38 (**c**) phosphorylation status in epididymal adipose tissue of male mice. ***p<0.005 Main Effect SCD vs. HFD. Data are mean ± SD. White bars are *wt* mice, black bars are *dusp2*$^{-/-}$ mice. Ns are 5, 7, 8 and 8 for *wt* SCD, *dusp2*$^{-/-}$ SCD, *wt* HFD and *dusp2*$^{-/-}$ HFD, respectively.

tion. Not only does DUSP2 share overlapping substrate specificity for MAPKs with certain of these other nuclear DUSPs [26,27], it also has a similar pattern of expression with other nuclear DUSPs in activated leukocytes, in particular DUSP4 and DUSP5 [18]. Support for functional redundancy amongst the nuclear DUSPs comes from the recent report showing that in contrast to mice lacking either DUSP1 or DUSP4, which exhibit no cardiac pathology, mice missing both of these DUSPs develop cardiomyopathy due to unrestrained p38 activation [28].

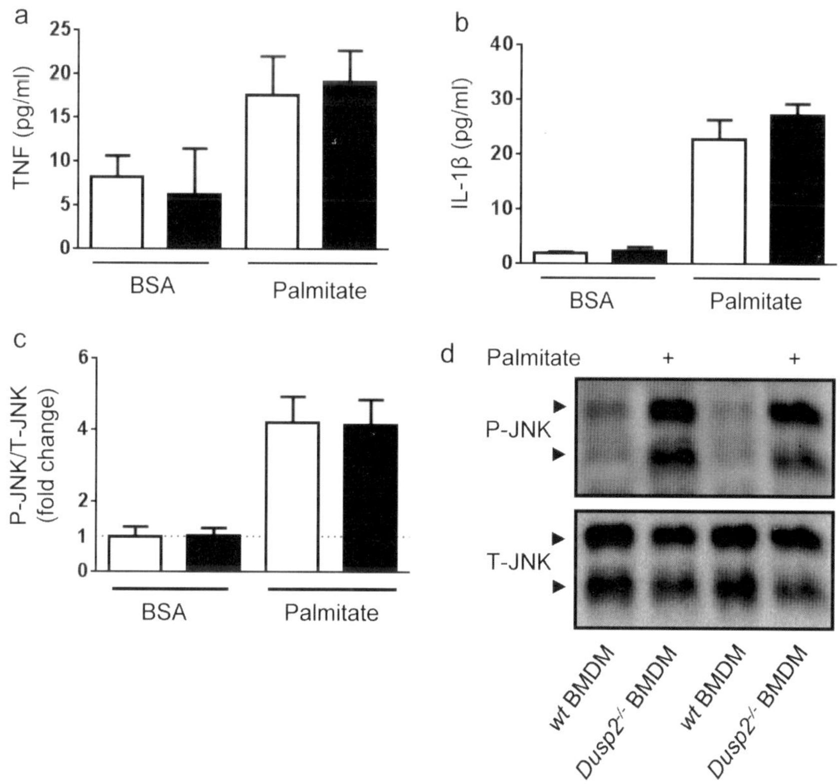

Figure 7. Treatment of BMDM from *wt* and *dusp2*$^{-/-}$ mice with the free fatty acid palmitate. BMDM were treated for 8 h (**a** and **b**) or 4 h (**c** and **d**) with either a control stimulus (BSA; white bars) or 1 mM Palmitate (black bars). **d** shows representative western blots from the quantifications shown in **c**. Data represent 3 separate mice per genotype each performed with 3 technical replicates. Data are mean ± SD.

While the absence of DUSP2 had no impact on obesity-associated inflammation and insulin resistance in male mice, we did observe a small, but significant improvement in the insulin sensitivity of female DUSP2-deficient mice fed the HFD. Of note, this improvement occurred irrespective of the absence of DUSP2 having no impact on HFD-induced obesity, immune cell recruitment or inflammation in the WAT. The increased insulin sensitivity in HF fed female *dusp2*$^{-/-}$ mice was modest, with these mice remaining markedly glucose intolerant and insulin resistant compared to mice fed the SCD. Irrespective of diet, we also observed that IL-10 gene expression was significantly lower in *dusp2*$^{-/-}$ female mice when compared to their *wt* counterparts. These changes while reproducible, were small, and in the absence of any other DUSP2-associated effect on other parameters of inflammation, suggests that this difference in IL-10 expression is unlikely to be of physiological significance.

With various PTPs, such as PTP1B [29], currently the subject of intense drug discovery efforts in the context of obesity and insulin resistance, specific DUSP family members found to control MAPK dependent obesity, inflammation and insulin resistance may represent potential targets in the treatment of metabolic disease. Using mice that lack DUSP2, a nuclear phosphatase shown to promote the production of pro-inflammatory cytokines, nitric oxide and prostaglandin E_2 by activated macrophages and mast cells [18], we assessed whether DUSP2 represented a therapeutic target by which MAPK-dependent inflammatory gene expression associated with obesity could be suppressed. Our data provide compelling evidence that DUSP2 does not play a non-redundant role in the development of obesity or obesity-associated inflammation and its related pathologies, despite these conditions being underpinned by a strong inflammatory component.

Acknowledgments

The authors gratefully acknowledge the team at AMREP animal services for their assistance with the maintenance of the animals during the study as well as Emma Roney at Monash Animal Services for assistance with the breeding of the mice.

Author Contributions

Conceived and designed the experiments: GIL MAF SG AB. Performed the experiments: GIL MJK HLK KGL EE. Analyzed the data: GIL MJK HLK EE. Contributed reagents/materials/analysis tools: RJG SG. Wrote the paper: GIL MJK HLK KLG AB MAF SG.

References

1. Hotamisligil GS (2006) Inflammation and metabolic disorders. Nature 444: 860–867.
2. Osborn O, Olefsky JM (2012) The cellular and signaling networks linking the immune system and metabolism in disease. Nat Med 18: 363–374.
3. Feuerer M, Herrero L, Cipolletta D, Naaz A, Wong J, et al. (2009) Lean, but not obese, fat is enriched for a unique population of regulatory T cells that affect metabolic parameters. Nat Med 15: 930–939.
4. Nishimura S, Manabe I, Nagasaki M, Eto K, Yamashita H, et al. (2009) CD8+ effector T cells contribute to macrophage recruitment and adipose tissue inflammation in obesity. Nat Med 15: 914–920.
5. Talukdar S, Oh da Y, Bandyopadhyay G, Li D, Xu J, et al. (2012) Neutrophils mediate insulin resistance in mice fed a high-fat diet through secreted elastase. Nat Med 18: 1407–1412.
6. Winer DA, Winer S, Shen L, Wadia PP, Yantha J, et al. (2011) B cells promote insulin resistance through modulation of T cells and production of pathogenic IgG antibodies. Nat Med 17: 610–617.
7. Wu D, Molofsky AB, Liang HE, Ricardo-Gonzalez RR, Jouihan HA, et al. (2011) Eosinophils sustain adipose alternatively activated macrophages associated with glucose homeostasis. Science 332: 243–247.
8. Patsouris D, Li PP, Thapar D, Chapman J, Olefsky JM, et al. (2008) Ablation of CD11c-positive cells normalizes insulin sensitivity in obese insulin resistant animals. Cell Metab 8: 301–309.
9. Xu E, Schwab M, Marette A (2014) Role of protein tyrosine phosphatases in the modulation of insulin signaling and their implication in the pathogenesis of obesity-linked insulin resistance. Rev Endocr Metab Disord 15: 79–97.
10. Jeffrey KL, Camps M, Rommel C, Mackay CR (2007) Targeting dual-specificity phosphatases: manipulating MAP kinase signalling and immune responses. Nat Rev Drug Discov 6: 391–403.
11. Elchebly M, Payette P, Michaliszyn E, Cromlish W, Collins S, et al. (1999) Increased insulin sensitivity and obesity resistance in mice lacking the protein tyrosine phosphatase-1B gene. Science 283: 1544–1548.
12. Fukushima A, Loh K, Galic S, Fam B, Shields B, et al. (2010) T-cell protein tyrosine phosphatase attenuates STAT3 and insulin signaling in the liver to regulate gluconeogenesis. Diabetes 59: 1906–1914.
13. Loh K, Fukushima A, Zhang X, Galic S, Briggs D, et al. (2011) Elevated hypothalamic TCPTP in obesity contributes to cellular leptin resistance. Cell Metab 14: 684–699.
14. Zabolotny JM, Bence-Hanulec KK, Stricker-Krongrad A, Haj F, Wang Y, et al. (2002) PTP1B regulates leptin signal transduction in vivo. Dev Cell 2: 489–495.
15. Patterson KI, Brummer T, O'Brien PM, Daly RJ (2009) Dual-specificity phosphatases: critical regulators with diverse cellular targets. Biochem J 418: 475–489.
16. Zhao Q, Wang X, Nelin LD, Yao Y, Matta R, et al. (2006) MAP kinase phosphatase 1 controls innate immune responses and suppresses endotoxic shock. J Exp Med 203: 131–140.
17. Zhang Y, Blattman JN, Kennedy NJ, Duong J, Nguyen T, et al. (2004) Regulation of innate and adaptive immune responses by MAP kinase phosphatase 5. Nature 430: 793–797.
18. Jeffrey KL, Brummer T, Rolph MS, Liu SM, Callejas NA, et al. (2006) Positive regulation of immune cell function and inflammatory responses by phosphatase PAC-1. Nat Immunol 7: 274–283.
19. Emanuelli B, Eberle D, Suzuki R, Kahn CR (2008) Overexpression of the dual-specificity phosphatase MKP-4/DUSP-9 protects against stress-induced insulin resistance. Proc Natl Acad Sci U S A 105: 3545–3550.
20. Wu JJ, Roth RJ, Anderson EJ, Hong EG, Lee MK, et al. (2006) Mice lacking MAP kinase phosphatase-1 have enhanced MAP kinase activity and resistance to diet-induced obesity. Cell Metab 4: 61–73.
21. Rohan PJ, Davis P, Moskaluk CA, Kearns M, Krutzsch H, et al. (1993) PAC-1: a mitogen-induced nuclear protein tyrosine phosphatase. Science 259: 1763–1766.
22. Grumont RJ, Rasko JE, Strasser A, Gerondakis S (1996) Activation of the mitogen-activated protein kinase pathway induces transcription of the PAC-1 phosphatase gene. Mol Cell Biol 16: 2913–2921.
23. Lancaster GI, Skiba B, Yang C, Nicholls HT, Langley KG, et al. (2012) IkappaB kinase beta (IKKbeta) does not mediate feedback inhibition of the insulin signalling cascade. Biochem J 442: 723–732.
24. Ghisletti S, Meda C, Maggi A, Vegeto E (2005) 17beta-estradiol inhibits inflammatory gene expression by controlling NF-kappaB intracellular localization. Mol Cell Biol 25: 2957–2968.
25. Ribas V, Drew BG, Le JA, Soleymani T, Daraei P, et al. (2011) Myeloid-specific estrogen receptor alpha deficiency impairs metabolic homeostasis and accelerates atherosclerotic lesion development. Proc Natl Acad Sci U S A 108: 16457–16462.
26. Chu Y, Solski PA, Khosravi-Far R, Der CJ, Kelly K (1996) The mitogen-activated protein kinase phosphatases PAC1, MKP-1, and MKP-2 have unique substrate specificities and reduced activity in vivo toward the ERK2 sevenmaker mutation. J Biol Chem 271: 6497–6501.
27. Caunt CJ, Keyse SM (2013) Dual-specificity MAP kinase phosphatases (MKPs): shaping the outcome of MAP kinase signalling. FEBS J 280: 489–504.
28. Auger-Messier M, Accornero F, Goonasekera SA, Bueno OF, Lorenz JN, et al. (2013) Unrestrained p38 MAPK activation in Dusp1/4 double-null mice induces cardiomyopathy. Circ Res 112: 48–56.
29. Haque A, Andersen JN, Salmeen A, Barford D, Tonks NK (2011) Conformation-sensing antibodies stabilize the oxidized form of PTP1B and inhibit its phosphatase activity. Cell 147: 185–198.

Factors Associated with Beta-Cell Dysfunction in Type 2 Diabetes

Giuseppina T. Russo[1]*, Carlo Bruno Giorda[2], Stefania Cercone[3], Antonio Nicolucci[4], Domenico Cucinotta[1], on behalf of BetaDecline Study Group¶

1 Department of Clinical and Experimental Medicine, University of Messina, Messina, Italy, **2** Metabolism and Diabetes Unit ASL TO5, Chieri, Italy, **3** MSD, Rome, Italy, **4** Department of Clinical Pharmacology and Epidemiology Fondazione Mario Negri Sud, S. Maria Imbaro, Italy

Abstract

Aims: Beta-cell dysfunction is an early event in the natural history of type 2 diabetes. However, its progression is variable and potentially influenced by several clinical factors. We report the baseline data of the BetaDecline study, an Italian prospective multicenter study on clinical predictors of beta-cell dysfunction in type 2 diabetes.

Materials and Methods: Clinical, lifestyle, and laboratory data, including circulating levels of inflammatory markers and non-esterified fatty acids, were collected in 507 type 2 diabetic outpatients on stable treatment with oral hypoglycemic drugs or diet for more than 1 year. Beta-cell dysfunction was evaluated by calculating the proinsulin/insulin ratio (P/I).

Results: At baseline, the subjects in the upper PI/I ratio quartile were more likely to be men and receiving secretagogue drugs; they also showed a borderline longer diabetes duration (P = 0.06) and higher serum levels of glycated hemoglobin (HbA_{1c}), fasting blood glucose, and triglycerides. An inverse trend across all PI/I quartiles was noted for BMI and serum levels of total cholesterol (T-C), LDL-C, HDL-C and C reactive protein (CRP), and with homeostatic model assessment (HOMA-B) and HOMA of insulin resistance (HOMA-IR) values ($P<0.05$ for all). At multivariate analysis, the risk of having a P/I ratio in the upper quartile was higher in the subjects on secretagogue drugs (odds ratio [OR] 4.2; 95% confidence interval [CI], 2.6–6.9) and in the males (OR 1.8; 95% CI, 1.1–2.9).

Conclusions: In the BetaDecline study population, baseline higher PI/I values, a marker of beta-cell dysfunction, were more frequent in men and in patients on secretagogues drugs. Follow-up of this cohort will allow the identification of clinical predictors of beta-cell failure in type 2 diabetic outpatients.

Editor: Franco Folli, University of Texas Health Science Center at San Antonio, United States of America

Funding: This study was organized by AMD Foundation Rome, and was in part funded by Merck Sharp & Dohme Corp. The funds are used for the costs of laboratory and data monitoring. There is no one outside of the author SC who is employed or has relationships with Merck Sharp & Dohme. SC's contribution is in data analysis and interpretation. No additional funding was received for this study. The funders had no role in study design, data collection and analysis, decision to publish, or preparation of the manuscript.

Competing Interests: One of the authors is employed by a commercial company (MSD, Rome, Italy).

* Email: Giuseppina.russo@unime.it

¶ Membership of the BetaDecline Study Group is provided in the Acknowledgments.

Introduction

The prevalence of type 2 diabetes mellitus (T2DM) is increasing worldwide [1]. T2DM is sustained by insulin resistance and impaired insulin secretion. Impaired insulin secretion due to either beta-cell dysfunction and/or beta-cell loss is now recognized in the pathogenesis and progression of diabetes. The loss of beta-cell mass and the progressive decline in beta-cell function is an early feature of the natural history of diabetes and it is detectable prior to diagnosis [2]. The United Kingdom Prospective Diabetes Study (UKPDS) showed that beta-cell function, as evaluated by the homeostatic model assessment (HOMA-B) index, was already decreased by 50% by the time of the diagnosis and that it continued to decline over the 6-year observation period, even with on-going hypoglycemic therapy [3].

The relative increase of α-cells mass, another typical defect on Langerhans islets of diabetic subjects, may even precede beta-cells loss, being already observed in normoglycaemic baboons with different degrees of obesity [4].

Beta-cell mass is influenced by a balance between proliferative and pro-apoptotic signals, which may be modulated by various growth factors, cytokines, and hormones, whose specific role in the rate of beta-cell decline remains unclear.

High levels of glucose and free fatty acids (gluco-and lipotoxicity), islet amyloid polypeptide deposition, and circulating inflammatory cytokines have been all implicated in beta-cell apoptosis [4–15] Thus, *in vitro* studies have demonstrated that high glucose levels induce an over-expression of pro-apoptotic genes of the Bcl family in cultured pancreatic Islets of Langerhans [8], and the important role of islet amyloid (IA) in the pathogenesis of beta cell dysfunction has been demonstrated in rodent models, non human primates, as well as in human studies [9,10,11,12]; also the influence of inflammation on beta cell function and peripheral insulin resistance has been increasingly recognized [13,14,15]

At any rate, whenever it appears, impaired beta-cell function leads to the progressive failure of islet cells to secrete sufficient amounts of insulin to overcome peripheral insulin resistance, ultimately resulting in failure to maintain normal glucose homeostasis over time. However, the rate of beta-cell failure is unpredictable and not all persons with T2DM will need insulin therapy to maintain their blood glucose levels.

Several factors may have a bearing on beta-cell function, including lifestyle, clinical, and metabolic factors, as well as ongoing therapies. The early identification of these clinical predictors could provide clues to developing strategies to ameliorate the long-term management of T2DM.

Here, we report the baseline data of the BetaDecline Study, that will prospectively evaluate the principal clinical and biochemical predictors of beta-cell dysfunction in a cohort of outpatients with T2DM, on stable treatment with oral hypoglycemic agents (OHAs) or diet only, over a 4-year follow-up period.

Methods

Subjects

BetaDecline is a prospective, longitudinal multicenter study with the aim to evaluate the rate and clinical predictors of beta-cell decline in T2DM over time. The study population was 507 T2DM outpatients regularly attending nine diabetes care centers. At each center, the fifth eligible patient seen per day was enrolled in the study, after giving written informed consent to participate in the study.

Data were collected from retrospective chart review, laboratory analysis of blood samples taken during visits to a diabetes center as part of routine care, and responses to a questionnaire. At the first and last visits, after 4 years of follow-up, fasting blood samples were taken. At the intermediate visit (after 2 years) only clinical data were collected.

Inclusion criteria were: a physician's diagnosis of T2DM by American Diabetes Association criteria [16]stable treatment with OHAs or diet for ≥1 year; age >40 years at enrolment; continuous care at the clinic (at least 2 visits) for at least 1 year; medical records with a minimum core data set; and completed consent form. All patients meeting these inclusion criteria were considered eligible for participation in the study.

Exclusion criteria were: type 1 diabetes; pregnancy; inability to understand the study purposes or fill out the consent form; participation in a clinical trial in the previous 3 years; current use of insulin or incretin-based therapies (DPP4 inhibitors and/or GLP1 receptor agonists).

All patients were on stable treatment for ≥1 year with dietary therapy and/or on an OHA (metformin, sulfonylureas, glinides, glytazones, acarbose), alone or in combination; none were receiving incretin-based or insulin therapy during the course of the study.

Ethics statements

Written informed consent was obtained from all participants; the study was conducted in accordance with the Declaration of Helsinki and approved by the local ethics committees:Ethics Committee of the University Hospital Saint Luigi Gonzaga of Orbassano, Turin.

Committee entered in the Register of the Regional Ethics Committees with the order number 7 in the section on committees set up under 'Article 5 of DPGR 16/11/2001 Piedmont region and D.G.R. n. 4/12/2006 78-4807 of operating in compliance with the Decree 24/06/2003 n. 211 and Good Clinical Practice. The Ethics Committee approved the study on 30/06/2008.

Measurements

Standardized questionnaires were administered to collect lifestyle and clinical data. Potential risk factors for beta-cell dysfunction were classified as follows: co-morbidities - dyslipidemia, hypertension, cardiac disease, long-term micro- and macro-vascular complications of diabetes; treatment variables - current antidiabetic drug treatments (name, starting date, dosage), history of antidiabetic drug treatment, antihypertensive therapy, continuous aspirin treatment, statin therapy.

BMI and blood pressure (BP) were measured according to standard procedures. Hypertension was defined as a systolic and/or diastolic BP value ≥130/80 mm Hg, and/or current use of antihypertensive medications. Use of hypolipidemic drugs and/or aspirin was also recorded.

Alcohol consumption was recorded as grams of alcohol/day. Subjects were defined as non-smokers or current smokers; those who had quit within 1 year prior to entry in the study were defined as current smokers.

Metabolic parameters

At baseline and final visits, blood samples after 12–14 hour fasting were drawn for the determination of blood chemistry parameters, which was performed centrally. After collection, plasma and serum were separated and the aliquots were stored at −20°C until analysis. Fasting blood glucose (FBG) was measured using the glucose oxidase-peroxidase (GOD-POD) method (normal laboratory reference range, 65–110 mg/dL).

Total serum cholesterol, high-density lipoprotein cholesterol (HDL-C), triglycerides, and creatinine levels were measured using standard automated laboratory methods (Roche Diagnostics, Milan, Italy). Low-density lipoprotein cholesterol (LDL-C) concentration was calculated by the Friedwald formula [17].

Glycated hemoglobin (HbA_{1c}) was measured on an automated high-performance liquid chromatography (HPLC) analyzer (normal laboratory reference range, 4–6%). Fasting insulin concentration was measured using an automated microparticle enzyme immunosorbent assay (MEIA) (normal reference range, 5–23 MU/L). Plasma proinsulin levels were measured using an enzyme-linked immunosorbent assay (ELISA) (normal reference values, >5.10 pmol/L), and the fasting proinsulin to insulin ratio (PI/I) was calculated. Insulin secretion was assessed with the HOMA-B model and insulin resistance was calculated using the HOMA-IR model [18,19].

Serum C-reactive protein (CRP) was measured using a turbidimetric assay (reference values, <3.0 mg/L), interleukin 6 (IL-6) by an enzymatic method using Acyl-CoA oxidase (ACS-ACOD-POD) (reference range, 0.0–2.3 ng/L), fasting non-esterified fatty acids (NEFA) by an enzymatic assay (reference range, 0.28–0.89 mmol/L), (CV % and %, respectively). The mean values for self-monitored 2-h post-prandial glucose (2-h PPG) were also recorded.

Statistical analysis

Data are given as mean ± SD or crude numbers and percentages. Patient characteristics according to gender were compared using unpaired Student's t-test or Mann-Whitney U-test or χ^2 test. Patient characteristics according to PI/I ratio quartiles were compared using ANOVA for linear trend (normally distributed variables), Kruskall-Wallis one-way ANOVA (continuous variables with non-normal distribution) or χ^2 test for linear trend (categorical variables). Bivariate associations were estimated using Spearman's rank correlation coefficient. Independent correlates of PI/I values in the upper quartile were evaluated using multiple logistic regression analysis with backward variable selection. Results are expressed as odds ratios (OR) with their respective 95% confidence intervals (95% CI). All statistical comparisons are two-tailed, and a P value<0.05 was considered significant. Statistical analysis was performed using the SPSS program, version 11.0 for Windows (SPSS Inc. Chicago, IL).

Results

Baseline clinical characteristics

Study subjects (507, 59% men) were overweight or obese (mean BMI 29.2 kg/m^2; mean waist circumference 102 cm), with acceptable glucose control, despite the relatively long duration of diabetes (**Table 1**). The FBG levels were high but the 2-h postprandial glucose (PPG) levels were within the recommended targets. BP and lipid profile were close to the target values. Mean serum fasting insulin and proinsulin levels were 10.1 mIU/L and 9.1 pmol/L, respectively. Mean circulating levels of serum CRP, IL-6, and NEFA were within the reference range (**Table 1**).

During the course of the study, 69% of the subjects were on antihypertensive drugs, 61% on lipid-lowering medications (either statins or fibrates), and 45% were regularly taking aspirin. The majority (84%) was on stable treatment with metformin alone or in combination with other OHAs, 51% were on secretagogues (sulfonylureas and glinides), and only 5% on diet therapy alone.

Questionnaire response to the items investigating lifestyle showed that 18% were current smokers, 20% reported habitual alcohol consumption, and 69% were sedentary, never or only occasionally engaging in physical activity (**Table 1**).

Comparison of baseline data of men versus women (**Table 1**) showed that the women were more often obese (BMI, P<0.0001) and had significantly higher serum levels of HbA1c (P = 0.05), fasting insulin (P = 0.003), total cholesterol (P = 0.002), HDL-C (P<0.0001) and LDL-C (P = 0.017), CRP (P<0.0001), and NEFA (P = 0.002), whereas FBG and fasting proinsulin values were higher in the men (P = 0.03 and P = 0.001, respectively).

The men reported a lower use of antihypertensive medications and a higher use of aspirin; no differences between the sexes were noted for use of lipid-lowering drugs or current treatment with hypoglycemic medications. Tobacco and alcohol use (both P< 0.0001) was more frequent among the men; regular physical activity was lower among the women (P = 0.002).

Baseline clinical characteristics according to Proinsulin/Insulin ratio values

Beta-cell dysfunction was estimated by the the proinsulin/insulin ratio (PI/I); HOMA-B and the degree of insulin resistance (HOMA-IR) were also evaluated. When the study subjects characteristics were stratified according to quartiles of the PI/I ratio, almost 70% of those in the upper PI/I quartile, indicating the highest degree of beta-cell dysfunction, were males. Overall, a higher degree of beta-cell dysfunction was also associated with poorer glucose control; thus, as shown in **Figure 1**, the number of subjects with out-of-target HbA1c values increased with increasing PI/I quartiles (HbA$_{1c}$ ≥7.0%; chi square for linear trend P< 0.0001).

To evaluate which factors were associated with beta-cell dysfunction, we stratified the clinical and laboratory characteristics according to PI/I quartiles (**Table 2**); because of the higher prevalence of male subjects among those with the highest PI/I quartile, p-values for comparisons in men and women separately are also presented (**Table 2**).

In the whole study population, the subjects in the highest PI/I ratio quartile (those with the highest degree of beta-cell dysfunction) were more likely to be smokers and to have a longer duration of diabetes than those in the lower quartiles (P = 0.02 and P = 0.06, respectively). Furthermore, the subjects in the upper PI/I quartile had a lower BMI (P<0.0001) and waist circumference (P<0.06), poorer metabolic control, evaluated as both HbA$_{1c}$ (P< 0.004) and FBG values (P<0.0001), without any significant difference in PPG levels. Those in the upper quartile also showed differences in lipid profile, with lower total cholesterol (P = 0.02), LDL-C (P = 0.01), and HDL-C concentrations (P = 0.007), and higher serum triglycerides levels (P = 0.01) (**Table 2**). The CRP values were significantly lower in the subjects in the upper PI/I quartile (P = 0.001), whereas no significant differences in IL-6 or NEFA or systolic and diastolic blood pressure values were noted according to the PI/I ratio in the whole study population. The insulin-sensitivity (HOMA-IR) and secretion indexes (HOMA-B) were both significantly lower in the highest PI/I quartile (P< 0.0001).

Among glucose-lowering drugs, the use of secretagogues (sulfonylureas and glinides) was significantly more frequent among subjects with the worst baseline insulin secretory capacity (P< 0.0001); conversely, no significant differences in the use of other drugs according to PI/I values were noted. Similarly, no differences were noted for use of antihypertensive and lipid-lowering drugs, whereas a larger number of subjects on aspirin were found in the highest PI/I quartile (P = 0.03).

When men and women were analyzed separately (Table 2), metabolic control as evaluated by FBG and HbA1c levels, as well as fasting insulin, proinsulin, HOMA-B, and HOMA-IR values, the use of sulphonilureas, glinides and overall secretagogues showed the same significant trend across PI/I quartiles observed in the whole population, without any gender-difference (**see File S1**). HDL-C levels were related with PI/I ratio with a borderline significance in both men and women, whereas, waist circumference, BMI, CRP levels significantly decreased across PI/I quartiles only in males. In women, when comparing the lowest with the highest PI/I quartile, higher PI/I values were also associated with slightly lower IL-6 concentrations (1.1 ng/L vs. 1.3 ng/L) and a lower percentage of subjects on diet only (2.4% vs. 8.1% in the highest vs. the lowest PI/I ratio quartile, respectively).

Factors associated with beta-cell dysfunction at univariate and multivariate analyses

At univariate correlation analysis (**Table 3**), the PI/I ratio negatively correlated with waist circumference, BMI,, CRP,, and positively with HbA$_{1c}$ and FBG,. Significant correlations were also noted for FBG in both sexes when the men and women were considered separately, whereas the inverse correlation with waist circumference and CRP remained significant only for the men.

At multivariate analysis, when age, gender, BMI, HbA$_{1c}$, total cholesterol, HDL-C, LDL-C, triglycerides, diabetes duration, CRP, IL-6, NEFA, metformin, secretagogues, thiazolidinediones (TZDs) were included in the model, male gender was associated with a 1.8-fold (OR 1.8; 95% CI, 1.1–2.9) higher probability of having beta-cell dysfunction (a PI/I ratio in the upper quartile), whereas the use of secretagogues was associated with a more than 4-fold higher risk (OR 4.20; 95% CI, 2.55–6.91). All other baseline

Table 1. Baseline clinical characteristics of BetaDecline study participants.

	Total	Men	Women	*P*-value men *vs.* women
No. (%)	507	298 (58.7)	209 (41.3)	
Age (years)	62.8±8.1	62.7±8.1	63.0±8.2	0.96 (NS)
BMI	29.2±4.9	28.4±4.3	30.2±5.5	<0.0001
Waist circumference (cm)	102±11	102±11	101±11	0.27 (NS)
Diabetes duration (years)	8.8±6.9	9.1±6.6	8.4±7.2	0.08 (NS)
HbA1c (%)	7.2±1.1	7.2±1.0	7.3±1.3	0.05
FBG (mg/dl)	164±59	168±60	160±59	0.03
PPG (mg/dl)	149±39	148±38	151±41	0.49 (NS)
Fasting insulin (mIU/L)	10.1±7.0	9.6±7.3	10.8±6.5	0.003
Fasting proinsulin (pmol/L)	9.1±11.3	10.1±13.1	7.8±7.9	0.001
Systolic blood pressure (mm Hg)	133±16	133±16	133±16	0.69 (NS)
Diastolic blood pressure (mm Hg)	78±8	78±8	79±8	0.62 (NS)
Total cholesterol (mg/dL)	177±41	172±37	184±44	0.002
HDL-cholesterol (mg/dL)	49.6±12.9	46.9±12.1	53.3±13.1	<0.0001
LDL-cholesterol (mg/dL)	103±33	99±32	107±34	0.017
Triglycerides (mg/dL)	132±79	134±83	132±74	0.79 (NS)
CRP (mg/L)	2.8±4.1	2.4±4.2	3.5±3.9	<0.0001
IL-6 (ng/L)	1.46±3.32	1.58±4.23	1.29±1.17	0.65 (NS)
NEFA (mmol/L)	0.6±0.3	0.6±0.2	0.6±0.2	0.002
Antihypertensive drugs – *no.* (%)	350 (69.0)	194 (65.1)	156 (74.6)	0.007
Lipid-lowering drugs - *no.* (%)	309 (60.9)	182 (61.1)	127 (60.8)	0.79 (NS)
Aspirin use – *no.* (%)	228 (45.0)	145 (48.7)	83 (39.7)	0.015
Hypoglicemic drugs – *no.* (%)				
Metformin	425 (83.8)	243 (81.5)	182 (87.1)	0.10 (NS)
Sulfonylureas	179 (35.3)	99 (33.2)	80 (38.3)	0.24 (NS)
TZD	50 (9.9)	29 (9.7)	21 (10.0)	0.91 (NS)
Glinides	81 (16.0)	53 (17.8)	28 (13.4)	0.18 (NS)
Acarbose	11 (2.2)	7 (2.3)	4 (1.9)	1.0 (NS)
Diet only	28 (5.5)	18 (6.0)	10 (4.8)	0.54 (NS)
Current tobacco use – *no.* (%)	90 (17.8)	77 (26.0)	13 (6.2)	<0.0001
Regular alcohol consumption - *no.* (%)	101 (20.0)	89 (30)	12 (5.7)	<0.0001
Physical activity (%)				0.002
No/Occasionally	347 (69.1)	190 (64.9)	157 (75.1)	
<3 times per week	57 (11.4)	40 (13.7)	17 (8.1)	
3–5 times per week	67 (13.3)	39 (13.3)	28 (13.4)	
>5 times per week	28 (5.6)	21 (7.2)	7 (3.3)	

Data are no. (%) and means ± SD. FBG, fasting blood glucose; PPG, postprandial blood glucose; CRP, C-reactive protein; IL-6, interleukin-6; NEFA, non-esterified fatty acids; PI, proinsulin; TZD thiazolidinediones.

clinical characteristics, including BMI, waist circumference, diabetes duration, metabolic control, gluco- and lipotoxicity measures, and inflammatory markers were not independently associated with beta-cell dysfunction in this population.

Discussion

T2DM is characterized by insulin resistance and various degrees of beta-cell impairment. Several lines of evidence strongly suggest that preserving beta-cell function is critical to prevent loss of glucose control and progression from prediabetes to overt diabetes [20,21,22] or from use of OHAs to insulin therapy in subjects with long-standing disease [3,23,24,25].Nonetheless, insulin therapy is not an inexorable end, and the rate of progression in T2DM appears to differ individually. Because such unpredictability may reflect individual variability in the rate of beta-cell decline, identifying the clinical factors that can predict it holds importance for diabetes management.

In this analysis of baseline data from the BetaDecline study, we examined the degree of beta-cell dysfunction and its potential associations with demographic, clinical, treatment variables, and markers of inflammation and lipotoxicity in a large cohort of

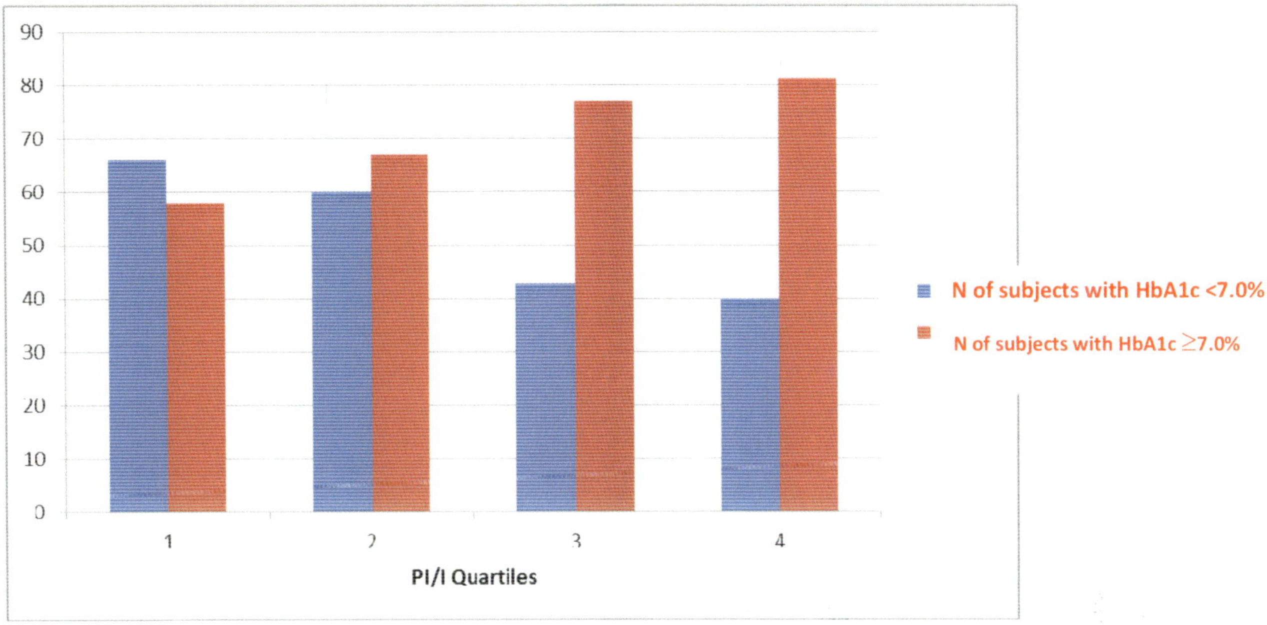

Figure 1. Type 2 diabetic subjects with HbA1c≥7.0% or <7.0% according to the degree of beta-cell dysfunction.

T2DM outpatients on stable treatment with diet and/or OHAs for more than 1 year.

Determining beta-cell failure is problematic in clinical practice, as there is no convenient and reliable way to quantify it. Furthermore, beta-cell decline may ensue from an impairment of their mass or function, and these two aspects may not necessarily coincide [19,26] Several static and dynamic methods are today available to estimate beta-cells functionality, such as HOMA-B, the acute insulin response 5 min after an i.v. glucose load (AIRg), the ratio between the increment in plasma insulin and plasma glucose 30 min after an OGTT (insulinogenic index, ΔI/ΔG-30), as well as more complex methods evaluating the response of plasma insulin to mixed meals during the day or the deconvolution of plasma C-peptide curve using kinetic parameters [24,27,28]. Although some of these methods are considered more reliable for the evaluation of beta-cell secretion, most of them are not easily applicable in the clinical practice. In the BetaDecline, beta-cell dysfunction was evaluated by calculating the PI/I ratio, which estimates the capacity of beta cells to convert proinsulin to insulin and may represent an acceptable method to indicate the degree of beta-cell secretion [19], whereas the role of the HOMA-B index, although still used in epidemiological studies, has been largely questioned [19,28].

In our cohort, the PI/I values were generally within the diabetic range and roughly double than those reported in normo-glycemic subjects [29,30,31],confirming the 2–3 fold increase in PI/I values usually observed in diabetic individuals [19,28].

The first finding of our study is that up to 70% of subjects in the upper quartile of PI/I ratio (those with a greater deficit in beta-cell secretion) were men. This gender-related difference merits deeper analysis since previous experimental and epidemiological studies indicate that women may be partially protected against beta-cell failure, probably thanks to the estrogens influence. Thus, metabolic diseases are less prevalent among premenopausal women [32] and hormone-related differences in regional fat distribution and function obviously play a crucial role in this context [33] Furthermore, two hormonal intervention studies, the Women's Health Initiative Study [34] and the Heart and Oestrogen/Progestin Replacement Study [35], both found a significant reduction in diabetes incidence in subjects receiving estrogens. Convincing evidence also comes from experimental models of insulin-deficient diabetes, where the frequency of diabetes was consistently higher in the male than female animals [36,37]. The hypothesis that estrogens may be beneficial for pancreatic beta cells has been confirmed by several *in vitro* studies showing that estrogens may protect pancreatic beta cells against apoptosis and prevent insulin-deficient diabetes mellitus through an estrogen receptor-mediated signal or indirectly through the modulation of other hormones [36,37,38].

Although estrogen levels and menopausal status were not specifically measured in our study, the observed gender -differences in the degree of beta-cell dysfunction seem to be in line with these reports. Furthermore, since the mean age of the women participating in our study was ~60 years, with most of them probably post-menopausal, our data also suggest that this relative protection may be extended after menopause. However, the effects of natural menopause on insulin secretion in humans have been poorly studied [36,39], and the results obtained so far are difficult to interpret because of the complex hormonal and metabolic milieu following menopause and the confounding effect of ageing.Another finding of our study is that the PI/I ratio values are related to the type of ongoing hypoglycemic therapy. Although the cross-sectional nature of our analysis did not allow us to establish causal relationships, our baseline data indicate that the use of secretagogues, either sulfonylureas or glinides, was 4-fold more frequent in subjects having a PI/I ratio in the upper quartile. Several reasons may underline this association, including an indication bias, owing to diabetologists' preferential use of secretagogues in patients with already reduced beta-cell secretion, i.e. in those who are not in good metabolic control. An alternative interpretation could be that these drugs may be associated with baseline higher PI/I ratio also because of their specific mechanism of action [40,41]. Thus, by attaching to their specific receptor on beta-cells, secretagogues might stimulate not only insulin release,

Table 2. Patient characteristics according to quartiles of proinsulin/insulin (PI/I) ratio *in total population and by gender.*

	PI/I ratio quartiles						
Variables	**I° ≤0.485**	**II° 0.486–0.80**	**III° 0.81–1.355**	**IV° >1.355**	**P**	**P-value in men**	**P-value in women**
Males (%)	37.9	60.8	67.2	68.5	<0.0001		
Age (years)	62.9±8.1	62.4±7.6	62.4±8.7	63.7±8.2	0.51 (NS)	0.90 (NS)	0.21 (NS)
Current smokers (%)	12.1	21.6	22.3	16.3	0.02	0.44 (NS)	0.08 (NS)
Diabetes duration (years)	8.0±6.5	9.4±8.3	8.1±5.7	9.7±6.7	0.06 (NS)	0.14 (NS)	0.58 (NS)
BMI (kg/m^2)	30.5±5.2	29.5±5.4	28.3±4.2	28.3±4.5	<0.0001	0.04	0.13 (NS)
Waist circumference (cm)	102.7±10.0	101.6±13.3	102.1±10.6	99.4±10.0	0.06 (NS)	0.09 (NS)	0.26 (NS)
HbA1c (%)	7.1±1.1	7.2±1.2	7.3±1.2	7.4±0.9	0.004	0.008	0.04
FBG (mg/dL)	149±54	156±53	173±59	181±66	<0.0001	<0.0001	0.001
PPG (mg/dL)	149±37	152±53	148±31	148±36	0.83 (NS)	0.67 (NS)	0.52 (NS)
SBP (mm Hg)	133±15	132±16	133±16	133±16	0.78 (NS)	0.95 (NS)	1.0 (NS)
DBP (mm Hg)	78.4±8.2	78.4±8.0	78.5±8.0	78.8±9.2	0.68 (NS)	0.71 (NS)	0.95 (NS)
Total cholesterol (mg/dL)	184±42	177±45	173±39	172±36	0.02	0.89 (NS)	0.18 (NS)
HDL-cholesterol (mg/dL)	52.8±13.6	48.6±13.4	47.1±11.0	49.1±12.3	0.007	0.09 (NS)	0.08 (NS)
LDL-cholesterol (mg/dL)	109±32	103±37	99±31	98±29	0.01	0.89 (NS)	0.34 (NS)
Triglycerides (mg/dL)	126±78	135±76	134±76	137±88	0.01	0.34 (NS)	0.48 (NS)
CRP (mg/L)	3.4±3.7	2.7±4.1	3.0±5.2	2.3±3.3	0.001	0.03	0.16 (NS)
IL-6 (ng/L)	1.3±1.0	2.2±6.4	1.3±0.8	1.1±0.9	0.28 (NS)	0.26 (NS)	0.06 (NS)
NEFA (mmol/L)	0.58±0.26	0.58±0.24	0.58±0.25	0.55±0.25	0.64 (NS)	0.57 (NS)	0.31 (NS)
Fasting insulin (mIU/L)	12.7±9.1	11.0±6.5	9.3±5.8	7.4±5.0	<0.0001	<0.0001	0.001
PI (pmol/L)	3.8±2.5	7.0±4.3	9.8±6.4	16.7±19.0	<0.0001	<0.0001	<0.0001
HOMA-B	73.4±63.8	51.6±33.2	37.7±30.4	29.9±33.4	<0.0001	<0.0001	<0.0001
HOMA-IR	4.8±4.4	4.4±4.1	4.0±3.1	3.4±2.7	<0.0001	0.001	0.003
Diet alone (%)	8.1	3.9	7.4	2.4	0.14 (NS)	0.16 (NS)	0.05
Metformin (%)	84.7	85.0	83.6	83.1	0.67 (NS)	0.91 (NS)	0.77 (NS)
Sulfonylureas (%)	29.0	26.0	37.7	47.6	<0.0001	0.003	0.01
Glinides (%)	10.5	11.8	15.6	26.6	<0.0001	0.03	0.01
Any secretagogue (%)	37.9	37.0	53.3	71.0	<0.0001	<0.0001	<0.0001
TZDs (%)	8.9	9.4	13.1	8.1	0.92 (NS)	0.88 (NS)	0.72 (NS)
Acarbose (%)	0.8	1.6	4.1	2.4	0.21 (NS)	0.07 (NS)	0.72 (NS)
Antihypertensives (%)	76.5	71.0	70.1	72.6	0.49 (NS)	0.11 (NS)	0.65 (NS)
Lipid-lowering drugs (%)	59.0	70.4	64.1	60.9	0.97 (NS)	0.07 (NS)	0.38 (NS)
Aspirin (%)	39.8	47.2	44.7	58.5	0.03	0.35 (NS)	0.99 (NS)

Data are no. (%) and means ± SD. FBG, fasting blood glucose; PPG, postprandial blood glucose; SBP and DBP, systolic and diastolic blood pressure; CRP, C-reactive protein; IL-6, interleukin-6; NEFA, non-esterified fatty acids; PI, proinsulin; TZD thiazolidinediones.

Table 3. Significant univariate correlations (Pearson's test) of proinsulin/insulin (PI/I) ratio with study variables according to sex.

	Total		Men		Women	
	r	*P*	*r*	*P*	*r*	*P*
Waist circumference	−0.11	0.02	−0.16	0.01	−0.12	0.097(NS)
BMI	−0.18	<0.0001	−0.13	0.02	−0.17	0.02
HbA_{1c}	0.16	<0.0001	0.20	0.001	0.15	0.03
FBG	0.24	<0.0001	0.26	<0.0001	0.20	0.004
CRP	−0.17	<0.0001	−0.16	0.008	−0.15	0.22(NS)

FBG, fasting blood glucose; CRP, C-reactive protein.

but also its production, therefore leading to an increased production of proinsulin.

Although only the follow-up analysis of our cohort will allow definitive conclusions, similarly to our baseline results, the ADOPT study [42], after initial 6-months increase in the insulinogenic index, demonstrated a faster rate of decline in glyburide treated patients versus those on rosiglitazone or metformin. The initial change with glyburide has been attributed to the alleviation of gluco-toxicity.

Unfortunately, comparative data for the effect of commonly used hypoglycemic drugs on the rate of beta-cell decline are still insufficient [24,25,43]. On the other hand, the UKPDS study reported that the progressive worsening of glucose control over time was not influenced by the type of ongoing therapy [3], and consistent with this observation was the finding that other hypoglycemic and/or antihypertensive, lipid-lowering medications and aspirin use were unrelated to PI/I values in our analysis.

Our data also indicate that a higher PI/I ratio is associated with higher HbA_{1c} levels, confirming the major role of beta-cell dysfunction in the deterioration of glucose control.

However, these associations were no longer significant at multivariate analysis, indicating that other factors may have influenced glucose control in our cohort. Notably, when we compared the baseline data of the men versus the women, we found significantly higher serum HbA_{1c} levels among the women, a finding shared by a recently large Italian survey [44] demonstrating that diabetic women are more likely than men to have poorer glycemic control and elevated HbA_{1c} values. These results seem to partly contrast with the finding of fewer women in the group with higher PI/I values (those with the worst glycemic control). However, in the Italian survey [44], as well as in other reports [45] comparative data on beta-cell function in men and women with diabetes were lacking, and the reported gender-related differences in metabolic control were mainly attributed to a poorer quality of diabetes care in women than in men [44,45].

Our data also showed decreasing values of HOMA-IR across increasing PI/I ratio quartiles, similarly to other studies reporting different degrees of beta-cell dysfunction according to the level of insulin sensibility [20,21,22]. Furthermore, features of the metabolic syndrome, including degrees of obesity, showed an overall inverse trend across increasing quartiles of the PI/I ratio, paralleling that of HOMA-IR, indicating that extreme insulin resistance and insulin secretory deficit may depict different phenotypes.

Because insulin resistance is known to precede beta-cell dysfunction in the natural history of T2DM, stratifying individuals on the basis of insulin resistance and insulin secretion measures would ideally identify subjects at different stages of the disease. Subjects with higher baseline PI/I values had a longer diabetes duration and higher HbA1c values, suggesting as one would expect, that with a longer diabetes duration, beta cell function would decline and glucose control deteriorates. However our data indicate that such stratification is not feasible in clinical practice. And although both insulin sensitivity and insulin secretion tend to decline with ageing [30,46], in our cohort, ageing and duration of diabetes were not independently related to PI/I ratio. The relatively younger age of our study subjects and the lack of reliability of diabetes duration estimates may be likely explanations for these results. The finding that age and diabetes duration were partly unrelated to PI/I values may also indicate that the decline in beta-cell function does not follow a regular timeline but it is variable and potentially influenced by different individual factors instead.

Among such factors, the level of gluco- and lipotoxicity and/or subclinical inflammation may play a role. Added to these, several growth factors, cytokines, hormones, including free fatty acids and inflammatory markers may induce beta-cell apoptosis [4–15]. In our study, circulating levels of IL-6, CRP, and NEFA were not related to beta-cell dysfunction at multivariate analysis, and blood sample collection in the fasting state may also have played a role, since circulating NEFA levels may be elevated in the post-absorptive period in diabetic subjects.

Furthermore, there was an overall decreasing trend for circulating levels of these inflammatory and lipotoxicity markers with increasing PI/I ratio values, although with gender-specific associations, which is likely explained by the stronger association of central obesity and chronic subclinical inflammation with the insulin-resistant phenotype. The different strength of the association of PI/I values with obesity and CRP levels in men and with IL-6 in women is difficult to be interpreted and would be likely clarified at the follow-up analysis.

Also, the proportion of smokers was higher in subjects in the top PI/I quartiles, but this association was no longer confirmed at multivariate analysis.

This study has several limitations principally related to its cross-sectional nature. Furthermore, other factors such as lifestyle measures [47] and genetic variants [48]potentially associated with beta-cell decline were not specifically assessed in the current analysis. Another limitation of our study is that we did not use more sophisticated and precise measures of insulin secretion. At this regard, it is important to note that PI/I ratio is a static measure, and its association with male sex and the use of secretagogues in a cross sectional study does not mean that these factors are "causally" related with the decline of beta cell function over time.

However, the aim of the BetaDecline study was to individuate tools to deal with the progressive decline of beta-cell secretion and its potential determinants in the clinical practice, and measuring PI/I ratio together with clinical information may be suitable to this purpose. At this regard, a strong point of the study is that the data were collected in a large outpatient population and so very likely reflect the real-world characteristics of diabetic patients attending a diabetes care center.

In conclusion, in this large cohort of type 2 diabetic outpatients, baseline higher PI/I values, a marker of beta-cell dysfunction, were more frequent in men and those using secretagogues.

These results need to be confirmed in the ongoing follow-up analysis of our study, since identifying specific metabolic and personal variables able to predict the degree of beta-cell loss over time will provide new tools to design better strategies for diabetes prevention and management.

Supporting Information

File S1 File containing Tables S1 and S2. Table S1: Patient characteristics according to quartiles of beta-cell insulin secretion, as evaluated by proinsulin/insulin (PI/I) ratio, **i**n male participants. Data are no. (%) and means ± SD. FBG, fasting blood glucose; PPG, postprandial blood glucose; SBP and DBP, systolic and diastolic blood pressure; CRP, C-reactive protein; IL-6, interleukin-6; NEFA, non-esterified fatty acids; PI, proinsulin; TZD thiazolidinediones. **Table S2**: Patient characteristics according to quartiles of beta-cell insulin secretion, as evaluated by proinsulin/insulin (PI/I) ratio, in female participants. Data are no. (%) and means ± SD. FBG, fasting blood glucose; PPG, postprandial blood glucose; SBP and DBP, systolic and diastolic blood pressure; CRP, C-reactive protein; IL-6, interleukin-6; NEFA, non-esterified fatty acids; PI, proinsulin; TZD thiazolidinediones.

Acknowledgments

GR is the guarantor of this work and, as such, had full access to all the data in the study and takes responsibility for the integrity of the data and the accuracy of the data analysis. All authors approved the final version.

Membership of the BetaDecline Group:

S. Leotta, A. Arcangeli, M. Calabrese, G. Vespasiani, S. De Cosmo A. Corda, L. Gentile, M. A. Pellegrini.

Author Contributions

Conceived and designed the experiments: GR CBG DC. Performed the experiments: GR CBG DC. Analyzed the data: AN SC. Contributed reagents/materials/analysis tools: AN SC. Wrote the paper: GR CBG DC.

References

1. Mokdad AH, Ford ES, Bowman BA, Dietz WH, Vinicor F, et al. (2001) Prevalence of obesity, diabetes, and obesity-related health risk factors. JAMA 289:76–9.
2. Kahn SE (2003) The relative contributions of insulin resistance and beta-cell dysfunction to the pathophysiology of Type 2 diabetes. Diabetologia 46:3–19.
3. Wright A, Burden AC, Paisey RB, Cull CA, Holman RR (2002) U.K. Prospective Diabetes Study Group. Sulfonylurea inadequacy: efficacy of addition of insulin over 6 years in patients with type 2 diabetes in the U.K. Prospective Diabetes Study (UKPDS 57). Diabetes Care 25:330–6.
4. Guardado-Mendoza R, Jimenez-Ceja L, Majluf-Cruz A, Kamath S, Fiorentino TV, et al. (2013) Impact of obesity severity and duration on pancreatic β- and α-cell dynamics in normoglycemic non-human primates. Int J Obes (Lond)37:1071–8.
5. Rhodes CJ (2005) Type 2 diabetes-a matter of beta-cell life and death? Science 307:380–384.
6. Lee SC, Pervaiz S (2007)Apoptosis in the pathophysiology of diabetes mellitus. Int J Biochem Cell Biol 39:497–504.
7. Folli F, Okada T, Perego C, Gunton J, Liew CW, et al. (2011) Altered insulin receptor signalling and β-cell cycle dynamics in type 2 diabetes mellitus. PLoS One 6(11):e28050.
8. Federici M, Hribal M, Perego L, Ranalli M, Caradonna Z, et al. (2001) High glucose causes apoptosis in cultured human pancreatic islets of Langerhans: a potential role for regulation of specific Bcl family genes toward an apoptotic cell death program. Diabetes 50:1290–301.
9. Verchere CB, D'Alessio DA, Palmiter RD, Weir GC, Bonner-Weir S, et al. (1996) Islet amyloid formation associated with hyperglycemia in transgenic mice with pancreatic beta cell expression of human islet amyloid polypeptide. Proc Natl Acad Sci U S A. 93:3492–6.
10. Guardado-Mendoza R, Davalli AM, Chavez AO, Hubbard GB, Dick EJ, et al. (2009) Pancreatic islet amyloidosis, beta-cell apoptosis, and alpha-cell proliferationare determinants of islet remodeling in type-2 diabetic baboons. Proc Natl Acad Sci U S A. 106:13992–7.
11. Jurgens CA, Toukatly MN, Fligner CL, Udayasankar J, Subramanian SL, et al. (2011) β-cell loss and β-cell apoptosis in human type 2 diabetes are related to islet amyloid deposition. Am J Pathol 178:2632–40.
12. Westermark P, Andersson A, Westermark GT (2011) Islet amyloid polypeptide, islet amyloid, and diabetes mellitus. Physiol Rev. 91:795–826.
13. Federici M, Hribal ML, Menghini R, Kanno H, Marchetti V, et al. (2005) Timp3 deficiency in insulin receptor-haploinsufficient mice promotes diabetes and vascular inflammation via increased TNF-alpha. J Clin Invest 115:3494–505.
14. Monroy A, Kamath S, Chavez AO, Centonze VE, Veerasamy M, et al. (2009) Impaired regulation of the TNF-alpha converting enzyme/tissue inhibitor of metalloproteinase 3 proteolytic system in skeletal muscle of obese type 2 diabetic patients: a new mechanism of insulin resistance in humans. Diabetologia 52:2169–81.
15. Tripathy D, Daniele G, Fiorentino TV, Perez-Cadena Z, Chavez-Velasquez A, et al. (2013) Pioglitazone improves glucose metabolism and modulates skeletal muscle TIMP-3-TACE dyad in type 2 diabetes mellitus: a randomised, double-blind, placebo-controlled, mechanistic study Diabetologia 56:2153–63.
16. The Expert Committee on the Diagnosis and Classification of Diabetes Mellitus (1997) Report of the Expert Committee on the Diagnosis and Classification of Diabetes Mellitus. Diabetes Care 20: 1183–97.
17. Friedewald WT, Levy RI, Fredrickson DS (1972) Estimation of the concentration of low-density lipoprotein cholesterol in plasma, without use of the preparative ultracentrifuge. Clin Chem 18:499–502.
18. Wallace TM, Levy JC, Matthews DR (2004) Use and abuse of HOMA modeling. Diabetes Care 27(6):1487–95.
19. Kahn SE, Carr DB, Faulenbach MV, Utzschneider KM (2008) An examination of beta-cell function measures and their potential use for estimating beta-cell mass. Diabetes Obes Metab 10 Suppl 4:63–76.
20. Kitabchi AE, Temprosa M, Knowler WC, Kahn SE, Fowler SE, et al. (2005) Diabetes Prevention Program Research Group. Role of insulin secretion and sensitivity in the evolution of type 2 diabetes in the diabetes prevention program: effects of lifestyle intervention and metformin. Diabetes 54:2404–14.
21. Weyer C, Bogardus C, Mott DM, Pratley RE (1999) The natural history of insulin secretory dysfunction and insulin resistance in the pathogenesis of type 2 diabetes mellitus. J Clin Invest 104:787–94.
22. DeFronzo RA, Banerji MA, Bray GA, Buchanan TA, Clement S, et al. (2010)ACT NOW Study Group. Determinants of glucose tolerance in impaired glucose tolerance at baseline in the Actos Now for Prevention of Diabetes (ACT NOW) study. Diabetologia 53: 435–45.
23. Kahn SE, Haffner SM, Heise MA, Herman WH, Holman RR, et al. (2006) ADOPT Study Group. Glycemic durability of rosiglitazone, metformin, or glyburide monotherapy. N Engl J Med 355:2427–43.
24. Bonora E (2008) Protection of pancreatic beta-cells: is it feasible? Nutr Metab Cardiovasc Dis 18:74–83.
25. Mudaliar S (2013) Choice of early treatment regimen and impact on β-cell preservation in type 2 diabetes. Int J Clin Pract 67: 876–87.
26. Brunzell JD, Robertson RP, Lerner RL, Hazzard WR, Ensinck JW, et al. (1976) Relationships between fasting plasma glucose levels and insulin secretion during intravenous glucose tolerance tests. J Clin Endocrinol Metab 42:222–9.
27. Phillips DI, Clark PM, Hales CN, Osmond C (1994) Understanding oral glucose tolerance: comparison of glucose or insulin measurements during the oral glucose tolerance test with specific measurements of insulin resistance and insulin secretion. Diabet Med 11:286–92.
28. Reaven GM (2009) Insulin secretory function in type 2 diabetes: Does it matter how you measure it? J Diabetes 1:142–50.
29. Festa A, Williams K, Hanley AJ, Haffner SM (2008) Beta-cell dysfunction in subjects with impaired glucose tolerance and early type 2 diabetes: comparison of surrogate markers with first-phase insulin secretion from an intravenous glucose tolerance test. Diabetes 57:1638–44.
30. Bryhni B, Arnesen E, Jenssen TG (2010) Associations of age with serum insulin, proinsulin and the proinsulin-to-insulin ratio: a cross-sectional study. BMC Endocr Disord 10:21.

31. Roder ME, Dinesen B, Hartling SG, Houssa P, Vestergaard H, et al. (1999) Intact proinsulin and beta-cell function in lean and obese subjects with and without type 2 diabetes. Diabetes Care 22: 609–14.
32. Ford ES (2005) Prevalence of the metabolic syndrome defined by the International Diabetes Federation among adults in the U.S. Diabetes Care 28:2745–49.
33. Shi H, Seeley RJ, Clegg DJ (2009) Sexual differences in the control of energy homeostasis. Front Neuroendocrinol 30:396–404.
34. Margolis KL, Bonds DE, Rodabough RJ, Tinker L, Phillips LS, et al. (2004) Women's Health Initiative Investigators. Effect of oestrogen plus progestin on the incidence of diabetes in postmenopausal women: results from the Women's Health Initiative Hormone Trial. Diabetologia 47:1175–87.
35. Kanaya AM, Herrington D, Vittinghoff E, Lin F, Grady D, et al. (2003) Heart and Estrogen/progestin Replacement Study. Glycemic effects of postmenopausal hormone therapy: the Heart and Estrogen/progestin Replacement Study. A randomized, double-blind, placebo-controlled trial. Ann Intern Med 138:1–9.
36. Godsland IF(2005) Oestrogens and insulin secretion. Diabetologia 48:2213–20
37. Tiano JP, Mauvais-Jarvis F (2012) Importance of oestrogen receptors to preserve functional β-cell mass in diabetes. Nat Rev Endocrinol 8:342–51.
38. Le May C, Chu K, Hu M, Ortega CS, Simpson ER, et al. (2006) Estrogens protect pancreatic beta-cells from apoptosis and prevent insulin-deficient diabetes mellitus in mice. Proc Natl Acad Sci U S A. 103:9232–37.
39. Chandler Laney PC, Phadke RP, Granger WM, Muñoz JA, Man CD, et al. (2010) Adiposity and β-cell function: relationships differ with ethnicity and age. Obesity 18:2086–92.
40. Dworacka M, Abramczyk M, Winiarska H, Kuczynski S, Borowska M, et al. (2006) Disproportionately elevated proinsulin levels in type 2 diabetic patients treated with sulfonylurea. Int J Clin Pharmacol Ther 44:14–21.
41. Pfützner A, Lorra B, Abdollahnia MR, Kann PH, Mathieu D, et al. (2006) The switch from sulfonylurea to preprandial short-acting insulin analog substitution has an immediate and comprehensive beta-cell protective effect in patients with type 2 diabetes mellitus. Diabetes Technol Ther 8:375–84.
42. Kahn SE, Lachin JM, Zinman B, Haffner SM, Aftring RP, et al. (2011) ADOPT Study. Effects of rosiglitazone, glyburide, and metformin on β-cell function and insulin sensitivity in ADOPT. Diabetes 60: 1552–60.
43. Pfützner A, Forst T (2011) Elevated intact proinsulin levels are indicative of Beta-cell dysfunction, insulin resistance, and cardiovascular risk: impact of the antidiabetic agent pioglitazone. J Diabetes Sci Technol 5:784–93.
44. Rossi MC, Cristofaro MR, Gentile S, Lucisano G, Manicardi V, et al. (2013)Sex Disparities in the Quality of Diabetes Care: Biological and Cultural Factors May Play a Different Role for Different Outcomes: A cross-sectional observational study from the AMD Annals initiative. Diabetes Care 36:3162–68.
45. Rivellese AA, Riccardi G, Vaccaro O (2010) Cardiovascular risk in women with diabetes. Nutr Metab Cardiovasc Dis.20:474–80.
46. Basu R, Breda E, Oberg AL, Powell CC, Dalla Man C, et al. (2003) Mechanisms of the age-associated deterioration in glucose tolerance: contribution of alterations in insulin secretion, action, and clearance. Diabetes 52:1738–48.
47. De Mello VD, Lindström J, Eriksson J, Ilanne-Parikka P, Keinänen-Kiukaanniemi S, et al. (2012) Insulin secretion and its determinants in the progression of impaired glucose tolerance to type 2 diabetes in impaired glucose-tolerant individuals: the Finnish Diabetes Prevention Study.Diabetes Care 35: 211–17.
48. Strawbridge RJ, Dupuis J, Prokopenko I, Barker A, Ahlqvist E, et al. (2011) Genome-wide association identifies nine common variants associated with fasting proinsulin levels and provides new insights into the pathophysiology of type 2 diabetes. Diabetes 60:2624–34.

Diabetes, Glucose Metabolism, and Glaucoma

Di Zhao[1,¶], **Juhee Cho**[2,¶], **Myung Hun Kim**[3*], **David Friedman**[4], **Eliseo Guallar**[1]

1 Department of Epidemiology and Welch Center for Prevention, Epidemiology, and Clinical Research, Johns Hopkins University Bloomberg School of Public Health, Baltimore, Maryland, United States of America, **2** Department of Health Sciences and Technology, Samsung Advanced Institute for Health Sciences and Technology, Sungkyunkwan University, Seoul, Korea, **3** Saevit Eye Hospital, Goyang, Gyeonggi-do, Korea, **4** Department of Ophthalmology, Johns Hopkins University School of Medicine, Baltimore, Maryland, United States of America

Abstract

Background: Diabetes may affect vascular autoregulation of the retina and optic nerve and may be associated with an increased risk of glaucoma,but the association of prediabetes, insulin resistance, markers of glucose metabolismwith glaucoma has not beenevaluated in general population samples.

Objective: To examine the relation between diabetes, pre-diabetes, metabolic syndrome and its components and the levels of fasting glucose, HbA1c and HOMA-IR with the prevalence of glaucoma in the general U.S. population.

Methods: Cross-sectional study of 3,299 adult men and women from the 2005–2008 National Health and NutritionExamination Survey (NHANES). The presence of diabetes, prediabetes, the metabolic syndrome and its individual components and biomarkers of glucose metabolisms were based on standardized questionnaire and physical exam data and laboratory tests. The history of glaucoma was assessed through questionnaire during the home interview.

Results: Diabetes was strongly associated with prevalent glaucoma.In fully adjusted models, the odds ratiofor glaucoma comparing participants with diabetes with participants in the reference group with neither pre-diabetes nor diabetes was 2.12 (95% CI: 1.23, 3.67). The corresponding odd ratio comparing participants with pre-diabetes to those in the reference group was 1.01 (95% CI: 0.57, 1.82). Patients with 5 or more years of diabetes duration hadan OR for glaucoma of 3.90 (95% CI: 1.63, 9.32) compared with patients with <5 years of diabetes duration. We also found a hockey-stick shaped associations between biomarkers of glucose metabolisms and the prevalence of glaucoma.

Conclusions: Diabetes was associated with higher risk of glaucoma. Participants without diabetes but at the higher levels of fasting glucose, fasting insulin, HbA1c and HOMA-IR spectrum may also be at greater risk of glaucoma.

Editor: Sanjoy Bhattacharya, Bascom Palmer Eye Institute, University of Miami School of Medicine;, United States of America

Funding: The authors have no support or funding to report.

Competing Interests: The authors have declared that no competing interests exist.

* Email: philip.mhkim@gmail.com

¶ DZ and JC are co-first authors on this work.

Introduction

Diabetes is a common chronic disease worldwide with a dramatic increase in incidence in recent decades [1]. Diabetes is associated with a variety of ocular complications, including retinopathy, cataracts, uveitis and neovascularization [2]. Several studies also suggested that diabetes may be associated with an increased risk of glaucoma [3–5].A meta-analysis of 12 studies published prior to 2004 found a pooled odds ratio for primary open angle glaucoma (POAG) comparing participants with diabetes to those without diabetes of 1.50 (95% confidence interval [CI] 1.16–1.93) [6], but there was significant heterogeneity and many studies reported non-significant associations [7–11] or negative point estimates [12–15].

Other abnormalities of glucose metabolism, including prediabetes, metabolic syndrome, insulin resistance, and elevated fasting glucose or hemoglobin A1c (HbA1c), may also be associated with glaucoma risk, but few studies have examined this issue, with conflicting results [16–19].The objective of this study was thus to examine the relation between diabetes, pre-diabetes, metabolic syndrome, and markers of glucose metabolism with the prevalence of glaucoma in the U.S. populationaged 40 years and older using data from the 2005–2008 National Health and Nutrition Examination Survey (NHANES).

Research Design and Methods

Study population

The National Health and Nutrition Examination Survey (NHANES) is a nationally representative study of the non-institutionalized US population, obtained by using a stratified multistage probability design with planned oversampling of certain age and minority groups. NHANES is conducted by the National Center of Health Statistics of the Centers for Disease Control and Prevention [20]. Information on glaucoma prevalence was only available in the 2005–2008 survey waves, and fasting glucose and insulin levels were only assessed in participants who were examined in the morning session. Therefore, we restricted our analysis to NHANES 2005–2008 participants 40 years of age or older who were examined in the morning session (N = 3,299). We then excluded 255 participants whose duration of fasting was < 8 h (if they didn't have a prior diagnosis of diabetes), 17 participants who had missing information regarding glaucoma in the questionnaire, and 1 participant with missing data in all exposure variables of interest. The final analysis was based on3,026 participants (1,501 men and 1,525 women).

The 2005–2008 NHANES study protocols were approved by the Institutional Review Board of the National Center for Health Statistics. Written informed consent was obtained from all participants.

Measurements

NHANES included a standardized questionnaire administered at home by a trained interviewer and a detailed physical examination at a mobile examination center. Self-reported glaucoma status was ascertained via the question "Have you ever been told by an eye doctor that you have glaucoma, sometimes called high pressure in your eyes?" Demographic information, education, smoking history, physical activity levels, alcohol consumption, medication use, health history, and age of diabetes onset were also determined by self-report. Leisure-time physical activities were coded and classified according to the rate of energy expenditure (<7.5, 7.5 to <15, and ≥15 metabolic equivalent hours per week) to correspond with cut points in the 2008 US federal physical activity guidelines [21] and the 2010 World Health Organization (WHO) guidelines. [22] Height, weight, and blood pressure were measured at the mobile examination center using standard procedures by trained health technicians [23,24]. Body mass index (BMI) was calculated as weight in kilograms divided by height in meters squared.

The average (SD) Fasting time was 12.3 (2.6) hours. Fasting blood samples were centrifuged and plasma was separated within 30 minutes from blood collection. Plasma glucose was analyzed using the hexokinase method in a Roche/Hitachi 911 (Roche Diagnostics, 9115 Hague Road, Indianapolis, IN) and a Roche Modular P chemistry analyzer (Roche Diagnostics, 9115 Hague Road, Indianapolis, IN) in 2005–2006 and 2007–2008, respectively [25]. Fasting insulin was analyzed using Merocodia Insulin ELISA kits [20]. HbA1cwas measured using high-performance liquid chromatography on an A1c 2.2 Plus Glycohemoglobin Analyzer (Tosoh Medics, Inc., San Francisco, Ca) in 2005–2006 and on an A1c G7 HPLC Glycohemoglobin Analyzer (Tosoh Medics, Inc., San Francisco, Ca) in 2007–2008 [26].

Diabetes was defined as a fasting plasma glucose level ≥ 126 mg/dL, an HbA1c level ≥6.5%, a self-reported diagnosis of diabetes (excluding gestational diabetes mellitus), or a self-report of current insulin or diabetes medication use. Pre-diabetes was defined in participants without diabetes as a fasting plasma glucose level between 100 mg/dL and 126 mg/dL, an HbA1c level between 5.7 and 6.5%, or a self-report of a diagnosis of borderline diabetes. Additional analyses were conducted defining diabetes and pre-diabetes using fasting plasma glucose or HbA1 ccriteria separately. Diabetes duration was calculated as the age at interview minus the age at the first time that the participant was told to have diabetes.

Metabolic syndrome components were defined as detailed in the Adult Treatment Panel (ATP) III report [27]: 1) waist circumference ≥102 cm in men and ≥88 cm in women; 2) fasting triglycerides ≥150 mg/dL; 3) HDL cholesterol <40 mg/dL in men and <50 mg/dL in women; 4) blood pressure ≥130/85 mm Hg; and 5) fasting glucose ≥110 mg/dL or use of antidiabetic medication. Persons with at least 3 of these characteristics were defined as having metabolic syndrome. We also calculated the homeostatic model assessment of insulin resistance (HOMA-IR) as fasting glucose (mg/dl) x fasting Insulin (uU/mL)/405 and defined insulin resistance as HOMA-IR >2.6 [28].

Statistical analysis

All statistical analyses were performed using NHANES weights and *svy* commands in STATA (version 12; Stata Corp., College Station, TX) to account for the complex multistage probability sampling design. Analyses of fasting glucose, fasting insulin, HOMA-IR, and HbA1 clevels were restricted to participants not taking insulin or antidiabetic medications (N = 2,509). Fasting glucose, fasting insulin, HOMA-IR, and HbA1 clevels were categorized into quartiles based on the weighted population distribution.

We used multivariable logistic regression models to calculate odds ratios (OR) and 95% CI for the prevalence of glaucoma associated with glucose metabolism variables. Diabetes and pre-diabetes were included as exposures in the same model, and we fitted separate models for diabetes duration, metabolic syndrome and each its components, insulin resistance, fasting glucose, fasting insulin, HOMA-IR, and HbA1c. For each exposure, we used 3 models with progressive degrees of adjustment. Initial models were crude and then we adjusted for age, sex (male, female) and race/ethnicity (non-Hispanic, white, non-Hispanic black, Mexican American, and other). Finally, fully adjusted models further included education (< high school, high school, > high school), smoking (never, former, current), average physical activity level (low, medium, vigorous), alcohol drinking (<1 drink/week, 1 to < 3 drinks/week, ≥3 drinks/week) and BMI (continuous).

For dose-response analyses of the associations of fasting glucose, fasting insulin, HOMA-IR, and HbA1c levels with the prevalence of glaucoma, we calculated OR and 95% CI comparing quartiles 2–4 with the first quartile in categorical analyses, as well as OR and 95% CI comparing the 80th to the 20th percentiles of markers of glucose metabolism modeled as log-transformed continuous variables. In addition, we used restricted cubic spline models with knots at the 10th, 50th and 90th percentiles of the distribution of fasting glucose, fasting insulin, HOMA-IR, and HbA1c concentrations to provide a smooth yet flexible description of the shape of dose-response relationship. Tests for non-linear trends computed by log likelihood ratio tests comparing nested models with and without non-linear spline terms.

Results

The study population had a weighted mean (SE) age of 57.0(0.4) years (**Table 1**). The prevalence of diabetes, pre-diabetes, metabolic syndrome, and insulin resistance were 17.1, 49.0, 32.1, and 43.4%, respectively, and the prevalence of glaucoma was 4.2% (95% CI 3.3–5.3%). The average duration of diabetes was

Table 1. Characteristics of study participants by glaucoma status.*

		Glaucoma		p-value[†]
	Overall N = 3,026	No N = 2,835	Yes N = 191	
Age, year	57.0 (0.4)	56.5 (0.4)	68.7 (1.5)	<0.001
Female, %	53.2 (1.2)	53.2 (1.1)	52.3 (4.9)	0.87
Race, %				0.009
Mexican American	5.6 (0.8)	5.7 (0.8)	4.5 (1.6)	
NonHispanic white	76.2 (2.1)	76.4 (2.1)	71.6 (4.8)	
NonHispanic black	10.2 (1.4)	9.8 (1.4)	17.8 (3.7)	
Others	8.0 (1.1)	8.1 (1.1)	6.2 (2.5)	
Education, %				0.005
<High school	18.5 (1.2)	18.0 (1.1)	29.0 (5)	
High school	27.0 (1.3)	26.9 (1.3)	30.6 (5.2)	
>High school	54.5 (2.1)	55.1 (2.1)	40.4 (4.9)	
Waist circumference, cm	100.3 (0.4)	100.2 (0.4)	103 (1.3)	0.04
Systolic blood pressure, mm Hg	126.9 (0.5)	126.4 (0.5)	136.3 (2.2)	<0.001
Diastolic blood pressure, mm Hg	70.7 (0.4)	70.9 (0.4)	65.7 (1.7)	0.005
Body mass index, kg/m^2	29.0 (0.1)	29.0 (0.1)	29.7 (0.5)	0.15
Insulin, uU/mL[‡]	11.2 (0.3)	11.2 (0.3)	11.9 (1.1)	0.54
Serum fasting glucose, mg/dL[‡]	103.5 (0.7)	103.4 (0.7)	108.6 (2.0)	0.01
HDL, mg/dL	55.5 (0.3)	55.5 (0.3)	55.4 (1.5)	0.97
Triglycerides, mg/dL	146.0 (2.7)	145.6 (2.7)	154.0 (12.7)	0.52
HbA1c, %[‡]	5.5 (0.02)	5.5 (0.02)	5.7 (0.08)	0.01
HOMA-IR[‡]	3.0 (0.1)	3.0 (0.1)	3.3 (0.4)	0.40

*Data are means (SEs) or percentages (SEs).
[†]P value for homogeneity of means or proportions comparing participants with to those without glaucoma.
[‡]Values are based on the subsample of participants not taking insulin or medication for diabetes (N = 2,409).

11.8 years. Participants with prevalent glaucoma were more likely to be older, non-Hispanic black, less educated, and had higher waist circumference, blood pressure, fasting glucose and HbA1c levels (**Table 1**) and to have a significantly higher prevalence of diabetes, elevated blood pressure, and elevated fasting glucose (**Table 2**).

The prevalence of glaucoma in participants with diabetes, with pre-diabetes, and without diabetes or pre-diabetes was 9.5, 3.5, and 2.6%, respectively (P<0.001).In age-, sex-, and race/ethnicity-adjusted models, the OR for glaucoma comparing participants with diabetes to those without diabetes or pre-diabetes was 2.09 (95% CI 1.11 to 3.92) (**Table 3**). The corresponding OR

Table 2. Prevalence of glucose metabolism abnormalities by glaucoma status.*

		Glaucoma		p-value[†]
	Overall N = 3,026	No N = 2,835	Yes N = 191	
Diabetes, %	17.1 (0.9)	16.1 (0.9)	38.8 (4.1)	<0.001
Prediabetes, %	49.0 (1.4)	49.4 (1.4)	40.4 (3.7)	0.34
Insulin resistance, %	43.4 (1.5)	43.1 (1.5)	49.8 (4.7)	0.13
Metabolic syndrome, %	32.1 (1.2)	31.7 (1.2)	41.1 (5.4)	0.06
Elevated waist circumference, %	60.3 (1.4)	60.0 (1.4)	66.4 (4.1)	0.14
Elevated blood pressure, %	42.1 (1.1)	41.1 (1.1)	63.3 (4.1)	<0.001
Elevated triglyceride, %	33.7 (0.9)	33.7 (1.0)	33.6 (5.5)	0.98
Reduced HDL, %	24.0 (0.8)	24.2 (0.8)	18.0 (3.9)	0.17
Elevated fasting glucose, %	28.8 (1.4)	28.2 (1.4)	43.3 (3.7)	<0.001
Duration of diabetes, years	11.7 (0.6)	11.3 (0.6)	15.2 (1.8)	0.04

*Data are percentages or means (SEs).
[†]P value for homogeneity of means or proportions comparing participants with to those without glaucoma.

in fully adjusted models was 1.80 (95% CI 0.93 to 3.47). The association of diabetes with glaucoma prevalence was stronger when the definition of diabetes was based on either fasting glucose or HbA1c levels only, with ORs of 2.12 (95% CI 1.23 to 3.67) and 2.10 (95% CI 1.19 to 3.71), respectively. The fully adjusted OR (95% CI) for glaucoma comparing participants with pre-diabetes to those without diabetes or pre-diabetes was 0.88 (95% CI 0.45 to 1.75). Diabetes duration was also significantly associated with glaucoma. Among participants with diabetes, the multivariable-adjusted OR for glaucoma comparing participants with a duration of disease ≥5 years to those with a duration of disease <5 years was3.90 (95% CI 1.63 to 9.32).

The prevalence of glaucoma in patients with and without metabolic syndrome was 5.3 and 3.6%, respectively (P = 0.06). The OR for glaucoma comparing participants with to those without metabolic syndrome was 1.30 (95% CI 0.83 to 2.03) in age-, sex-, and race/ethnicity-adjusted models and 1.13 (95% CI 0.60 to 2.16) in fully adjusted models (**Table 3**). In fully adjusted models, none of the individual components of the metabolic syndrome or the presence of insulin resistance were significantly associated with the prevalence of glaucoma (**Table 3**).

In dose-response models with glucose biomarkers modeled as continuous variables or categorized in quartiles, the prevalence of glaucoma increased with increasing biomarker levels but the trends were only statistically significant for fasting glucose (**Table 4**). In fully adjusted models, the OR for glaucoma comparing the fourth to the first quartiles of fasting glucose, insulin, HOMA-IR, and HbA1C were 1.20 (95% CI 0.67 to 2.13; P trend 0.27), 1.22 (95% CI 0.54 to 2.75; P trend 0.75), 1.37 (95% CI 0.57 to 3.27; P trend 0.19) and 1.55 (95% CI 0.59 to 4.08; P trend 0.48), respectively. In spline models, however, the dose-response relationships between markers of glucose metabolism and the prevalence of glaucoma were hockey-stick shaped for insulin, HOMA-IR, and HbA1C and J-shaped for fasting glucose (**Figure 1**).The P values for the non-linear spline terms in the restricted cubic models were significant for all glucose biomarkers ($p<0.001$ for all).

Discussion

In a large sample representative of the general US population, the prevalence of glaucoma was higher in participants with diabetes compared to those with no glucose abnormality, even after controlling for multiple potential confounders. Pre-diabetes and the metabolic syndrome and its components were not consistently associated with the prevalence of glaucoma. However, markers of glucose metabolism showed significant non-linear associations with glaucoma prevalence, including hockey-stick shaped associations for fasting insulin, HbA1c and HOMA-IR, and a J-shaped association for fasting glucose. These non-linear relationships suggest threshold effects for the association of glucose metabolism markers and glaucoma.

The association between diabetes and glaucoma has been evaluated in many studies [9,13–15,17,29,30]. An increased risk of glaucoma in persons with diabetes compared to those who did not have diabetes was also observed in the Beaver Dam Eye study, the Blue Mountains Eye study, the Los Angeles Latino Eye Study and several other population-based studies [3,5,16,19,31–35], but some well-known cohorts did not show statistically significant associations [9,14,17]. The discrepancy with these studies may be attributed to study population, sample size, methods to assess diabetes or glaucoma, or drop-out rates. The Baltimore Eye

Table 3. Odds ratio and 95% CIs for the presence of glaucoma.

	Crude model	Model 1†	Model 2‡
Diabetes			
HbA1c or fasting glucose*	3.99 (2.05, 7.76)	2.09 (1.11, 3.92)	1.80 (0.93, 3.47)
Fasting glucose only§	3.83 (2.24, 6.55)	2.28 (1.37, 3.81)	2.12 (1.23, 3.67)
HbA1c only†	4.52 (2.65, 7.68)	2.65 (1.49, 4.71)	2.10 (1.19, 3.71)
Prediabetes			
HbA1c or fasting glucose*	1.36 (0.72, 2.56)	0.96 (0.52, 1.75)	0.88 (0.45, 1.75)
Fasting glucose only§	1.23 (0.75, 2.02)	1.02 (0.63, 1.66)	1.01 (0.57, 1.82)
HbA1c only†	2.63 (1.53, 4.51)	1.72 (0.98, 3.05)	1.57 (0.85, 2.92)
Metabolic syndrome	1.50 (0.98, 2.29)	1.30 (0.83, 2.03)	1.13 (0.60, 2.16)
Elevated waist circumference	1.31 (0.91, 1.90)	1.19 (0.81, 1.75)	0.89 (0.55, 1.45)
Elevated blood pressure	2.47 (1.71, 3.56)	1.38 (0.97, 1.97)	1.39 (0.92, 2.09)
Elevated triglyceride	0.99 (0.59, 1.68)	1.09 (0.65, 1.81)	0.90 (0.52, 1.57)
Reduced HDL	0.69 (0.40, 1.18)	0.83 (0.47, 1.47)	0.73 (0.35, 1.52)
Elevated fasting glucose	1.95 (1.40, 2.70)	1.35 (1.00, 1.83)	1.29 (0.85, 1.95)
Diabetes duration >5 years	2.48 (1.06, 5.76)	2.20 (1.02, 4.73)	3.90 (1.63, 9.32)
Insulin resistance‖	1.19 (0.78, 1.81)	1.22 (0.78, 1.90)	1.14 (0.64, 2.01)

†Adjusted for age, gender, and ethnicity.
‡Further adjusted for smoking, physical activity, alcohol intake, education, and BMI.
*Diabetes defined as self-report, HbA1c ≥6.5%, fasting glucose ≥126 mg/dL, or taking diabetic medications.Pre-diabetes defined as self-report, HbA1c ≥5.7% to < 6.5%, or fasting glucose ≥100 mg/dL to <126 mg/dL.
§Diabetes defined as self-report, HbA1c ≥6.5%, or taking diabetic medications. Pre-diabetes defined as self-report or HbA1c ≥5.7% to <6.5%.
†Diabetes defined as self-report, fasting glucose ≥126 mg/dL or taking diabetic medications. Pre-diabetes defined as self-report or fasting glucose ≥100 mg/dL to < 126 mg/dL.
‖Values are based on the subsample of participants not taking insulin or medication for diabetes.

Table 4. Association between markers of glucose metabolism and the presence of glaucoma*

	Odds ratio for glaucoma					P value for quadratic trend
	80th vs. 20th	**Quartile 1**	**Quartile 2**	**Quartile 3**	**Quartile 4**	
Fasting glucose						
Crude Model	1.37 (1.13, 1.64)	1.00 (reference)	0.71 (0.37, 1.34)	1.06 (0.55, 2.06)	1.56 (0.96, 2.56)	0.02
Model 1†	1.22 (0.97, 1.54)	1.00 (reference)	0.67 (0.35, 1.29)	0.98 (0.51, 1.88)	1.05 (0.64, 1.72)	0.47
Model 2‡	1.30 (1.00, 1.68)	1.00 (reference)	0.67 (0.34, 1.34)	1.08 (0.47, 2.47)	1.20 (0.67, 2.13)	0.26
Fasting Insulin						
Crude Model	1.06 (0.65, 1.73)	1.00 (reference)	1.00 (0.55, 1.81)	0.96 (0.44, 2.06)	1.14 (0.61, 2.15)	0.83
Model 1†	1.16 (0.67, 2.01)	1.00 (reference)	1.02 (0.54, 1.90)	0.97 (0.44, 2.11)	1.32 (0.70, 2.49)	0.54
Model 2‡	1.13 (0.53, 2.41)	1.00 (reference)	0.92 (0.43, 1.98)	0.80 (0.30, 2.14)	1.22 (0.54, 2.75)	0.56
HOMA-IR						
Crude Model	1.16 (0.70, 1.92)	1.00 (reference)	0.67 (0.34, 1.35)	1.36 (0.67, 2.76)	1.15 (0.61, 2.17)	0.24
Model 1†	1.21 (0.70, 2.11)	1.00 (reference)	0.68 (0.34, 1.39)	1.39 (0.71, 2.71)	1.22 (0.64, 2.34)	0.17
Model 2‡	1.25 (0.57, 2.72)	1.00 (reference)	0.61 (0.28, 1.34)	1.27 (0.53, 3.05)	1.37 (0.57, 3.27)	0.22
HbA1C						
Crude Model	1.43 (1.16, 1.77)	1.00 (reference)	1.43 (0.62, 3.31)	2.35 (0.95, 5.85)	3.91 (1.75, 8.71)	0.003
Model 1†	1.23 (0.94, 1.60)	1.00 (reference)	1.10 (0.48, 2.51)	1.60 (0.61, 4.21)	1.86 (0.80, 4.28)	0.21
Model 2‡	1.15 (0.85, 1.55)	1.00 (reference)	0.96 (0.38, 2.40)	1.51 (0.53, 4.30)	1.55 (0.59, 4.08)	0.32

*Conducted in people not taking diabetes medications.
†Adjusted for age, gender, and ethnicity.
‡Further adjusted for smoking, physical activity, alcohol intake, education, and BMI.

Survey was primarily composed of African Americans and used self-report to define diabetes [9].The Rotterdam Study used a prospective cohort design, but had few participants with diabetes and a high drop-out rate, so that the results were based only on 5 incident cases of glaucoma among 264 participants with diabetes [14].The Singapore Malay Eye Study used random serum glucose measurements instead of fasting glucose to define diabetes, which may result in substantial underdiagnosis, and had also limited power to identify an association between diabetes and glaucoma [17]. In spite of these negative studies, the majority of the epidemiological evidence points to an increased prevalence of glaucoma in patients with diabetes.

Few studies have evaluated the association between metabolic syndrome or glucose metabolism biomarkers and glaucoma, with conflicting results [16–19]. In the Singapore Malay Eye Study, participants with metabolic syndrome had a lower prevalence of

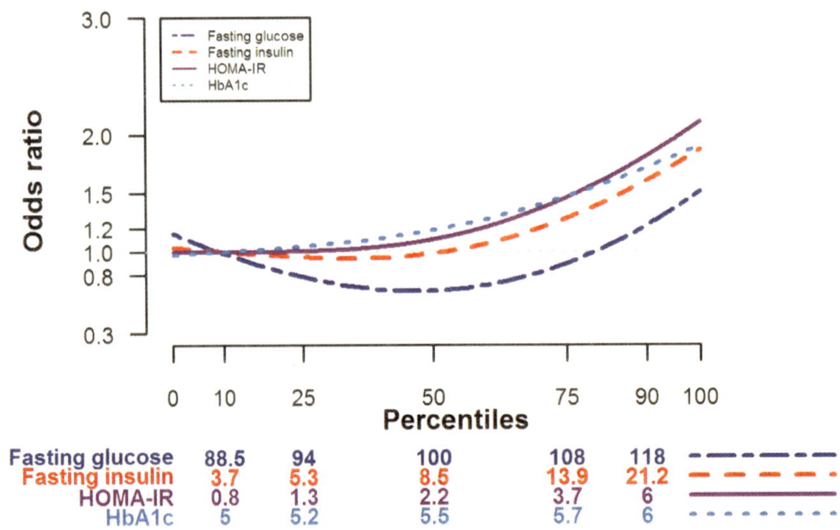

Figure 1. Adjusted odds ratio for glaucoma by levels of markers of glucose metabolism. Adjusted odds ratios were estimated using restricted cubic splines with knots at the 10th, 50th, and 90th percentiles of the distribution of each marker of glucose metabolism. The reference value (odds ratio = 1) was set at the 10th percentile of each parameter. Odds ratios were adjusted for age, sex, race, education, smoking status, physical activity, alcohol consumption, and body mass index (see text for details).

glaucoma [17], while the number of metabolic syndrome components was positively associated with the hazard of open-angle glaucoma in a US cohort [19]. As for HbA1c and glucose, the Singapore Malay Eye Study showed an elevated but non-significant trend while a case-control study in Europe showed a significantly positive association between increased HbA1c levels and glaucoma [16]. In our study, the association between glucose metabolism biomarkers and the prevalence of glaucoma was non-linear and affected only to participants in the higher half of the distribution of glucose metabolism parameters. These findings suggest that a certain degree of impairment in glucose metabolism is needed before glaucoma appears as a complication of insulin resistance.

In addition to the level of glucose metabolism biomarkers, the duration of the metabolic abnormalities may also be important in determining glaucoma risk. We found that duration of diabetes was significantly associated with an increased prevalence of glaucoma, but we did not have information on the duration of the elevations in glucose metabolism biomarkers or on their trajectories over time. Additional research is needed to confirm these thresholds and to understand the increase in glaucoma risk with increasing duration in glucose metabolism abnormalities.

Several biological mechanisms could explain an increased risk of glaucoma in patients with diabetes. Diabetes may induce structural and functional abnormalities to the small blood vessels feeding the optic nerve, resulting in damage to the optic nerve and the retinal nerve fiber layer [36]. Besides the vascular implications, diabetes may also exacerbate glaucomatous optic neuropathy by increasing the susceptibility of retinal ganglion cells to apoptosis due to elevated intraocular pressure (IOP) [37]. This mechanism may also explain progressive optic nerve injury and neuronal damage with a longer duration of diabetes. Furthermore, diabetic retinopathy may also compromise the glial and neuronal elements, impair retinal function and metabolism, and result in accelerated degeneration of retinal inner neurons [38].

The potential mechanisms underlying the association between glucose metabolism abnormalities and the prevalence of glaucoma in subjects without diabetes are unclear. The presence of the metabolic syndrome and elevated levels of glucose, HOMA-IR and glycosylated hemoglobin may be associated with increased levels of IOP, a key causal factor for glaucoma [31,39–44]. Hyperglycemia increased fibronectin production in the bovine trabecular meshwork, which may increase the resistance to aqueous humor outflow and lead to elevated IOP [45]. Moreover, hyperglycemia could induce apoptosis in retinal neuronal cells through the hexosamine biosynthetic pathway [46]. Additionally, hyperglycemia-induced oxidative stress and advanced glycation end products may increase apoptotic death in retinal neurons [47,48].

Several limitations need to be considered in the interpretation of our findings. First, the cross-sectional nature of this study limited our ability to establish the causality of the observed associations. Second, while we used high quality laboratory methods and fasting plasma samples to assess glucose metabolism status, the prevalence of glaucoma was assessed by self-report without an ophthalmologic exam. Although the prevalence of glaucoma in NHANES was similar to that reported in other US studies [49], the lack of a clinical assessment of glaucoma may have resulted in under-diagnosis and recall bias. Previous studies of the validity of self-report of glaucoma have shown low sensitivity and very high specificity when compared to eye examinations, and substantial agreement when compared to medical records [50,51]. Additional studies with high quality measurements of both glucose metabolism parameters and glaucoma status are needed to confirm our findings. Third, the increased prevalence of glaucoma in patients with diabetes and in those with longer duration of diabetes may have been overestimated because of more frequent ophthalmology visits in persons with compared to those without diabetes. We did not have information on the frequency of eye examinations in study participants, but other studies suggested that this type of surveillance bias could not completely account for the positive association between diabetes and glaucoma risk [5,31]. In the Blue Mountains Eye study, most cases of glaucoma had been diagnosed before the diabetes diagnosis [5], and the Nurses' Health Study also showed that the prospective association between diabetes and glaucoma was unaltered when adjusting for factors related with the number of eye examinations [31]. In spite of these limitations, the large sample size, the standardization and rigorous quality control procedures of NHANES, and the generalizability of the findings to the general US population are important strengths that add to the relevance of our findings.

Glaucoma has a long latency period, in which glaucomatous optic nerve damage is ongoing but remains asymptomatic until later stages. Since vision loss is irreversible, screening and early detection of glaucoma is important in persons with diabetes, given the increased risk for glaucoma and the high frequency coexistence of other mechanisms for vision loss. The adherence to regular ophthalmological exams should be emphasized in diabetic patients, especially among those with long duration of diabetes, regardless of age. Our results also indicate that ophthalmologist referral may be considered for adults without diabetes but with elevated levels of glucose biomarkers.

In conclusion, data from NHANES 2005–2008, a large sample representative of the general US population, showed a higher prevalence of glaucoma in patients with diabetes, particularly in those with longer duration of disease, as well as an increased prevalence of glaucoma with increasing levels of glucose metabolism abnormalities in participants in the higher end of the distribution of glucose metabolism parameters. The mechanisms underlying these associations and the impact of the duration of glucose abnormalities on glaucoma risk need to be established in future studies. Our results support the recommendation that patients with diabetes, as well as those with elevated levels of glucose metabolism parameters, undergo regular ophthalmological exams to monitor for the onset or progression of glaucoma.

Author Contributions

Conceived and designed the experiments: MK EG. Analyzed the data: DZ JC. Wrote the paper: DZ JC. Interpretation of data and reviewed and edited the manuscript: EG DF MK. Supervision of data analysis: EG.

References

1. Wild S, Roglic G, Green A, Sicree R, King H (2004) Global prevalence of diabetes: estimates for the year 2000 and projections for 2030. Diabetes Care 27: 1047–1053.
2. Stanga PE, Boyd SR, Hamilton AM (1999) Ocular manifestations of diabetes mellitus. CurrOpinOphthalmol 10: 483–489.
3. Klein BE, Klein R, Jensen SC (1994) Open-angle glaucoma and older-onset diabetes. The Beaver Dam Eye Study. Ophthalmology 101: 1173–1177.
4. Dielemans I, de Jong PT, Stolk R, Vingerling JR, Grobbee DE, et al. (1996) Primary open-angle glaucoma, intraocular pressure, and diabetes mellitus in the general elderly population. The Rotterdam Study. Ophthalmology 103: 1271–1275.
5. Mitchell P, Smith W, Chey T, Healey PR (1997) Open-angle glaucoma and diabetes: the Blue Mountains eye study, Australia. Ophthalmology 104: 712–718.

6. Bonovas S, Peponis V, Filioussi K (2004) Diabetes mellitus as a risk factor for primary open-angle glaucoma: a meta-analysis. Diabet Med 21: 609–614. doi:10.1111/j.1464-5491.2004.01173.x.
7. Kaimbo DK, Buntinx F, Missotten L (2001) Risk factors for open-angle glaucoma: a case-control study. J ClinEpidemiol 54: 166–171.
8. KaimboWaKaimbo D, Missotten L (1997) Risk factors for open-angle glaucoma in 260 black subjects in Congo. Bull SocBelgeOphtalmol 267: 29–34.
9. Tielsch JM, Katz J, Sommer A, Quigley HA, Javitt JC (1995) Hypertension, perfusion pressure, and primary open-angle glaucoma. A population-based assessment. Arch Ophthalmol 113: 216–221.
10. Leske MC, Connell AMS, Wu S-Y, Hyman LG, Schachat AP, et al. (1995) Risk Factors for Open-angle Glaucoma: The Barbados Eye Study. Arch Ophthalmol 113: 918–924. doi:10.1001/archopht.1995.01100070092031.
11. Quigley HA, West SK, Rodriguez J, Munoz B, Klein R, et al. (2001) The prevalence of glaucoma in a population-based study of Hispanic subjects: Proyecto VER. Arch Ophthalmol 119: 1819–1826.
12. Charliat G, Jolly D, Blanchard F (1994) Genetic risk factor in primary open-angle glaucoma: a case-control study. Ophthalmic Epidemiol 1: 131–138.
13. Jonas JB, Gründler AE (1998) Prevalence of diabetes mellitus and arterial hypertension in primary and secondary open-angle glaucomas. Graefes Arch ClinExpOphthalmol 236: 202–206.
14. De Voogd S, Ikram MK, Wolfs RCW, Jansonius NM, Witteman JCM, et al. (2006) Is diabetes mellitus a risk factor for open-angle glaucoma? The Rotterdam Study. Ophthalmology 113: 1827–1831. doi:10.1016/j.ophtha.2006.03.063.
15. Howard DL, Kim MM, Hartnett ME (2011) Predicting glaucoma diagnosis in an elderly sample: revisiting the established populations for epidemiologic studies of the elderly. J Natl Med Assoc 103: 332–341.
16. Welinder LG, Riis AH, Knudsen LL, Thomsen RW (2009) Diabetes, glycemic control and risk of medical glaucoma treatment: A population-based case-control study. ClinEpidemiol 1: 125–131.
17. Tan GS, Wong TY, Fong C-W, Aung T (2009) Diabetes, metabolic abnormalities, and glaucoma. Arch Ophthalmol 127: 1354–1361.
18. Elisaf M, Kitsos G, Bairaktari E, Kalaitzidis R, Kalogeropoulos C, et al. (2001) Metabolic abnormalities in patients with primary open-angle glaucoma. ActaOphthalmolScand 79: 129–132.
19. Newman-Casey PA, Talwar N, Nan B, Musch DC, Stein JD (2011) The relationship between components of metabolic syndrome and open-angle glaucoma. Ophthalmology 118: 1318–1326. doi:10.1016/j.ophtha.2010.11.022.
20. Centers for Disease Control and Prevention. National Health and Nutrition Examination Survey: questionnaires, datasets, and related documentation (n.d.). Available: http://www.cdc.gov/nchs/nhanes/nhanes_questionnaires.htm. Accessed 26 March 2013.
21. Physical Activity Guidelines for Americans (n.d.). Available: http://www.health.gov/paguidelines/guidelines/. Accessed 6 July 2013.
22. WHO | Global recommendations on physical activity for health (n.d.). WHO. Available: http://www.who.int/dietphysicalactivity/publications/9789241599979/en/. Accessed 6 July 2013.
23. Centers for Disease Control and Prevention. 2005–2006 National Health and Nutrition Examination Survey: survey operations manuals, brochures, consent documents (n.d.). Available: http://www.cdc.gov/nchs/nhanes/nhanes2005-2006/current_nhanes_05_06.htm. Accessed 26 March 2013.
24. Centers for Disease Control and Prevention. 2007–2008 National Health and Nutrition Examination Survey: survey operations manuals, brochures, consent documents (n.d.). Available: http://www.cdc.gov/nchs/nhanes/nhanes2007-2008/current_nhanes_07_08.htm. Accessed 26 March 2013.
25. NHANES 2007–2008: Plasma Fasting Glucose and Insulin Data Documentation, Codebook, and Frequencies (n.d.). Available: http://www.cdc.gov/nchs/nhanes/nhanes2007-2008/Glu_E.htm. Accessed 26 March 2013.
26. NHANES 2007–2008: Glycohemoglobin Data Documentation, Codebook, and Frequencies (n.d.). Available: http://www.cdc.gov/nchs/nhanes/nhanes2007-2008/GHB_E.htm. Accessed 7 July 2013.
27. Third Report of the National Cholesterol Education Program (NCEP) Expert Panel on Detection, Evaluation, and Treatment of High Blood Cholesterol in Adults (Adult Treatment Panel III) final report (2002). Circulation 106: 3143–3421.
28. Ascaso JF, Pardo S, Real JT, Lorente RI, Priego A, et al. (2003) Diagnosing Insulin Resistance by Simple Quantitative Methods in Subjects With Normal Glucose Metabolism. Dia Care 26: 3320–3325. doi:10.2337/diacare.26.12.3320.
29. Uhm KB, Shin DH (1992) Glaucoma risk factors in primary open-angle glaucoma patients compared to ocular hypertensives and control subjects. Korean J Ophthalmol 6: 91–99.
30. Orzalesi N, Rossetti L, Omboni S (2007) Vascular risk factors in glaucoma: the results of a national survey. Graefes Arch ClinExpOphthalmol 245: 795–802. doi:10.1007/s00417-006-0457-5.
31. Pasquale LR, Kang JH, Manson JE, Willett WC, Rosner BA, et al. (2006) Prospective Study of Type 2 Diabetes Mellitus and Risk of Primary Open-Angle Glaucoma in Women. Ophthalmology 113: 1081–1086. doi:10.1016/j.ophtha.2006.01.066.
32. Chopra V, Varma R, Francis BA, Wu J, Torres M, et al. (2008) Type 2 Diabetes Mellitus and the Risk of Open-angle Glaucoma: The Los Angeles Latino Eye Study. Ophthalmology 115: 227–232.e1. doi:10.1016/j.ophtha.2007.04.049.
33. Graw J, Welzl G, Ahmad N, Klopp N, Heier M, et al. (2011) The KORA Eye Study: a population-based study on eye diseases in Southern Germany (KORA F4). Invest Ophthalmol Vis Sci 52: 7778–7786. doi:10.1167/iovs.10-7113.
34. Ellis JD, Evans JM, Ruta DA, Baines PS, Leese G, et al. (2000) Glaucoma incidence in an unselected cohort of diabetic patients: is diabetes mellitus a risk factor for glaucoma? DARTS/MEMO collaboration. Diabetes Audit and Research in Tayside Study. Medicines Monitoring Unit. Br J Ophthalmol 84: 1218–1224.
35. Wise LA, Rosenberg L, Radin RG, Mattox C, Yang EB, et al. (2011) A prospective study of diabetes, lifestyle factors, and glaucoma among African-American women. Ann Epidemiol 21: 430–439. doi:10.1016/j.annepidem.2011.03.006.
36. Szaflik JP, Rusin P, Zaleska-Zmijewska A, Kowalski M, Majsterek I, et al. (2010) Reactive oxygen species promote localized DNA damage in glaucoma-iris tissues of elderly patients vulnerable to diabetic injury. Mutat Res 697: 19–23. doi:10.1016/j.mrgentox.2010.02.003.
37. Kanamori A, Nakamura M, Mukuno H, Maeda H, Negi A (2004) Diabetes has an additive effect on neural apoptosis in rat retina with chronically elevated intraocular pressure. Curr Eye Res 28: 47–54. doi:10.1076/ceyr.28.1.47.23487.
38. Nakamura M, Kanamori A, Negi A (2005) Diabetes mellitus as a risk factor for glaucomatous optic neuropathy. Ophthalmologica 219: 1–10. doi:10.1159/000081775.
39. Oh SW, Lee S, Park C, Kim DJ (2005) Elevated intraocular pressure is associated with insulin resistance and metabolic syndrome. Diabetes Metab Res Rev 21: 434–440. doi:10.1002/dmrr.529.
40. Chen H-Y, Lai S-W (2005) Relation between intraocular pressure and systemic health parameters in Taiwan. South Med J 98: 28–32.
41. Xu L, Xie XW, Wang YX, Jonas JB (2009) Ocular and systemic factors associated with diabetes mellitus in the adult population in rural and urban China. The Beijing Eye Study. Eye (Lond) 23: 676–682. doi:10.1038/sj.eye.6703104.
42. Chang YC, Lin J-W, Wang LC, Chen HM, Hwang JJ, et al. (2010) Association of intraocular pressure with the metabolic syndrome and novel cardiometabolic risk factors. Eye (Lond) 24: 1037–1043.
43. Lin C-P, Lin Y-S, Wu S-C, Ko Y-S (2012) Age- and gender-specific association between intraocular pressure and metabolic variables in a Taiwanese population. Eur J Intern Med 23: 76–82. doi:10.1016/j.ejim.2011.06.002.
44. Park S, Lee E-H, Jargal G, Paek D, Cho S (2010) The distribution of intraocular pressure and its association with metabolic syndrome in a community. J Prev Med Public Health 43: 125–130.
45. Sato T, Roy S (2002) Effect of high glucose on fibronectin expression and cell proliferation in trabecular meshwork cells. Invest Ophthalmol Vis Sci 43: 170–175.
46. Nakamura M, Barber AJ, Antonetti DA, LaNoue KF, Robinson KA, et al. (2001) Excessive hexosamines block the neuroprotective effect of insulin and induce apoptosis in retinal neurons. J BiolChem 276: 43748–43755. doi:10.1074/jbc.M108594200.
47. King GL, Brownlee M (1996) The cellular and molecular mechanisms of diabetic complications. EndocrinolMetabClin North Am 25: 255–270.
48. Van Dam PS (2002) Oxidative stress and diabetic neuropathy: pathophysiological mechanisms and treatment perspectives. Diabetes Metab Res Rev 18: 176–184. doi:10.1002/dmrr.287.
49. Leske MC (2007) Open-angle glaucoma — an epidemiologic overview. Ophthalmic Epidemiol 14: 166–172. doi:10.1080/09286580701501931.
50. Patty L, Wu C, Torres M, Azen S, Varma R, et al. (2012) Validity of self-reported eye disease and treatment in a population-based study: the Los Angeles Latino Eye Study. Ophthalmology 119: 1725–1730. doi:10.1016/j.ophtha.2012.02.029.
51. MacLennan PA, McGwin G, Searcey K, Owsley C (2013) Medical record validation of self-reported eye diseases and eye care utilization among older adults. Curr Eye Res 38: 1–8. doi:10.3109/02713683.2012.733054.

MR Quantification of Total Liver Fat in Patients with Impaired Glucose Tolerance and Healthy Subjects

Zhi Dong[1,¶], Yanji Luo[1,¶], Zhongwei Zhang[2], Huasong Cai[1], Yanbing Li[3], Tao Chan[4], Ling Wu[5], Zi-Ping Li[1]*, Shi-Ting Feng[1]*

1 Department of Radiology, The First Affiliated Hospital of Sun Yat-Sen University, Guangzhou, China, **2** Department of Radiology, The University of Texas Southwestern Medical Center, Dallas, Texas, United States of America, **3** Department of Endocrinology and Diabetes Center, The First Affiliated Hospital of Sun Yat-sen University, Guangzhou, China, **4** Medical Imaging Department, Union Hospital, Hong Kong, **5** Department of Radiology, Kiang Wu Hospital, Macao

Abstract

Objective: To explore the correlations between liver fat content and clinical index in patients with impaired glucose tolerance (IGT) and healthy subjects.

Materials and Methods: 56 subjects were enrolled and each of them underwent upper-abdominal MRI examination that involved a T1 VIBE Dixon sequence. 14 was clinically diagnosed with IGT (collectively as IGT group) while 42 showed normal glucose tolerance,(collectively as NGT group). NGT group was further divided into NGTFat (BMI≥25, 18 subjects) and NGTLean (BMI<25, 24 subjects). The total liver fat contents was measured and compared with clinical findings and laboratory results in order to determine statistical correlations between these parameters. Differences among IGT, NGTFat and NGTLean groups were evaluated.

Results: For all the subjects, fat volume fractions (FVFs) ranged from 4.2% to 24.2%, positive correlations was observed with BMI, waist hip ratio(WHR), low density lipoprotein(LDL), fasting plasma insulin(FPI), homeostasis model assessment insulin resistance (HOMA-IR) and homeostasis model assessment β(HOMAβ). FVFs of IGT group (p = 0.004) and NGTFat group (p = 0.006) were significantly higher than those of NGTLean group.

Conclusions: People with higher BMI, WHR and LDL levels tend to have higher liver fat content. Patients with BMI≥25 are more likely to develop IGT. Patients with higher FVF showed higher resistance to insulin, thus obtained a higher risk of developing type 2 diabetes mellitus.

Editor: Melania Manco, Scientific Directorate, Bambino Hospital, Italy

Funding: This work was funded by National Natural Science Foundation of China (81000626), Natural Science Foundation of Guangdong Province (S2013010016004), Zhujiang Scientific and Technological New Star Foundation (2012J2200084), and the Fundamental Research Funds for the Central Universities (10ykpy11). The funders had no role in study design, data collection and analysis, decision to publish, or preparation of the manuscript.

Competing Interests: The authors have declared that no competing interests exist.

* Email: fst1977@163.com (STF); liziping163@163.com (ZL)

These authors contributed equally to this work.

¶ ZD and YJL are co-first authors on this work

Introduction

Ectopic fat deposition is commonly seen in many diseases, especially in metabolic disorders, such as obesity, insulin resistance, and other components of metabolic syndrome. It plays an important role in the development and progression of nonalcoholic fatty liver disease (NAFLD) [1–3]. It is thought to have direct positive impact on the increasing rate of obesity and NAFLD prevalence across the world [4]. According to some researchers, about 10~20% patients with NAFLD are affected by the progressive form of NAFLD, otherwise known as nonalcoholic steatohepatitis (NASH) where 20~30% of patients with NASH will develop cirrhosis and end-stage liver disease [5–7].

Liver fat content is an essential indicator for the progression of NAFLD [8]. So far, many techniques and methods have been developed for diagnosing fatty liver disease and quantifying liver fat content. This can be achieved by techniques such as liver biopsy/pathology, computed tomography (CT) scanning, ultrasound, and magnetic resonance imaging (MRI). However, all these techniques have various shortcomings. For example, the gold standard for assessing fat content in liver, biopsy/pathology, is invasive and subjective to sampling error [9–12]. CT can only be used to detect the existence of fat but not to measure the total amount of the fat content. Furthermore, the accumulative radiation exposure from repeated CT scans can be harmful which limits its role in evaluating disease progression during long term follow up. In comparison, Magnetic resonance (MR) spectroscopy has been widely-applied and can provide accurate evaluation of hepatic fat content, however, it is time consuming and evaluation only limits to part of the liver [13–15].

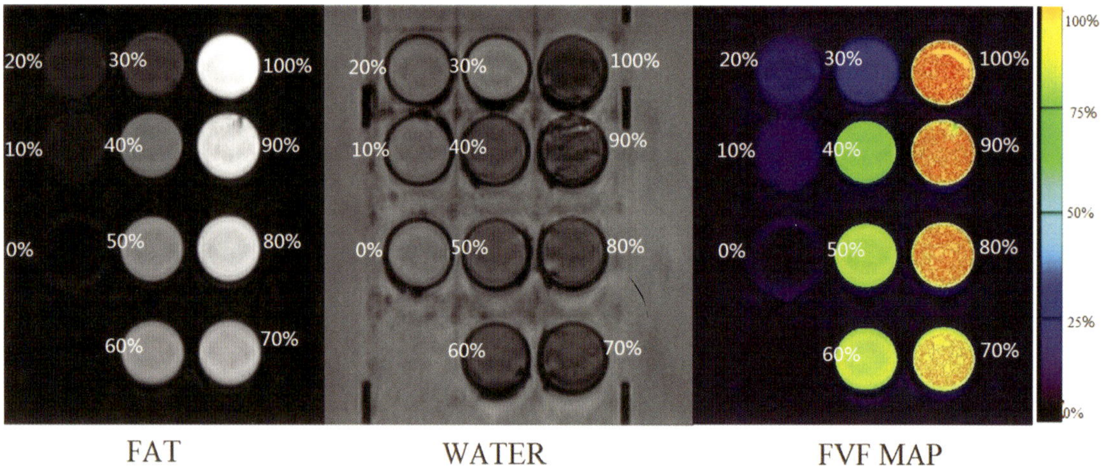

Figure 1. Results of phantom experiment. The bottle on the lower left side is filled with pure water (fat content: 0%), and the upper right one is filled with 100% peanut oil, while others have fat content ranging from 10% to 90% in sequence. In the fat phase image, the higher the fat content is, the higher signal intensity can be seen. But in water phase, the signal intensity of each bottle turned opposite to that of fat phase. The fat volume fraction (FVF) map demonstrates clear differences for different amounts of fat and water through the change of color.

MR technique for quantifying fat content is based on chemical shift imaging. It is one of the most promising techniques due to its non-invasive, radiation-free and easy-to-perform characteristics [14,16]. Dixon technique is a two-point chemical shift-based fat-water separation method described by Dixon in 1984 [17]. It acquires two images with different echo times (TE) to separate the fat signals from the water signals in the same voxel (in-phase and out-of-phase). Pure fat image and water image are obtained by the following equation:

$$W = \frac{SIP + SOP}{2}$$

$$F = \frac{SIP - SOP}{2}$$

(W: water phase; F: fat phase; SIP: signal of in-phase; SOP: signal of out-of-phase).

With this technique, the map of fat deposition in the liver can be displayed, and the fat content across the entire liver can be measured.

Clinical and laboratory parameters such as body mass index (BMI), waist hip ratio (WHR), serum triglycerides (TG), and low density lipoprotein (LDL) levels are thought to be related to extent of fat accumulation in liver [18,19]. Accurate fat quantification of the entire liver, and the investigations of the relationship between liver fat content and clinical parameters may provide information for future clinical interventions. This study aims to validate the use of Dixon technique in total liver fat content quantification, as well as to explore the correlations between liver fat content and clinical paremeters in both healthy subjects and those with impaired glucose tolerance.

Materials and Methods

Ethic statement

The study was conducted in accordance with ethical guidelines for human research, the Health Insurance Portability and Accountability Act (HIPAA) and was approved by the research ethical committee of The First Affiliated Hospital of Sun Yat-sen University. Written informed consent was obtained from all patients, and legal guardian if the patients were younger than 18 years old. Permission was obtained from the hospital for the publications of medical images seen in the Figures.

Phantom validation

We first evaluated the accuracy of the fat-quantifying technique with some fat-water phantoms. Homogeneous emulsions consisting of vegetable (peanut) oil and distilled water were prepared in 50 ml bottles, with fat volume fractions (FVF) of 0%, 10%, 20%, 30%, 40%, 50%, 60%, 70%, 80%, 90%, 100%, using a magnetic stirrer hotplate heated to 50°C. Agar gel (2% by weight) and dioctyl sulfosuccinate sodium salt (15 mmol/L) were added in each bottle to stabilize the emulsions (Figure 1) [20]. All the bottles were placed in a water tank with a temperature of 37°C (mimic the temperature of normal human body).

MR images were obtained using a 3-Tesla whole-body human MRI scanner (SIEMENS 3.0T MAGNETOM Verio). A head coil was used and T1 volumetric interpolated breath-hold examination (VIBE) Dixon sequence was applied with the following parameters: TE, 2.5 ms, 3.7 ms; TR, 5.62 ms; flip angle, 5°; receiver bandwidth, ±504.0 kHz; slice thickness, 3.0 mm. Four images of the phantoms were generated, including in-phase and out-of-phase, as well as fat and water phase images.

Subjects and clinical data

Fifty-six subjects were enrolled in the study. Oral glucose tolerance test was conducted subjects were divided into either impaired glucose tolerance (IGT) group or normal glucose tolerance (NGT) group accordingly. 14 were clinically diagnosed with impaired glucose tolerance (2 males, 12 females, age range 47~58 years old, average age was 53 years old) and 42 with normal glucose tolerance (18 males, 24 females, age range 43~57

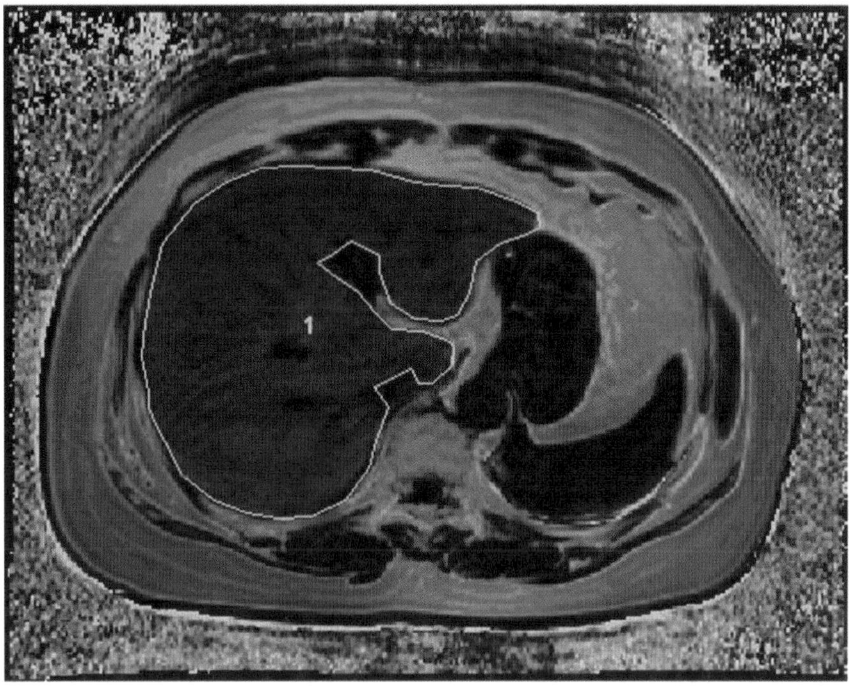

Figure 2. Irregular-shaped Regions of Interest (ROI) (1) covering the entire liver was placed in 21 consecutive slices (max-area centered) on the fat volume fraction (FVF) map of a typical patient. The average FVF in the ROI was recorded.

years old, average age 50 years old). Other clinical parameters and laboratory tests were also measured: BMI, WHR, body fat content (BFC), total cholesterol (CHOL), TG, LDL, fasting plasma insulin (FPI), homeostasis model assessment IR (HOMA-IR), homeostasis model assessmentβ (HOMAβ). NGT group was further divided into two groups according to BMI: NGTFat group, BMI >25 (the upper-limit in healthy people), 18 subjects (BMI: 26.6±1.4); NGTLean group, BMI <25, 24 subjects (BMI: 23.0±1.4). The BMI of all 14 patients in IGT group were higher than 25(BMI: 28.0±2.2).

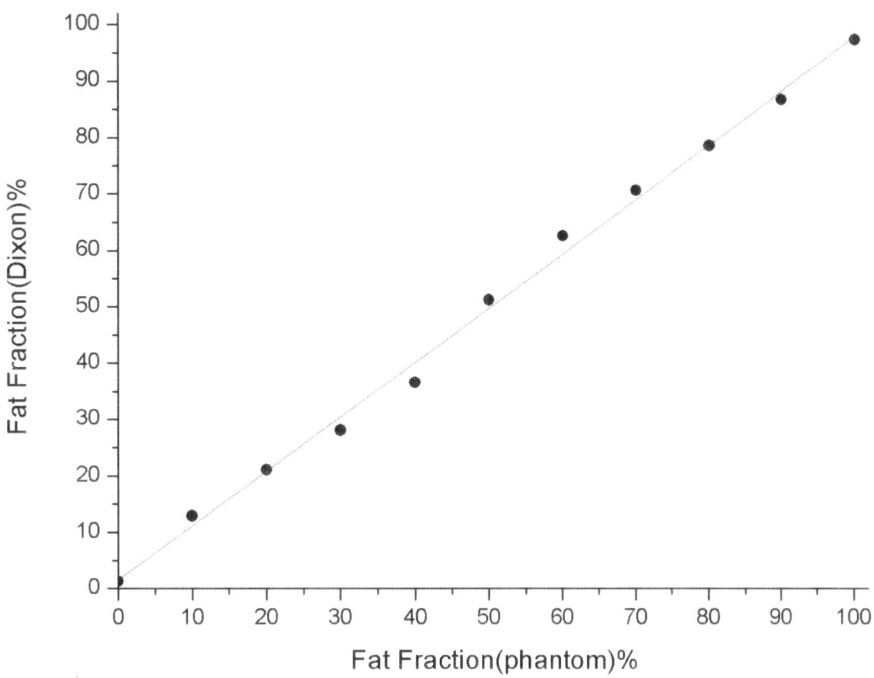

Figure 3. Correlation of actual fat volume fraction (FVF) of the water/fat phantoms against the mean fat fraction computed from Dixon technique. The best-fit-line was displayed. (r2 = 0.994, p = 0.000).

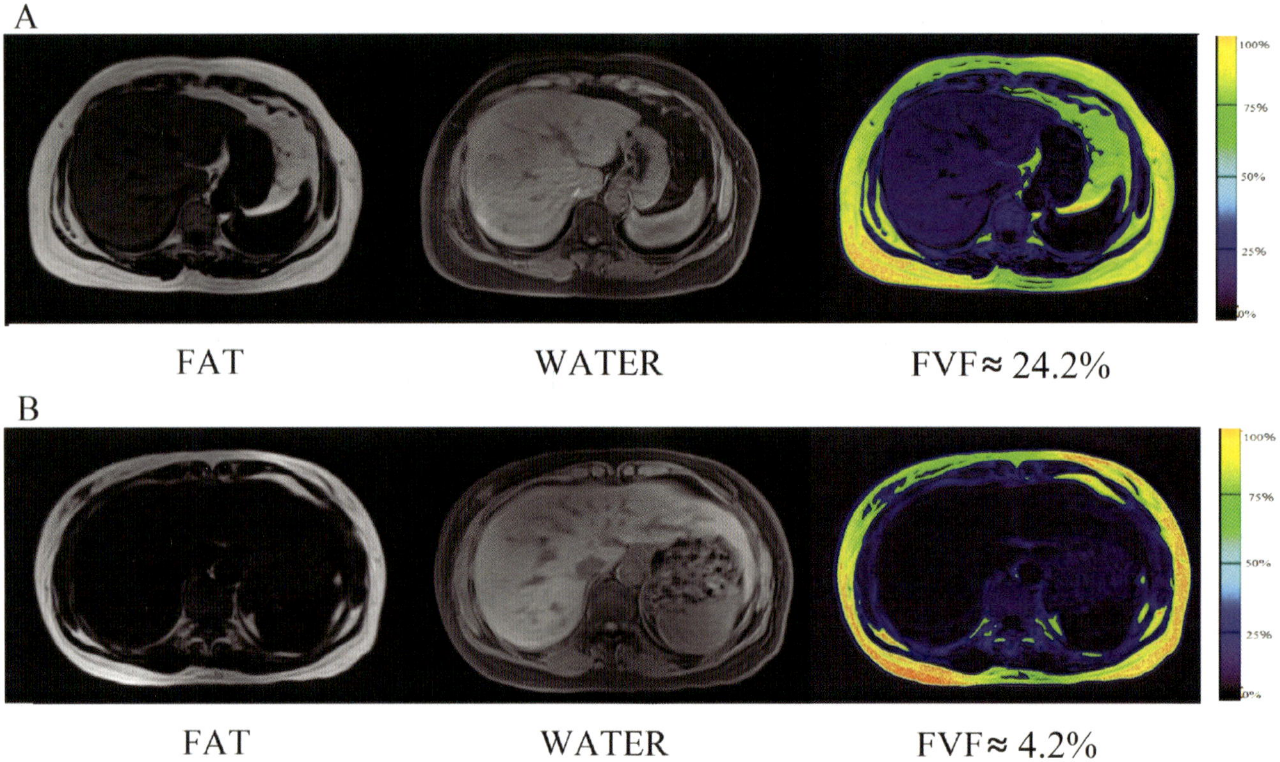

Figure 4. FVF maps of two typical subjects from IGT group (A) and NGTLean group (B). A: a 58 years old female who was diagnosed as IGT (BMI = 31.85), with a mean FVF of 24.23%. The fat phase and FVF map demonstrated that the deposition of fat is homogeneous. B: a 50 years old female (BMI = 23.13) with a mean FVF of 4.15%. The color of the liver in case B is much darker than that in case A, indicating a lower fat content.

Each subject underwent an upper-abdominal MRI examination that involved an initial set of localizer images and then a T1 VIBE Dixon sequence. The imaging parameters were the same as those in the phantom study, with TE of 2.5/3.7 ms and TR of 5.47 ms. All the subjects were imaged in supine position and carefully instructed to breath hold during end inspiration to ensure consistency amongst subjects. Four images, in-phase, out-of-phase, fat-phase and water-phase, were obtained at the same time within a single breath-hold for each patient.

MR Image post processing and analysis

Fat volume fraction (FVF) map was generated by combining the MR images obtained during both fat-phase and water-phase of each subject. This was done by using a newly designed plug-in algorithm created under MATLAB platform (MATLAB r2011b,

Table 1. Correlations between the liver FVF values and clinical parameters in all subjects as determined by Spearman correlation test.[a,b]

Variables	Correlation Coefficient	*P*
BMI	0.595	0.004
BFC	−0.024	0.915
WHR	0.432	0.045
CHOL	0.352	0.108
TG	0.689	0.019
LDL	0.455	0.033
FPI	0.886	0.019
HOMA-IR	0.886	0.019
HOMAβ	0.943	0.005

[a]FVFs have positive correlation with BMI, WHR, TG, LDL, FPI, HOMA-IR and HOMAβ, while BFC and CHOL were found to have no statistical correlation with liver fat content.
[b]FVF, fat volume fraction; BMI, body mass index; BFC, body fat content; WHR, waist hip rate; CHOL, cholesterol; TG, triglyceride; LDL, low density lipoprotein; FPI, fasting plasma insulin; HOMA-IR, homeostasis model assessment insulin resistance; HOMAβ, homeostasis model assessmentβ.

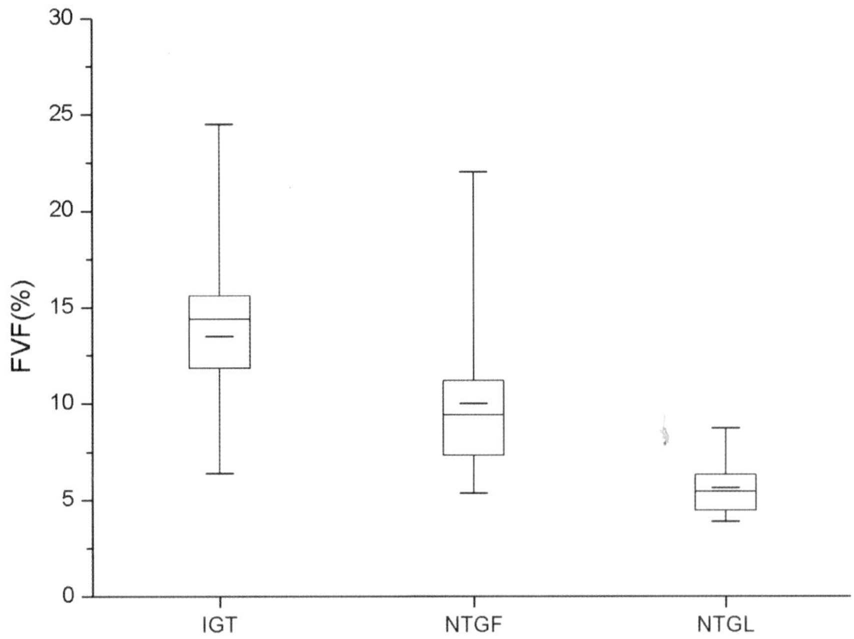

Figure 5. Boxplots of FVF values for the IFT, NGTFat and NGTLean groups. Significant differences was found between IGT group and NGTLean group (p = 0.004), as well as the NGTFat group and NGTLean group (p = 0.006). But there was no significant difference between IGT group and NGTFat group (p = 0.359).

MathWorks, America), using the following equation:

$$FVF = \frac{F}{W+F} \times 100\%$$

(FVF: fat volume fraction; F: fat volume; W: water volume).

In phantom study, two trained radiologists manually traced a round-shaped region of interest (ROI) on each bottle, and recorded the results of FVFs. The diameter of ROI is 3 cm, the size of the transverse section of the bottles. Average FVFs of each bottle were acquired.

In vivo study, two trained radiologists manually placed an irregular-shaped ROI covering the entire liver in 21 consecutive slices (max-area centered) of each patient (Figure 2). The mean FVF in the ROI of each subject was recorded.

Statistical analysis

FVF values were calculated using the Dixon technique and compared to true FVFs in the phantom experiment using linear correlation. In vivo study, statistical correlations between FVFs and results of clinical and laboratory tests were determined by using the Spearman's rank correlation. The difference in FVF between three groups was evaluated using the Wilcoxon test. A p value lower than 0.05 was considered as statistically significant. All the analyses were performed in SPSS (SPSS, Version 13.0, Chicago, IL, USA).

Results

Phantom study

Figure 1 summarizes the results from the phantom study. The bottle on the lower left side is filled will pure water (fat content: 0%), and the upper right one is filled with 100% peanut oil. Others contain fat content ranging from 10% to 90%. During the fat phase image, higher fat content was associated with a higher signal intensity. The opposite was observed during the water phase image where higher fat content was associated with a lower signal intensity. FVF map demonstrated different amounts of water/fat in the emulsions ranging from 0% to 100% with changing color. A graph comparing the actual FVF against fat fraction calculated by Dixon technique also showed excellent correlation (Figure 3, $r2 = 0.994$, $p = 0.000$)). This result indicates that Dixon technique is applicable for measuring the actual fat content of the liver.

In vivo results

For each subject, FVF maps were generated from the source images of both fat phase and water phase. Figure 4 shows the FVF maps of two typical subjects from IGT group (A) and NGTLean group (B) respectively. The darker color of the liver seen in Figure 4B indicates lower fat content in NGTLean group when compared to the IGT group as seen in Figure 4A. Furthermore, in both fat phase image and FVF map (Fig. 4A), the distribution of fat in liver in people with metabolic disorders tended to be homogeneous, which is different from fat accumulation caused by inflammation [21].

For all the subjects, FVFs ranged from 4.2% to 24.2%, and had positive correlation with BMI ($p = 0.004$), WHR ($p = 0.045$), TG ($p = 0.019$), LDL ($p = 0.033$), FPI ($p = 0.019$), HOMA-IR ($p = 0.019$) and HOMAβ ($p = 0.005$) (Table 1, Spearman's rank correlation). For IGT group, FVFs positively correlated with FPI ($p = 0.019$), HOMA-IR ($p = 0.019$), HOMAβ ($p = 0.005$), while the FVFs of healthy groups did not show significant correlation with any of these clinical parameters.

FVFs of IGT group were significantly different from those of NGTLean group ($p = 0.004$), but no significant difference was found between IGT group and NGTFat group ($p > 0.05$). FVFs of NGTLean group were also significantly different from those of NGTFat group ($p = 0.006$) (Figure 5).

Discussion

The amount of the liver fat content is essential in monitoring the progression of NAFLD and it acts as a potential indicator of underlying metabolic disorders [22]. Unlike MR spectroscopy, Dixon technique provides us with separate fat and water phase images within a single breath-hold. Dxion technique is easier to perform than MRS; and the image analysis is also more straightforward. Liver fat content measurement and detection using Dixon technique have been reported in previous studies [23–27]. For example, D'Assignies, G. et al. have evaluated the ability of MRS, Dixon technique and diffusion-weighted MR imaging (DWI) to detect liver steatosis using histopathology as a reference [23]. They have also evaluated the correlations between fat fraction (FF) measured by MRS, Dixon technique and clinical parameters such as LDL and cholesterol concentrations, which showed consistent result with our study. However, their study mainly focuses on the sensitivity, specificity and accuracy in diagnosis of liver steatosis for three different noninvasive MR techniques, MRS, Dixon technique and DWI. In another study, Houchun H. Hu and colleagues have demonstrated a strong potential for IDEAL technique (Iterative Decomposition with Echo Asymmetry and Least squares estimation, a modified Dixon technique) as a liver fat quantification tool and a valuable method for obesity research [24]. However, in the studies mentioned above, only a small oval- or square-shaped ROI on the liver was studied, hence could not appropriately evaluate the total amount of the liver fat content.

In this study, from the separate fat and water phase images, a 3D voxel-wise fat fraction map of the entire abdomen was generated which showed the spatial pattern of ectopic fat, and mean FVF of the entire liver on the map was calculated. For each subject, 21 consecutive slices (max-area centered) of the FVF map was used to generate the liver ROI, and the mean value was recorded to stand for the FVF of this subject. Proved to be dependable by the phantom study, FVFs obtained via the Dixon technique is found to approximately equate to the actual fat content throughout the liver. The spatial information of the liver fat is also readily available (Fig. 1 and Fig. 4).

Under normal circumstance, liver plays an important role in the lipid metabolism. It is involved in free fatty acid uptake from the blood to synthesize TG, essential in the lipoprotein transportation by combining different types of lipids with lipid-carrying protein. When the efficiency of TG synthesis exceeds the transporting capacity of lipoproteins, TG and other types of lipids accumulates in the liver, resulting in fatty liver, or otherwise known as, ectopic fat deposition [1,2]. Unlike fat accumulation resulted from inflammation [21], people with metabolic disorders tend to have homogeneous fat deposition, and this is demonstrated in the FVF maps. Fat accumulation caused by acute hepatitis, for instance, demonstrates focal fat content from local hepatocyte necrosis and proliferation of fibrous connective tissue. However, fat accumulation due to metabolism disorders is a systematic process, and has no region-specific predisposition. Therefore, the possible cause of liver fat deposition may be diagnosed based on the pattern of fat distribution seen in FVF map.

In our study, it was found that FVFs have positive correlations with many clinical and laboratory results such as BMI, WHR, TG and LDL, which are consistent with some previous reports [18,19]. Besides, FVFs in IGT group is significantly higher than those of NGTLean group, while there is no significant difference seen between IGT group and NGTFat group. This indicates that fat people (BMI≥25) tend to have a higher fat content in liver due to increased burden on the liver from high free fatty acids in the blood. When the burden overwhelms the ability of processing fatty acids in liver, the fat will gradually accumulate in liver and this deposition may cause fatty liver diseases. In addition, high serum free fatty acid will slow down the utilization of glucose and stimulate the secretion of insulin. This leads to increased insulin resistance over time, which may eventually progress into IGT. Thus it is possible that the subjects of NGTFat group are at higher risk of developing IGT than people with normal BMI. This can be further supported by the lack of significant differences seen in lier fat content between the IGT and NGTFat subjects where BMIs of subjects in both groups were greater than 25.

On the other hand, we have found that liver fat content did not statistically correlate with BFC. One possible explanation is that high BFC does not equate to high viscera fat content, and the latter contributes much more to the liver fat content than BFC. Instead, WHR provided better reflection regarding the fat distribution of the body. People with high WHR have more fat deposition around the abdomen and in the viscera. Therefore, the higher WHR, the higher viscera fat deposition, and the higher the fat content in liver, as well.

This study also demonstrated that liver fat content has a positive correlation with FPI, HOMA-IR and HOMAβ. That means people with higher liver fat content tend to have higher FPI, HOMA-IR and HOMAβ levels. FPI reflects the body's sensitivity to insulin. Higher FPI is associated with lower insulin sensitivity. HOMA-IR can be calculated from FPI, which reflects insulin resistance. Thus, our results may indicate that people with high HOMA-IR levels are more resistant to insulin. Insulin resistance is recognized as a main risk factor for many metabolic disorders, and it especially increases the probability to develop type 2 diabetes [28]. In our study, FVFs of IGT group was positively correlated with FPI and HOMA-IR. In other words, IGT patients with higher FVFs are more resistant to insulin, and may have a higher risk to develop type 2 diabetes mellitus. Therefore, fat content quantification using Dixon technique has its value as a prognostic tool for IGT patients.

To summarize, this study has verified an accurate, noninvasive and easy-to-perform method based on Dixon technique to quantify the fat content across the entire liver. FVF calculated with the technique reflects the actual liver fat content. The significant correlations of FVF with some other clinical parameters indicate further investigations are necessary for the epidemiology and pathophysiology of NAFLD as well as other metabolism disorders.

Acknowledgments

This work was funded by National Natural Science Foundation of China (81000626), Natural Science Foundation of Guangdong Province (S2013010016004), Zhujiang Scientific and Technological New Star Foundation (2012J2200084), and the Fundamental Research Funds for the Central Universities (10ykpy11).

Author Contributions

Conceived and designed the experiments: ZL STF. Performed the experiments: HSC ZD YJL TC LW ZWZ. Analyzed the data: ZD YJL. Contributed reagents/materials/analysis tools: HSC TC LW. Contributed to the writing of the manuscript: ZD YJL ZL STF HSC YBL TC LW ZWZ.

References

1. Clark JM (2006) The epidemiology of nonalcoholic fatty liver disease in adults. Journal of Clinical Gastroenterology 40: S5–10.
2. Kotronen A, Peltonen M, Hakkarainen A, Sevastianova K, Bergholm R, et al. (2009) Prediction of non-alcoholic fatty liver disease and liver fat using metabolic and genetic factors. Gastroenterology 137: 865–72.
3. Marchesini G, Bugianesi E, Forlani G, Cerrelli F, Lenzi M, et al. (2003) Nonalcoholic fatty liver, steatohepatitis, and the metabolic syndrome. Hepatology 37: 917–23.
4. Vernon G, Baranova A, Younossi ZM (2011) Systematic review: the epidemiology and natural history of non-alcoholic fatty liver disease and non-alcoholic steatohepatitis in adults. Alimentary Pharmacology and herapeutics 34: 274–85.
5. Bacon BR, Farahvash MJ, Janney CG, Neuschwander-Tetri BA (1994) Nonalcoholic steatohepatitis: an expanding clinical entity. Gastroenterology 107: 1103–9.
6. Angulo P (2002) Nonalcoholic fatty liver disease. N Engl J Med 346: 1221–31.
7. Wieckowska A, McCullough AJ, Feldstein AE (2007) Noninvasive diagnosis and monitoring of nonalcoholic steatohepatitis: present and future. Hepatology 46: 582–9.
8. Ligabue G, Besutti G, Scaglioni R, Stentarelli C, Guaraldi G (2013) MR quantitative biomarkers of non alcoholic fatty liver disease: technical evolutions and future trends. Quant Imaging Med Surg 3: 192–5.
9. Fernández-Salazar L, Velayos B, Aller R, Lozano F, Garrote JA (2011) Percutaneous liver biopsy: patients' point of view. Scand J Gastroenterol 46: 727–31.
10. El-Badry AM, Breitenstein S, Jochum W, Washington K, Paradis V, et al. (2009) Assessment of hepatic steatosis by expert pathologists: the end of a gold standard. Ann Surg 250: 691–7.
11. Bedossa P, Dargère D, Paradis V (2003) Sampling variability of liver fibrosis in chronic hepatitis C Hepatology 38: 1449–57.
12. Ratziu V, Charlotte F, Heurtier A, Gombert S, Giral P, et al. (2005) Sampling variability of liver biopsy in nonalcoholic fatty liver disease. Gastroenterology 128: 1898–906.
13. Bydder M, Yokoo T, Hamilton G, Middleton MS, Chavez AD, et al. (2008) Relaxation effects in the quantification of fat using gradient echo imaging. Magn Reson Imaging 26: 347–59.
14. Guiu B, Petit JM, Loffroy R, Ben Salem D, Aho S, et al. (2009) Quantification of liver fat content: comparison of triple-echo chemical shift gradient-echo imaging and in vivo proton MR spectroscopy. Radiology 250: 95–102.
15. Reeder SB, Robson PM, Yu H, Shimakawa A, Hines CD, et al. (2009) Quantification of hepatic steatosis with MRI: the effects of accurate fat spectral modeling. J Magn Reson Imaging 29: 1332–9.
16. Meisamy S, Hines CD, Hamilton G, Sirlin CB, McKenzie CA, et al. (2011) Quantification of hepatic steatosis with T1-independent, T2-corrected MR imaging with spectral modeling of fat: blinded comparison with MR spectroscopy. Radiology 258: 767–75.
17. Dixon WT (1984) Simple proton spectroscopic imaging. Radiology 153: 189–194.
18. Petta S, Amato MC, Di Marco V, Cammà C, Pizzolanti G, et al. (2012) Visceral adiposity index is associated with significant fibrosis in patients with non-alcoholic fatty liver disease. Aliment Pharmacol Ther 35: 238–47.
19. Monteiro PA, Mota J, Silveira LS, Cayres SU, Antunes BdM, et al. (2013) Morphological and metabolic determinants of nonalcoholic fatty liver disease in obese youth: a pilot study. BMC Res Notes 6: 89.
20. Bernard CP, Liney GP, Manton DJ, Turnbull LW, Langton CM (2008) Comparison of Fat Quantification Methods: A Phantom Study at 3.0T. Journal of magnetic resonance imaging 27: 192–7.
21. Kammen BF, Pacharn P, Thoeni RF, Lu Y, Qayyum A, et al. (2001) Focal fatty infiltration of the liver: analysis of prevalence and CT findings in children and young adults. Am J Roentgenol 177: 1035–9.
22. Reeder SB, Cruite I, Hamilton G, Sirlin CB (2011) Quantitative assessment of liver fat with magnetic resonance imaging and spectroscopy. J Magn Reson Imaging 34: 729–49.
23. D'Assignies G, Martin R, Abdesslem K, Luigi L, Miguel C, et al. (2009) Noninvasive quantitation of human liver steatosis using magnetic resonance and bioassay methods. Eur. Radiol 19: 2033–40.
24. Hu HH, Kim HW, Nayak KS, Goran MI (2010) Comparison of fat–water MRI and single-voxel MRS in the assessment of hepatic and pancreatic fat fractions in humans. Obesity (Silver Spring) 18: 841–7.
25. Leporq B, Ratiney H, Pilleul F, Beuf O (2013) Liver fat volume fraction quantification with fat and water T1 and T2* estimation and accounting for NMR multiple components in patients with chronic liver disease at 1.5 and 3.0 T. Eur Radiol 23: 2175–86.
26. Yokoo T, Shiehmorteza M, Hamilton G, Wolfson T, Schroeder ME, et al. (2011) Estimation of hepatic proton-density fat fraction by using MR imaging at 3.0 T. Radiology 258: 749–59.
27. Yokoo T, Bydder M, Hamilton G, Middleton MS, Gamst AC, et al. (2009) Nonalcoholic fatty liver disease: diagnostic and fat grading accuracy of low-flip-angle multiecho gradient-recalled-echo MR imaging at 1.5 T. Radiology 251: 67–6.
28. Cusi K (2009) Nonalcoholic fatty liver disease in type 2 diabetes mellitus. Curr Opin Endocrinol Diabetes Obes 16: 141–9.

Chronic Maternal Vitamin B12 Restriction Induced Changes in Body Composition & Glucose Metabolism in the Wistar Rat Offspring Are Partly Correctable by Rehabilitation

Kalle Anand Kumar[1], Anumula Lalitha[1], Umakar Reddy[2], Giriraj Ratan Chandak[2], Shantanu Sengupta[3], Manchala Raghunath[1]*

1 Division of Endocrinology and Metabolism, National Institute of Nutrition, Indian Council of Medical Research (ICMR), Hyderabad, Telangana, India, **2** Centre for Cellular and Molecular Biology (CCMB), Council of Scientific and Industrial Research (CSIR), Hyderabad, Telangana, India, **3** Institute of Genomics and Integrative Biology, Council of Scientific and Industrial Research (CSIR), New Delhi, India

Abstract

Maternal under-nutrition increases the risk of developing metabolic diseases. We studied the effects of chronic maternal dietary vitamin B12 restriction on lean body mass (LBM), fat free mass (FFM), muscle function, glucose tolerance and metabolism in Wistar rat offspring. Prevention/reversibility of changes by rehabilitating restricted mothers from conception or parturition and their offspring from weaning was assessed. Female weaning Wistar rats (n = 30) were fed *ad libitum* for 12 weeks, a control diet (n = 6) or the same with 40% restriction of vitamin B12 (B12R) (n = 24); after confirming deficiency, were mated with control males. Six each of pregnant B12R dams were rehabilitated from conception and parturition and their offspring weaned to control diet. While offspring of six B12R dams were weaned to control diet, those of the remaining six B12R dams continued on B12R diet. Biochemical parameters and body composition were determined in dams before mating and in male offspring at 3, 6, 9 and 12 months of their age. Dietary vitamin B12 restriction increased body weight but decreased LBM% and FFM% but not the percent of tissue associated fat (TAF%) in dams. Maternal B12R decreased LBM% and FFM% in the male offspring, but their TAF%, basal and insulin stimulated glucose uptake by diaphragm were unaltered. At 12 months age, B12R offspring had higher (than controls) fasting plasma glucose, insulin, HOMA-IR and impaired glucose tolerance. Their hepatic gluconeogenic enzyme activities were increased. B12R offspring had increased oxidative stress and decreased antioxidant status. Changes in body composition, glucose metabolism and stress were reversed by rehabilitating B12R dams from conception, whereas rehabilitation from parturition and weaning corrected them partially, highlighting the importance of vitamin B12 during pregnancy and lactation on growth, muscle development, glucose tolerance and metabolism in the offspring.

Editor: Cheryl S. Rosenfeld, University of Missouri, United States of America

Funding: This work was supported by a research grant (# BT/PR-7506/PID/20/294/2006) to Manchala Raghunath, Giriraj Ratan Chandak and Shantanu Sengupta, from the Department of Biotechnology, Government of India, New Delhi, India (URL: http://dbtindia.nic.in/index.asp). The authors acknowledge the support and encouragement received from the Directors of National Institute of Nutrition and the Centre for Cellular and Molecular Biology, Hyderabad in the conduct of these studies. Kalle Anand Kumar is grateful to the Indian Council of Medical Research (ICMR), India, for awarding a senior research fellowship. The funders had no role in study design, data collection and analysis, decision to publish, or preparation of the manuscript.

Competing Interests: The authors have declared that no competing interests exist.

* Email: mraghunath55@yahoo.com

Introduction

Under-nutrition continues to be a major problem in the developing world, particularly among women and children. Its adverse health effects are frequently compounded by deficiencies of micronutrients: iodine, iron, zinc, vitamin A, folic acid and vitamin B12 in particular. Chiun et al [1] reported that vitamin B12 administration to young vitamin B12 deficient female rats increased food intake, enhanced their growth rate and suggested that it may play a role in carbohydrate or fat metabolism. Conditions in the maternal womb program fetal physiology [2] and nutrition is the major intrauterine environmental factor that alters the expression of the fetal genome which may have life-long consequences. Indeed, Emerson et al [3] showed that maternal vitamin B12 deficiency decreased litter size and birth weight of the offspring compared to control diet fed rats.

Vitamin B12 is essential for neural development, myelination of nervous system and its deficiency results in neurological complications [4]. It is an important component of one carbon metabolism which modulates methylation of DNA and proteins [5]. Its deficiency increases plasma homocysteine, an independent risk factor for recurrent, spontaneous, early pregnancy losses [6]. That in patients with metabolic syndrome, folate and vitamin B12 treatment improved insulin resistance (IR) and endothelial dysfunction, in addition to decreasing homocysteine levels, suggests its importance to metabolic syndrome [7]. However, the role of maternal vitamin B12 deficiency in the development of adiposity, IR and associated diseases like type 2 diabetes (T2D) and cardio vascular diseases (CVD) in the offspring is not known.

We recently reported low birth weight in the offspring born to vitamin B12 restricted (but not folate or folate and vitamin B12 dual restricted) rat dams and that offspring of folate and/or vitamin B12 restricted rat dams weighed higher than controls at/from weaning [8]. They had higher body fat% (especially visceral fat) at/from three months of age and at 12 months had altered lipid metabolism, adipocytokine levels and were dyslipidemic. Lawlor [9] reported that birth weight of the offspring is inversely related to maternal insulin resistance and we observed earlier that after 3 months of dietary vitamin B12 restriction, female Wistar rats had increased body fat% and dyslipidemia [8], which usually precede IR. It therefore appears that B12R dams may have developed IR during pregnancy and hence the lower birth weight of the offspring.

Considering that during fetal growth, decreased muscle and soft tissue development is compensated by/associated with increased body fat [10] and we reported similar findings earlier in the offspring of rat dams deficient in a variety of micronutrients [11–15], it was considered pertinent to assess changes in the LBM and FFM in the B12R offspring and their reversibility/prevention by rehabilitation.

Growing evidence suggests that epigenetics links genetics and environment in framing endocrine function [16] and that maternal nutritional status can alter the epigenetic state of the fetal genome and imprint gene expression [17]. Epigenetic alterations in early embryos may be carried forward to subsequent developmental stages [18]. DNA methylation, histone tail modification and chromatin remodeling are the known mechanisms mediating epigenetics which affect gene expression [19]. Kevin et al [20] reported that insulin resistance and blood pressure in offspring are determined by maternal folate and methionine status during the peri-conceptional periods that would lead to epigenetic alterations like DNA methylation. Indeed, Michal et al [21] reported that pre or peri-conceptional supplementation of folic acid and vitamin B6 to mothers with history of fetal growth restriction and hyperhomocytenemia resulted in favorable perinatal outcome.

Considering that i) vitamin B12 deficiency is a significant public health problem among Indians [22], ii) maternal vitamin B12 restriction impaired body adiposity and adipose tissue function in rat offspring [8] and iii) adipose and muscle are the two insulin sensitive tissues primarily responsible for the postprandial clearance of glucose [23] we have now assessed the effects of chronic maternal vitamin B12 restriction on the development and function of muscle in Wistar rat offspring. In addition, prevention/reversibility of the changes by appropriate rehabilitation and the role if any of altered oxidative stress and antioxidant status in the changes seen in offspring were also evaluated.

Materials and Methods

Ethics statement

The experiment was conducted in outbred Wistar rats at the animal house in Centre for Cellular and Molecular Biology, Hyderabad, India, in accordance with 'principles of laboratory animal care' [24] and with the approval of the 'Institute's Ethical Committee on Animal Experiments'.

Justification for using a Wistar rat model

Rodents have been important models in fetal and neonatal studies because of the strong similarities between murine and human placentae [25]. Conventionally, albino rats have been in use to assess the effects of nutrition on development, physiology and function [25]. Therefore, we have used the Wistar rat model to assess the effects of maternal vitamin B12 restriction on the development and function of muscle (LBM) and impairment if any in IR, glucose tolerance and metabolism.

Feeding and maintenance of animals

The study design of the animal experiment is given schematically in figure 1. Outbred, weanling, female Wistar rats (n = 30) were housed individually in polypropylene cages with wire mesh bottom and maintained at 22°C±2, under standard lighting conditions (12- hour light/dark cycle). The animals were divided in to two groups and fed *ad libitum* for 12 weeks, a casein based (20% protein) (AIN 76 A) control diet (n = 6) or the same diet restricted in vitamin B12 (B12R) (n = 24). The control and vitamin B12 restricted diets were purchased from M/S Research Diets Inc., USA and all animals had free access to deionized water. Vitamin B12 content of the restricted diet was approximately 60% of that of control diet (0.006 vs 0.010 mg/kg diet); B12R diet contained 50 g pectin/kg diet (in addition to cellulose), because it has been shown earlier that pectin binds vitamin B12 in the intestine and makes it less bioavailable [26]. Daily food intake and weekly body weights were monitored till 12 weeks of feeding and their plasma folate, vitamin B12 and homocysteine levels were determined at the end of 12 weeks of feeding.

Mating of animals, pregnancy, lactation and weaning

After ensuring deficiency in B12R rats (low plasma vitamin B12 levels), they were mated with control males (@ two females per male). The day on which a vaginal plug was detected was counted as day 1 of conception/pregnancy and six pregnant B12R rats were rehabilitated with control diet from conception and their offspring were weaned on to control diet (B12RC). The remaining B12R dams (n = 18) continued on restricted diet throughout pregnancy and at/from parturition, six B12R dams were switched over to control diet and their offspring were weaned on to control diet (B12RP). At/from weaning, offspring born to six B12R dams were switched to control diet (B12RW), while the offspring born to the remaining six B12R dams continued on restricted diet (B12R). To ensure comparable nutrition to the offspring in all the groups, a uniform litter size of eight pups (equal number of males and females wherever possible) was maintained with each mother from day 3 of lactation till weaning on postnatal day 21. Considering that estrogens influence insulin action, glucose homeostasis and insulin sensitivity [27–29], we have monitored the effects in only the male offspring (n = 24 for each group) to avoid the interference of estrogens on the parameters studied and to assess the effects of maternal vitamin B12 restriction *per se* in the offspring. The plasma homocysteine and vitamin B12 status were monitored in the offspring at quarterly intervals starting from 3 months of their age.

Body composition

Body composition was determined as described by us earlier [11,12], in the female Wistar rats after three months of feeding their respective diets (just before mating) and in the offspring at 3,6,9 and 12 months of their age using total body electrical conductivity (TOBEC), a small animal body composition analysis system (model SA 3000 multi-detector; EMSCAN, Springfield,

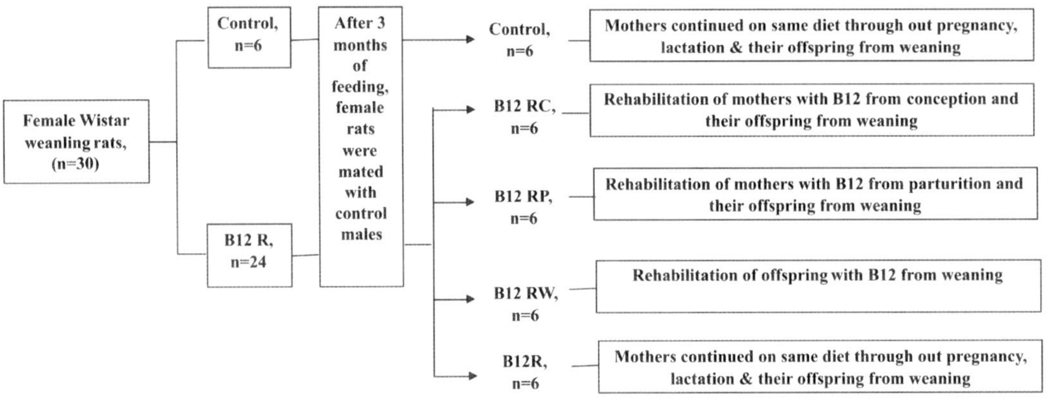

Figure 1. Feeding protocol for different groups of Wistar female rats and their male offspring. Schematic representation of the feeding protocol. Control (C), B12 restricted (B12R), B12 rehabilitation from conception (B12RC), B12 rehabilitation from parturition (B12RP), B12 rehabilitation from weaning (B12RW).

IL). Lean body mass% (LBM%) and fat free mass% (FFM%) were computed according to Morbach and Brans [30]. Difference between the LBM% and FFM% was calculated and considered to reflect the percent of tissue associated fat (TAF%).

Biochemical parameters

Plasma vitamin B12 levels were determined by RIA kit (SIEMENS Medical Solutions Diagnostics) based on a dual count, solid phase no boil assay and homocysteine concentrations were analyzed in plasma by HPLC equipped with a fluorescence detector as described earlier [31].

i) Glucose metabolism

a. Fasting glucose, insulin and insulin resistance: To assess the animals' IR status, they were fasted overnight and blood samples were collected from tail vein. Plasma glucose was estimated using an enzymatic kit (glucose-oxidase/peroxidase kit, Biosystems, Spain); plasma insulin using the RIA kit (for rat insulin from Linco Research, USA) and HOMA IR was computed as mentioned earlier [11,12] in the offspring at 3,6,9 and 12 months of their age.

b. Oral glucose tolerance and post prandial insulin resistance: At the time points mentioned above, oral glucose tolerance test was conducted in six rats (fasted overnight) from each group, by administering through oral gavage, a glucose solution (40 g/dl) @ 2.5 g/Kg body weight and blood samples were drawn before and at 30, 60 and 120 minutes after the glucose load. Plasma glucose and insulin were determined and the rats' insulin response to glucose challenge and its post-prandial insulin resistance were evaluated from the area under curve (AUC) for insulin and the ratio of AUC glucose to AUC insulin as described by us earlier [11,12].

c. Basal and insulin stimulated glucose uptake by muscle (diaphragm): Diaphragm is considered a skeletal muscle rather than smooth muscle because the cells cannot transfer nerve impulses from one to another and each cell is indeed connected to a neuron [32]. Also, GLUT1 (in membrane) and GLUT4 (in intracellular compartments), the two glucose transporters important in postprandial blood glucose clearance, are expressed both in skeletal muscle and diaphragm and diaphragm has been used commonly for determining glucose uptake by skeletal muscle [33,34]. Therefore in the present study, diaphragm has been used to study the effect of maternal vitamin B12 restriction on glucose uptake (basal and inulin stimulated) by skeletal muscle in the offspring. Briefly, intact diaphragm was isolated from the offspring of different groups at the time points mentioned earlier and the uptake of ^{3}H labeled 3-O- methyl D glucose (basal and insulin stimulated) was determined according to Kipnis and Cori [35] as described by us earlier [36].

d. Intra cellular glucose metabolism: To assess whether increased gluconeogenesis underlies the high fasting glucose levels in B12R offspring, we determined the activities of the key, rate limiting enzymes: glucokinase (GK), pyruvate-kinase (PK), fructose-1,6-bisphosphatase (FBPase) and phosphoenolpyruvate-carboxykinase (PEPCK) in the cytosolic fraction of liver using standard methods [37–40]. Activity of glucose 6 phosphatase (G6Pase) was determined in the microsomal fraction (100,000 g pellet) according to Gierow and Jergil [41].

ii) Determination of oxidative stress. Considering that i) Urakawa [42] proposed greater oxidative stress and/or decreased anti-oxidant status to be one of the mechanisms by which obesity, insulin resistance and metabolic syndrome lead to T2DM in humans and ii) we observed them earlier to be associated with maternal micronutrient deficiency induced changes in rat offspring [11,14,15], oxidative stress was determined in the liver by measuring lipid peroxidation (Malondialdehyde), protein carbonyls, reduced/oxidized glutathione (GSH/GSSG) and activity of catalase in post mitochondrial supernatant (20,000 g supernatant) as described earlier [36]. Activities of superoxide dismutase (SOD) and glutathione peroxidase were determined in the cytosol fraction according to Padmavathi et al [14].

Statistical analysis

The results are presented as mean ± SEM and the data was analyzed using SPSS statistics package (version 21.0). Values for different parameters in the offspring are given only at 3 and 12 months of age for simplicity. All parameters in B12R female rats (before mating) and their pups were compared with respective controls. Differences between control and B12R female Wistar rats (just before mating) were analyzed using the Student's 't' test. One-way ANOVA followed by post hoc least significant difference test was used to analyze the differences among the offspring of different groups at a given time point. Differences were considered significant if 'p' was at least ≤ 0.05.

Results

Effects in female Wistar rats

Food intake was comparable among control and B12R diet fed female Wistar rats. (Table 1). After 3 months of feeding, B12R rats had ~75% lower levels of plasma vitamin B12 and significantly higher plasma homocysteine levels than control rats. Although B12R rats weighed significantly heavier than controls at the end of 3 months of feeding, they had lower LBM% and FFM% than controls. However, TAF% (Table 1) and reproductive performance were comparable between the two groups of rats. (Table S1).

Effects in offspring

Body weight at birth, weaning and later. At birth, B12R offspring weighed significantly lower than controls and rehabilitation from conception (B12RC) prevented this change (Table 2). Interestingly B12R offspring weighed significantly higher than controls at/from weaning, whereas the weaning weights of B12RC, B12RP offspring were comparable to that of control offspring (Table 2). Food intake was comparable among all the groups at all the time points studied (Table S2). B12RC and B12RP prevented the increase in offspring's body weight (compared to B12R) at all the time points studied (Table 2), whereas rehabilitation from weaning (B12RW) mitigated the change *albeit* partly.

Plasma Vitamin B12 and homocysteine. As expected, B12R offspring had significantly lower (than control) levels of plasma vitamin B12 till their sacrifice at 12 months of age (Table 2). Although B12RC, B12RP and B12RW offspring had higher levels of plasma vitamin B12 than B12R, their levels were significantly lower than those of controls at all time-points studied (Table 2). Though higher in B12R offspring than controls, plasma homocysteine levels were comparable between the two groups at 12 months of age. As a corollary, plasma homocysteine levels in the rehabilitation groups were also comparable to those of control and B12R offspring at 12 months of age (Table 2).

Body composition. Both at three and twelve months of their age, LBM% and FFM% of B12R offspring were lower than those of controls (Figure 2). Although all three rehabilitation regimes appeared to correct these changes at three months of age, only B12RC and B12RP but not B12RW appeared to do so at twelve months of age. These findings suggest the importance of dams' vitamin B12 status during pregnancy and lactation in programming/modulating the body composition of the offspring.

TAF% was higher in B12R than control offspring at 3 months of age; B12RC and B12RP but not B12RW appeared to correct this change at this time point. However, TAF% was comparable among groups at twelve months of age, probably suggesting the transient nature of the change.

Glucose uptake by diaphragm. For reasons mentioned earlier (materials and methods section) diaphragm was used in this study to determine the effects if any, of maternal vitamin B12 status on glucose uptake (basal and insulin stimulated) by skeletal muscle in the offspring. No significant difference was observed among different groups either in the basal or insulin stimulated glucose uptake by diaphragm (muscle) at any of the time points studied, suggesting that maternal vitamin B12 status may not affect the function of the muscle (glucose uptake). (Table S3).

Oral glucose tolerance and insulin response to glucose challenge. Fasting hyperglycemia and hyperinsulinemia were seen in B12R offspring at 12 months of age (but not earlier). Vitamin B12 rehabilitation from conception mitigated these changes whereas rehabilitation from parturition and weaning did so *albeit* partly (Figure 3). Accordingly, HOMA IR was higher (than controls) in B12R offspring at twelve months of age and B12RC restored the values to control levels, whereas B12RP and B12RW could correct the change only partially (Figure 3).

In line with fasting hyperglycemia and hyperinsulinemia B12R offspring had higher (than controls) AUC for glucose and insulin during the oral glucose tolerance test, at 12 months of age but not earlier. While none of the rehabilitation regimes corrected the increase in AUC glucose during the OGTT (Figure 4), the increased insulin AUC was reversed by B12RC, but the mitigation was only partial by B12RP and B12RW (Figure 4). The ratio of AUC glucose and AUC insulin was comparable among groups at all-time points tested (Table S4).

Hepatic gluconeogenic enzyme activities. Phosphoenolpyruvate-carboxykinase (PEPCK) activity was higher (than controls) in B12R offspring; B12RC and B12RP but not B12RW corrected this change (Table 3). Increased activity of fructose-1-6-bisphosphotase observed in B12R offspring was corrected partially by B12RC and B12RW but it was curious that B12RP could reverse this change. Interestingly, the activities of Glucokinase and Glucose-6-phosphotase were comparable among all the groups. However, a decreased activity of pyruvate kinase was observed in B12R offspring and this was corrected by B12RC and B12RP but not by B12RW (Table 3).

Oxidative Stress in B12R rats. Increased protein carbonyl and MDA levels were observed in the liver of B12R compared to

Table 1. Food intake, plasma vitamin B12, homocysteine concentrations and body composition in female rats after 3 months of Feeding.

Parameter	Control	B12R
Food intake (g/day)	12.9±0.466	13.5±0.340
Vitamin B12 (pg/ml)	1164±8.1	277±4.54*
Homocysteine (μM)	4.89±0.358	8.03±0.208*
Body weight (g)	184±4.46	213±7.82*
LBM (%)	90.5±0.919	87.5±0.685*
FFM (%)	57.3±0.764	53.6±0.752*
TAF (%)	33.2±0.277	33.7±0.321

Food intake, plasma vitamin B12 and homocysteine concentrations, body weights, percentages of (Lean Body Mass) LBM, (Fat Free Mass) FFM and Tissue Associated Fat (TAF) in Wistar female rats fed control and vitamin B12 restricted (B12R) diets for 3 months from weaning. Values are mean ± SE (n=6).
*Significantly different from controls by Student's 't' test ($p<0.05$).

Table 2. Plasma vitamin B12, homocysteine concentrations and body weight changes in male offspring at various time points of age.

Group	Time point	Control	B12R	B12RC	B12RP	B12RW
Vitamin B12 (pg/ml)	3 months	1142 ± 60.5^{a}	32.2 ± 11.6^{b}	275 ± 29.1^{c}	301 ± 18.5^{c}	363 ± 61.5^{c}
	9 months	958 ± 17.3^{a}	132 ± 11.3^{b}	665 ± 48.6^{c}	589 ± 29.7^{c}	735 ± 49.1^{c}
	12 months	925 ± 14.2^{a}	87.0 ± 7.44^{b}	610 ± 28.9^{c}	673 ± 11.3^{c}	741 ± 15.4^{c}
Homocysteine (μM)	12 months	12.6 ± 1.80	18.5 ± 2.52	12.7 ± 2.13	13.2 ± 0.955	16.0 ± 3.55
Body weight (g)	Birth	6.41 ± 0.407^{a}	5.61 ± 0.212^{b}	6.15 ± 0.241^{a}	-	-
	Weaning	36.0 ± 2.72^{a}	51.1 ± 4.64^{b}	35.4 ± 2.51^{a}	36.0 ± 2.00^{a}	51.1 ± 4.64^{b}
	3 months	227 ± 13.7^{a}	356 ± 5.42^{b}	165 ± 9.36^{c}	223 ± 19.2^{a}	283 ± 6.66^{d}
	9 months	390 ± 16.1^{a}	546 ± 19.4^{b}	398 ± 13.7^{a}	431 ± 10.1^{c}	446 ± 4.51^{c}
	12 months	391 ± 18.8^{a}	577 ± 9.93^{b}	418 ± 15.5^{a}	406 ± 17.5^{a}	431 ± 10.4^{a}

Plasma vitamin B12 and homocysteine concentrations and body weight changes in male offspring fed different diets at different time points; control, B12 restriction (B12R), B12 rehabilitation from conception (B12RC), B12 rehabilitation from parturition (B12RP), B12 rehabilitation from weaning (B12RW). Values are mean ± SE (n = 6). **Values in a row with different superscripts (a/b/c/d) are significantly different from others at $p<0.05$ by one way ANOVA/LSD tests.**

controls. The changes were corrected *albeit* partially, by the rehabilitation regimes. Decreased concentration of reduced glutathione and increased concentration of oxidised glutathione were observed in B12R rat offspring (compared to controls) and these were also corrected partially by B12 rehabilitation. Interestingly, the ratio of reduced and oxidised glutathione (GSH/GSSG) that was significantly lowered in B12R was restored to control levels by B12RC alone, whereas the other rehabilitations showed only partial correction of the change (Table 4).

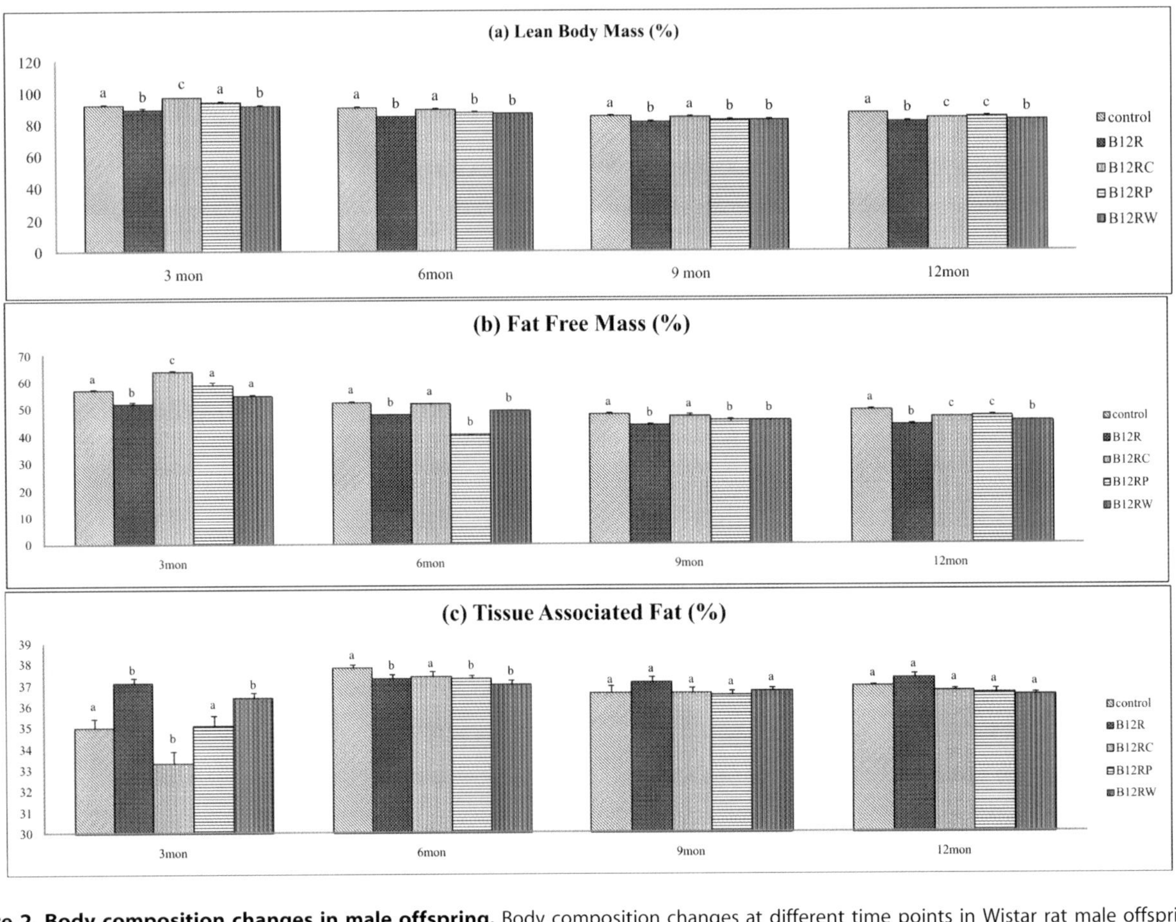

Figure 2. Body composition changes in male offspring. Body composition changes at different time points in Wistar rat male offspring fed different diets: Control (C), B12 restricted (B12R), B12 rehabilitation from conception (B12RC), B12 rehabilitation from parturition (B12RP) and B12 rehabilitation from weaning (B12RW). (a) Lean Body Mass%, (b) Fat Free Mass% (c) Tissue Associated fat%. Values are mean ± SE (n = 6). Bars with different superscripts (a/b/c) are significantly different from one another at $p<0.05$ by one way ANOVA/LSD test.

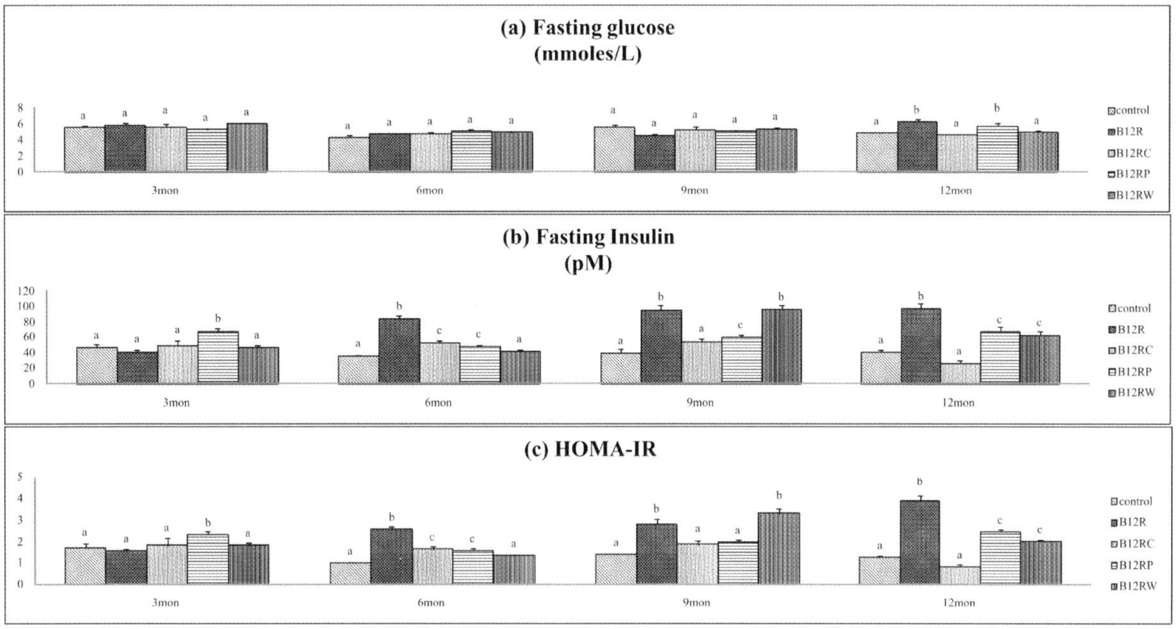

Figure 3. Glucose tolerance and insulin resistance parameters in male offspring. Glucose tolerance and insulin resistance parameters at different time points in Wistar rat male offspring fed different diets: Control (C), B12 restricted (B12R), B12 rehabilitation from conception (B12RC), B12 rehabilitation from parturition (B12RP) and B12 rehabilitation from weaning (B12RW). (a) Fasting glucose (mmol/L), (b) Fasting insulin (pM), (c) HOMA-IR. Values are mean ± SE (n = 6). Bars with different superscripts (a/b/c) are significantly different from one another at $p<0.05$ by one way ANOVA/LSD test.

A significant decrease was observed in the activity of superoxide dismutase (SOD) and catalase in B12R rats and this was corrected/restored to control levels by all three rehabilitation regimes. However, glutathione peroxidase activity was comparable among all the groups (Table 4).

Discussion

Micronutrients are well known to be associated with metabolic diseases like Type 2 diabetes, Coronary artery disease etc. We had shown earlier that chronic dietary vitamin B12 restriction *per se* increased the body weight and body fat specially the visceral adiposity [8] in female Wistar rats. We now report here for the first time to the best of our knowledge that chronic dietary vitamin B12 restriction *per se* decreased the % of LBM and FFM without affecting their TAF%. Taken together with our earlier report the present findings indicate that chronic vitamin B12 restriction in rats increased only central adiposity but not tissue associated fat, implying that the decrease observed in LBM% and FFM% could be due to decreased soft tissue (muscle?) mass.

In line with decreased litter size and birth weight reported earlier in the offspring of vitamin B12 deficient mothers [3], maternal vitamin B12 restriction decreased the birth weight of the offspring highlighting the importance of maternal vitamin B12

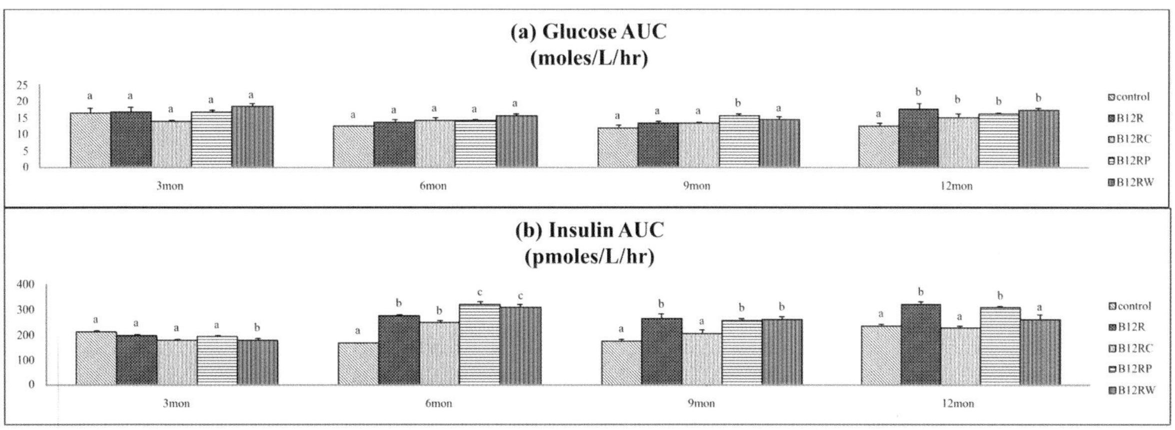

Figure 4. Glucose and insulin AUC during oral glucose tolerance test. Area Under Curves (AUC) of Glucose and insulin at different time points in Wistar rat male offspring fed different diets: Control (C), B12 restricted (B12R), B12 rehabilitation from conception (B12RC), B12 rehabilitation from parturition (B12RP) and B12 rehabilitation from weaning (B12RW). (a) Glucose AUC (moles/L/hr), (b) Insulin AUC (pmoles/L/hr). Values are mean ± SE (n = 6). Bars with different superscripts (a/b/c) are significantly different from one another at $p<0.05$ by one way ANOVA/LSD test.

Table 3. Specific activities of rate limiting enzymes involved in carbohydrate metabolism in male offspring.

Enzyme (units/ml/mg protein)	Control	B12R	B12RC	B12RP	B12RW
Phosphoenol-pyruvate-carboxykinase	1.54±0.253[a]	3.47±0.604[b]	1.68±0.221[a]	2.61±0.609[a]	3.07±0.309[b]
Fructose-1,6-bisphosphotase	1.26±0.114[a]	2.99±0.519[b]	2.28±0.131[c]	1.23±0.209[a]	2.00±0.138[c]
Glucose-6-phosphotase	3.17±0.250	3.22±0.129	3.21±0.132	3.86±0.439	3.39±0.118
Glucokinase	1.22±0.283	1.08±0.209	1.16±0.237	1.12±0.200	1.02±0.093
Pyruvatekinase	3.11±0.249[a]	1.54±0.278[b]	2.96±0.786[a]	2.61±0.512[a]	1.30±0.341[b]

Specific activities of rate limiting enzymes involved in carbohydrate metabolism in male offspring fed different diets at 12 months of age; control, B12 restriction (B12R), B12 rehabilitation from conception (B12RC), B12 rehabilitation from parturition (B12RP), B12 rehabilitation from weaning (B12RW). **Values are mean ± SE (n = 6). Values in a row with different superscripts (a/b/c) are significantly different from one another at p<0.05 by one way ANOVA/LSD tests.**

status in fetal development. Our findings are in line with recent studies demonstrating strong association between vitamin B12 and intrauterine growth retardation [43] and the influence of erythrocyte folate and serum vitamin B12 status on birth weight [44]. They also agree with the Pune maternal nutritional study which demonstrated micronutrient deficiencies to be important limiting factors for fetal growth in undernourished communities [45]. That rehabilitation of pregnant B12R dams from conception restored the offspring's birth weight to controls appears to validate this inference and is in agreement with the report that maternal iron supplementation improved the birth weight [46].

Rehabilitating vitamin B12 restricted dams from conception/ parturition or their offspring from weaning improved the plasma vitamin B12 levels of the offspring, but the levels were lower than those of controls even at twelve months of their age, perhaps suggesting that vitamin B12 deficiency created in dams may not be mitigated completely even on long term rehabilitation. Nevertheless, rehabilitation could prevent the marginal increase in plasma homocysteine levels in B12R offspring, perhaps be due to the fact that there was no concurrent folate deficiency in the animals. Although the higher body weights (than controls) of B12R dams and their offspring from weaning onwards seems to suggest greater feed efficiency in B12R rats, our finding that the increased weight was associated with increased body fat rather than LBM or FFM negates such an inference.

Abundant literature indicates altered body adiposity and lipid metabolism to be the earliest changes seen, much before tissue insulin resistance manifests [47,48]. We reported earlier that although the birth weight in B12R pups were lower than the controls, the body weight increased with age and was significantly higher than that of controls at 12 months. Further, the increased body weight of the B12R offspring was associated with increased body fat percentage (especially central adiposity) [8]. We now report the decrease in the % of LBM and FFM (but not TAF%) in the B12R dams and offspring suggesting that the decreased LBM% and FFM% could indeed be due to an absolute decrease in the soft tissue (muscle?) mass. Considering that adipose and muscle are the two insulin sensitive tissues primarily responsible for the postprandial clearance of glucose [23], it is evident from these results that maternal vitamin B12 restriction altered the offspring's body composition (specially of adipose and muscle) in a way suggestive of their predisposal to insulin resistance in later life. It was interesting that though maternal vitamin B12 restriction decreased LBM% and FFM% suggestive of decreased muscle mass, it did not affect the muscle function as indicated by our finding that basal or insulin stimulated glucose uptake by the muscle (diaphragm) were not affected in B12R offspring.

Our findings are in line with the following literature: i) Skeletal muscle develops in the early and mid-gestation and nutritional insult at this stage might impair muscle development affecting muscle fiber number and composition, which may predispose the

Table 4. Oxidative stress markers, specific activity of antioxidant enzymes in liver tissues of male offspring at 12 months of their age.

Parameter	Control	B12R	B12RC	B12RP	B12RW
Proteincarbonyls (nmoles/mg protein)	1.05±0.156[a]	2.77±0.148[b]	1.92±0.405[c]	1.83±0.366[a]	2.02±0.445[b]
Malondialdehyde (nmoles/mg protein)	0.413±0.079[a]	0.990±0.135[b]	0.847±0.222[b]	0.751±0.195[a]	0.524±0.108[a]
Reduced glutathione (μmol/mg protein)	0.764±0.097[a]	0.278±0.035[b]	0.605±0.082[a]	0.652±0.097[a]	0.521±0.100[c]
Oxidised glutathione (μmol/mg protein)	4.05±0.165[a]	6.81±0.311[b]	3.42±0.195[a]	5.68±0.249[c]	5.61±0.170[c]
Reduced glutathione (GSH)/oxidized glutathione (GSSG)	0.191±0.027[a]	0.041±0.005[b]	0.174±0.020[a]	0.112±0.012[c]	0.092±0.018[c]
Superoxidedismutase (units/ml/mg protein)	0.820±0.057[a]	0.302±0.045[b]	0.743±0.052[a]	0.707±0.101[a]	0.987±0.182[a]
Glutathioneperoxidase (units/ml/mg protein)	0.223±0.020	0.238±0.038	0.228±0.027	0.220±0.023	0.294±0.039
Catalase (units/ml/mg protein)	0.079±0.006[a]	0.030±0.003[b]	0.055±0.008[a]	0.062±0.018[a]	0.055±0.006[a]

Oxidative stress and specific activities of antioxidant enzymes in male offspring fed different diets at 12 months of age; control, B12 restriction (B12R), B12 rehabilitation from conception (B12RC), B12 rehabilitation from parturition (B12RP), B12 rehabilitation from weaning (B12RW). Values are mean ± SE (n = 6). **Values in a row with different superscripts (a/b/c) are significantly different from others at p<0.05 by one way ANOVA/LSD tests.**

offspring to obesity and type 2 diabetes [49], ii) Nutrient deficiencies in ruminants during midgestation reduce the secondary muscle fiber formation [10] and iii) Children born to vitamin B12 deficient mothers were reported to have a reduced cardiac sympathetic activity [50]. Considering that up-regulation of Wnt/β-catenin pathway promotes myogenesis and down-regulation enhances adipogenesis [10], it will be interesting to decipher the role if any of this mechanism in mediating the maternal Vitamin B12 restriction induced changes in adipose and muscle development in the offspring. That changes in LBM% and FFM% were at least partially corrected by B12RC and B12RP but not by B12RW again seems to confirm the importance of vitamin B12 during pregnancy and lactation in determining/programming the soft tissue development in the offspring. This finding is in line with a previous report that maternal zinc supplementation improved lean tissue mass accretion in the offspring [51]. It is also supported by the report that maternal folate supplementation reduced the risk of developing cardiovascular diseases in their offspring [52].

Maternal vitamin B12 deficiency is associated with gestational diabetes and later T2D in mothers and offspring [53]. Yajnik et al [54] proposed that low maternal vitamin B12 with high folate levels could be an important contributor to the epidemic of adiposity and type 2 diabetes in India. In line with these reports maternal vitamin B12 restriction induced fasting hyper-insulinemia and insulin resistance (increased HOMA-IR) in the offspring as early as six months of age, whereas fasting hyper-glycemia and impaired glucose tolerance were observed at 12 months of age. Indeed at 12 months of age, B12R offspring were insulin resistant both under fasting (high HOMA IR) and fed conditions (higher AUC insulin during OGTT). These observations are also in agreement with reports that maternal vitamin D deficiency was associated with poor muscle mass and higher insulin resistance in their offspring [55]. The importance of maternal vitamin B12 status in modulating insulin sensitivity/resistance in the offspring and their probable causal relationship is apparent from the finding that the changes were corrected by B12RC. Further, these findings corroborate our recent observations in maternal Cr restricted offspring [14] and partly agree partially with those in MgR offspring [12].

That the fasting hyperglycemia in B12R offspring could be due to altered intracellular glucose metabolism was studied next. Indeed, the increase in the activities of phosphoenolpyruvate-carboxykinase (PEPCK) and fructose-1-6-bisphosphotase in the liver of the B12R rat offspring appears to suggest increased gluconeogenesis in B12R offspring. That activity of PEPCK was reversed by B12RC but only partly by B12RP and B12RW, whereas that of fructose-1-6-bisphosphotase was reversed by B12RP and partly by B12RC and B12RW, not only suggest their causal relationship but also the differential effects of vitamin B12 on these enzymes of gluconeogenic pathway. In line with these findings, there was a decreased activity of *pyruvatekinase* in B12R offspring and was reversed by B12RC and B12RP but not by B12RW. It was however intriguing that glucokinase and glucose-6-phosphatase activities were unaffected in B12R offspring. These findings thus reiterate the importance of maternal vitamin B12 status during pregnancy and lactation in modulating/programming intracellular glucose metabolism (e.g., increasing gluconeogenesis) in the offspring.

Inflammation and oxidative stress play a key role in the development of adiposity in the offspring, while the restoration of antioxidant status improved the condition [56]. Oxidative stress is proposed to be a mechanism through which obesity, insulin resistance and metabolic syndrome lead to T2DM in humans [42]. Considering that maternal dietary restriction of a variety of micronutrients resulted in similar phenotypic changes in rat offspring [57], the present findings of similar nature in B12R offspring prompted us to decipher the probable associated/underlying common mechanism(s). The observed increase in the levels of MDA, protein carbonyls, oxidized glutathione and decreased levels of reduced glutathione along with decreased activities of SOD and catalase strongly indicate that increased oxidative stress probably due to decreased antioxidant capacity could be a common underlying/associated mechanism. That these changes also were corrected by rehabilitation *albeit* partially probably suggest a causal relationship between maternal vitamin B12 status and oxidative stress in the offspring. Unlike the SOD and catalase activities, glutathione-peroxidase activity was increased in B12R offspring corroborating the differential modulation of antioxidant enzyme activities by maternal vitamin B12 restriction, probably to cope up with increased oxidative stress. These findings are in general agreement with earlier observations in the offspring of various vitamin and mineral restricted rats [11,14,15,58–62].

We recently identified 38 differentially expressed proteins in the liver of B12R offspring that were enriched in pathways regulating amino acid, lipid and carbohydrate metabolism [63] and also reported the age dependent differential expression of peroxisome proliferator activated receptor (PPAR) α and γ in the liver of B12R pups. Vitamin B12, folic acid and DHA play an important role in one carbon metabolism and influence global DNA methylation in placenta [64] altering gene expression. Thus it seems possible that the changes observed in the expression of various proteins/genes could be due to the modulation of epigenetics by the maternal vitamin B12 status. Indeed Ian et al [65] demonstrated the reversal of maternally inherent epigenomic marks through methyl supplementation in adult offspring suggesting the importance of one carbon metabolic pathway and hence vitamin B12 status. Studies are in progress in B12R offspring to assess the epigenetic changes if any that underlie the altered gene expression and their modulation by rehabilitation.

In conclusion, maternal vitamin B12 restriction decreased the % of LBM and FFM in the offspring but had no effect on their TAF% or glucose uptake (basal and insulin stimulated) by the muscle. Nevertheless the offspring were insulin resistant, impaired glucose tolerant and increased hepatic gluconeogenesis appeared to be a mechanism underlying fasting hyperglycemia. Increased oxidative stress perhaps due to reduced anti-oxidant enzyme activity seems to underlie the effects of maternal vitamin B12 restriction, while differential regulation of gene expression by modulating epigenetics may be another mechanism. That rehabilitation from conception and parturition but not weaning, corrected maternal vitamin B12 restriction induced changes (including those in oxidative stress) in the offspring not only highlight the role of oxidative stress in mediating these changes but also the importance of vitamin B12 in fetal programming of the body composition and glucose metabolism in their later life. Our findings are in line with the hypothesis that improved environmental conditions (e.g., maternal nutrition) would eventually lead to a decline in the prevalence of type 2 diabetes and other cardiovascular risk factors, as better maternal health and nutrition result in improved fetal growth [66].

Supporting Information

Table S1 Reproductive Performance of Wistar female rats fed control and vitamin B12 restricted diets (B12R) for 3 months from weaning.

Table S2 Food intake (grams/day) by male offspring at different time points. Food intake by male offspring at different time points; control, B12 restriction (B12R), B12 rehabilitation from conception (B12RC), B12 rehabilitation from parturition (B12RP), B12 rehabilitation from weaning (B12RW). Values are mean ± SE (n = 6).

Table S3 Glucose uptake by diaphragm (nmol/hour/gram tissue) of male offspring of different groups at 12 months of age. Glucose uptake by diaphragm in male offspring at 12 months of age. Control, B12 restriction (B12R), B12 rehabilitation from conception (B12RC), B12 rehabilitation from parturition (B12RP), B12 rehabilitation from weaning (B12RW). Values are mean ± SE (n = 6).

Table S4 AUC glucose: AUC insulin ratio in the offspring during oral glucose tolerance test. Area Under Curve (AUC) ratio of glucose and insulin at different time points of their age. Control, B12 restriction (B12R), B12 rehabilitation from conception (B12RC), B12 rehabilitation from parturition (B12RP), B12 rehabilitation from weaning (B12RW). Values are mean ± SE (n = 6). Values in a column (a,b) with different superscripts are significantly different from one another at $p<0.05$ by one way ANOVA/LSD tests.

Acknowledgments

The authors acknowledge the support and encouragement received from the Directors of National Institute of Nutrition and the Centre for Cellular and Molecular Biology, Hyderabad, India, in the conduct of these studies.

Author Contributions

Conceived and designed the experiments: MR GRC SS. Performed the experiments: KAK AL UR. Analyzed the data: KAK MR. Contributed reagents/materials/analysis tools: GRC SS. Contributed to the writing of the manuscript: KAK MR.

References

1. Ling CT, Chow BF (1952) Effect of vitamin B12 on the body composition of rats. J Biol Chem 198: 439–444.
2. Barker DJ (2004) The developmental origins of adult disease. J Am Coll Nutr 23: 588S–595S.
3. Emerson G, Wurtz E, Zanetti ME (1949) Vitamin B12-a growth factor for young rats. Fed Proc 8: 381–382.
4. Bourre JM (2006) Effects of nutrients (in food) on the structure and function of the nervous system: update on dietary requirements for brain Part 1: Micronutrients. J Nutr Health Aging 10: 377–385.
5. Selhub J (2002) Folate, vitamin B12 and vitamin B6 and one carbon metabolism. J Nutr Health Aging 6: 39–42.
6. Nelen W, Blom H, Steegers E, Den HM, Thomas C, et al. (2000) Homocysteine and folate levels as risk factors for recurrent early pregnancy loss. Obstet Gynecol 95: 519–524.
7. Setola E, Monti LD, Galluccio E, Palloshi A, Fragasso G, et al. (2004) Insulin resistance and endothelial function are improved after folate and vitamin B12 therapy in patients with metabolic syndrome: relationship between homocysteine levels and hyperinsulinemia. Eur J Endocrinol 151: 483–9.
8. Kalle AK, Lalitha A, Pavithra D, Padmavathi IJN, Manisha G, et al. (2013) Maternal dietary folate and/or vitamin B12 restrictions alter body composition (adiposity) and lipid metabolism in Wistar rat offspring. J Nutr Biochem 24: 25–31. doi:10.1016/j.jnutbio.2012.01.004.
9. Lawlor DA, George DS, Shah E (2002) Birth weight of offspring and insulin resistance in late adulthood: cross sectional survey. BMJ 325: 359. doi:http://dx.doi.org/10.1136/bmj.325.7360.359.
10. Du M, Tong J, Zhao J, Underwood KR, Zhu M, et al. (2010) Fetal programming of skeletal muscle development in ruminant animals. J Anim Sci 88: E51–E60. doi:10.2527/jas.2009-2311.
11. Venu L, Harishankar N, Prasanna TK, Raghunath M (2004a) Maternal dietary vitamin restriction increases body fat content but not insulin resistance in WNIN rat offspring up to 6 months of age. Diabetologia 47: 1493–1501.
12. Venu L, Harishankar N, Prasanna KT, Raghunath M (2004b) Does maternal dietary mineral restriction per se predispose the offspring to insulin resistance? Eur J Endocrinol 151: 287–294.
13. Padmavathi IJN, Kishore YD, Venu L, Manisha G, Harishankar N, et al. (2009) Prenatal and perinatal zinc restriction: effects on body composition, glucose tolerance and insulin response in rat offspring. Exp Physiol 94: 761–769. doi:10.1113/expphysiol.2008.045856.
14. Padmavathi IJN, Rao KR, Venu L, Manisha G, Kalle AK, et al. (2010) Chronic Maternal Dietary Chromium Restriction Modulates Visceral Adiposity. Probable Underlying Mechanisms. Diabetes 59: 98–104. doi:10.2337/db09-0779.
15. Manisha G, Sainath PB, Padmavathi IJN, Venu L, Kalle AK, et al. (2011) Maternal manganese restriction increases susceptibility to high fat diet induced dyslipidemia and altered adipose function in WNIN male rat offspring. Exp Diabetes Res 2011: 486316. (doi:10.1155/2011/486316).
16. Zhang X, Ho SM (2011) Epigenetics meets endocrinology. J Mol Endocrinol 46: R11–32.
17. Heijmans BT, Tobi EW, Stein AD, Putter H, Blauw GJ, et al. (2008) Persistent epigenetic differences associated with prenatal exposure to famine in humans. PNAS 105: 17046–49.
18. Waterland RA, Jirtle RL (2004) Early nutrition, epigenetic changes at transposons and imprinted genes, and enhanced susceptibility to adult chronic diseases. Nutrition 20: 63–68.
19. Jaenisch R, Bird A (2003) Epigenetic regulation of gene expression: how the genome integrates intrinsic and environmental signals. Nat Genet (Suppl.) 33: 245–254.
20. Sinclair KD, Allegrucci C, Singh R, Gardner DS, Sebastian S, et al. (2007) DNA methylation, insulin resistance and blood pressure in offspring determined by maternal periconceptional B vitamin and methionine status. PNAS 104: 19351–19356.
21. Leeda M, Riyazi N, De Vries JIP, Jakobs C, Van Geijn HP, et al. (1998) Effects of folic acid and vitamin B6 supplementation on women with hyperhomocysteinemia and a history of preeclampsia or fetal growth restriction. Am J Obstet Gynecol 179: 135–9.
22. Sargoor RV, Krishnaveni GV, Srinivasan K, Wills AK, Sumithra M, et al. (2010) Higher Maternal Plasma Folate but Not Vitamin B-12 Concentrations during Pregnancy Are Associated with Better Cognitive Function Scores in 9- to 10- Year-Old Children in South India. J Nutr 140: 1014–1022. doi:10.3945/jn.109.118075.
23. Panayota M, Raptis SA George D (2010) Insulin action in hyperthyroidism: A focus on muscle and adipose tissue. Endocrine Reviews 31: 663–79. doi:10.1210/er.2009-0046.
24. US Department of Health, Education and Welfare: *Guide for the Care and Use of Laboratory Animals*. (1985) Washington, DC, U.S. Govt. Printing Office, (NIH publ. no. 85–23).
25. Caroline EB, Mark AH (2001) Animal models and programming of the metabolic syndrome. Br Med Bull 60: 103–121. doi:10.1093/bmb/60.1.103.
26. Choi SW, Simonetta F, Haifa G, Pamela JB, Jacob S, et al. (2004) Vitamin B-12 Deficiency Induces Anomalies of Base Substitution and Methylation in the DNA of Rat Colonic Epithelium. J Nutr 134: 750–755.
27. Nuutila P, Knuuti MJ, Maki M, Laine H, Ruotsalainen U, et al. (1995) Gender and insulin sensitivity in the heart and in skeletal muscles. Studies using positron emission tomography. Diabetes 44: 31–36.
28. Donahue RP, Bean JA, Donahue RA, Goldberg RB, Prineas RJ (1997) Insulin response in a triethnic population: effects of sex, ethnic origin, and body fat. Miami Community Health Study. Diabetes Care 20: 1670–1676.
29. Louet JF, LeMay C, Mauvais-Jarvis F (2004) Antidiabetic actions of estrogen: insight from human and genetic mouse models. Curr Atheroscler Rep 6: 180–185. DOI:10.1007/s11883-004-0030-9.
30. Morbach CA, Brans YW (1992) Determination of body composition in growing rats by total body electrical conductivity. J Pediatr Gastroenterol Nutr 14: 283–292.
31. Shantanu S, Chen H, Toqawa T, DiBello PM, Majors AK, et al. (2001) Albumin thiolate anion is an intermediate in the formation of albumin-S S-homocysteine. J BiolChem 276: 30111–30117.
32. Geraldine FG, Helen AP (1966) Cytological studies of fiber types in skeletal muscle. A comparative study of the mammalian diaphragm. J Cell Biol 28: 333–354. Doi:10.1083/Jcb.28.2.333.
33. Wardzala LJ, Jeanrenaud B (1983) Identification of the D-glucose-inhibitable cytochalasin B binding site as the glucose transporter in rat diaphragm plasma and microsomal membranes. Biochem Biophys Acta 730: 49–56.
34. Karen LY (1999) Engagement Of The Insulin-Sensitive Pathway In The Stimulation Of Glucose Transport By A-Lipoic Acid. M. Sc. Thesis. University Of Toronto. Available at Government of Canada website: http://www.collectionscanada.gc.ca/obj/s4/f2/dsk1/tape7/PQDD_0020/MQ45881.pdf. Accessed 2014 Oct 3.
35. Kipnis DM, Cori CF (1957) Studies of tissue permeability. III. The effect of insulin on pentose uptake by the diaphragm. J Biol Chem 224: 681–693.

36. Venu L, Padmavathi IJN, Kishore YD, Bhanu NV, Rao KR, et al. (2008) Long-term effects of maternal magnesium restriction on adiposity and insulin resistance in rat pups. Obesity 16: 1270–6. doi:10.1038/oby.2008.72.
37. Pilkis SJ (1975) Glucokinase of rat liver. Methods Enzymol 42: 31–39.
38. Bucher T, Pfleiderer G (1955) Pyruvate kinase from muscle. Methods Enzymol 1: 435–440.
39. Marcus F, Rittenhouse J, Chatterjee T, Hosey MM (1982) Fructose-1,6-bisphosphatase from rat liver. Methods Enzymol 90: 352–357.
40. Burgess SC, He T, Yan Z, Lindner J, Sherry AD, et al. (2007) Cytosolic phosphoenolpyruvatecarboxykinase does not solely control the rate of hepatic gluconeogenesis in the intact mouse liver. Cell Metab 5: 313–20.
41. Gierow P, Jergil B (1982) Spectrophotometric method for glucose-6-phosphate phosphatase. Methods Enzymol 89: 44–47.
42. Urakawa H, Akira K, Yasuhiro S, Gabazza EC, Murashima S, et al. (2003) Oxidative Stress Is Associated with Adiposity and Insulin Resistance in Men. J Clin Endocrinol Metab 88: 4673–4676.
43. Muthayya S, Kurpad AV, Duggan CP, Bosch RJ, Dwarkanath P, et al. (2006) Low maternal vitamin B12 status is associated with intrauterine growth retardation in urban South Indians. Eur J Clin Nutr 60: 791–801. doi:10.1038/sj.ejcn.1602383.
44. Caroline LR, Mark SP, Parker L (2005) The influence of erythrocyte folate and serum vitamin B12 status on birth weight. Br J Nutr 93: 593–599.
45. Shobha R, Yajnik CS, Asawari K, Fall CHD, Margetts BM, et al. (2001) Intake of micronutrient-rich foods in rural Indian mothers is associated with the size of their babies at birth: Pune maternal nutrition study. J Nutr 131: 1217–1224.
46. Usha R (2004) Nutrition and low birth weight: from research to practice. Am J ClinNutr 79: 17–21.
47. Jones AP, Friedman MI (1982) Obesity and adipocyte abnormalities in offspring of rats undernourished during pregnancy. Science 215: 1518–9.
48. Smith U (2002) Impaired ('diabetic') insulin signaling and action occur in fat cells long before glucose intolerance- is insulin resistance initiated in the adipose tissue? Int. J. Obes.Relat. Metab. Disord. 26: 897–904. DOI:10.1038/sj.ijo.0802028.
49. Zhu MJ, Ford SP, Means WJ, Hess BW, Nathanielsz PW, et al. (2006) Maternal nutrient restriction affects properties of skeletal muscle in offspring. J Physiol 575: 241–250.
50. Sucharita S, Pratibha D, Tinku T, Krishnamachari S, Kurpad AV, et al. (2014) Low maternal vitamin B12 status during pregnancy is associated with reduced heart rate variability indices in young children. Matern Child Nutr 10: 226–233.
51. Lora LI, Zavaleta N, Zulema L, Anuraj HS, Caulfield LE (2008) Maternal zinc supplementation and growth in Peruvian infants. Am J Clin Nutr 88: 154–160.
52. Torrens C, Brawley L, Anthony FW, Dance CS, Rebecca U, et al. (2006) Folate Supplementation During Pregnancy Improves Offspring Cardiovascular Dysfunction Induced by Protein Restriction. Hypertension 47: 982–987.
53. Krishnaveni GV, Hill JC, Veena SR, Bhat DS, Wills AK, et al. (2009) Low plasma vitamin B12 in pregnancy is associated with gestational 'diabesity' and later diabetes. Diabetologia 52: 2350–2358.
54. Yajnik CS, Deshpande SS, Jackson AA, Refsum H, Rao S, et al. (2008) Vitamin B_{12} and folate concentrations during pregnancy and insulin resistance in the offspring: the Pune Maternal Nutrition Study. Diabetologia 51: 29–38.
55. Krishnaveni GV, Veena SR, Winder NR, Hill JC, Noonan K, et al. (2011) Maternal vitamin D status during pregnancy and body composition and cardiovascular risk markers in Indian children: the Mysore Parthenon Study. Am J Clin Nutr 93: 628–35.
56. Sarbattama S, Rebecca AS (2010) Maternal Antioxidant Supplementation Prevents Adiposity in the Offspring of Western Diet Fed Rats. Diabetes 59: 3058–3065.
57. Raghunath M, Venu L, Padmavathi IJN, Kishore YD, Ganeshan M, et al. (2009) Modulation of macronutrient metabolism in the offspring by maternal micronutrient deficiency in experimental animals. Indian J Med Res 130: 655–65.
58. Casanueva E, Viteri EF (2003) Iron and Oxidative Stress in Pregnancy. J Nutr 133: 1700S–1708S.
59. Yih FL, Hsiu-Ling T, Lee YC, Chang SJ (2005) Maternal Vitamin E Supplementation Affects the Antioxidant Capability and Oxidative Status of Hatching Chicks. J Nutr 135: 2457–2461.
60. Devrim E, Tarhan I, Erquder IB, Durak I (2006) Oxidant/Antioxidant Status of Placenta, Blood, and Cord Blood Samples From Pregnant Women Supplemented With Iron. J Soc Gynecol Investig 13: 502–505. doi:10.1016/j.jsgi.2006.07.004.
61. Amy LF, Ruchira TN, Ekström EC, Rasmussen KM, Frongillo EA (2009) Micronutrient supplementation affects maternal-infant feeding interactions and maternal distress in Bangladesh. Am J Clin Nutr 90: 141–148. doi:10.3945/ajcn.2008.26817.
62. Nisreen AA, Greenwood DC, Simpson NAB, McArdle HJ, Godfrey KM, et al. (2011) Dietary iron intake during early pregnancy and birth outcomes in a cohort of British women. Hum Reprod 26: 911–919. doi:10.1093/humrep/der005.
63. Ahmad S, Kalle AK, Trayambak B, Gourav B, Dilip Y, et al. (2013) PPAR Signalling Pathway is a Key Modulator of Liver Proteome in Pups Born to Vitamin B12 Deficient Rats. J proteomics 91: 297–308.
64. Asmita K, Kamini D, Anvita K, Pratiksha S, Preeti CG, et al. (2011) Effects of Altered Maternal Folic Acid, Vitamin B12 and Docosahexaenoic Acid on Placental Global DNA Methylation Patterns in Wistar Rats. PLoS One 6: e17706. DOI:10.1371/journal.pone.0017706.
65. Ian CGW, Frances AC, Shelley EB, Sergiy D, Shakti S, et al. (2005) Reversal of maternal programming of stress responses in adult offspring through methyl supplementation: Altering epigenetic marking later in life. J Neurosci 25: 11045–11054; doi:10.1523/JNEUROSCI.3652-05.2005.
66. Drake AJ, Walker BR (2004) The intergenerational effects of fetal programming: non-genomic mechanisms for the inheritance of low birth weight and cardiovascular risk. J Endocrinol 180: 1–16.

25

Effect of Vitamin D Supplementation on Cardiometabolic Risks and Health-Related Quality of Life among Urban Premenopausal Women in a Tropical Country

Mazliza Ramly[1]*, Moy Foong Ming[2], Karuthan Chinna[1], Suhaili Suboh[1], Rokiah Pendek[3]

1 Department of Social and Preventive Medicine, Faculty of Medicine, University of Malaya, Kuala Lumpur, Malaysia, **2** Julius Centre University of Malaya, Department of Social and Preventive Medicine, Faculty of Medicine, University of Malaya, Kuala Lumpur, Malaysia, **3** Department of Medicine, Faculty of Medicine, University of Malaya, Kuala Lumpur, Malaysia

Abstract

Background: Many observational studies linked vitamin D to cardiometabolic risks besides its pivotal role in musculoskeletal diseases, but evidence from trials is lacking and inconsistent.

Aim: To determine whether Vitamin D supplementation in urban premenopausal women with vitamin D deficiency can improve cardiometabolic risks and health-related quality of life (HRQOL).

Design: A double-blind randomized controlled trial was conducted in Kuala Lumpur, Malaysia. A total of 192 vitamin D deficient (<50 nmol/l) premenopausal women were randomized to receive either vitamin D 50,000 IU or placebo once a week for 2 months and then monthly for 10 months. Primary outcomes were serum 25(OH)D, serum lipid profiles, blood pressure and HOMA-IR measured at baseline, 6 months and 12 months. HRQOL was assessed with SF-36 at baseline and 12 months.

Results: Ninety three and ninety-nine women were randomised into intervention and placebo groups respectively. After 12 months, there were significant differences in the serum 25(OH)D concentration (mean difference: 49.54; 95% CI: 43.94 to 55.14) nmol/l) and PTH levels (mean difference: −1.02; 95% CI: −1.67 to −0.38 pmol/l) in the intervention group compared to placebo group. There was significant difference between treatment group in both serum 25(OH)D and PTH. There was no effect of supplementation on HOMA-IR, serum lipid profiles and blood pressure (all $p>0.05$) between two groups. There was a small but significant improvement in HRQOL in the components of vitality (mean difference: 5.041; 95% CI: 0.709 to 9.374) and mental component score (mean difference: 2.951; 95% CI: 0.573 to 5.329) in the intervention group compared to placebo group.

Conclusion: Large and less frequent dosage vitamin D supplementation was safe and effective in the achievement of vitamin D sufficiency. However, there was no improvement in measured cardiometabolic risk factors in premenopausal women. Conversely vitamin D supplementation improves some components of HRQOL.

Editor: D. W. Cameron, University of Ottawa, Canada

Funding: The study was funded by the University Malaya (Post Graduate Research Grant, PV080/2012A) and the Ministry of Education High Impact Research Grant (MOE HIR No. E 2000069-20001). The funders had no role in study design, data collection and analysis, decision to publish or preparation of the manuscript.

Competing Interests: The authors have declared that no competing interests exist.

* Email: drmazliza@siswa.um.edu.my

Introduction

Vitamin D is well known for its fundamental role in bone mechanism and calcium homeostasis [1,2]. More recently, many studies found that vitamin D may play an important role in the prevention of cardiovascular diseases and metabolic syndrome risk factors [2–6]. The mechanisms in which vitamin D may protect against these diseases include activation of the renin-angiotensin-aldosterone systems, increase arterial intimae thickness, enhancement in insulin secretion and insulin sensitivity and inflammatory cytokines [2]. Many observational studies have shown that vitamin D deficiency, defined as serum 25(OH)D<50 nmol/l or 20 ng/ml [7] is associated with cardiometabolic diseases [4,8–10]. A meta-analysis of prospective studies by Khan et al [5] evaluated association between vitamin D levels and metabolic outcomes in healthy adults, demonstrated a significant inverse association of vitamin D status with metabolic syndrome. However, findings from this review were not able to establish causality, which required robust evidence from clinical trials. Clinical trials on the other hand produced inconsistent results [11–17]. These trials had marked study design variation in terms of samples size, study duration, participants' characteristics, primary outcomes, intervention dosage and formulation. Furthermore, existing randomized controlled trials were generally short duration (less than one year), insufficient dosage or underpowered.

Vitamin D deficiency is established risk factors for osteoporosis, falls and fractures and all these may impair HRQOL. Vitamin D deficiency can occur to any individuals regardless of age or health condition. Yet, assessment of HRQOL in vitamin D deficiency was only performed in elderly population. These observational studies found vitamin D deficiency to be inversely associated with mental and physical HRQOL [18–24]. Furthermore, most studies were restricted to disease-specific populations such as the postmenopausal osteoporotic women [18,19,22,23], elderly with heart failure [25] and elderly on dialysis [20]. Nevertheless, one observational study was found to examine the association between vitamin D and HRQOL among healthy premenopausal women [26] and another assessed the association between vitamin D and HRQOL among elderly in community setting [24]. Both studies observed inverse association between vitamin D and HRQOL. To our best knowledge, so far there are no other clinical trials evaluating the effect of vitamin D supplements on HRQOL in a healthy population.

Therefore, we designed this double-blind randomized placebo-controlled trial to determine whether vitamin D supplement can improve cardiometabolic risk factors such as blood pressure (BP), homeostasis model assessment insulin resistance (HOMA IR), triglycerides (TG) and high-density lipoprotein cholesterol (HDL) as well as HRQOL in urban pre-menopausal women who were vitamin D deficient.

Method

The protocol for this trial is reported in full details in the published protocol [27]. The CONSORT checklist and Table S1 and Table S2 are available as supporting information; see Checklist S1, Table S1 and Table S2.

This was a randomized placebo-controlled, doubled-blind parallel trial. All premenopausal women aged 30 years old and above, working in a public university in Kuala Lumpur, Malaysia ($n = 389$) were screened for vitamin D deficiency (serum 25(OH)D≤20 ng/ml or ≤50 nmol/l). Exclusion criteria included abnormal serum PTH level (reference range for healthy adult was 1.1–7.3 pmol/l) and serum calcium (>2.7 nmol/l), known to have illnesses such as granuloma forming disorder, lymphoma, sarcoidosis or any types of cancer and taking daily vitamin D supplementation >1000 IU/day as well as pregnant women. Finally, 192 subjects were recruited in this trial (Figure 1).

The study was divided into two phases. Recruitment and screening including baseline clinical and anthropometry measurements were obtained in Phase one. All selected participants who meet the inclusion criteria in Phase one was ultimately invited to participate in this trial and proceed to Phase two. Written informed consent was obtained from these selected participants at this phase. The randomization and intervention of the first cohort ($n = 110$) commenced in October 2012 while the second cohort ($n = 82$) commenced in January 2013 (Phase two) (Figure 1). Intervention consisted of 50,000 IU (0.5 gram) of cholecalciferol (25(OH)D3) powder or placebo (0.5 gram) taken orally by diluting the powder into warm water before consumption. The consumption frequency was once a week for 8 weeks (equivalent to 7142 IU/day) and then once a month for 10 months (equivalent to 1667 IU/day) [7]. The consumption of 50,000 IU of vitamin D per week or per month is considered to be safe as the tolerable upper intake level for vitamin D is 10,000 IU per day [28]. We provided treatment for participants in the placebo group for 4 months after the trial completed, as it was unethical to withhold treatment. To ensure compliance with the intervention, participants were required to consume the active supplements or placebo in front of researcher during every follow-up. For those who did not attend the appointment, the researcher visited them at their workplace to give them the active supplements or placebo personally.

The randomization sequence was created using GraphPad Software with a 1:1 allocation by a staff (AC) with no involvement in the trial. The participant's names were matched with the random number sequence. The names of participants from intervention and placebo were printed and pasted on to the tubes filled with either vitamin D powder or placebo. The contents were not labelled on the bottles to maintain the allocation concealment. The tubes used were identical for both active intervention and placebo. Allocation sequence data was kept by AC in a secure place so that it could not be accessed or influenced by anyone, including the researchers. Outcomes measurements, randomization and allocation were fully concealed from the researchers, staffs involved in the trial and participants until the completion of data collection.

The primary outcome measures were serum 25(OH)D, systolic blood pressure, diastolic blood pressure, fasting blood insulin, fasting blood glucose, HOMA-IR, triglycerides, high-density lipoprotein cholesterol, low-density lipoprotein cholesterol and HRQOL using the SF-36 questionnaire.

Participants were recalled for clinical and anthropometry measurements at 6 months and 12 months. Serum calcium results at 6 months were checked for abnormality to detect any adverse reaction due to high dose of vitamin D supplementation. Participants were also advised to contact the researchers immediately if they suspected a reaction to supplements. Participants who were found to be pregnant at some point in the trial were also excluded in view of ethical consideration.

Methods for all measurements, questionnaires and laboratory analysis are reported in full details in the published protocol [27]. Homeostasis model assessment of insulin resistance (HOMA-IR) was used to establish a measure for insulin resistance. It can be calculated from a simple linear equation based on pairing FBS and Fasting Blood Insulin to establish a measure for insulin resistance: HOMA-IR = FBS(mmol/L)×Fasting Blood Insulin/22.5 [21]. Vitamin D concentration was analyzed using electrochemiluminescence immunoassay (ECLIA) vitamin D3 (25-OH) method on the Cobas E-411 analyzer. All tests and analyses were carried out by the Clinical Diagnostic Laboratory, University Malaya Medical Centre.

Statistical methods

A minimum of 88 subjects was required for each arm of the trial to demonstrate a significant difference at 80% power and a two-sided 5% significance. The calculations were based on the results by Zittermann et al. [29] which achieved a reduction in triglycerides of 0.19±0.54 mmol/L in vitamin D group while there is an increment of 0.03±0.50 in placebo group. Assuming a drop-out rate of 10%, 97 subjects would need to be recruited per arm. Sample size calculation was conducted using the OpenEpi Software version 2.3.1.

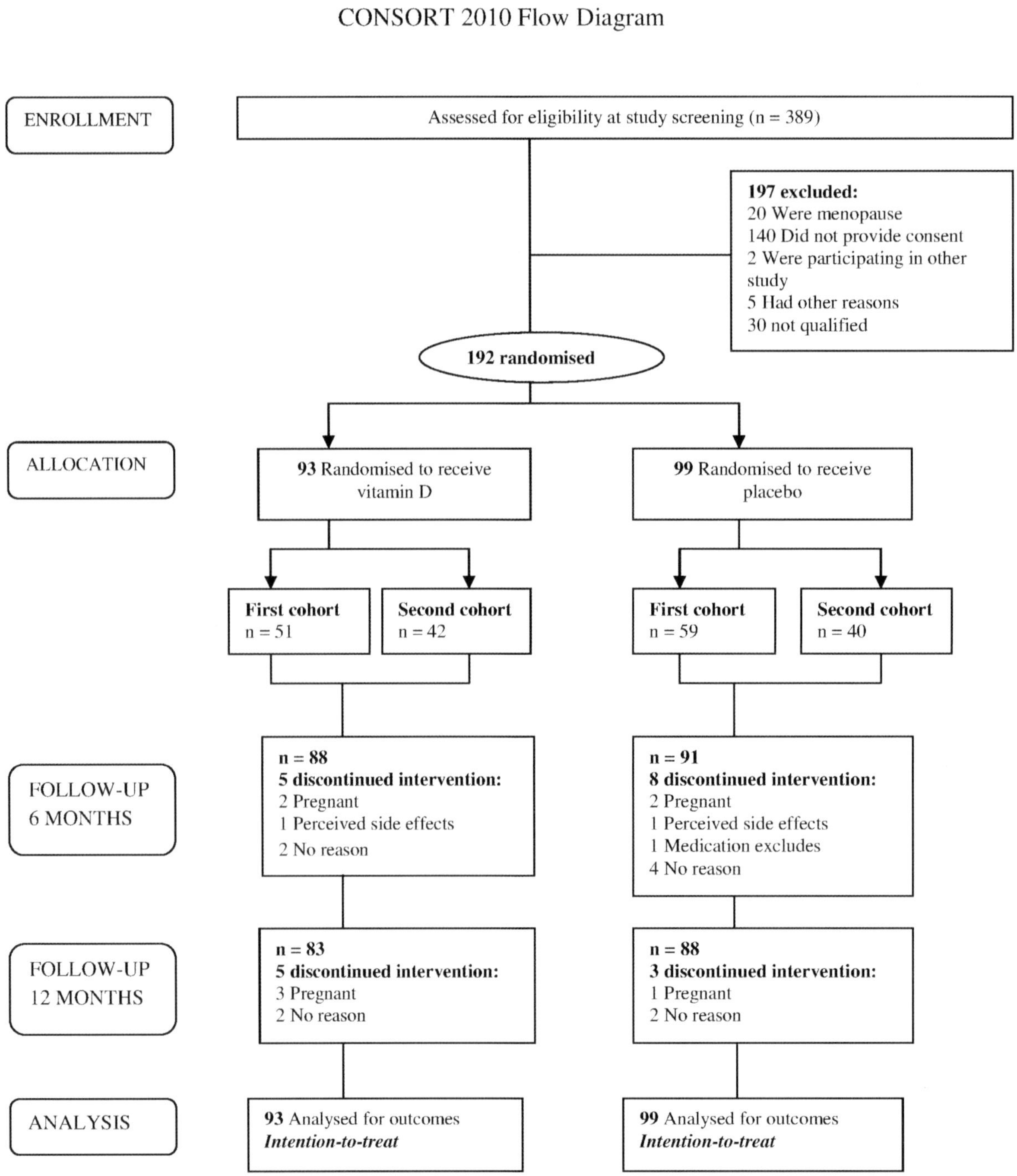

Figure 1. Flow diagram of the study, showing numbers of participants who were randomly assigned, received the intended treatment and were analyzed for the primary outcomes.

For baseline characteristics, descriptive statistics were used. Categorical data was described using count and percentages. All numerical data was checked for normality. Normally distributed variables were presented as mean ± standard deviation while abnormally distributed variables were presented as median ± interquartile range. Statistical comparisons were performed with independent *t-test*, Mann-Whitney U test or Chi-square test as appropriate. P-value was preset at 0.05. Some of the cases were loss to follow-up, therefore linear mixed effects procedure was used to test the differences in primary outcomes from baseline to follow-up at 6 months and 12 months. Data were analyzed according to the intention-to-treat principle. We also performed a linear mixed effects sensitivity analysis using complete cases. All statistical analysis was performed using the SPSS software version 16.0 (SPSS Inc, 2009, Chicago, Illinois).

Ethical approval

This trial was approved by the Medical Ethics Committee of University Malaya Medical Centre (reference number 907.22).

Results

Figure 1 shows the flow of participants in the trial. Three hundred eighty-nine potentially suitable participants were identified and invited for screening. Of these, a total of 192 women were randomly assigned to either intervention or placebo group. In total 21 women withdrew from the trial due to pregnancy, perceived side effects (amenorrhea) or no particular reasons. There were no reports of vitamin D intoxication or adverse reaction. A total of 171 participants completed the follow-up of 12 months.

Baseline data

Baseline characteristics of the participants are shown in Table 1. Both groups were similar in all the reported measures ($P>0.05$). Their mean age was 42±5 years, majority were Malays (>89%) and had at least secondary education (92%). A total of 15.6% of the participants had high cholesterol, 8.9% had hypertension and only 1% had diabetes mellitus. The mean scores for the HRQOL components were in the range of 60 to 70.

Effects of vitamin D supplements on cardiometabolic risk factors

Primary outcomes for both groups at baseline, 6 months and 12 months are presented (Table 2). Mean serum 25(OH)D concentrations in the intervention group increased drastically in the first 6 months (mean difference: 53.72; 95% CI: 49.23 to 58.18 nmol/l) followed with a small increment after that (mean difference: 1.83; 95% CI: −0.94 to 4.61 nmol/l). There was also significant increase in the mean serum 25(OH)D in the placebo group after 6 months (mean difference: 7.17, 95% CI: 1.46 to 12.85 nmol/l), however the level was still in the deficient category (<50 nmol/l). A total of 91.6% of the intervention group achieved 25(OH)D more than 50 nmol/l (20 ng/ml) and 63.4% achieved a level of 75 nmol/l (30 ng/ml) or higher. In contrast, 13.1% of the placebo group had 25(OH)D above 50 nmol/l and only 1% had a value of 75 nmol/l or higher. Mean PTH concentration remained suppressed in the intervention group as the mean serum 25(OH)D increased, however the change in PTH was not statistically significant. In the placebo group, the mean PTH concentration increased from baseline to 6 months (mean difference: 1.04; 95% CI: 0.49 to 1.60 pmol/l) but declined slightly at 12 months (mean difference: −0.58, 95% CI: −1.12 to −0.05 pmol/l). There were significant differences in mean concentrations of total 25(OH)D and PTH between treatment groups after 12 months of treatment.

BMI did not declined in the intervention group between baseline to 6 months (mean difference: 0.85, 95% CI: −1.07 to 2.77 kg/m^2), however these changes were not clinically significant and did not differ between treatment groups. There were significant differences in the change in serum calcium, systolic blood pressure and LDL within the intervention group ($p<0.05$). Serum calcium and LDL were significantly different over time within the placebo group ($p<0.05$). However, these changes did not differ between treatment groups and were not clinically significant. An increase in serum 25(OH)D in the intervention group induced a reduction in HOMA-IR whereas the reverse was observed in the placebo group. However, these changes were not statistically significant between treatment groups. Sensitivity analysis using complete cases showed similar results (Table S1).

There was a reduction in proportion of metabolic syndrome from 28% to 25.8% in the intervention group, while in placebo group, the proportion increased from 22.2% to 23.2%. There was no difference between groups ($p=0.762$). Among participants with metabolic risks at baseline ($n=26$ for intervention group and $n=22$ for placebo group), there was a small but significant improvement ($p=0.021$) in the proportion of low HDL in the intervention group at the end of the trial. Similar improvement was also noted in the proportions of high blood pressure, abdominal obesity and elevated glucose, however all these were not statistically significant (data not shown).

Effects of vitamin D supplements on health-related quality of life

The health-related quality of life (HRQOL) of the intervention and placebo groups is presented in Table 3. At baseline, the mean scores of HRQOL components in the SF-36 were in between 60 to 70. Vitamin D supplement improved general health of the intervention group (mean difference: 3.65; 95% CI: 0.57 to 7.73). However, there was no significant difference when compared to the placebo group. Apparently there was a small but significant improvement in vitality (mean difference: 5.041; 95% CI: 0.709 to 9.374) and mental component score (mean difference: 2.951; 95% CI: 0.573 to 5.329) in the intervention group compared to placebo group. Sensitivity analysis using complete cases were also performed for HRQOL and it also showed similar results (Table S2).

Discussion

Our participants were urban, premenopausal women working in a public university in the capital city of Malaysia. Although they were vitamin D deficient, the proportion of them having non-communicable diseases (NCD) such as hypertension and diabetes was relatively low compared to the general population [30]. However, more than 20% of them had metabolic syndrome. Their mean BMI was in the overweight category. This reflected that our participants were at risks for CVD in the future. As expected, the participants' scores for some of the HRQOL components, namely the physical functioning, role physical and social functioning were found to be lower than the general population [31].

In the present study, we demonstrated 12 months of vitamin D supplementation at a dosage of 50,000 IU per week for the first 2 months and 50,000 IU per month for the next 10 months increased serum 25(OH)D to sufficient level among our participants. However, correction of vitamin D deficiency did not improve HOMA-IR, HDL, LDL or triglycerides. Nevertheless, among participants with metabolic syndrome, vitamin D supplementation improved HDL level, offering a promising non-pharmacologic intervention in the prevention of metabolic syndrome. We also found that vitamin D supplements improved the HRQOL among the participants particularly in vitality and mental component scores.

Our results also showed the dosage and frequency of Vitamin D supplementation was safe and effective. More than 80% of participants from the intervention group achieved serum 25(OH)D above 50 nmol/l compared to only 13% from placebo group. These results were comparable with other studies which used daily dosage of vitamin D3 [16,17]. Although all women in the intervention group received the same dosage of vitamin D, a small proportion did not achieve a sufficient level of circulating vitamin D. This could be due to heterogeneity among women such as obesity. On further exploration of data, 6 out of 7 of these women were obese (>25 kg/m^2). This is probably because of a decreased in bioavailability of vitamin D that is sequestered in the fat of individuals with excess adipose tissue. Monthly dosage had

Table 1. Baseline socio-demographic characteristics of the intervention and placebo groups.

Characteristics	Intervention (n = 93)	Placebo (n = 99)	P-value[a]
	N (%)	N (%)	N (%)
Ethnicity			
Malay	83 (89.3%)	89 (89.9%)	0.777
Chinese	3 (3.2%)	3 (3.0%)	
Indian	7 (7.5%)	6 (6.1%)	
Others	0 (0%)	1 (1.0%)	
Level of education			
Primary	6 (6.5%)	8 (8.1%)	0.496
Secondary	43 (46.2%)	38 (38.4%)	
Tertiary	44 (47.3%)	53 (53.5%)	
History of CVD			
Diabetes mellitus	1 (1.1%)	1 (1.0%)	0.965
Hypertension	9 (9.7%)	8 (8.1%)	0.697
High cholesterol	15 (16.1%)	15 (15.2%)	0.852
Metabolic syndrome	26 (28%)	22 (22.2%)	0.359
	Mean ± SD	**Mean ± SD**	
Age (years)	42.58±5.35	42.88±4.99	0.69
BMI (kg/m^2)	27.23±5.49	27.23±5.09	0.99
Blood pressure			
Systolic (mmHg)	121.61±16.19	118.90±14.85	0.23
Diastolic (mmHg)	77.77±10.64	76.80±10.99	0.53
Serum 25(OH)D (nmol/l)	30.19±8.71	29.99±9.70	0.88
Serum calcium (mmol/l)	2.18±0.07	2.19±0.08	0.246
Serum PTH (pmol/l)	4.60±2.19	4.76±2.05	0.611
Lipid values (mmol/l)			
Total cholesterol	5.17±0.99	5.28±0.83	0.425
HDL - Cholesterol	1.45±0.49	1.44±0.35	0.846
LDL - Cholesterol	3.26±0.76	3.34±0.71	0.457
Triglycerides	1.15±0.53	1.17±0.62	0.770
HRQOL (SF-36)			
Physical functioning	74.68±20.23	70.96±24.24	0.252
Role physical	74.35±22.98	72.27±24.40	0.544
Bodily pain	73.13±19.64	71.13±18.31	0.467
General health	66.77±16.87	66.12±17.13	0.791
Vitality	65.27±11.98	61.76±13.88	0.063
Social functioning	78.77±19.50	74.26±21.85	0.134
Role emotional	78.92±22.37	76.26±23.99	0.428
Mental health	73.12±12.11	71.06±16.62	0.331
PCS	49.57±6.78	48.80±7.41	0.453
MCS	50.09±6.69	48.65±9.17	0.218
	Median; IQR	**Median, IQR**	
Insulin resistance			
Serum glucose (mmol/l)	4.80; 0.65	4.80; 0.70	0.871
Serum insulin (mU/L)	9.30; 9.95	9.20; 8.80	0.874
HOMA-IR	2.00; 2.28	2.00; 2.00	0.908

HOMA-IR, homeostasis model assessment insulin resistance; CVD, cardiovascular disease; PTH, parathyroid hormone; 25(OH)D, 25-hydroxyvitamin D; IQR, Interquartile range; PCS, Physical component score; MCS, Mental component score; BMI was calculated as weight (kilogram) divided by height (m^2).
[a]Determined with independent t-test or Mann-Whitney test for continuous variables as appropriate and with χ^2 test for categorical data.

Table 2. Summary of the outcome measurements overtime (baseline, 6 months and 12 months) – Intention-to-treat analysis.

	Intervention (n = 93)	Placebo (n = 99)	Mean difference (95% CI) between treatment group[a]
	Mean (95% CI)	**Mean (95% CI)**	
Se 25(OH)D (nmol/l)			
Baseline	30.19 (28.56 to 31.82)	29.98 (27.20 to 32.78)	0.19 (–2.43 to 2.82
6 month	83.91 (79.84 to 87.97)	37.15 (34.39 to 39.90)	**46.92 (42.42 to 51.43)**
12 months	85.74 (81.25 to 90.22)	36.09 (33.63 to 38.55)	**49.54 (43.94 to 55.14)***
Se PTH (pmol/l)			
Baseline	4.60 (4.18 to 5.03)	4.76 (4.34 to 5.18)	–0.16 (–0.76 to 0.45)
6 month	4.58 (4.05 to 5.10)	5.86 (5.34 to 6.38)	**–1.28 (–2.02 to –0.55)***
12 months	4.19 (3.74 to 4.66)	5.22 (4.77 to 5.67)	**–1.02 (–1.67 to –0.38)***
Se calcium (mmol/l)			
Baseline	2.18 (2.17 to 2.19)	2.19 (2.18 to 2.21)	–0.01 (–0.03 to 0.009)
6 month	2.23 (2.21 to 2.26)	2.24 (2.21 to 2.26)	–0.005 (–0.04 to 0.03)
12 months	2.24 (2.22 to 2.26)	2.22 (2.20 to 2.24)	0.02 (–0.01 to 0.05)
BMI			
Baseline	27.22 (26.14 to 28.31)	27.23 (26.18 to 28.28)	–0.005 (–1.511 to 1.500)
6 month	28.08 (26.96 to 29.19)	27.76 (26.67 to 28.86)	0.313 (–1.251 to 1.877)
12 months	27.63 (26.45 to 28.78)	27.84 (26.73 to 28.95)	–0.209 (–1.807 to 1.389)
Systolic BP			
Baseline	121.6 (118.4 to 124.8)	118.9 (115.8 to 121.9)	2.71 (–1.71 to 7.13)
6 month	126.3 (122.9 to 129.6)	123.9 (120.7 to 127.2)	2.38 (–2.27 to 7.04)
12 months	125.8 (122.6 to 128.9)	123.9 (120.8 to 126.9)	1.89 (–2.56 to 6.35)
Diastolic BP			
Baseline	77.77 (75.56 to 79.99)	76.79 (74.65 to 78.94)	0.976 (–2.107 to 4.059)
6 month	79.74 (77.38 to 82.10)	79.23 (76.97 to 81.55)	0.508 (–2.805 to 3.820)
12 months	77.52 (75.22 to 79.81)	76.76 (74.53 to 78.99)	0.757 (–2.441 to 3.954)
Se Glucose (mmol/l)			
Baseline	5.07 (4.88 to 5.25)	4.93 (4.75 to 5.12)	0.13 (–0.13 to 0.39)
6 month	5.14 (4.97 to 5.32)	5.07 (4.89 to 5.24)	0.07 (–0.17 to 0.32)
12 months	5.04 (4.83 to 5.26)	5.11 (4.90 to 5.32)	–0.07 (–0.37 to 0.23)
Se insulin (mU/L			
Baseline	13.81 (10.38 to 17.24)	11.07 (7.74 to 14.39)	2.74 (–2.04 to 7.51)
6 month	13.11 (11.18 to 15.04)	12.17 (10.27 to 14.06)	0.943 (–1.75 to 3.65)
12 months	13.93 (11.47 to 16.38)	12.74 (10.36 to 15.12)	1.19 (–2.23 to 4.61)
HOMA-IR			
Baseline	3.72 (2.25 to 5.19)	2.47 (1.04 to 3.91)	1.25 (–0.81 to 3.31)
6 month	3.12 (2.57 to 3.67)	2.84 (2.29 to 3.38)	0.28 (–0.49 to 1.05)
12 months	3.19 (2.61 to 3.78)	2.99 (2.42 to 3.56)	0.21 (–0.61 to 1.03)
TG (mmol/l)			
Baseline	1.15 (1.03 to 1.26)	1.17 (1.06 to 1.29)	–0.03 (–0.19 to 0.14)
6 month	1.38 (1.25 to 1.51)	1.19 (1.07 to 1.32)	**0.19 (0.01 to 0.37)***
12 months	1.36 (1.23 to 1.49)	1.22 (1.09 to 1.35)	0.14 (–0.33 to 0.33)
HDL-C (mmol/l)			
Baseline	1.45 (1.36 to 1.54)	1.44 (1.35 to 1.52)	0.01 (–0.11 to 0.13)
6 month	1.43 (1.36 to 1.49)	1.50 (1.44 to 1.57)	–0.08 (–0.18 to 0.02)
12 months	1.52 (1.44 to 1.59)	1.53 1.50 (1.43 to 1.58)	0.02 (–0.09 to 0.13)
LDL-C (mmol/l)			
Baseline	3.26 (3.11 to 3.41)	3.34 (3.19 to 3.48)	–0.08 (–0.29 to 0.13)
6 month	3.25 (3.09 to 3.39)	3.31 (3.17 to 3.46)	–0.07 (–0.28 to 0.15)

Table 2. Cont.

	Intervention (n = 93)	Placebo (n = 99)	Mean difference (95% CI) between treatment group[a]
	Mean (95% CI)	Mean (95% CI)	
12 months	3.62 (3.44 to 3.79)	3.63 (3.46 to 3.80)	–0.01 (–0.26 to 0.23)

*Significant at $p<0.05$.
[a]Determined with linear mixed effect.

advantage in terms of compliance. Von Hurst et al [16] reported that their participants found it difficult to comply with daily dosage of vitamin D. None of our participants reported any adverse effects of vitamin D clinically or biochemically.

Evidences from epidemiologic studies showed vitamin D deficiency was linked with cardiometabolic risks [9,10,32–40].

Table 3. Summary of the health-related quality of life parameters overtime (baseline and 12 months) – Intention-to-treat analysis.

	Intervention (n = 93)	Placebo (n = 99)	Mean difference (95% CI) between treatment group[a]
	Mean (95% CI)	Mean (95% CI)	
Physical functioning			
Baseline	74.68 (70.81 to 78.84)	70.96 (66.13 to 75.79)	3.718 (–2.624 to 10.06)
12 months	71.81 (66.53 to 77.09)	71.48 (66.62 to 76.33)	0.330 (–6.792 to 7.452)
Role physical			
Baseline	74.36 (69.62 to 79.09)	72.27 (67.41 to 77.14)	2.082 (–4.662 to 8.826)
12 months	73.45 (67.94 to 78.95)	72.84 (67.78 to 77.90)	0.605 (–6.820–8.029)
Bodily pain			
Baseline	73.13 (69.09 to 77.17)	71.13 (67.48 to 74.78)	1.998 (–3.416 to 7.411)
12 months	72.93 (67.76 to 77.09)	69.31 (65.64 to 72.97)	3.621 (–1.891 to 9.132)
General health			
Baseline	66.77 (63.29 to 70.25)	66.12 (62.71 to 69.54)	0.653 (–4.188 to 5.494)
12 months	70.42 (66.85 to 73.99)	68.66 (65.57 to 71.75)	1.763 (–2.924 to 6.449)
Vitality			
Baseline	65.27 (62.80 to 67.74)	61.76 (58.99 to 64.53)	3.511 (–0.173 to 7.196)
12 months	65.53 (62.45 to 68.61)	60.49 (57.39 to 63.58)	**5.041 (0.709 to 9.374)***
Social functioning			
Baseline	78.77 (74.76 to 82.79)	74.26 (69.91 to 78.62)	4.512 (–1.377 to 10.401)
12 months	80.27 (76.24 to 84.29)	75.11 (70.66 to 79.56)	5.151 (–0.804 to 11.107)
Role emotional			
Baseline	78.93 (74.32 to 85.53)	76.26 (71.48 to 79.62)	2.662 (–3.938 to 9.262)
12 months	80.52 (75.45 to 85.58)	74.52 (69.43 to 79.62)	5.995 (–1.138 to 13.129)
Mental health			
Baseline	73.12 (70.63 to 75.61)	71.06 (67.74 to 74.37)	2.058 (–2.065 to 6.180)
12 months	75.12 (72.16 to 78.08)	71.53 (68.25 to 74.82)	3.586 (–0.806 to 7.979)
Physical component score			
Baseline	49.57 (48.17 to 50.97)	48.80 (47.32 to 50.28)	0.772 (–1.249 to 2.793)
12 months	48.99 (47.51 to 50.47)	49.06 (47.79 to 50.32)	–0.069 (–1.997 to 1.860)
Mental component score			
Baseline	50.09 (48.71 to 51.46)	48.65 (46.82 to 50.48)	1.440 (–0.835 to 3.715)
12 months	51.34 (49.81 to 52.86)	48.39 (46.54 to 50.23)	**2.951 (0.573 to 5.329)***

*Significant at $p<0.05$.
[a]Determined with linear mixed effect.

Vitamin D insufficiency induced alterations in the calcium flux of pancreatic b-cells thus reduced insulin secretion [41,42] and this might influence on insulin resistance (IR). In addition, vitamin D insufficiency also induced elevations in PTH, which could adversely affect glucose metabolism. As expected, PTH levels decreased within the intervention group. On the other hand, the PTH levels also decreased within the placebo group. This could possibly due to unintentional increased consumption of dietary calcium in the placebo group because of Hawthorne effect. This could be the reason for no significant differences in insulin resistance or glucose levels between groups.

They were many clinical trials trying to establish the role of vitamin D deficiency in the pathogenesis of type 2 diabetes mellitus [11,12,14–17,33,34,43]. However, the results had been inconsistent. Most of these trials failed to detect any improvement in the glucose levels and insulin resistance. Our findings were consistent with results of many other published studies, in which the vitamin D supplements appeared to have no effect on fasting glucose and HOMA-IR [11,12,14,15,17]. Reasons for these negative results could be due to the studies were short duration, had small sample size and different dosage used in vitamin D formulations. On the contrary, data from two clinical trials showed that vitamin D supplementation improved plasma glucose and insulin resistance [16,43].

Systematic reviews and observational studies found associations between vitamin D deficiency and triglycerides, HDL and LDL [44–47]. However, results from trials had been inconsistent. Clinical trials by Brevlasky et al [11] and Wood et al [17] found an absence of improvement in lipid profiles, similar with our findings. On the other hand, two other clinical trials [13,29] found significant decrease in lipid in the treatment group. Major et al [13] reported that total cholesterol:HDL and LDL:HDL ratio in the treatment group were significantly decreased. Whereas, in study by Zitterman et al [29] the serum triglycerides and LDL ($p< 0.001$) were reduced after one year of treatment with 3320 IU of vitamin D daily among healthy overweight individuals with inadequate vitamin D levels. These inconsistent results could be due to variations in sample size, dosage and formulation of vitamin D supplement, characteristics of participants and duration of trials.

Our participants were generally healthy premenopausal women with vitamin D deficiency. Although 26% of them had history of CVD, majority had normal glucose and lipid values, which may be difficult to improve further with vitamin D supplement. However, individuals with higher baseline metabolic risks may benefit from vitamin D supplementation. Analysis on a subset of our participants with metabolic risks at baseline demonstrated an improvement in HDL among the intervention group. However, the null effect of vitamin D supplementation on other metabolic risk factors may be due to the small sample size of our participants with metabolic risks. Therefore, there might be inadequate power to detect the effectiveness of vitamin D on these components. Future studies should recruit women with vitamin D deficiency and at risks for metabolic syndrome or CVD.

The increase levels in some of the clinical indicators (systolic blood pressure, triglycerides, LDL-cholesterol) within both intervention and placebo groups was probably due to the advancing age that affected the pathogenesis of these indicators [48]. Twelve months of treatment with vitamin D may not be sufficient to produce a significant reduction in the cardiometabolic risk factors as more time may be needed for the vitamin D to correct the metabolic risks back to normal.

The optimal dose for vitamin D supplementation on cardiometabolic risk could also influence our results. Expert opinions for daily vitamin D dosage ranged from 600 to 2000 IU for prevention of cardiovascular or metabolic risk [28,49,50]. The Institute of Medicine Report [28] concluded that due to lack of evidence, they could not make any recommendation for non-skeletal outcomes. The method of vitamin D supplementation in our study (50,000 IU weekly for 2 months and once a month after that) differed from the daily doses (400–4000 IU) used in majority of other studies [12,15–17,43,51]. We used the recommendation by Holick [7] which stated that for an effective vitamin D deficiency treatment, higher dosage was needed at initial stage to correct the vitamin D deficient status. However, this recommendation only corrected the vitamin D deficiency. There is no current recommendation on the optimum dosage needed for improvement of cardiometabolic outcomes. There are few other studies using similar dosage [52] or larger dose of vitamin D supplementation [14,25,53] but in shorter duration (less than 6 months). Although we did not find any effect of vitamin D supplementation on cardiometabolic risks, we cannot exclude the possibility that higher dosage of supplementation for a longer duration might help in the prevention of cardiometabolic risks among individuals with existing co-morbidities or cardiometabolic events such as myocardial infarct or stroke. However, a review article has indicate that negative outcomes could be predicted due to failure to maintain circulating vitamin D over time as with monthly, quarterly or yearly bolus vitamin D dosing [54]. It appears that for the optimal benefits of vitamin D supplementation, sufficient amount of vitamin D should be provided on a daily basis to ensure that stable circulating concentrations are maintained over time as vitamin D has short circulating half-life of vitamin D. These particular reasons might explain the varying results of clinical trials. Therefore, a large-scale prospective clinical trial is needed to examine large dosage of daily versus weekly and monthly vitamin D with the same primary outcome measures.

On the other hand, we found vitamin D supplements improved the HRQOL of participants particularly in vitality and mental component score. These improvements were statistically significant but clinically insignificant. However, it has some clinical relevance as vitality assessed energy and fatigue; and women with vitamin D deficiency usually feel tired, low energy and worn out. Vitamin D is a nuclear steroid hormone which thought to be involved in brain health and function as well as neuromuscular functions. Vitamin D receptors in the cell's nucleus regulate the expression of target genes when bound to 1,25(OH)D. These receptors are expressed in areas of the brain important to behavioural regulation [55]. An observational study by Ecemis et al [26] found physical component score, mental component score, physical functioning score and vitality score were impaired in vitamin D deficient and insufficient healthy premenopausal women. Other studies did relate vitamin D status with depression [56–59] and mental component score [19]. Another observational study also concluded that women who were on daily vitamin D supplementation had higher mental HRQOL scores [19].

At baseline, our study showed slightly higher scores in bodily pain components compared to the general population [20]. Although muscle and bone pain was a common symptom of vitamin D deficiency, we did not find any significant improvement for physical components score. This may be due to non-specific definition of pain was used in the SF-36 questionnaire which we administered. For example, Huang et al [21] used VR-36 (Veteran Rand 36 items) questionnaire as well as VAS (visual analog scale) to evaluate bodily pain and found that vitamin D supplementation was effective to alleviate pain and improve other components of HRQOL. Similarly, Sakalli et al [60] used VAS and SF-36 questionnaire to detect the level of pain and they reported that single megadose of vitamin D was effective to increase QOL particularly physical functioning, role physical, bodily pain, general health, social functioning and also decrease non-specific musculoskeletal pain. On the contrary, another study that used a disease-specific tool (Minnesota Living with Heart Failure questionnaire) did not find any improvement in physical function or HRQOL in older patients with heart failure [25].

To date, very few studies examined the relationship of vitamin D and HRQOL among healthy premenopausal women without osteoporosis as the study population. So far, we only found study by Ecemis et al [26] on Vitamin D and HRQOL among the healthy premenopausal women. They reported significant association between vitamin D and HRQOL.

It is difficult to recommend sunlight exposure to improve vitamin D levels due to interpersonal variations in sunlight exposure as well as the risks of skin cancer due to excessive UV radiation. However, skin cancer is a rare disease in Asia as compared to Caucasians [61]. A study by Nurbazlin et al. [62] has found that urban women in Malaysia had significantly lower sunlight exposure and vitamin D status compared to rural women. This study shown that sun index were the major factors influencing vitamin D status in Malaysian women. A trial study on the effect of nutrition education and sun exposure on vitamin D status among postmenopausal Malay women also found serum vitamin D level was increased through nutrition education and sunlight exposure [63]. Therefore it is sensible to recommend additional sunlight exposure for Malaysian women especially those living in the urban. Besides that, the best way of preventing vitamin D deficiency is by food fortification. Food fortification has the dual advantage of being able to deliver nutrients to large segments of the population without requiring radical changes in food consumption patterns. A recent review study found vitamin D fortification using vegetable oil can be the efficacious way to increase intake of daily vitamin D in Southeast Asian countries [64]. In addition to fortification, supplementation can be the alternative solution with high and less frequent doses are advisable especially to high risk population such as elderly. Nevertheless, we need to learn more about the long term safety and efficacy of the high dosage, less frequent vitamin D supplementation.

Limitations and Strength

Although all of our participants were vitamin D deficient, only small proportion of them was at risk for CVD as our study was conducted in a non-clinical setting. From the National Health and Morbidity Survey IV (NHMS IV) conducted in 2011, only 14.5% of women age more than 18 years old were diabetic while 31.6% were hypertensive [65]. Therefore, we had difficulty recruiting women with vitamin D deficiency as those with CVD risk. So, our study was not powered to detect the effect of vitamin D supplementation on cardiometabolic risks. We were also not able to examine the incidence of cardiovascular events due to the short duration. A larger sample size of high risk population for CVD with longer follow-up and higher intakes of vitamin D supplementation may be needed to establish whether steady normalization of vitamin D levels will translate to decrease in cardiovascular event incidence. An article by Heaney [66] has indicated that inadequate intakes of vitamin D may produce more than one disease by more than one mechanisms and may require several years for the consequent morbidity to be sufficiently evident to be clinically recognizable as "disease". Similarly more established evident are needed to prove that higher intakes of vitamin D are required for its prevention. For example, preventing the osteoporosis requires almost 4 times the amount of vitamin D needed to prevent rickets and this knowledge takes years to be established.

Nevertheless, our study has several strengths that worth mention. One of them is its high quality of randomisation where there was concealment of allocation, double-blinding among the participant and researchers and placebo controlled design. This reduced bias in term of selection and information bias as self-reported HRQOL was subjective. Larger but less frequent dosage of vitamin D may be advantageous from a compliance perspective compared to daily doses. There was also no problem with seasonal confounders as Malaysia is blessed with sufficient sunshine all year round necessary for cutaneous synthesis of vitamin D. Both groups were comparable in outdoor physical activity, sunlight exposure activity and diet at baseline and there were no changes pre and post intervention. In addition, our participants' retention rate was good with only 11% drop-out from the study.

Conclusion

This trial showed that Vitamin D supplementation over one year to premenopausal vitamin D deficient women living in an urban tropical country had no meaningful effect on measured cardiometabolic risk factors, but it did improve some components of HRQOL. Our findings provided evidence for the larger dosage but lower frequency to be effective in improving serum vitamin D levels. Further long term trials of this intervention versus daily and weekly vitamin D dosing especially among the high risk individuals with existing co-morbidities are needed.

Acknowledgments

The authors would like to acknowledge all participants of the trial and the management of the University of Malaya for supporting this study.

Author Contributions

Conceived and designed the experiments: MR MFM RP. Performed the experiments: MR SS. Analyzed the data: MR MFM. Contributed to the writing of the manuscript: MR MFM.

References

1. Wacker M, Holick MF (2013) Vitamin D - effects on skeletal and extraskeletal health and the need for supplementation. Nutrients 5: 111–148.
2. Holick MF (2011) Vitamin D: A D-Lightful Solution for Health. Journal of Investigative Medicine 59: 9.
3. Holick MF (2004) Vitamin D: importance in the prevention of cancers, type 1 diabetes, heart disease, and osteoporosis. Am J Clin Nutr 79: 362–371.
4. Hosseinpanah F, Yarjanli M, Sheikholeslami F, Heibatollahi M, Eskandary PS, et al. (2011) Associations between vitamin D and cardiovascular outcomes; Tehran Lipid and Glucose Study. Atherosclerosis 218: 238–242.

5. Khan H, Kunutsor S, Franco OH, Chowdhury R (2013) Vitamin D, type 2 diabetes and other metabolic outcomes: a systematic review and meta-analysis of prospective studies. Proc Nutr Soc 72: 89–97.
6. Lee JH, O'Keefe JH, Bell D, Hensrud DD, Holick MF (2008) Vitamin D Deficiency: An Important, Common, and Easily Treatable Cardiovascular Risk Factor? Journal of the American College of Cardiology 52: 1949–1956.
7. Holick MF (2009) Vitamin D Status: Measurement, Interpretation, and Clinical Application. Annals of Epidemiology 19: 73–78.
8. Anderson JL, May HT, Horne BD, Bair TL, Hall NL, et al. (2010) Relation of Vitamin D Deficiency to Cardiovascular Risk Factors, Disease Status, and Incident Events in a General Healthcare Population. The American Journal of Cardiology 106: 963–968.
9. Chacko SA, Song Y, Manson JE, Van Horn L, Eaton C, et al. (2011) Serum 25-hydroxyvitamin D concentrations in relation to cardiometabolic risk factors and metabolic syndrome in postmenopausal women. American Journal of Clinical Nutrition 94: 209–217.
10. El-Menyar A, Rahil A, Dousa K, Ibrahim W, Ibrahim T, et al. (2012) Low vitamin D and cardiovascular risk factors in males and females from a sunny, rich country. Open Cardiovascular Medicine Journal 6: 76–80.
11. Breslavsky A, Frand J, Matas Z, Boaz M, Barnea Z, et al. (2013) Effect of high doses of vitamin D on arterial properties, adiponectin, leptin and glucose homeostasis in type 2 diabetic patients. Clin Nutr 32: 970–975.
12. Harris SS, Pittas AG, Palermo NJ (2012) A randomized, placebo-controlled trial of vitamin D supplementation to improve glycaemia in overweight and obese African Americans. Diabetes Obes Metab 14: 789–794.
13. Major GC, Alaric F, Dore J, Phouttama S, Tremblay A (2007) Supplementation with calcium + vitamin D enhances the beneficial effect of weight loss on plasma lipid and lipoprotein concentrations. Am J Clin Nutr 85: 54–59.
14. Nagpal J, Pande JN, Bhartia A (2009) A double-blind, randomized, placebo-controlled trial of the short-term effect of vitamin D3 supplementation on insulin sensitivity in apparently healthy, middle-aged, centrally obese men. Diabet Med 26: 19–27.
15. Ryu OH, Lee S, Yu J, Choi MG, Yoo HJ, et al. (2013) A prospective randomized controlled trial of the effects of vitamin D supplementation on long-term glycemic control in type 2 diabetes mellitus of Korea. Endocr J.
16. von Hurst PR, Stonehouse W, Coad J (2010) Vitamin D supplementation reduces insulin resistance in South Asian women living in New Zealand who are insulin resistant and vitamin D deficient - a randomised, placebo-controlled trial. Br J Nutr 103: 549–555.
17. Wood AD, Secombes KR, Thies F, Aucott L, Black AJ, et al. (2012) Vitamin D3 supplementation has no effect on conventional cardiovascular risk factors: a parallel-group, double-blind, placebo-controlled RCT. J Clin Endocrinol Metab 97: 3557–3568.
18. Basaran S, Guzel R, Coskun-Benlidayi I, Guler-Uysal F (2007) Vitamin D status: effects on quality of life in osteoporosis among Turkish women. Quality of Life Research 16: 1491–1499.
19. Motsinger S, Lazovich D, MacLehose RF, Torkelson CJ, Robien K (2012) Vitamin D intake and mental health-related quality of life in older women: the Iowa Women's Health Study. Maturitas 71: 267–273.
20. Anand S, Kaysen GA, Chertow GM, Johansen KL, Grimes B, et al. (2011) Vitamin D deficiency, self-reported physical activity and health-related quality of life: the Comprehensive Dialysis Study. Nephrol Dial Transplant 26: 3683–3688.
21. Huang W, Shah S, Long Q, Crankshaw AK, Tangpricha V (2013) Improvement of pain, sleep, and quality of life in chronic pain patients with vitamin D supplementation. Clin J Pain 29: 341–347.
22. Michael YL, Smit E, Seguin R, Curb JD, Phillips LS, et al. (2011) Serum 25-hydroxyvitamin D and physical performance in postmenopausal women. J Womens Health (Larchmt) 20: 1603–1608.
23. Ohta H, Uemura Y, Nakamura T, Fukunaga M, Ohashi Y, et al. (2014) Serum 25-hydroxyvitamin D level as an independent determinant of quality of life in osteoporosis with a high risk for fracture. Clinical Therapeutics 36: 225–235.
24. Chao YS, Ekwaru JP, Ohinmaa A, Griener G, Veugelers PJ (2014) Vitamin D and health-related quality of life in a community sample of older Canadians. Qual Life Res.
25. Witham MD, Crighton LJ, Gillespie ND, Struthers AD, McMurdo MET (2010) The Effects of Vitamin D Supplementation on Physical Function and Quality of Life in Older Patients With Heart Failure: A Randomized Controlled Trial. Circulation: Heart Failure 3: 195–201.
26. Ecemis GC, Atmaca A (2013) Quality of life is impaired not only in vitamin D deficient but also in vitamin D-insufficient pre-menopausal women. J Endocrinol Invest 36: 622–627.
27. Ramly M, Moy FM, Pendek R, Suboh S, Tan Tong Boon A (2013) Study protocol: the effect of vitamin D supplements on cardiometabolic risk factors among urban premenopausal women in a tropical country – a randomized controlled trial. BMC Public Health 13: 416.
28. Ross AC, Manson JE, Abrams SA, Aloia JF, Brannon PM, et al. (2011) The 2011 report on dietary reference intakes for calcium and vitamin D from the Institute of Medicine: what clinicians need to know. J Clin Endocrinol Metab 96: 53–58.
29. Zittermann A, Frisch S, Berthold HK, Gotting C, Kuhn J, et al. (2009) Vitamin D supplementation enhances the beneficial effects of weight loss on cardiovascular disease risk markers. Am J Clin Nutr 89: 1321–1327.
30. Begg GA, Cleland JG, Witte KK (2010) Letter by Begg, et al regarding article, "The effects of vitamin d supplementation on physical function and quality of life in older heart failure patients: a randomized controlled trial". Circ Heart Fail 3: e24; author reply e25.
31. Azman AB, Sararaks S, Rugayah B, Low LL, Azian AA, et al. (2003) Quality of life of the Malaysian general population: results from a postal survey using the SF-36. Med J Malaysia 58: 694–711.
32. Alam U, Najam O, Al-Himdani S, Benoliel S, Jinadev P, et al. (2012) Marked vitamin D deficiency in patients with diabetes in the UK: ethnic and seasonal differences and an association with dyslipidaemia. Diabet Med 29: 1343–1345.
33. Al-Daghri N (2010) Serum 25-hydroxy-vitamin D is associated with insulin resistance and adiponectin levels in diabetic Saudi adults. Osteoporosis International 21: S726.
34. Al-Daghri NM, Alkharfy KM, Al-Saleh Y, Al-Attas OS, Alokail MS, et al. (2012) Modest reversal of metabolic syndrome manifestations with vitamin D status correction: A 12-month prospective study. Metabolism: Clinical and Experimental 61: 661–666.
35. Botella-Carretero JI, Alvarez-Blasco F, Villafruela JJ, Balsa JA, Vázquez C, et al. (2007) Vitamin D deficiency is associated with the metabolic syndrome in morbid obesity. Clinical Nutrition 26: 573–580.
36. Chailurkit LO, Aekplakorn W, Ongphiphadhanakul B (2012) The association between vitamin D status and type 2 diabetes in a Thai population, a cross-sectional study. Clin Endocrinol (Oxf) 77: 658–664.
37. Moy FM, Bulgiba A (2011) High prevalence of vitamin D insufficiency and its association with obesity and metabolic syndrome among Malay adults in Kuala Lumpur, Malaysia. BMC Public Health 11: 735.
38. Kayaniyil S, Vieth R, Harris SB, Retnakaran R, Knight JA, et al. (2011) Association of 25(OH)D and PTH with metabolic syndrome and its traditional and nontraditional components. Journal of Clinical Endocrinology and Metabolism 96: 168–175.
39. Mark F M (2009) Poor vitamin D status may contribute to high risk for insulin resistance, obesity, and cardiovascular disease in Asian Indians. Medical Hypotheses 72: 647–651.
40. Siadat ZD, Kiani K, Sadeghi M, Shariat AS, Farajzadegan Z, et al. (2012) Association of vitamin D deficiency and coronary artery disease with cardiovascular risk factors. Journal of Research in Medical Sciences 17: 1052–1055.
41. Zhou QG, Hou FF, Guo ZJ, Liang M, Wang GB, et al. (2008) 1,25-Dihydroxyvitamin D improved the free fatty-acid-induced insulin resistance in cultured C2C12 cells. Diabetes Metab Res Rev 24: 459–464.
42. Manna P, Jain SK (2012) Vitamin D up-regulates glucose transporter 4 (GLUT4) translocation and glucose utilization mediated by cystathionine-gamma-lyase (CSE) activation and H2S formation in 3T3L1 adipocytes. J Biol Chem 287: 42324–42332.
43. Pittas AG, Harris SS, Stark PC, Dawson-Hughes B (2007) The effects of calcium and vitamin D supplementation on blood glucose and markers of inflammation in nondiabetic adults. Diabetes Care 30: 980–986.
44. Maki KC, Rubin MR, Wong LG, McManus JF, Jensen CD, et al. (2009) Serum 25-hydroxyvitamin D is independently associated with high-density lipoprotein cholesterol and the metabolic syndrome in men and women. Journal of Clinical Lipidology 3: 289–296.
45. Minambres I, Sanchez-Quesada JL, Sanchez-Hernandez J, Rodriguez J, De Leiva A, et al. (2014) Vitamin D concentrations in familial combined hyperlipidemia: Effects of lipid lowering treatment. Diabetology and Metabolic Syndrome 6.
46. Rejnmark L, Vestergaard P, Heickendorff L, Mosekilde L (2010) Simvastatin does not affect vitamin d status, but low vitamin d levels are associated with dyslipidemia: results from a randomised, controlled trial. Int J Endocrinol 2010: 957174.
47. Jorde R, Grimnes G (2011) Vitamin D and metabolic health with special reference to the effect of vitamin D on serum lipids. Progress in Lipid Research 50: 303–312.
48. Ford ES, Giles WH, Dietz WH (2002) Prevalence of the metabolic syndrome among US adults: Findings from the Third National Health and Nutrition Examination Survey. Journal of the American Medical Association 287: 356–359.
49. Vacek JL, Vanga SR, Good M, Lai SM, Lakkireddy D, et al. (2012) Vitamin D Deficiency and Supplementation and Relation to Cardiovascular Health. The American Journal of Cardiology 109: 359–363.
50. Whiting S, Evans C, Foo L (2013) Recent systematic reviews indicate adults need (greater-than or equal to) 800 iu vitamin D to reduce risk of disease. Annals of Nutrition and Metabolism 63: 347.
51. Mitri J, Dawson-Hughes B, Hu FB, Pittas AG (2011) Effects of vitamin D and calcium supplementation on pancreatic beta cell function, insulin sensitivity, and glycemia in adults at high risk of diabetes: the Calcium and Vitamin D for Diabetes Mellitus (CaDDM) randomized controlled trial. Am J Clin Nutr 94: 486–494.
52. Talaei A, Mohamadi M, Adgi Z (2013) The effect of vitamin D on insulin resistance in patients with type 2 diabetes. Diabetol Metab Syndr 5: 8.
53. Tai K, Need AG, Horowitz M, Chapman IM (2008) Glucose tolerance and vitamin D: effects of treating vitamin D deficiency. Nutrition 24: 950–956.
54. Hollis BW, Wagner CL (2013) Clinical review: The role of the parent compound vitamin D with respect to metabolism and function: Why clinical dose intervals can affect clinical outcomes. J Clin Endocrinol Metab 98: 4619–4628.

55. Kalueff AV, Tuohimaa P (2007) Neurosteroid hormone vitamin D and its utility in clinical nutrition. Curr Opin Clin Nutr Metab Care 10: 12–19.
56. Ju SY, Lee YJ, Jeong SN (2013) Serum 25-hydroxyvitamin D levels and the risk of depression: a systematic review and meta-analysis. J Nutr Health Aging 17: 447–455.
57. May HT, Bair TL, Lappe DL, Anderson JL, Horne BD, et al. (2010) Association of vitamin D levels with incident depression among a general cardiovascular population. Am Heart J 159: 1037–1043.
58. Penckofer S, Kouba J, Byrn M, Estwing Ferrans C (2010) Vitamin D and depression: where is all the sunshine? Issues Ment Health Nurs 31: 385–393.
59. Shaffer JA, Edmondson D, Wasson LT, Falzon L, Homma K, et al. (2014) Vitamin D Supplementation for Depressive Symptoms: A Systematic Review and Meta-Analysis of Randomized Controlled Trials. Psychosom Med.
60. Sakalli H, Arslan D, Yucel AE (2012) The effect of oral and parenteral vitamin D supplementation in the elderly: a prospective, double-blinded, randomized, placebo-controlled study. Rheumatol Int 32: 2279–2283.
61. Lee HY, Chay WY, Tang MB, Chio MT, Tan SH (2012) Melanoma: differences between Asian and Caucasian patients. Ann Acad Med Singapore 41: 17–20.
62. Nurbazlin M, Chee WS, Rokiah P, Tan AT, Chew YY, et al. (2013) Effects of sun exposure on 25(OH) vitamin D concentration in urban and rural women in Malaysia. Asia Pac J Clin Nutr 22: 391–399.
63. Istiany A, Rahman SA, Kasim ZM, Swee WCS, Yassin Z, et al. (2012) Effect Of Nutrition Education And Sun Exposure On Vitamin D Status Among Postmenopausal Malay Women. International Journal of Science and Engineering Investigations 1: 91–97.
64. Yang Z, Laillou A, Smith G, Schofield D, Moench-Pfanner R (2013) A review of vitamin D fortification: implications for nutrition programming in Southeast Asia. Food Nutr Bull 34: S81–89.
65. Ministry of Health M (2011) National Health and Morbidity Survey (NHMS) 2011. 15th NIH Scientific Meeting incorporating NHMS 2011 and GATS conference, 2012. Holiday Villa, Subang Jaya, Selangor.
66. Heaney RP (2003) Long-latency deficiency disease: insights from calcium and vitamin D. Am J Clin Nutr 78: 912–919.

Permissions

All chapters in this book were first published in PLOS ONE, by The Public Library of Science; hereby published with permission under the Creative Commons Attribution License or equivalent. Every chapter published in this book has been scrutinized by our experts. Their significance has been extensively debated. The topics covered herein carry significant findings which will fuel the growth of the discipline. They may even be implemented as practical applications or may be referred to as a beginning point for another development.

The contributors of this book come from diverse backgrounds, making this book a truly international effort. This book will bring forth new frontiers with its revolutionizing research information and detailed analysis of the nascent developments around the world.

We would like to thank all the contributing authors for lending their expertise to make the book truly unique. They have played a crucial role in the development of this book. Without their invaluable contributions this book wouldn't have been possible. They have made vital efforts to compile up to date information on the varied aspects of this subject to make this book a valuable addition to the collection of many professionals and students.

This book was conceptualized with the vision of imparting up-to-date information and advanced data in this field. To ensure the same, a matchless editorial board was set up. Every individual on the board went through rigorous rounds of assessment to prove their worth. After which they invested a large part of their time researching and compiling the most relevant data for our readers.

The editorial board has been involved in producing this book since its inception. They have spent rigorous hours researching and exploring the diverse topics which have resulted in the successful publishing of this book. They have passed on their knowledge of decades through this book. To expedite this challenging task, the publisher supported the team at every step. A small team of assistant editors was also appointed to further simplify the editing procedure and attain best results for the readers.

Apart from the editorial board, the designing team has also invested a significant amount of their time in understanding the subject and creating the most relevant covers. They scrutinized every image to scout for the most suitable representation of the subject and create an appropriate cover for the book.

The publishing team has been an ardent support to the editorial, designing and production team. Their endless efforts to recruit the best for this project, has resulted in the accomplishment of this book. They are a veteran in the field of academics and their pool of knowledge is as vast as their experience in printing. Their expertise and guidance has proved useful at every step. Their uncompromising quality standards have made this book an exceptional effort. Their encouragement from time to time has been an inspiration for everyone.

The publisher and the editorial board hope that this book will prove to be a valuable piece of knowledge for researchers, students, practitioners and scholars across the globe.

List of Contributors

Rocco Barazzoni, Gianluca Gortan Cappellari, Annamaria Semolic, Enrico Chendi, Mario Ius, Roberta Situlin, Michela Zanetti, Pierandrea Vinci and Gianfranco Guarnieri
Internal Medicine, Department of Medical, Surgical and Health Sciences, University of Trieste, Trieste, Italy

Milos Lazic, Davide Povero and Ariel E. Feldstein
Department of Pediatrics, University of California San Diego, La Jolla, California, United States of America

Maria Eugenia Inzaugarat and Alejandra C. Cherñavsky
Institute of Immunology, Genetics and Metabolism, CONICET-UBA, Buenos Aires, Argentina

Iris C. Zhao
Skaggs School of Pharmacy and Pharmaceutical Sciences, University of California San Diego, La Jolla, California, United States of America

Mark Chen, Madlena Nalbandian, Yury I. Miller and Dorothy D. Sears
Department of Medicine, University of California San Diego, La Jolla, California, United States of America

Michele La Merrill
Department of Environmental Toxicology, University of California Davis, Davis, California, United States of America
Department of Preventive Medicine, Mount Sinai School of Medicine, New York, New York, United States of America
Metabolism Institute, Mount Sinai School of Medicine, New York, New York, United States of America

Emma Karey
Department of Environmental Toxicology, University of California Davis, Davis, California, United States of America

Erin Moshier
Department of Preventive Medicine, Mount Sinai School of Medicine, New York, New York, United States of America

Claudia Lindtner and Christoph Buettner
Metabolism Institute, Mount Sinai School of Medicine, New York, New York, United States of America
Division of Endocrinology, Diabetes and Bone Disease, Mount Sinai School of Medicine, New York, New York, United States of America

Michael R. La Frano
West Coast Metabolomic Center, University of California Davis, Davis, California, United States of America
Department of Nutrition, University of California Davis, Davis, California, United States of America

John W. Newman
West Coast Metabolomic Center, University of California Davis, Davis, California, United States of America
Department of Nutrition, University of California Davis, Davis, California, United States of America
Obesity and Metabolism Research Unit, USDA-ARS-Western Human Nutrition Research Center, Davis, California, United States of America

Cecilia Vecoli, Daniela Giacopelli and Pascale Beffy
Istituto di Fisiologia Clinica-CNR, Pisa, Italy

Michela Novelli and Pellegrino Masiello
Dipartimento di Ricerca Traslazionale e delle Nuove Tecnologie in Medicina e Chirurgia, Università di Pisa, Pisa, Italy

Anna Pippa
Institute of Life Sciences, Scuola Superiore Sant'Anna, Pisa, Italy

Antonio L'Abbate
Istituto di Fisiologia Clinica-CNR, Pisa, Italy
Institute of Life Sciences, Scuola Superiore Sant'Anna, Pisa, Italy

Danilo Neglia
Istituto di Fisiologia Clinica-CNR, Pisa, Italy
Fondazione Toscana G. Monasterio-CNR, Pisa, Italy

Jan Freark de Boer, Arne Dikkers, Angelika Jurdzinski and Uwe J. F. Tietge
Department of Pediatrics, Center for Liver, Digestive and Metabolic Diseases, University of Groningen, University Medical Center Groningen, Groningen, The Netherlands

Johann von Felden and Udo Bavendiek
Clinic of Cardiology and Angiology, Hannover Medical School, Hannover, Germany

Matthias Gaestel
Institute of Biochemistry, Hannover Medical School, Hannover, Germany

Erik J. M. Toonen and Dov B. Ballak
Department of Internal Medicine, Radboud University Medical Centre, Nijmegen, The Netherlands

Anke J. Laskewitz and Aycha Bleeker
Department of Pediatrics, University of Groningen, University Medical Center Groningen, Groningen, The Netherlands

Theo H. van Dijk
Department of Laboratory Medicine, University of Groningen, University Medical Center Groningen, Groningen, The Netherlands

Albert K. Groen
Department of Pediatrics, University of Groningen, University Medical Center Groningen, Groningen, The Netherlands
Department of Laboratory Medicine, University of Groningen, University Medical Center Groningen, Groningen, The Netherlands

Aldo Grefhorst
Department of Internal Medicine, Erasmus MC, University Medical Center Rotterdam, Rotterdam, The Netherlands

Annelies E. Schouten, Ellen A. J. Bastiaanssen, Cindy van Doorn, Monique A. J. van der Vleuten, Marie-Jose C. van Lierop and Wim H. A. Dokter
Department of Immune Therapeutics, MSD Research Laboratories, Oss, The Netherlands

Marije I. Koenders
Department of Experimental Rheumatology, Radboud Institute for Molecular Life Sciences (RIMLS), Radboud University Medical Centre, Nijmegen, The Netherlands

Ved Prakash Meena and Naval K. Vikram
Department of Medicine, All India Institute of Medical Sciences, New Delhi, India

V. Seenu
Department of Surgical Disciplines, All India Institute of Medical Sciences, New Delhi, India

M. C. Sharma and Saumya Ranjan Mallic
Department of Pathology, All India Institute of Medical Sciences, New Delhi, India

Ashu Seith Bhalla
Department of Radiodiagnosis, All India Institute of Medical Sciences, New Delhi, India

Nandita Gupta
Department of Endocrinology and Metabolism, All India Institute of Medical Sciences, New Delhi, India

Anant Mohan and Randeep Guleria
Departments of Pulmonary Medicine and Sleep Disorders, All India Institute of Medical Sciences, New Delhi, India

Ravindra M. Pandey
Department of Biostatistics, All India Institute of Medical Sciences, New Delhi, India,

Kalpana Luthra
Department of Biochemistry, All India Institute of Medical Sciences, New Delhi, India

Laura Diesse
Department of Paediatrics, University of Chieti, Chieti, Italy

Valentina Chiavaroli, Maria Loredana Marcovecchio, Tommaso de Giorgis, Francesco Chiarelli and Angelika Mohn
Department of Paediatrics, University of Chieti, Chieti, Italy
Center of Excellence on Aging, "G. d'Annunzio" University Foundation, University of Chieti, Chieti, Italy

Karyn J. Catalano, Jaroslaw Szary and Fred Schaufele
Department of Obstetrics and Gynecology and the Diabetes Center, University of California San Francisco, San Francisco, California, United States of America,

Jack F. Youngren and Ira D. Goldfine
Division of Endocrinology and Metabolism, University of California San Francisco, San Francisco, California, United States of America

Betty A. Maddux
Department of Obstetrics and Gynecology and the Diabetes Center, University of California San Francisco, San Francisco, California, United States of America,
Division of Endocrinology and Metabolism, University of California San Francisco, San Francisco, California, United States of America

Anete S. Mecenas, Priscila A. Maranhão and Eliete Bouskela
Laboratory for Clinical and Experimental Research on Vascular Biology (BioVasc), Biomedical Center, State University of Rio de Janeiro, Rio de Janeiro, Brazil

Ruth Clapauch
Laboratory for Clinical and Experimental Research on Vascular Biology (BioVasc), Biomedical Center, State University of Rio de Janeiro, Rio de Janeiro, Brazil
Hospital da Lagoa, Endocrinology Sector, Health Ministry, Rio de Janeiro, Brazil

André Felipe Mourão and Ana Rossini
Departamento de Bioquímica, IBRAG, State University of Rio de Janeiro, Rio de Janeiro, Brazil

Dianjianyi Sun
Department of Epidemiology and Biostatistics, School of Public Health, Peking University Health Science Center, Beijing, China
Department of Epidemiology, Tulane University, New Orleans, Louisiana, United States of America

Shengxu Li, Xiaotao Zhang, Camilo Fernandez, Wei Chen, Sathanur R. Srinivasan and Gerald S. Berenson
Department of Epidemiology, Tulane University, New Orleans, Louisiana, United States of America

Jaswinder K. Sethi and Krisztina Hegyi
The Department of Clinical Biochemistry, University of Cambridge Metabolic Research Laboratories, Institute of Metabolic Science, Addenbrooke's Hospital, Cambridge, United Kingdom

Katherine A. Robinson and Maria G. Buse
The Departments of Biochemistry and Molecular Biology and Medicine, Division Diabetes, Endocrinology and Medical Genetics, Medical University of South Carolina, Charleston, South Carolina, United States of America

Yusuf A. Hannun
The Department of Medicine and the Stony Brook Cancer Center, Stony Brook University, Stony Brook, New York, United States of America

Leonardo B. Leiria, José M. Dora, Simone M. Wajner, Aline A. F. Estivalet, Daisy Crispim and Ana Luiza Maia
Thyroid Section, Endocrine Division, Hospital de Clínicas de Porto Alegre, Universidade Federal do Rio Grande do Sul, Porto Alegre, RS, Brazil

Rana Mahfouz, Rhéa Khoury, Pascal Ferré, Fabienne Foufelle and Eric Hajduch
INSERM, UMR-S 1138, Centre de Recherche des Cordeliers, Paris, France
Université Pierre et Marie Curie - Paris 6, UMR-S 1138, Paris, France
Université Paris Descartes, UMR-S 1138, Paris, France

Agnieszka Blachnio-Zabielska
Department of Physiology, Medical University of Bialystok, Bialystok, Poland

Sophie Turban, Christopher Lipina, Clare Stretton and Harinder S. Hundal
Division of Cell Signalling and Immunology, College of Life Sciences, University of Dundee, Dundee, United Kingdom

Nicolas Loiseau
INRA, UMR1331 Toxalim, Research Centre in Food Toxicology, Toulouse, France

Olivier Bourron
INSERM, UMR-S 1138, Centre de Recherche des Cordeliers, Paris, France
Université Pierre et Marie Curie - Paris 6, UMR-S 1138, Paris, France
Université Paris Descartes, UMR-S 1138, Paris, France
Département de Diabétologie et Maladies métaboliques, AP-HP, Hôpital Pitié-Salpêtrière, Paris, France

Michael Maris
Division of Endocrinology and Metabolism, Department of Medicine, University of California San Diego, La Jolla, California, United States of America
Clinical and Experimental Endocrinology, Catholic University Leuven, Leuven, Belgium

Sarah Nalbandian, Olivia Osborn and Niclas Franck
Division of Endocrinology and Metabolism, Department of Medicine, University of California San Diego, La Jolla, California, United States of America

Saswata Talukdar, Hans-Peter Hofmann and David Bullough
Pfizer Inc. Research Laboratories, Cambridge, Massachusetts, United States of America

Simon Schenk
Department of Orthopedic Surgery, University of California San Diego, La Jolla, California, United States of America

Nattayaporn Apaijai and Kroekkiat Chinda
Cardiac Electrophysiology Research and Training Center, Faculty of Medicine, Chiang Mai University, Chiang Mai, Thailand
Cardiac Electrophysiology Unit, Department of Physiology, Faculty of Medicine, Chiang Mai University, Chiang Mai, Thailand

Siripong Palee
Cardiac Electrophysiology Research and Training Center, Faculty of Medicine, Chiang Mai University, Chiang Mai, Thailand
School of Medicine, Mae FahLuang University, Chiang Rai, Thailand

Siriporn Chattipakorn
Cardiac Electrophysiology Research and Training Center, Faculty of Medicine, Chiang Mai University, Chiang Mai, Thailand
Department of Oral Biology and Diagnostic Sciences, Faculty of Dentistry, Chiang Mai University, Chiang Mai, Thailand

Nipon Chattipakorn
Cardiac Electrophysiology Research and Training Center, Faculty of Medicine, Chiang Mai University, Chiang Mai, Thailand
Cardiac Electrophysiology Unit, Department of Physiology, Faculty of Medicine, Chiang Mai University, Chiang Mai, Thailand
Biomedical Engineering Center, Chiang Mai University, Chiang Mai, Thailand

Michelle M. Averill
Department of Environmental and Occupational Health, University of Washington, Seattle, Washington, United States of America

Eung Ju Kim, Leela Goodspeed, Shari Wang, Savitha Subramanian, Laura J. Den Hartigh, Chongren Tang, Yilei Ding and Alan Chait
Department of Medicine, University of Washington, Seattle, Washington, United States of America

Catherine A. Reardon and Godfrey S. Getz
Department of Pathology, University of Chicago, Chicago, Illinois, United States of America

Naoto Tsuda
Discovery Research, Mochida Pharmaceutical Company Limited, Shizuoka, Japan
Department of Molecular Endocrinology and Metabolism, Graduate School of Medical and Dental Sciences, Tokyo Medical and Dental University, Tokyo, Japan

Shin Kumadaki, Chika Higashi, Makoto Ozawa, Mikihiko Shinozaki, Yutaka Kato, Koutarou Hoshida, Satomi Kikuchi, Yoshihisa Nakano and Shoji Furusako
Discovery Research, Mochida Pharmaceutical Company Limited, Shizuoka, Japan

Yoshihiro Ogawa
Department of Molecular Endocrinology and Metabolism, Graduate School of Medical and Dental Sciences, Tokyo Medical and Dental University, Tokyo, Japan

Chin-Hsiao Tseng
Department of Internal Medicine, National Taiwan University College of Medicine, Taipei, Taiwan
Division of Endocrinology and Metabolism, Department of Internal Medicine, National Taiwan University Hospital, Taipei, Taiwan
Division of Environmental Health and Occupational Medicine of the National Health Research Institutes, Taipei, Taiwan

Xuan-Han Koh
Department of Biological Sciences, National University of Singapore, Singapore

Xuanyao Liu
NUS Graduate School for Integrative Science and Engineering, National University of Singapore, Singapore
Saw Swee Hock School of Public Health, National University of Singapore, Singapore

Yik-Ying Teo
NUS Graduate School for Integrative Science and Engineering, National University of Singapore, Singapore
Saw Swee Hock School of Public Health, National University of Singapore, Singapore
Life Sciences Institute, National University of Singapore, Singapore
Department of Statistics and Applied Probability, National University of Singapore, Singapore
Genome Institute of Singapore, Agency for Science, Technology and Research, Singapore

Graeme I. Lancaster, Michael J. Kraakman, Helene L. Kammoun, Katherine G. Langley, Emma Estevez and Mark A. Febbraio
Cellular and Molecular Metabolism Laboratory, Baker IDI Heart and Diabetes Institute, Melbourne, Victoria, Australia

Raelene J. Grumont and Steve Gerondakis
The Australian Centre for Blood Diseases and Department of Clinical Hematology, Monash University Central Clinical School, Melbourne, Victoria, Australia

Ashish Banerjee
Centre for Cancer Research, MIMR-PHI Institute of Medical Research, Monash University, Victoria, Australia

Giuseppina T. Russo and Domenico Cucinotta
Department of Clinical and Experimental Medicine, University of Messina, Messina, Italy

Carlo Bruno Giorda
Metabolism and Diabetes Unit ASL TO5, Chieri, Italy

Stefania Cercone
MSD, Rome, Italy

Antonio Nicolucci
Department of Clinical Pharmacology and Epidemiology Fondazione Mario Negri Sud, S. Maria Imbaro, Italy

Di Zhao and Eliseo Guallar
Department of Epidemiology and Welch Center for Prevention, Epidemiology, and Clinical Research, Johns Hopkins University Bloomberg School of Public Health, Baltimore, Maryland, United States of America

Juhee Cho
Department of Health Sciences and Technology, Samsung Advanced Institute for Health Sciences and Technology, Sungkyunkwan University, Seoul, Korea

Myung Hun Kim
Saevit Eye Hospital, Goyang, Gyeonggi-do, Korea

David Friedman
Department of Ophthalmology, Johns Hopkins University School of Medicine, Baltimore, Maryland, United States of America

Zhi Dong, Yanji Luo, Huasong Cai Zi-Ping Li and Shi-Ting Feng
Department of Radiology, The First Affiliated Hospital of Sun Yat-Sen University, Guangzhou, China

Zhongwei Zhang
Department of Radiology, The University of Texas Southwestern Medical Center, Dallas, Texas, United States of America

Yanbing Li
Department of Endocrinology and Diabetes Center, The First Affiliated Hospital of Sun Yat-sen University, Guangzhou, China

Tao Chan
Medical Imaging Department, Union Hospital, Hong Kong

Ling Wu
Department of Radiology, Kiang Wu Hospital, Macao

Kalle Anand Kumar, Anumula Lalitha and Manchala Raghunath
Division of Endocrinology and Metabolism, National Institute of Nutrition, Indian Council of Medical Research (ICMR), Hyderabad, Telangana, India

Umakar Reddy and Giriraj Ratan Chandak
Centre for Cellular and Molecular Biology (CCMB), Council of Scientific and Industrial Research (CSIR), Hyderabad, Telangana, India

Shantanu Sengupta
Institute of Genomics and Integrative Biology, Council of Scientific and Industrial Research (CSIR), New Delhi, India

Mária Fízel'ová, Alena Stančáková and Jagadish Vangipurapu
Department of Medicine, University of Eastern Finland, Kuopio, Finland

Henna Cederberg, Raimo Jauhiainen, Johanna Kuusisto and Markku Laakso
Department of Medicine, University of Eastern Finland and Kuopio University Hospital, Kuopio, Finland

Rokiah Pendek
Department of Medicine, Faculty of Medicine, University of Malaya, Kuala Lumpur, Malaysia

Hanpeng Huang
Department of Respirology, Affiliated Hospital of Jiangsu University, Zhenjiang, China

Xiufeng Jiang
Department of Respirology, Nanjing Medical University affiliated Wuxi People's Hospital, Wuxi, China

Yanbin Dong, Xiaofeng Zhang, Ning Ding and Xilong Zhang
Department of Respirology, The First Affiliated Hospital with Nanjing Medical University, Nanjing, China

Jiannan Liu and Gan Lu
Department of Respiratory Diseases, Jangsu Geriatric Hospital, Nanjing, China

Sean Z. Hutchinson
Morsani College of Medicine, Tampa, FL, United States of America

Lorena del Rocío Ibarra-Reynoso, Liudmila Pisarchyk, Elva Leticia Pérez-Luque, Ma. Eugenia Garay-Sevilla and Juan Manuel Malacara
Department of Medical Sciences, University of Guanajuato, Campus León, 20 de Enero 929, León Guanajuato, México

Ying Li and Changhao Sun
Department of Nutrition and Food Hygiene, Public Health College, Harbin Medical University, Harbin, Heilongjiang, People's Republic of China

Yonghan He
Department of Nutrition and Food Hygiene, Public Health College, Harbin Medical University, Harbin, Heilongjiang, People's Republic of China
Aquatic and Crop Resource Development, Life Sciences Branch, National Research Council Canada, Charlottetown, Prince Edward Island, Canada

State Key Laboratory of Genetic Resources and Evolution, Kunming Institute of Zoology, Chinese Academy of Sciences, Kunming, Yunnan, People's Republic of China

Wen Li
Department of Endocrinology, Third People's Hospital of Yunnan Province, Kunming, Yunnan, People's Republic of China

Shuocheng Zhang and Yanwen Wang
Aquatic and Crop Resource Development, Life Sciences Branch, National Research Council Canada, Charlottetown, Prince Edward Island, Canada

Department of Biomedical Sciences, University of Prince Edward Island, Charlottetown, Prince Edward Island, Canada

Mazliza Ramly, Karuthan Chinna and Suhaili Suboh
Department of Social and Preventive Medicine, Faculty of Medicine, University of Malaya, Kuala Lumpur, Malaysia

Moy Foong Ming
Julius Centre University of Malaya, Department of Social and Preventive Medicine, Faculty of Medicine, University of Malaya, Kuala Lumpur, Malaysia,

Index